Review Editic

This review edition has been prepared for discussion and consultation during the Hungarian Council Presidency, 2011. We would be grateful if you could share your comments with us. Please send them to us before 15 May 2011 (mwi@obs.euro.who.int). The final edition of the book will be published the following month."

Health Professional Mobility and Health Systems

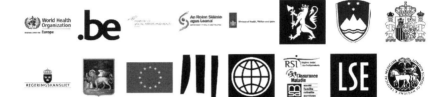

The European Observatory on Health Systems and Policies supports and promotes evidence-based health policy-making through comprehensive and rigorous analysis of health systems in Europe. It brings together a wide range of policy-makers, academics and practitioners to analyse trends in health reform, drawing on experience from across Europe to illuminate policy issues.

The European Observatory on Health Systems and Policies is a partnership between the World Health Organization Regional Office for Europe, the Governments of Belgium, Finland, Ireland, the Netherlands, Norway, Slovenia, Spain, Sweden and the Veneto Region of Italy, the European Commission, the European Investment Bank, the World Bank, UNCAM (French National Union of Health Insurance Funds), the London School of Economics and Political Science, and the London School of Hygiene & Tropical Medicine.

Health Professional Mobility and Health Systems

Evidence from 17 European countries

Edited by

**Matthias Wismar, Claudia B. Maier, Irene A. Glinos,
Gilles Dussault, Josep Figueras**

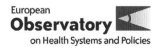

European
Observatory
on Health Systems and Policies

Contents

Foreword

This work contributes a great deal to the current reflection of the Commission and Member States about the future of the European Union health workforce. The Europe 2020 Strategy for smart, sustainable and inclusive growth highlights the need to reform labour markets, upgrade skills and match them with market demand. In parallel we also need to plan for our ageing society and the additional health care which will be needed in the future. It is estimated that by 2020 there will be a shortfall of 1 000 000 health professionals in the European Union. We need to work together with all actors, national authorities, health professionals and civil society to address this challenge.

When the Commission published its Green Paper on the European Workforce for Health, it emerged from the public consultation that one of the most significant barriers to effective workforce planning is the lack of data and information. Of this, the biggest challenge for planners has been the lack of data on mobility of health professionals - where they go; how long they stay away, whether they come back or not.

Indeed, the need for better quantitative and qualitative data to support decision-making proved to be one of the most pertinent issues. It is the human face, the case histories which provide us with greater understanding of motivations, aspirations and personal circumstances that influence health professionals. The testimonials in this book illustrate this point.

I therefore commend this book as a contribution to addressing the bigger picture and putting a human face to some of the challenges we need to overcome. I hope readers will derive inspiration from it.

Paola Testori Coggi
Director-General, Directorate General for Health and Consumers

Foreword

Migration of health professionals has globally increased over the last decades. By losing health workers, already fragile health systems in low- and middle-income countries may be further weakened. In the context of the global health workforce crisis these migratory flows became a matter of global policy concern. To respond to this challenge the World Health Assembly adopted in 2010 the WHO Global Code of Practice for the International Recruitment of Health Personnel. The Code discourages recruitment from countries with workforce shortages and provides guidance to strengthen the workforce and health systems across the globe, including an emphasis on improving staff retention, workforce sustainability and effective workforce planning.

The WHO Regional Office for Europe and the Member States strongly supported the development and adoption of the Code, building on their experience with national and regional codes, ethical workforce policies and other instruments for steering and managing health professional mobility, as well as broader aspects of health workforce policy and planning. The Code has relevance for Europe and the European Union and provides a framework for health workforce development and health system sustainability. It stresses the strengthening and further development of education and training, the monitoring and coordination of labour market activities; it addresses maldistribution of health professionals through educational measures, financial incentives, regulatory measures and social and professional support.

This volume gives a comprehensive analysis of mobility patterns, the impacts of migration on health systems and its relevance for policy-making and policy responses across Europe. It will enhance our knowledge not only on health workforce mobility but also on workforce development. I appreciate the insights given by the inclusion of a wide range of countries across the European region, both within and outside the European Union.

I therefore welcome this volume with its emphasis on the need to put health professional mobility into the wider country and health systems context.

Zsuzsanna Jakab, WHO Regional Director for Europe

Acknowledgements

This volume is one of a series of books produced by the European Observatory on Health Systems and Policies. We would like to express our gratitude to the country authors for their dedication and expertise; to Jonathan North for his patience and support in the production process; to Jo Woodhead for her diligence and precision in language editing; and to Peter Powell for his professionalism and typesetting skill. This book would not have been possible without their outstanding work and persistence.

For Chapter 2, the authors would like to thank Mr Sohaïb Azibou, Ms Caroline Jadot, Mr Henk Vandenbroele and Mr Toon De Geest (FPS Public Health); Mr Chris Segaert and Mr Pascal Meert (NIHDI); Mr Daniël De Schrijver (NARIC-Vlaanderen); Ms Anne Hellemans and Mr Julien Boudart (Ministry of the French Community); and Ms Hellen Sjerps-de Boer and Mr Jurian Luiten (Dutch Ministry of Public Health). This research would not have been possible without their help in providing us with data and/or valuable information.

For Chapter 4, the authors would like to thank G Le Breton-Lerouvillois, F Montané and O Uguen (CNOM); DHD Bui (Center for Sociology and Medical Demography); E Quillet (DHOS, Ministère de la Santé et des Sports); S Guigner and A Le Vigouroux (EHESP); M Millan (Ministère de la Santé et des Sports), P Garel (European Hospital and Healthcare Federation), J-C Dumont and G Lafortune (OECD); C Aguilella and C Couzinou (ONCD); and M Burdillat (ONDPS).

For Chapter 7, the authors thank Jaime Pinilla and Sara Santiago for their help.

For Chapter 9, the authors are grateful to Evi Lindmäe (Head, Department of Registers and Licences, Health Board), Erna Mering (Head, Bureau of Registries, Health Board) and Eero Mõttus (Chief Specialist, Information- and Communication Technology Department, Ministry of Social Affairs of Estonia) for their assistance in providing statistical information. The authors are also grateful to Taavi Lai (Senior Analyst, Health Information and Analysis Department, Ministry of Social Affairs of Estonia) and Triin Habicht (Head, Health Economics Department, Estonian Health Insurance Fund) for their valuable feedback and comments during the report review process.

For Chapter 10, we would like to thank Dr Péter Balázs who was a special contributor to this study. We used data, analytical results and studies from his relevant publications and consulted with him on some issues that arose.

For Chapter 12, the authors would like to acknowledge the valuable contribution of Agata Grudzień, Marcin Mikos and Dariusz Poznański in the process of collecting data and supporting information on the migration of Polish health professionals.

For Chapter 13, the authors are grateful to Ioana Pertache (Deputy Director, NCOEHIS, Bucharest) for providing valuable input about the National Registry of Physicians. They are also grateful to Professor Vasile *Astărăstoae* (President of the Romanian College of Physicians); Mircea Timofte (President of the Order of Nurses and Midwives); Professor Alexandru Rafila (University of Medicine and Pharmacy Bucharest, former Adviser for Health Policies, Ministry of Health); Beatrice Nimereanu (Head, Human Resources Department, Ministry of Health); Cassandra Butu (Technical Officer, WHO Country Office); and Cezar Popa-Canache (Legal Adviser, Institute of Public Health, Bucharest) for their useful information, comments and revisions.

For Chapter 16, the authors would like to express their gratitude to the following institutions and their representatives who contributed valuable insights and data on health professionals: Dr Ivana Mišić (Assistant Minister and Head of Department of Health Service Organization, Ministry of Health); Dr Tanja Radosavljević (President, Serbian Chamber of Physicians); Mr Dragan *Šašić* (Director, Serbian Chamber of Nurses and Health Technicians); Mrs Radmila Nešić (President, Association of Health Workers of Serbia); Mrs Verica Milovanović (President) and Mrs Živka Mitić (Association of Nurses, Technicians and Midwives of Serbia); Serbian Chamber of Dentists, Serbian Medical Association, Institute of Public Health "Dr Milan Jovanovic Batut", Clinical Center of Serbia, Belgrade and others. Professor Vladimir Grečić (School of Economics, University of Belgrade), a renowned expert in the field of migration, gave us valuable expert opinion. Special thanks to Ms Miroslava Narančić for data entry and formatting.

List of tables, figures and boxes

Boxes

List of abbreviations

ADELI	*Automatisation des Listes*
AFS	Attestation of specialized training (*Attestation de formation spécialisée*)
AFSA	Attestation of specialized training, advanced level (*Attestation de formation spécialisée approfondie*)
AMS	Public Employment Service Austria (*Arbeitsmarktservice Österreich*)
AO	hospital public enterprises (*aziende ospedaliere*)
APSEP	Association of Spanish Health Professionals in Portugal (*Associação de Profissionais da Saúde Espanhóis em Portugal*)
azM	University Hospital of Maastricht
BMG	Austrian Federal Ministry of Health (*Bundesministerium für Gesundheit*)
CEE	central and eastern Europe
CGS	certificate of good standing
CNEL	National Council for Economics and Labour (*Consiglio Nazionale Economia e Lavoro*)
CNOM	National Medical Council (*Conseil National de l'Ordre des Médecins*)
ÇSGB	Ministry of Labour and Social Security (*Çalışma ve Sosyal Güvenlik Bakanlığı*)
CSP	*Code de la santé publique*
DBfK	German Nursing Association (*Deutscher Berufsverband für Pflegeberufe*)
DDASS	*Direction Départementale des Affaires Sanitaires et Socials*
DPR	German Nursing Council (*Deutscher Pflegerat*)
DREES	Directorate of Research, Studies, Evaluation and Statistics (*Direction de la Recherche, des Etudes, de l'Evaluation et des Statistiques*)
DRG	diagnosis related group
FNOMCeO	Order of Medical Surgeons and Dentists (*Federazione Nazionale Ordini Medici Chirurghi e Odontoiatri*)
GDC	General Dental Council
GMC	General Medical Council
GUS	Central Statistical Office of Poland (*Glówny Urząd Statystynzny*)
EAPS	Economically Active Population Survey
EEA	European Economic Area
EEIG	European Economic Interest Grouping
EHIF	Estonian Health Insurance Fund
ERDF	European Regional Development Fund
ESF	European Social Fund
EU	European Union
EURES	National Employment Agency (Romania)

FPS	Federal Public Service
GDP	gross domestic product
GSP	Great Student Project
HB	Health Board (known as Health Care Board before 2010)
HCB	Health Care Board (became Health Board in 2010)
HIIS	Health Insurance Institute of Slovenia
HMC	Hungarian Medical Chamber
HPC	Health Professions Council
HTP	Health Transformation Programme
IDE	*Infirmier diplômé d'Etat*
INAIL	Italian Workers Compensation Authority (*Istituto Nazionale per l'Assicurazione contro gli Infortuni sul Lavoro*)
INE	National Statistics Institute (*Instituto Nacional de Estadística*)
IPASVI	National Board of Nursing (*Federazione Nazionale Collegi Infermieri*)
IRDES	Institute for Research and Information in Health Economics (*Institut de Recherche et Documentation en Economie de la Santé*)
Istat	National Institute of Statistics (*Istituto Nazionale di Statistica*)
KASTE Programme	National Development Programme for Social Welfare and Health Care
MCS	Medical Chamber of Slovenia
Migri	Finnish Immigration Service
MIR	specialist resident (*médico interno residente*)
MVZ	medical treatment centres (*Medizinisches Versorgungszentrum*)
NCOEHIS	National Centre for Organising and Ensuring the Health Information System
NCS	Nursing Chamber of Slovenia
NHCPD	National Health Care Providers Database
NHIC	National Health Information Centre
NHS	National Health Service
NIHD	National Institute for Health Development
NIHDI	National Institute for Health and Disability Insurance
NIS	National Immigrant Survey
NMC	Nursing and Midwifery Council
NÖGUS	Lower Austria Health and Social Capital Fund (*Niederösterreichischer Gesundheits- und Sozialfonds*)
ÖÄK	Austrian Medical Chamber (*Österreichische Ärztekammer*)
OAMMR	Order of Nurses and Midwives (*Ordinul Asistenților Medicali și Moașelor din România*)
ÖBIG	Austrian Federal Institute for Health Care (*Österreichisches Bundesinstitut für Gesundheit*)
OECD	Organisation for Economic Co-operation and Development
ÖGKV	Austrian Health Nurses Association (*Österreichischer Gesundheits- und Krankenpflegeverband*)
OHAAP	Office of Health Authorisation and Administrative Procedures
ÖHG	Austrian Association of Midwives (*Österreichisches Hebammengremium*)

OMC	Organization of Medical Colleges
ONCD	National Order of Dental Surgeons (*Ordre National des Chirurgiens Dentistes*)
ONDPS	National Observatory on the Demography of Health Professions (*Observatoire National de la Démographie des Professions de Santé*)
ORF	Austrian Broadcast Association (*Österreichischer Rundfunk*)
ÖSG	Austrian Structural Plan for Health (*Österreichischer Strukturplan Gesundheit*)
PAC	associate practitioner (*Praticiens adjoints contractuels*)
PADHUE	*Praticiens à diplôme Hors Union Européenne*
RCP	Romanian College of Physicians
RPSGB	Royal Pharmaceutical Society of Great Britain
RSG	Regional structural plan for health (*Regionaler Strukturplan Gesundheit*)
SHU	Slovak Health University in Bratislava
SIP	Italian Society of Psychiatry (*Società Italiana Psichiatria*)
SU HSMTC	Semmelweis University Health Services Management Training Centre
THL	National Institute for Health and Welfare
TMA	Turkish Medical Association
UCL	*Université catholique de Louvain*
ULSS	local health authorities (*unita locale socio sanitaria*)
UZA	University Hospital of Antwerp
Valvira	National Supervisory Authority for Welfare and Health
WHO	World Health Organization (WHO)
WIFO	Austrian Institute of Economic Research (*Österreichisches Institut für Wirtschaftsforschung*)
WRT	Workforce Review Team
WTD	Working Time Directive

List of contributors

Chapter 1. Austria

Guido Offermanns, Associate Professor, Faculty of Management and Economics, University of Klagenfurt, Austria

Eva Maria Malle, Research Assistant, Faculty of Management and Economics, University of Klagenfurt, Austria

Mirela Jusic, Research Assistant, Faculty of Management and Economics, University of Klagenfurt, Austria

Chapter 2. Belgium

Anna Safuta, former Researcher, European Social Observatory, Belgium and PhD student, Catholic University of Louvain-la-Neuve, Belgium

Rita Baeten, Senior Policy Analyst, European Social Observatory, Belgium

Chapter 3. Finland

Hannamaria Kuusio, Researcher, National Institute for Health and Welfare (THL), Finland

Meri Koivusalo, Senior Researcher, THL, Finland

Marko Elovainio, Research Professor, THL, Finland

Tarja Heponiemi, Senior Researcher, THL, Finland

Anna-Mari Aalto, Head of Unit, THL, Finland

Ilmo Keskimäki, Research Professor, THL, Finland

Chapter 4. France

Marie-Laure Delamaire, Associate Researcher, Ecole des Hautes Etudes en Santé Publique (EHESP), France

François-Xavier Schweyer, Senior Lecturer, EHESP, France

Chapter 5. Germany

Diana Ognyanova, Research Fellow, Department of Health Care Management, Berlin University of Technology, Germany

Reinhard Busse, Professor of Health Care Management, Berlin University of Technology and Associate Head for Research Policy, European Observatory on Health Systems and Policies, Germany

Chapter 6. Italy

Luigi Bertinato, Director of Service for International, Social and Health Relations, ULSS 20 Veneto Region, Italy

Irene A Glinos, researcher, European Observatory on Health Systems and Policies, Belgium

Elisa Boscolo, EU Policy Adviser, ULSS 5 Veneto Region, Italy

Leopoldo Ciato, Director of Human Resources, ULSS 5 Veneto Region, Italy

Chapter 7. Spain

Beatriz González López-Valcárcel, Professor, University of Las Palmas de Gran Canaria, Spain

Patricia Barber Pérez, Associate Professor, University of Las Palmas de Gran Canaria, Spain

Carmen Delia Dávila Quintana, Associate Professor, University of Las Palmas de Gran Canaria, Spain

Chapter 8. United Kingdom

Ruth Young, Reader in Health Policy Evaluation, Florence Nightingale School of Nursing and Midwifery, King's College, London, United Kingdom

Chapter 9. Estonia

Pille Saar, Adviser, Health Care Department, Ministry of Social Affairs of Estonia, Estonia

Jarno Habicht, WHO Representative/Head of Country Office, Republic of Moldova (Head, WHO Country Office, Estonia until end 2010)

Chapter 10. Hungary

Edit Eke, Edmond Girasek, Miklós Szócska

Edit Eke, Human Resources for Health Expert, at Health Services Management Training Centre, Semmelweis University, Hungary

Edmond Girasek, Assistant Lecturer, Health Services Management Training Centre, Semmelweis University, Hungary

Miklós Szócska, Minister of State for Health, Ministry of National Resources, Hungary; formerly Director and Associate Professor, Health Services Management Training Centre, Semmelweis University, Hungary

Chapter 11. Lithuania

Žilvinas Padaiga, Professor of Public Health, Department of Preventive Medicine and Dean of International Relations and Study Centre, Medical Academy, Lithuanian University of Health Sciences, Lithuania

Liudvika Starkienė, Associate Professor, Department of Preventive Medicine, Medical Academy, Lithuanian University of Health Sciences, Lithuania

Martynas Pukas, PhD student, Department of Preventive Medicine, Medical Academy, Lithuanian University of Health Sciences, Lithuania

Chapter 12. Poland

Marcin Kautsch, Katarzyna Czabanowska

Marcin Kautsch, Assistant Professor, Institute of Public Health, Jagiellonian University, Poland

Katarzyna Czabanowska, Assistant Professor, Department of International Health, Faculty of Health Medicine and Life Sciences, Maastricht University, Netherlands

Chapter 13. Romania

Adriana Galan, Public Health Consultant, National Institute of Public Health, Romania

Victor Olsavszky, Head of WHO Country Office, Romania

Cristian Vladescu, Professor of Public Health, University of Medicine and Pharmacy, Timisoara, Romania

Chapter 14. Slovakia

Kvetoslava Beňušová, Assistant Professor, St. Elizabeth University of Health and Social Sciences, Bratislava, Slovakia

Miloslava Kováčová, Senior Expert, Ministry of Health of the Slovak Republic, Slovakia

Marián Nagy, Senior Expert, Ministry of Health of the Slovak Republic, Slovakia

Matthias Wismar, Senior Health Policy Analyst, European Observatory on Health Systems and Policies, Belgium

Chapter 15. Slovenia

Tit Albreht, Head of the Department of Health System Analyses, National Institute of Public Health, Slovenia

Chapter 16. Serbia

Ivan M Jekić, National Coordinator/Health Services Expert, European Investment Bank Technical Assistant to the Ministry of Health Project for the Modernization of the Four Clinical Centres in Serbia, Serbia

Annette Katrava, International Consultant; Team Leader and Health Accreditation Expert, Delegation of the European Union to the Republic of Serbia; Technical Assistant to Ministry of Health Project for the Establishment of the Public Agency for Accreditation and Continuous Quality Improvement of Health Care in Serbia

Maja Vučković-Krčmar, Project Manager, Health & Social Affairs, Delegation of the European Union to the Republic of Serbia, Serbia

Chapter 17. Turkey

Hasan Hüseyin Yıldırım, Assistant Professor, Department of Health Care Management, Faculty of Economics and Administrative Sciences, Hacettepe University, Turkey

Sıdıka Kaya, Professor, Department of Health Care Management, Faculty of Economics and Administrative Sciences, Hacettepe University, Turkey

Part 1
Setting the scene, results and conclusions

Health professional mobility and health systems in Europe: an introduction

Claudia B Maier, Irene A Glinos, Matthias Wismar, Jeni Bremner,
Gilles Dussault, Josep Figueras

1. Introduction

This volume presents an analysis of health professional mobility in Europe from a health system perspective. The central policy issue is that health professional mobility impacts on the performance of health systems and that these impacts are increasing in line with increasing mobility in Europe.

Health professional mobility impacts on the performance of health systems by changing the composition of the health workforce in both sending and receiving countries. These gains and losses may strengthen or weaken the performance of health systems and, while they may seem negligible, produce visible impacts when numbers increase or through continuous mobility over years. Health professional mobility also affects the skill-mix since skills travel with the mobile health professional. When these skills are rare and essential, outflows of even small numbers of health professionals can impact on health system performance. Health professional mobility can also affect the distribution of health workers in a country. A disproportionately high outflow from a region may cause or aggravate maldistribution, resulting in under-supplied and underserved areas in which the local population is left without sufficient health workers. However, the impacts on health system performance are often indirect and part of a complex chain of causalities.

The EU enlargements in 2004 and 2007 introduced 100 million citizens from 12 new Member States and have caused substantial expansion of the pool of health professionals within the EU labour market. This has fuelled mobility as some of these health professionals have joined those already moving around

Europe in search of better career opportunities, better salaries and better working conditions. Migrants may be motivated by the desire to acquire new skills, by family reasons or by curiosity; they may commute for days or weekends; stay for short periods or several years; and may move on, return or settle permanently. In addition, enlargement has increased the economic diversity of the EU. Larger salary differentials and larger differences in infrastructures and in the use and availability of modern medical technology have further incentivized health professional mobility from the EU-12 countries.

But what do we know about this important phenomenon? Knowledge on health professional mobility in Europe is limited. For example, there are gaps in understanding of the magnitude of health professional mobility, particularly concerning EU enlargement. There is also no overview of the motivators that drive the mobile European health workforce (not just health workers from third countries) or any systematic mapping of the impacts of health professional mobility. By learning about responses to health professional mobility in other countries it will become possible to identify best practices.

This volume aims to enhance knowledge on the nature and extent of health professional mobility in the EU, assess its impact on country health systems and outline some major policy strategies to address mobility The book seeks to provide not only a rigorous and systematic analysis of the mobility patterns in Europe but also a series of evidence-base and policy-relevant lessons that contribute to the policy debate in the EU.

The analytical framework for the study is therefore structured around a set of key policy-makers' questions which will form the conceptual backbone of this volume.

- What are the scale and characteristics of health professional mobility in the EU?

- What have been the effects of EU enlargement on professional mobility?

- What are the motivations of the mobile workforce? Why do some health professionals leave their country while others stay or return?

- What positive or negative impacts on the performance of health systems result from mobility flows?

- What is the policy relevance of those impacts vis-à-vis other workforce challenges? In other words, should policy-makers address health professional mobility as a priority?

- What policy options and regulatory inventions (recruitment policies, international frameworks, workforce planning and general workforce measures) are needed to address health professional mobility issues? Is their evidence on their impact and applicability?

The analysis presented in this volume results from the Health PROMeTHEUS[1] project. This three-year research began in 2009 with the aim of addressing gaps in the knowledge on health professional mobility in order to generate recommendations for more effective human resources for health policies. The project is funded through the European Commission's Seventh Framework Programme.[2]

This publication will be followed by a second volume structured around a series of themes on health professional mobility including the changing dynamics, monitoring and measuring, the mobile individual and changing responses and will conclude with scenarios on the future of health professional mobility.

This chapter will first outline the policy context in which professional mobility takes place in EU countries. The next section will explain the conceptual framework employed to analyse country experiences and will be followed by a description of the study methodology. The final section will provide an outline of the rest of this volume.

2. The EU context

Health professional mobility impacts on the composition of the health workforce which in turn impacts on health system performance. This cannot be viewed in isolation as health professional mobility interacts with many other factors and challenges that also affect the health workforce. These include new technologies, globalization, feminization of the workforce, training capacities, working conditions and working environments (Dubois et al. 2006, Wiskow et al. 2010). Such interactions have to be taken into account in order to gain full understanding of the phenomenon and how best to address it. This study places health professional mobility in this broader context and needs to consider all these elements. Here we briefly illustrate the role of three of these contextual elements: (i) demographic transition; (ii) strategies addressing general workforce issues; and (iii) the unique EU context.

First, the ageing of the health workforce imposes some restrictions on policy responses as increases in training capacities or recruitment from other sectors are no longer effective in all countries. In Europe the pool of young people is decreasing at a fast pace (OECD 2007) and this will bring increasing competition for recruitment between different employers and sectors. Finland

---

1 Health PROMeTHEUS = Health PROfessional Mobility in THe European Union Study.
2 Grant agreement number 223383.

has already reacted to this development by introducing nationwide workforce planning (Dussault et al. 2010).

Second, health professional mobility needs to be understood within the wider strategies addressing the general workforce issues with which it interacts (Dubois et al. 2006). A Europewide debate on the topic was initiated by the European Commission's Green Paper on the European workforce for health (Commission of the European Communities 2008), followed by a consultation process (Directorate General for Health and Consumers 2009). Connected to this, the Belgium Council Presidency, together with the European Commission and the EU Member States have explored three topics: (i) assessing future health workforce needs; (ii) adapting skills and redistribution of tasks; and (iii) creating a supportive working environment to attract motivated health professionals.[3]

Health professional mobility can undermine attempts to forecast workforce needs if inflows and outflows are not well-understood and factored into the planning. Good understanding of the trends and early warnings of their fluctuations are even more essential in times of uncertainty. Similarly, inadequate monitoring or poor understanding of the inflows and outflows of skills will reduce the effectiveness of strategies to change the skill-mix and task distribution. Improvement of the working environment is an important strategy for retaining health professionals in health-care organizations and it is essential to understand whether retention strategies also work for health professionals with intentions to migrate.

Finally, several factors shape the unique conditions under which the EU can respond to health professional mobility. These include the free-movement framework, European social values and the policy instruments of the EU.

The formulation of any response to health professional mobility in the EU must take account of the very limited potential for imposing such restrictions on EU citizens. The **free movement** of workers is an economic imperative and a civil right enshrined in the Treaties, supported by a host of secondary legislation.[4] Most importantly, Directive 2005/36/EC on the recognition of professional qualifications ensures a high portability of qualifications for medical doctors, nurses and dentists by facilitating an automatic procedure in which qualifications are checked by the conformity of their qualification

---

3 In support of these activities policy briefs and summaries were published on forecasting (Dussault et al. 2010), skill-mix (Horsley et al. 2010), working conditions (Wiskow C et al. 2010) and quality and safety (Flottorp et al. 2010). Also, policy dialogues were conducted in Leuven, Belgium, 26–30 April 2010. Under the Belgium Council Presidency, the Member States adopted Council conclusions on investing in Europe's health workforce of tomorrow (Council of the European Union 2010).

4 This freedom of movement applies to the European Economic Area (EEA), which includes the EU 27 Member States and three European Free Trade Association (EFTA) members – Iceland, Liechtenstein and Norway. Switzerland is a member of the EFTA but not of the EEA and has a separate bilateral agreement on mobility with the EU.

levels and training periods rather than by individual assessment of the skills and competencies acquired (Peeters et al. 2010).

Research on European integration in health and health care has referred to the imbalance between the **social values** of the EU and the economic imperative of European integration (Mossialos et al. 2010). Yet these social values are relevant when formulating responses to health professional mobility. The European Court of Justice has found repeatedly that patient mobility (technically the mobility of services) can be restricted on the grounds that it may threaten the economic viability of hospitals by increasing the difficulty of human resource planning (Palm et al. 2011). It remains to be seen whether similar legal arguments will be made for concerns regarding quality and patient safety in health professional mobility.

The EU has a large set of **policy instruments** (including regulations, directives and decisions) with which to respond to health professional mobility issues. In addition, budgets for public health and research and for social development and social cohesion are available to address workforce issues within countries. This distinguishes the EU response to health professional mobility from the global response articulated in the *WHO Global Code of Practice on the International Recruitment of Health Personnel* (WHO 2010) which builds on voluntary commitments from Member States.

3. Conceptual framework

The analysis of professional mobility presented in this volume is structured around a series of policy questions (outlined in the introductory section) which form the basis for the presentation of main results in the following chapter. In turn, these results summarize the evidence drawn from the country case studies in Part II. This section will outline the policy questions and the policy relevance and highlight research gaps. It will conclude with a brief explanation of how we tackle the questions.

3.1 *Mobility profiles*

Policy-makers and stakeholders face a pressing question – what are the scale and characteristics of health professional mobility in the EU?

Quantification of health professional mobility is a centrepiece of the research because the magnitude of health professional mobility determines the magnitude of the impacts on health system performance. Policy responses and ethical concerns also require understanding of mobility patterns and the source regions of professionals, including the wider Europe (WHO European Region countries outside the free-movement area) and third countries.

But what do we know about health professional mobility in Europe? A World Health Organization (WHO) study (Dussault et al. 2009) reports that migratory flows of health workers are generally documented poorly. Currently, there is no mechanism to compile migration data and monitor flows in either the EU or the wider Europe and existing data tend to be fragmentary and unreliable since they do not represent direct measurement of migration (Dussault et al. 2009).

Some important international publications shed some light on the situation in Europe. A WHO study provides an overview of the 53 countries in the WHO European Region. Published in 2009, the data for most countries are for 2005 or earlier (Dussault et al. 2009). Three OECD studies provide relevant information. The first reports a (Dussault et al. 2009) substantial rise in health professional mobility between 1995 and 2005 in 12 selected OECD countries, including 8 European countries[5] (OECD 2007). The second is a comprehensive study of looming workforce crises which includes analysis of the reliance on foreign health professionals as well as some flow data (OECD 2008). The third examines how the financial and economic crisis has affected mobility trends. It includes the European free-movement area and makes reference to Norway, Poland, Switzerland and the United Kingdom. However, the results for those countries are inconclusive and do not explicitly refer to health professionals (OECD 2010). Finally, a joint OECD/WHO policy brief presents data on levels of reliance on foreign health professionals including 17 countries for medical doctors and 11 for nurses (WHO & OECD 2010).

At country level, some European countries are paying greater attention to health professional mobility and developing solid information bases through high-quality data collection and research. Case studies have been published on Member States that acceded to the EU before 2004, including France (Cash & Ulmann 2008), Italy (Chaloff 2008), Germany (Buchan 2006b), Ireland (Humphries et al. 2008) and the United Kingdom (Buchan 2002 & 2006a, Buchan & O'May 1999, Jinks et al. 2000). Other case studies cover the 2004 and 2007 accession countries including the Czech Republic (Angelovski et al. 2006), Poland (Leśniowska 2007), Estonia (Buchan & Pefilieva 2006), Lithuania (Buchan 2006b) and Romania (Galan 2006). There are also case studies on EU candidate countries such as Croatia (Džakula et al. 2006) and Serbia (Djikanovic 2006). Case studies on the United States (Cooper 2008) and New Zealand (Zurn & Dumont 2008) are also of value since these are destination countries for European health professionals. The case studies provide very important analysis but show wide variations in thematic focus, coverage

5 Denmark, Finland, Ireland, the Netherlands, Norway, Sweden, Switzerland and the United Kingdom.

of professions and analytical depth and it is difficult (if not impossible) to draw comparisons. Swift developments in the EU mean that there is insufficient coverage of EU enlargement and some countries have introduced major health policy reforms and changes to their workforce policies since publication of their case studies.

We address some of the knowledge gaps on the scale and characteristics of health professional mobility by analysing the levels of reliance on foreign health professionals and the scale of actual inflows and outflows, complemented by analysis of the geographical patterns of mobility and the source regions of the mobile workforce. The analysis will be based on a secondary data collection retrieved from different sources in the individual countries. To ensure comparability the coverage of the professions and the data will apply across all countries included in the volume.

3.2 *Role of EU enlargement*

What have been the effects of EU enlargement on professional mobility?

Analysis of the role of enlargement is important not only because of the impetus it has provided for the volume and diversity of health professional mobility in Europe but also for policy debate. The latter covers the concerns of the prospective EU-12 countries regarding expected brain drain and concerns in some EU-12 countries about disruptive impacts on their health system stemming from excessively high inflows. The question is also important for consideration of the likely effects of lifting remaining labour market restrictions and of future enlargements.

There is still no comprehensive analysis of mobility trends during the course of enlargement (OECD 2008, Wiskow 2006). A few of the reports and case studies mentioned in section 2.1 provide some insights but the Romanian case study was published before accession (Galan 2006). Other reports and case studies include only the first 12 to 18 months of EU accession in Estonia (Buchan & Pefilieva 2006) and Lithuania (Buchan 2006b). Data and analysis published on Polish nurses include the first quarter of 2007 (Leśniowska 2007& 2008).

We will respond to the question on the role of enlargement and address the knowledge gaps by analysing the outflows from the seven EU-12 countries included in this study and identifying these health professionals in the statistics of the destination countries. We will also assess the time trends notwithstanding the lack of data in many countries. Intention-to-leave data will be used to fill data gaps when quantifying outflows.

3.3 *Motivation of the mobile workforce*

What are the motivations of the mobile workforce? Why do some health professionals leave their country but others stay or return? Understanding of these motivations is an essential precondition for policy-makers seeking to develop adequate recruitment and retention policies.

Some existing studies in Europe provide some insights into motivations but huge gaps remain. The OECD (2008) has looked into these motivations and some studies focus on migrants from third countries (Nichols & Campbell 2010a & 2010b). In Lithuania, studies were conducted on intentions to leave among physicians and medical residents (Stankunas et al. 2004), nurses (Matuleviciute 2007) and pharmacists (Smigelskas 2007). Related to this research, the framework of the European NEXT-Study[6] has included extensive research on intention to leave the profession and another study has explored young doctors' willingness to work in rural areas (Girasek et al. 2010).

We have asked authors to address the motivations of the mobile workforce by researching specific motivational factors within their country based on surveys, qualitative interviews, focus groups, grey literature and expert observations. Specifically, we have asked the authors to consider instigating, activating and facilitating factors and encouraged them to identify research into the particular motivations driving health professionals intending to leave, to stay or to return.

3.4 *Impacts on performance*

What are the (positive or negative) impacts on the performance of health systems that result from mobility flows?

A central concern of our research and therefore of this volume is to analyse the impacts of health professional mobility on the performance of health systems. These are the lynchpin of the policy debate on health professional mobility. It is important to see whether both hopes and worries concerning health professional mobility are supported by the evidence reported from the countries. Also, there is a need for further examination of the distribution of effects between source and destination countries.

But what is known already about the impacts? Overall, there have been only a few attempts to identify impacts in Europe (Peeters et al. 2010), covering only a handful of countries including the United Kingdom (Ballard et al. 2004, Jinks et al. 2000), Germany (Hyde 2005), the Czech Republic (Mareckova 2006) and Poland (Leśniowska 2007). Some of the impacts relate to regional or local shortages, others to the training pipeline. There have also been reports

---

6 Nurses' early exit study (http://www.next.uni-wuppertal.de/EN/index.php?next-study, accessed 13 March 2011).

on the impact on workforce planning. Another example are the concerns about impacts on health system performance raised by the informal network of competent authorities for the recognition of qualifications for doctors. These concerns focused on the quality of care and patient safety linked to the professional skills and language knowledge of migrant doctors and to their integration within the host country's health system (Informal Network Competent Authorities for Doctors 2010).

In this study we pick up on the observation discussed earlier – that impacts may affect health system performance indirectly through complex chains of causality. In conceptual terms, we are analysing not only direct impacts on performance but also impacts on the functions contributing to the objectives of a health system. To this end we have adopted a broad health systems approach based on the WHO health systems model depicted in Fig. 0.1.

Fig. 0.1 *Categorizing the impacts of health professional of mobility according to the functions and objectives of the health system*

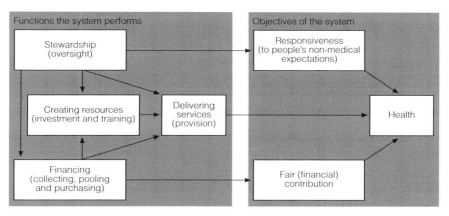

Source: World Health Organization 2000.

3.5 *Policy relevance*

What is the policy relevance of these impacts vis-à-vis other workforce challenges? In other words – should policy-makers address health professional mobility as a priority?

It is important to place health professional mobility within the context of other workforce issues in order to prioritize policy action. The results of such an examination can provide an overview to determine whether this is a pressing issue across Europe. It can also indicate whether health professional mobility requires specific policies or should be tackled in the context of other workforce measures.

In order to respond to these questions we have asked authors to qualitatively assess the relevance of health professional mobility in comparison to domestic workforce issues including the maldistribution of health workers over the territory, workforce shortages, attrition, demographic transition and problems with the training pipeline. In comparative terms we will classify countries in different levels of policy relevance.

3.6 *Policy and regulatory interventions*

What are the policy options for addressing health professional mobility issues?

Policy-makers aiming to tackle health professional mobility or to improve existing strategies will benefit from information on the use of policy and regulatory measures in other countries. Learning about the use of instruments individually and in conjunction with others may inspire solutions for their own country.

There is limited knowledge on policy development concerning health professional mobility and general workforce issues and there is no comprehensive overview, only selected frameworks. Interest in workforce planning as a centrepiece of workforce policy has grown only recently (Dussault et al 2010). Buchan's (2008) categorization of the instruments for managing health professional mobility (Table 0.1) provides a very useful starting point for further research but, apart from the research on bilateral agreements (Dhillon et al. 2010), knowledge remains patchy.

To address some of the knowledge gaps, case study authors were asked to search for explicit recruitment policies (international and self-sufficiency), international frameworks (see Table 0.1), workforce planning procedures and general workforce measures facilitating the retention of health professionals by improving working conditions and the working environment.

4. Methodology

This section will provide more details on the methodologies employed to research the evidence for this book, starting with a brief summary of the PROMeTHEUS project. This will be followed by a discussion of the challenges that faced the project and some of the strategies used to address the challenges: a good country sample, mechanisms to ensure comparability and a mix of research methodologies to develop analytically rich case studies.

Table 0.1 *Cross-border instruments and tools for steering and managing health professional mobility*

Instrument/tool	Description
Twinning	Links developed by health-care organizations in source and destination countries based on staff exchanges, staff support and flow of resources to source country
Staff exchange	Structured temporary move of staff to another organization, based on career and personal development opportunities or organizational development
Educational support	Educators and/or educational resources and/or funding in temporary move from destination to source organization
Compensation	Destination country provides some type of compensation to source country in recompense for the impact of active recruitment (much discussed but little evidence in practice)
Training for international recruitment	Government or private sector makes explicit decision to develop a training infrastructure to train health professionals for employment in other countries in order to generate remittances or fees
International code	Code of ethics on international recruitment. The best known codes are those from the United Kingdom (introduced 2001) and the WHO Global Code (adopted 2010).

Source: adapted from Buchan 2008.

Health PROMeTHEUS is a research project funded through the European Commission's Seventh Framework Programme on research and innovation and run by a consortium of 11 partners, supported by 7 country correspondents and a large number of country informants. Outputs of the project include several publications, conference workshops and policy dialogues. The acronym PROMeTHEUS was chosen because this titan of Greek mythology was a champion of mankind who stole fire from Zeus and gave it to mortals. Similarly, the aim of the project is to illuminate what would otherwise remain in the dark and compare the situation and trends of health mobility between countries in Europe.

The project has faced a number of daunting challenges. First, throughout the course of the project the analytical work of country case study authors was hindered by the lack of a commonly agreed definition of health professional mobility. A definition was deemed necessary to define the scope of research and is also a starting point for future categorization of different types of health professional mobility. Second, country coverage. How to ensure the capture of key developments and trends with a small sample? Time and resources would not allow the inclusion of all 31 countries from the European free-movement area, let alone reaching out to the wider Europe. Third, how to ensure the comparability of research results? Variations between European countries (in institutional settings, types of health systems and organizational peculiarities, for example) do not allow direct comparison. Also, diverse countries produce diverse stories. This may be appealing to the reader but offers limited scope for comparison if each case study emphasizes or omits different aspects. Fourth, how to ensure that the analytical quality of a country's case study is not undermined by variations in the availability of data and research literature? International studies and international databases have shown wide differences in data availability and time trend data. Some countries have well-established research on health professional mobility that provides a robust basis for developing a country case study but good literature is scarce in other countries. It is not claimed that such a multitude of challenges could be overcome completely but a set of strategies was employed to address these concerns.

To better define the focus of research and also to capture health professional mobility beyond the meaning of the foreign-trained, foreign-born and foreign-national indicators, an adequate definition of health professional mobility was discussed from the beginning of the project. This definition (Box 0.1) will also provide guidance for our future research by providing a starting point for the development of typologies of health professional mobility and assessing the validity of indicators.

Box 0.1 *Definition of health professional mobility emerging from the project*

Any intentional change of country after graduation with the purpose and effect of delivering health-related services, including during training periods

---

A country sample was established with the intention of capturing the situation in Europe and covering the major trends without the need to include all 31 countries in the research. Four criteria were used to determine country selection. First, the sample should be sufficiently diverse and represent every corner of the EU including larger and smaller countries, those with national health systems and those with social health insurance. Second, the sample should enable a particular focus on the 2004 and 2007 enlargement countries since their role in health professional mobility was under-researched. Third, the sample should include larger European labour markets in Europe since they have a high capacity to absorb large absolute numbers of mobile health professionals while showing relatively low reliance on foreign health professionals. Fourth, the sample should meet the need to build the bridge to a wider Europe and to understand mobility between countries within and outside the free-movement area (Table 0.2).

Table 0.2 *Country coverage*

Member States before 2004	Member States since 2004/2007	Countries having applied for EU membership
Austria	Estonia	Serbia
Belgium	Hungary	Turkey
Finland	Lithuania	
France	Poland	
Germany	Romania	
Italy	Slovakia	
Spain	Slovenia	
United Kingdom		

The analytical framework discussed above was the centrepiece for ensuring comparability of results. All country authors were asked to respond to the questions raised in the analytical framework which was supported by a resource package including a template, a conceptual background document. A user guide provided detailed instructions on the coverage of professions, data types and data time points.

A mix of methodologies has been employed to research health professional mobility. The basic methodology is the country case study because impacts, inflows, outflows and policy responses are hugely influenced by country context. Case studies provide a systematic way of looking at health professional mobility, collecting data, analysing information and reporting the results. For developing the country case studies several methodologies were applied. All case study authors conducted a literature review on the basis of the analytical framework using international and national publications, different databases and the World Wide Web. Secondary data collections were collated from data on the reliance on foreign health professionals and on actual flows. The time trend data requested were chosen to reflect flows before and after the profound geopolitical changes of 1989. Country case-study authors and country informants were asked to collect data for every year from 2000. Given the challenge of limited data and limited literature in some countries interviews were conducted where necessary and appropriate – interviews with individual mobile health professionals to enable better understanding of the practicalities of health professional mobility; with experts in order to complement the existing literature and data. All country case-study authors were asked to develop vignettes on health professional mobility to provide short summaries of individual experiences of health professional mobility.

4.1 *Limitations*

The data on health professional mobility have imposed restrictions on the case studies as many have come with long disclaimers. Data analysis has been limited by the availability of indicators and of data and by the data collection methods. Outflow data are disputed because they do not measure outflows directly and therefore impose serious limitations on the data analysis.

In addition, the time taken to develop a book of this magnitude and employ all the necessary quality measures means that some data collections were finalized a year before publication. Therefore, the impacts of the global financial crisis were not yet visible in many countries at the time when this research took place.

Country case studies provide the broad view and can put health professional mobility in context. This is essential for understanding the phenomenon but the reader is likely to want to know more about the details of the trends; the difficulties surrounding indicators, data and data collection; and many other topics. It is hoped that all these issues will be covered in much greater detail in the second volume.

5. Structure of the book

This book is divided into four parts. Part 1 comprises this introduction, the cross-country analysis and a conclusion. Based on the country case studies, the cross-country analysis starts by quantifying mobility in Europe. This is followed by sections on the geographical patterns of mobility, the role of EU enlargement and the motivational factors that drive the mobile workforce. The next section presents the impacts on health systems performance will be presented and is followed by an analysis of the workforce context and the relevance of health professional mobility. The chapter ends with policy and regulatory interventions and a summary of results.

The concluding chapter of Part 1 aims to address the needs of policy-makers by bringing together all the different threads of the research, beginning with some highlights of health professional mobility. These are followed by an examination of the importance of mobility that presents key observation from the research. Discussion of the risks and uncertainties related to health professional mobility is used to make the case for a proactive stance and to identify policy implications. The chapter ends with a brief conclusion linking the research to the policy processes in Europe.

Parts 2–4 contain the 17 country case studies on how health professional mobility impacts on health system performance. Each chapter follows the same structure. Part 2 includes eight country case studies from the EU-15 countries

– Austria, Belgium, Finland, France, Germany, Italy, Spain and the United Kingdom. Part 3 comprises seven country case studies from the 2004 and 2007 accession countries – Estonia, Hungary, Lithuania, Poland, Romania, Slovakia and Slovenia. Part 4 comprises two country case studies – one from a candidate country (Turkey) and one from a country that has applied for EU membership (Serbia).

The rationale for this structure is the geopolitical context of the EU and the resulting asymmetries. The research shows how the 2004 and 2007 enlargements have diversified and intensified health professional mobility in the EU, although the direction of flows has been from east to west. This is in line with other observable asymmetries. Almost all countries in the EU are losing health professionals to other countries but, while most countries in the EU-15 also have considerable inflows, inflows to the EU-12 are rather small. The same applies to reliance on foreign health professionals. Generally, EU-15 countries are much more reliant on foreign health professionals than those in the EU-12, with the notable exception of Slovenia. Turkey and Serbia have been placed in a separate section as they are not included in the free-movement framework.

References

Angelovski I et al. (2006). Health worker migration in selected CEE countries – Czech Republic. In: Wiskow C (ed.). *Health worker migration flows in Europe: overview and case studies in selected CEE countries – Romania, Czech Republic, Serbia and Croatia*. Geneva, International Labour Office (ILO Working Paper No. 245).

Ballard KD et al. (2004). Why do general practitioners from France choose to work in London practices? A qualitative study. *British Journal of General Practice*, 55(511):147–148.

Buchan J (2002). *International recruitment of nurses: United Kingdom case study*. Edinburgh, the World Health Organization, the International Council of Nurses and the Royal College of Nursing.

Buchan J (2006a). Filipino nurses in the UK: a case study in active international recruitment. *Harvard Health Policy Review*, 7(1):113–120.

Buchan J (2006b). Migration of health workers in Europe: policy problem or policy solution? In: Dubois C-A et al. (eds.). *Human resources for health in Europe*. Maidenhead, Open University Press.

Buchan J (2008). How can the migration of health service professionals be managed so as to reduce any negative effects on supply? Copenhagen, WHO Regional Office for Europe and European Observatory on Health Systems and Policies.

Buchan J, O'May F (1999). Globalisation and healthcare labour markets: a case study from the United Kingdom. *Human Resources for Health Development Journal*, 3(3):199–209.

Buchan J, Pefilieva G (2006). Health worker migration in the European Union: country case studies and policy implications. In: Wiskow C (ed.). *Health worker migration flows in Europe: overview and case studies in selected CEE countries – Romania, Czech Republic, Serbia and Croatia*. Geneva, International Labour Office (ILO Working Paper No. 245).

Cash R, Ulmann P (2008). *Projet OCDE sur la migration des professionnels de santé: le cas de la France*. Paris, Organisation for Economic Co-operation and Development (OECD Health Working Papers No. 36).

Chaloff J (2008). Mismatches in the formal sector, expansion of the informal sector: immigration of health professionals to Italy. Paris, Organisation for Economic Co-operation and Development (OECD Health Working Papers No. 34).

Commission of the European Communities (2008). *Green Paper on the European workforce for health*. Brussels (http://ec.europa.eu/health/ph_systems/docs/workforce_gp_en.pdf, accessed 14 March 2011).

Cooper RA (2008). *The US physician workforce: where do we stand?* Paris, Organisation for Economic Co-operation and Development.

Council of the European Union (2010). Council conclusions on investing in Europe's health workforce of tomorrow: scope for innovation and collaboration. Brussels (http://www.consilium.europa.eu/uedocs/cms_data/docs/pressdata/en/lsa/118280.pdf, accessed 19 February 2011.

Dhillon IS et al. (2010). Innovations in cooperation: a guidebook on bilateral agreements to address health worker migration. Washington DC, Aspen Institute (http://www.aspeninstitute.org/sites/default/files/content/docs/pubs/Bilateral%20Report_final%20code.pdf, accessed 20 February 2011).

Directorate General for Health and Consumers (2009). Report on the open consultation on the Green Paper on the European workforce for health. Luxembourg (http://ec.europa.eu/health/archive/ph_systems/docs/workforce_report.pdf, accessed 19 February 2011).

Djikanovic B (2006). Health worker migration in selected CEE countries: Serbia. In: Wiskow C (ed.). *Health worker migration flows in Europe: overview and case studies in selected CEE countries – Romania, Czech Republic, Serbia and Croatia*. Geneva, International Labour Office (ILO Working Paper No. 245).

Dubois C-A et al. (2006). Analysing trends, opportunities and challenges. In: Dubois C-A, et al. (eds.). *Human resources for health*. Maidenhead, Open University Press.

Dussault G et al. (2010). *Assessing future health workforce needs*. Copenhagen, WHO Regional Office for Europe and European Observatory on Health Systems and Policies.

Dussault G et al. (2009). *Migration of health personnel in the WHO European Region*. Copenhagen, WHO Regional Office for Europe (http://www.euro.who.int/ Document/E93039.pdf, accessed 30 March 2010).

Džakula A et al. (2006). Health worker migration in selected CEE countries: Croatia. In: Wiskow C (ed.). *Health worker migration flows in Europe: overview and case studies in selected CEE countries – Romania, Czech Republic, Serbia and Croatia*. Geneva, International Labour Office (ILO Working Paper No. 245).

Flottorp SA et al. (2010). *Using audit and feedback to health professionals to improve the quality and safety of health care*. Copenhagen, WHO Regional Office for Europe and European Observatory on Health Systems and Policies.

Galan A (2006). Health worker migration in selected CEE countries: Romania. In: Wiskow C (ed.). *Health worker migration flows in Europe: overview and case studies in selected CEE countries – Romania, Czech Republic, Serbia and Croatia*. Geneva, International Labour Office (ILO Working Paper No. 245).

Girasek E et al. (2010). Analysis of a survey on young doctors' willingness to work in rural Hungary. *Human Resources for Health*, 8:13.

Horsley T et al. (2010). How to create conditions for adapting physicians' skills to new needs and lifelong learning. Copenhagen, WHO Regional Office for Europe and European Observatory on Health Systems and Policies.

Humphries M et al. (2008). Overseas nurse recruitment: Ireland as an illustration of the dynamic nature of nurse migration. *Health Policy*, 87(2):264–272.

Hyde R (2005). Germany plans to lure doctors back from west to east. *The Lancet*, 366(9482):279–280.

Informal Network Competent Authorities for Doctors (2010). *Berlin statement, 13 September 2010*. Berlin (http://www.europarl.europa.eu/document/ activities/cont/201010/20101027 ATT90655/20101027ATT90655EN.pdf, accessed 20 February 2011).

Jinks C et al. (2000). Mobile medics? The mobility of doctors in the European Economic Area. *Health Policy*, 54(1):45–64.

Leśniowska J (2007). Migration patterns of Polish doctors within the EU. *Eurohealth*, 13(4):7–8.

Matuleviciute E (2007). Nurses' intentions to work abroad [thesis]. Kaunas, Kaunas University of Medicine.

Mareckova M (2006). Exodus of Czech doctors leaves gaps in health care. *The Lancet*, 363(9419):1443–1446.

Mossialos E et al. (2009). *Health systems governance in Europe. The role of European Union law and policy*. Cambridge, Cambridge University Press.

Nichols J, Campbell J (2010a). The experiences of internationally recruited nurses in the UK (1995–2007): an integrative review. *Journal of Clinical Nursing*, 19(19–20):2814–2823.

Nichols J, Campbell J (2010b). Experiences of overseas nurses recruited to the NHS. *Nursing Management*, 17(5):30–35.

OECD (2007). *International migration outlook 2007*. Paris, Organisation for Economic Co-operation and Development.

OECD (2008). *The looming crisis in the health workforce. How can OECD countries respond?* Paris, Organisation for Economic Co-operation and Development.

OECD (2010). *International migration outlook 2010*. Paris, Organisation for Economic Co-operation and Development.

Palm W et al. (2011). Towards a renewed Community framework for safe, high-quality and efficient cross-border health care within the European Union. In: Wismar M et al. (eds.). *Cross-border health care in the European Union: mapping and analysing practices and policies*. Copenhagen, WHO Regional Office for Europe on behalf of the European Observatory on Health Systems and Policies.

Peeters M et al. (2010). EU law and health professionals. In: Mossialos E et al. (eds.). *Health systems governance in Europe. The role of European Union law and policy*. Cambridge, Cambridge University Press.

Smigelskas et al. (2007). Do Lithuanian pharmacists intend to migrate? *Journal of Ethnic and Migration Studies*, 33(3):501–509.

Stankunas M et al. (2004). The survey of Lithuanian physicians and medical residents regarding possible migration to the European Union [in Lithuanian]. *Medicina (Kaunas)*, 40(1):68–74.

Wiskow C (2006). Moving westwards? Myths and facts on international migration of health workers in the European region. In: Wiskow C (ed.). *Health worker migration flows in Europe: overview and case studies in selected CEE countries – Romania, Czech Republic, Serbia and Croatia*. Geneva, International Labour Office (ILO Working Paper No. 245).

Wiskow C et al. (2010). How to create an attractive and supportive working environment for health professionals. Copenhagen, WHO Regional Office for Europe and European Observatory on Health Systems and Policies.

WHO (2010). *WHO global code of practice on the international recruitment of health personnel*. Geneva, World Health Organization (http://www.who.int/hrh/migration/code/code_en.pdf, 19 February 2011.

WHO (2000). The world health report 2000. Health systems: improving performance. Geneva, World Health Organization.

WHO/OECD (2010). *International migration of health workers. Improving international cooperation to address the global health workforce crisis*. Paris, Organisation for Economic Co-operation and Development (OECD Policy brief)   (http://www.who.int/hrh/resources/oecd-who_policy_brief_en.pdf, accessed 20 February 2011).

Zurn P, Dumont J-C (2008). *Health workforce and international migration: can New Zealand compete?* Paris, Organisation for Economic Co-operation and Development (OECD Health Working Paper No.33).

Cross-country analysis of health professional mobility in Europe: the results

1. Introduction

In this chapter we present a cross-country analysis of health professional mobility from a health system's perspective. The analysis brings to light time trends, geographical patterns, clusters of countries and horizontal issues in a comparative manner. The reader is taken through Europe to gain a picture of health professional mobility, its extent and implications that is as complete and accurate as possible.

The cross-country analysis is based on research results from case studies carried out in 17 countries.[1] As noted in the previous chapter, the sample of countries provides a sound basis on which to draw conclusions about health professional mobility in Europe. The presentation of the results will not strictly follow the order of the conceptual framework outlined but rather takes inspiration from the framework's broad thematic categories to systematize and analyse the case-study findings in a manner which highlights key issues for researchers and policy-makers.

The chapter is structured around seven main sections. It begins by quantifying health professional mobility in Europe in order to give the reader a clear sense of its magnitude (section 2). Two aspects are examined: (i) reliance on foreign medical doctors, nurses and dentists in order to illustrate the extent to which foreign health professionals contribute to a country's workforce; and (ii) mobility flows in order to measure the movements of health professionals which exit (outflows) and enter (inflows) the countries studied. The section concludes by raising a series of methodological issues relevant for quantifying mobility. To understand the directions of flows, section 3 looks at the geographical patterns of mobility in Europe. Three patterns are identified: (i) mobility within the European free-movement area;[2] (ii) mobility between neighbouring

---

1 Austria, Belgium, Estonia, Finland, France, Germany, Hungary, Italy, Lithuania, Poland, Romania, Serbia, Slovakia, Slovenia, Spain, Turkey, United Kingdom.

2 Throughout the text the term European free-movement area applies to European Union (EU) and European Economic Area (EEA) countries plus Switzerland.

countries; and (iii) the role of EU enlargements. The latter is of such importance that section 4 is dedicated to analysing the effects of the 2004 and 2007 enlargements in both source and destination countries.

Having presented mobility in quantitative and geographical terms, the chapter moves on to examine the motivational factors that influence individual health professionals to migrate (section 5). This is followed by an analysis of how health professional mobility impacts on health systems (section 6). Research findings on impacts are analysed according to the four health system functions of service delivery, resource creation, stewardship and financing. The impacts of mobility will also affect this issue's degree of relevance within the domestic context. Section 7 examines the relevance of mobility vis-à-vis other health workforce issues such as territorial maldistribution, shortages, attrition, ageing and production of the health workforce. It also suggests a classification of countries based on the (high, medium or lower) relevance of health professional mobility.

It is necessary to understand the impacts and relevance of mobility before considering the policy and regulatory interventions that countries employ to deal with health professional mobility. Section 8 explains policy and regulatory interventions covering international recruitment and self-sufficiency policies; workforce planning as a continuous process of aligning workforce size, skills and competences with the needs and priorities of the system; cross-border frameworks including codes of conduct and bilateral agreements. It also examines the effects of general workforce measures such as increasing salaries, improving working conditions and modernizing the health-care infrastructure on the mobility of health professionals. The key findings and results are summarized in section 9.

2. Quantifying mobility in Europe

Cross-border movements of health professionals affect the sizes of the health workforces in source and destination countries, their skill mix and distribution over the territory. These changes impact on health systems – the larger these movements the greater the likelihood of tangible impacts on health systems. Quantification of mobility is therefore the starting point for analysis of health professional mobility in Europe. This section will address two questions: (i) How much do health systems rely on foreign health professionals? and (ii) What is the magnitude of actual flows from and to countries?

Reliance on foreign health professionals is defined as the share of foreign health professionals within a country's health workforce in a given year, expressed as a percentage of the stock of the workforce. Health professional mobility is presented in a cumulative way as the statistics may not differentiate between foreign health professionals who moved to a country many years ago and those who moved very recently. Thus, the reliance changes only gradually over time despite policy changes or other events.

Flow is defined as the actual number of health professionals entering or leaving a country in a given year. It can also be expressed in percentages as the share of foreign health professionals newly entering the health system relative to all new entrants, providing an up-to-date measure of yearly intakes to the system. Likewise, outflows can be calculated by total numbers or the numbers of health professionals leaving the country as a proportion of the total workforce. Flows are measured against the migrating professionals. They can be subject to stark fluctuations and can react quickly to policy changes or changes in the geopolitical and economic contexts.

The section on quantifying mobility covers three professions – medical doctors, nurses and dentists. This is not only because of their importance for the health workforce but also because they fall under the automatic diploma recognition procedure specified in Directive 2005/36/EC on the recognition of professional qualifications which makes their qualifications highly portable across borders. Australia, Canada, Ireland, New Zealand, Switzerland and the United States of America have been added to the comparison in order to better understand the relative position of the countries included in the case study sample. Three indicators are used to measure foreign health professionals – foreign trained, foreign born and foreign national. The data on which the analysis builds were taken from the case studies. These include registry data, census data, labour market data, work permits and intention-to-leave data. OECD data were included for the countries outside the case study sample. The most recent year included in the analysis was 2008 since the data were collected in 2009 and 2010. The section presents a situation analysis and, where data were available, time trends. For the latter, data for 1988 and 2000 have been used to capture the situation before and after major geopolitical developments including the revolutions of 1989 and the dissolution of Yugoslavia (beginning in 1990), the USSR (1991) and Czechoslovakia (1993), respectively. Data for 2004 and later serve to describe health professional mobility in the times of EU enlargement.

The section starts with a comparative analysis of the reliance on foreign health professionals. within health systems This is followed by a flow analysis. The last section is a brief discussion of the data limitations caused by the unavailability or poor quality of the data.

2.1 *Reliance on foreign health professionals*

The analysis of reliance on foreign health professionals in the workforce starts with medical doctors and moves on to nurses and dentists. Countries are grouped according to their level of reliance on each profession: negligible to low reliance (less than 5%); moderate reliance (5–10%); high reliance (10–20%); and very high reliance (more than 20%). Differences between the EU-12 and the EU-15 will be discussed. The section ends with a comparison of the three professions.

Turkey, Estonia and Slovakia show negligible reliance on foreign medical doctors, ranging from 0.02% to 0.7%. Poland, Hungary, Italy and France also have relatively low reliance on medical doctors – less than 5% (see Fig. 0.2). Moderate reliance on foreign medical doctors can be observed for Germany and Finland (5.2% and 6.2% respectively). Belgium, Portugal, Spain, Austria, Canada, Norway and Sweden have a high reliance (11.1–18.4%). Ranging between 22.5% and 36.8%, Switzerland, Slovenia, Ireland and the United Kingdom are the European countries with very high reliance on foreign medical doctors.

Fig. 0.2 *Reliance on foreign medical doctors in selected European and non-European OECD countries, 2008 or latest year available*

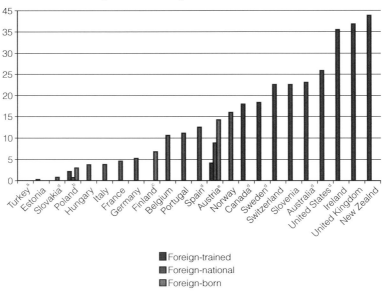

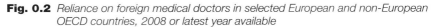

Sources: data sources from case studies[3] – Estonia: Health Care Board; Slovakia: National Health Information Centre, National Register of Health Professionals; Poland: Polish Chamber of Physicians and Dentists; Hungary: Office of Health Authorisation and Administrative Procedures (OHAAP); France: Conseil National de l'Ordre des Médecins (CNOM); Germany: Federal Chamber of Physicians; Finland: Statistics Finland; Belgium: Federal Database of Health Care Professions; Spain: Organization of Medical Colleges (OMC); Austria: Census data (foreign-born) ÖAK (foreign-national), OECD 2010 (foreign-trained); Slovenia: Medical Chamber of Slovenia; United Kingdom: General Medical Council (GMC). OECD (2010) data were used for the following countries: Turkey, Italy, Portugal, Norway, Canada, Sweden, Switzerland, Australia, United States, Ireland, New Zealand. *Note*: data not available in Romania, Serbia, Lithuania; [a] very low percentages [b] 2009 (all indicators); [c] 2006; [d]2007; [e] 2001 (applies only to indicator: foreign-born).

---

3 Full references are given in the reference lists of the individual country case studies.

No registry data on foreign medical doctors were available for Romania, Serbia and Lithuania. As a proxy, data on work permits for foreign medical doctors in Lithuania point to a negligible number of foreign health professionals, although issue of a work permit does not necessarily mean that the medical doctor will go on to join the health workforce.

Reliance on foreign medical doctors in Europe is characterized by large differences across countries. The United Kingdom is at one extreme, with more than one in three medical doctors being foreign trained. Reliance levels gradually decrease towards the eastern part of Europe (ranging between <1% and 2% in most 2004 and 2007 accession countries), pointing towards east-west asymmetries. Set in a global context, the scales of mobility in the "top three" European countries (United Kingdom, Ireland, Switzerland) are comparable to those in Australia, Canada, New Zealand and the United States, four of the major destinations worldwide.

Overall, it appears that Europe is less reliant on foreign nurses than on foreign doctors, although fewer countries in the sample can provide data. Reliance on foreign nurses is negligible in Turkey and Slovakia and relatively low in Spain,

Fig. 0.3 *Reliance on foreign nurses in selected European and non-European OECD countries, 2008 or latest year available*

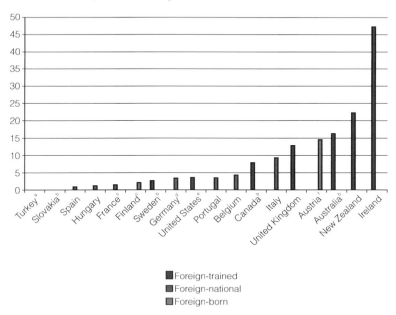

■ Foreign-trained
■ Foreign-national
■ Foreign-born

Sources: Slovakia: National Health Information Centre; Spain: Council of Nurses, EAPS; Hungary: Office of Health Authorisation and Administrative Procedures (OHAAP); France: Cash & Ullman 2008; Finland: Statistics Finland; Germany: Federal Employment Agency; Belgium: Federal Database of Health Care Professions; United Kingdom: Nursing and Midwifery Council (NMC); Austria: Census data. OECD (2010) data were used for the following countries: Turkey, Italy, Portugal, Norway, Canada, Sweden, Switzerland, Australia, United States of America, Ireland, New Zealand. *Notes*: no data provided for Estonia, Lithuania, Norway, Poland, Romania, Serbia, Slovenia, Switzerland. *Notes*: [a] 2005; [b] 2007, [c] 2006, [d] covers nurses and midwives subject to social insurance contributions; [e] 2004, [f] 2001.

Hungary, France, Finland, Sweden, Germany, the United States, Portugal and Belgium. Canada and Italy are the only countries in the cluster that has moderate reliance on foreign nurses. Within Europe, the United Kingdom, Austria and Ireland have high or very high reliance on foreign nurses – ranging between 10% and 47.1%.

EU-15 countries show much greater reliance on foreign nurses than those in the EU-12, mirroring the findings for medical doctors. Hungary is the EU-12 country with the highest reliance on foreign nurses (1.3%), a sharp contrast to Ireland (47%). However, Ireland seems to be an outlier as even the non-European OECD countries included in the analysis have lower reliance on foreign nurses (although high reliance on foreign medical doctors).

No data were available in eight countries – Estonia, Lithuania, Norway, Poland, Romania, Serbia, Slovenia and Switzerland. The case studies from Italy, Germany and Austria reveal a severe lack of data on a related issue – the numbers of foreign nurses and care workers working mainly in the provision of care to elderly people in private settings outside the official sector. This is predominantly an unofficial market either for non-EU nurses who are not eligible for diploma recognition or for EU nurses subject to labour market restrictions.

Fig. 0.4 *Reliance on foreign dentists in selected European and non-European OECD countries, 2008 or latest year available*

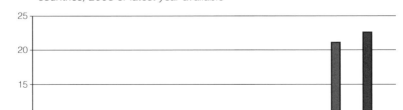

Foreign-trained
Foreign-national
Foreign-born

Sources: Slovakia: National Health Information Centre, National Register of Health Professions; Germany: Federal Chamber of Dentists; France: Ordre National des Chirurgiens Dentistes (ONCD); Poland: Polish Chamber of Physicians and Dentists; Hungary: Office of Health Authorisation and Administrative Procedures (OHAAP); Finland: Statistics Finland; Belgium: Federal Database of Health Care Professions; Austria: Austrian Chamber of Dentists; Slovenia: Medical and Dental Register, Medical Chamber of Slovenia. *Notes*: no data provided for Australia, Canada, Estonia, Ireland, Italy, Lithuania, New Zealand, Norway, Portugal, Romania, Serbia, Spain, Sweden, Switzerland, Turkey, United Kingdom, United States. [a] 2007, [b] 2009 (all indicators), [c] 2006.

Their working conditions give cause for concern and official information on the quality and nature of services they deliver is largely nonexistent.

With regard to dentists,[4] the findings from Slovakia, Germany, France, Poland, Hungary and Finland show negligible to relatively low reliance on foreign dentists (0.7%–4.0%); Belgium has moderate reliance (6.1%); Austria (21.3%) and Slovenia (22.7%) have very high reliance. Although no national data were presented for Spain, regional data from 2007 point to high and very high reliance on foreign dentists in Madrid and Valencia (approximately 20%) and Las Palmas (43%).

Analysis of the reliance on foreign dentists is limited by the lack of data. Only eight of the case studies included data on dentists and there were no OECD data to complement the analysis. In light of the paucity of quantitative information, no conclusions could be drawn or characteristics identified across Europe. However, it should be noted that the very high reliance on foreign dentists in Slovenia corresponds with the results for medical doctors.

2.2 *Flow analysis*

Flow analysis captures the dynamic of health professional mobility, quantifying the phenomenon by counting the numbers of health professionals leaving and entering countries. It can also be presented in terms of the share of foreign health professionals among all health professionals newly entering the health system or the share of health professionals leaving as a proportion of all health professionals in the service.

Inflow analysis plays an important role in monitoring not only the numbers of incoming health professionals but also their professions, specializations and geographical distribution. Ethical reasons require monitoring of the source country in order to avoid recruiting from countries facing workforce shortages. Inflow analysis is an important tool for ensuring the accuracy of workforce planning.

Outflow analysis is also relevant for workforce planning. If not factored in adequately, workforce planners may underestimate annual losses of the workforce and the loss of specific skills thereby producing inaccurate planning projections that may lead to inadequate decisions. Outflow analysis is also an early warning signal of health workers' dissatisfaction with their working conditions, working environment and work content. The signal can help to attract the attention of policy-makers, health-care managers and professional organizations and enable timely responses.

---

4 Dental doctors in Slovakia.

From a long-term perspective, mobility and migration in Europe appear to have increased. With the exception of the United Kingdom, most of the EU-15 countries for which data were available show a rise in yearly inflows of medical doctors and dentists over the last 10 to 20 years. Trends among nurses are inconclusive due to a severe lack of data. Outflows from the EU-12 countries appear to have increased since the EU enlargements but on a smaller scale than expected (see section 4). Moreover, even some of the EU-15 countries have experienced increasing outflows. All three of these developments point towards increasing levels of mobility on the whole. However, a degree of caution is required as the findings are based on a relatively small number of countries providing time series data,[5] often covering a shorter time period than requested[6] and reflecting the paucity of evidence available to show time trends.

Inflows

This section provides an analysis of the inflows of medical doctors, nurses and dentists. A situation analysis of inflows in 2008 will be presented for each profession. This will be followed by an analysis of the increases or decreases since 1988. Finally the continuities and discontinuities of these trends will be analysed. Differences between the EU-15 and the EU-12 will be discussed throughout the section.

Although based on a limited sample, the situation analysis for medical doctors in 2008 clearly shows that the EU-15 have experienced higher inflows than the EU-12 in both absolute numbers and in relative terms. In 2008, inflow data for medical doctors were reported for Austria, Finland, France, Germany, Hungary, Lithuania, Poland, Slovenia, Spain and the United Kingdom. In absolute numbers, the largest inflows of medical doctors were experienced by Spain (8282 foreign degrees recognized), the United Kingdom (5022 foreign-trained newly registered) and Germany (1583 foreign-national newly registered). Lithuania reported the lowest absolute number – 11 work permits issued to new entrants. Only a handful of country case studies reported on the share of foreign health professionals within all newly registered medical doctors. Of these countries, the United Kingdom reported by far the highest proportion (42.6%) followed by Austria (13.5%), Hungary (4.7%) and Poland (2.7%).

For the purpose of presentation, the time-trend figures were split between countries with inflows of fewer than 1000 foreign medical doctors per year (Fig. 0.5) and those with more (Fig. 0.6).

---

5 Data on time trends were retrieved from the 17 case studies and included in the analysis only when at least three points in time were covered.

6 Many case study authors could not provide data on long-term trends such as the 10 or 20 year time period requested and provided data for periods of only 6 to 8 years (e.g. 2003–2008).

Fig. 0.5 *Inflows of foreign medical doctors (countries with annual inflows below 1000) 1988–2008*

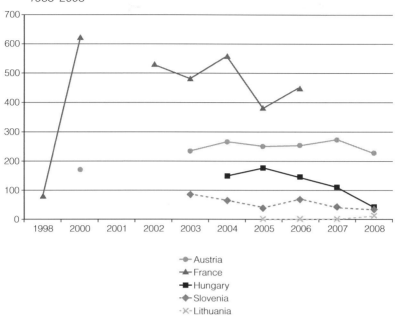

Notes: Austria: newly registered foreign-national medical doctors (data source: ÖÄK); France: newly registered foreign-national medical doctors (CNOM); Hungary: newly registered foreign-national medical doctors (OHAAP); Lithuania: work permits issued to foreign health professionals (Lithuanian Labour Exchange); Slovenia: foreign-trained newly registered medical doctors (Medical Chamber of Slovenia).

Fig. 0.6 *Inflows of foreign medical doctors (countries with annual inflows above 1000) 1988–2008*

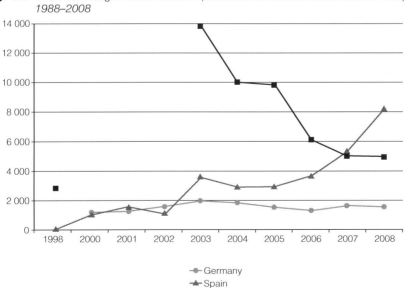

Notes: Germany: newly registered foreign-national medical doctors (source: Federal Chamber of Physicians); Spain: foreign degrees in general medicine recognized in Spain, not including speciality degrees (INE database, Ministry of Education); United Kingdom: newly registered foreign-trained medical doctors (GMC).

Not all countries could provide data for the whole reporting period starting in 1988. Based on the available data, inflows to EU-15 and EU-12 countries indicate diverging trends. The trends in Slovenia and Hungary are more difficult to interpret as the former covers only six years (since 2003) and the latter only five (since 2004). However, yearly inflows have decreased during these periods. The numbers for Lithuania are so low that no conclusions can be drawn.

In most EU-15 countries for which data were available, the inflows of foreign medical doctors appear to have increased or peaked. Inflows to Austria reached their highest numbers in 2004 and 2007 but showed an overall growth in total numbers in comparison to 2000. France reported stark fluctuations in yearly inflows but yearly inflows between 2002 and 2006 were higher than in 1988. Inflows to Germany increased from 2000 and peaked in 2003 but did not decrease substantially over the following years. Spain has experienced a continuous and, since 2004, an increasingly rapid growth in inflows. Inflows to the United Kingdom grew rapidly and must have peaked in or before 2003. A key reason for this is the change in recruitment policy from international recruitment to self-sufficiency (see section 8).

The situation analysis of inflows of foreign nurses in 2008 is based on data reported for Austria, Belgium, Finland, France, Hungary, Italy and the United Kingdom. Italy reported the highest number of foreign-trained nurses (9168), followed by the United Kingdom (3724 foreign-trained nurses). Finland reported a small number of foreign-born nurses (97). The share of foreign nurses among all newly registered nurses was markedly highest in Italy (28%), followed by the United Kingdom (14.7%) and Belgium (13.5%). In Hungary, only 2.4% of all newly registered nurses were foreign nationals.

Data on time trends for nurses showed major limitations and were available in only 4 of the 17 case studies: Austria, Belgium, Hungary and the United Kingdom. These cover time periods of four to six years[7] with the exception of the United Kingdom for which data dating back to 1988 were available. Austria and Belgium showed a clear upward trend of yearly inflows (Austria:[8] 428 in 2003 to 773 in 2008, Belgium:[9] 205 in 2005 to 565 in 2008). A decreasing trend emerged in Hungary, where numbers dropped from 439 in 2004 to 190 in 2008. In the United Kingdom, the effects of changes in its recruitment policy are clearly reflected in flow data: yearly inflows increased substantially from 1988 to 2004 (from 2808 to 15 065 foreign-trained nurses and midwives) and decreased considerably thereafter (to 3724 in 2008). Yet, given the limited country coverage of time-series data on nurses, no conclusions could be drawn on the patterns between EU-12 and EU-15 countries.

---

7 Austria: 2003–2008, Belgium: 2005–2008, Hungary: 2004–2008, United Kingdom: 1988 and 2003–2008.

8 Foreign-trained nurses having applied for diploma validation.

9 Newly licensed foreign-trained nurses.

The situation analysis for dentists in 2008 is based on data reported from Austria, Belgium, Finland, Hungary, Poland, Slovenia and Spain. Analogous with the results for medical doctors, EU-15 countries experienced higher inflows than those in the EU-12, both in absolute numbers and in the share of foreign dentists among all newly registered dentists. The highest absolute inflow number of foreign-trained dentists was reported in Spain (421), followed by Austria (100). All other countries reported much lower inflow numbers; Hungary reported the lowest (18). In Austria newly registered foreign national dentists comprised 40.8% of all newly registered dentists, followed by the United Kingdom (33.7%), Belgium (19%), Hungary (9.7%) and Poland (3%).

Fig. 0.7 *Inflows of foreign dentists 1988–2008*

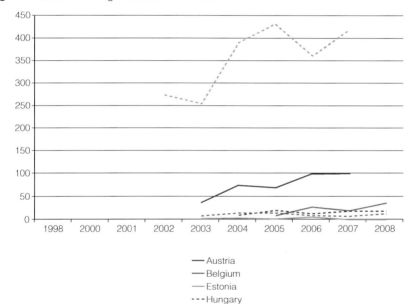

Sources: Austria: newly registered foreign-national dentists in Austria (Austrian Chamber of Dentists); Belgium: foreign-trained newly licensed dentists (Belgian Federal Database of Health Care Professionals; Estonia: practising foreign-trained registered dentists in Estonia (HCB); Hungary: foreign-national newly registered dentists in Hungary (OHAAP); Slovenia: foreign-trained newly registered dentists (Medical Chamber of Slovenia); Spain: non-EU and EEA degrees recognized in Spain (INE).

The analysis shows increases in the inflows of foreign dentists to Spain, Austria, and Belgium although there is a lack of trend data. The absolute numbers for Estonia, Hungary and Slovenia are so low that no conclusions on the trends can be drawn.

Outflows

Outflows reflect the numbers of health professionals leaving a country. They can be expressed in absolute or relative terms, the latter analysing the share of health professionals lost from the workforce. Measurement of outflows is a key challenge for workforce planners and policy-makers and in most countries the numbers are unknown and subject to speculation.

Outflows can be measured against registry data from receiving countries. However, not all countries hold registry data for all health professions and not all countries identify newly registered health professionals. Intention-to-leave data are used as proxies but do not equal actual cross-border mobility. The term "intention to leave" is self-explanatory, signalling health professionals' intentions to move as evidenced by active requests for confirmation of entitlement to practise abroad. These are data on requests for diploma recognition in other countries following the procedure of Directive 2005/36/EC on the recognition of professional qualifications. However, there are two main reasons why these data have limited accuracy. Firstly, the Belgian and Slovak case studies reported that not all countries systematically request these certificates and this may lead to an underestimate of actual outflows. Secondly, health professionals may apply but do not actually move or individuals may apply more than once and cause overestimates of actual flows.

Outflows are one of the most contentious policy issues in health professional mobility. The term brain drain was used widely to describe the exodus of health professionals from countries already facing labour shortages in the health system. Outflows are also a high-profile policy issue in the EU, since EU-12 countries are worried about systematic loss of their workforces to EU-15 countries.

According to the case studies, mobility has increased over time in terms of outflows too. However, the substantial lack of data on emigrating health professionals means that outflow data are only approximate – based on certificates of diploma recognition or of good standing which should be interpreted as outflow intentions.

Outflows from Estonia, Hungary, Poland, Romania, Slovakia and Slovenia increased substantially at the time of EU enlargements and then decreased but remained at a higher overall scale than before EU enlargement. Recent (2009 or 2010) data from Estonia, Hungary and Romania point towards new increases in outflows, possibly showing the effects of the global economic crisis. Some of the large destination countries, such as Austria, Germany, Italy and the United Kingdom also experienced increases in actual outflows and the outflow intentions of their workforces (discussed in detail in the section on enlargement). Between 1988 and 2007, the number of Austrian medical doctors on the German medical registry increased from 260 to 1613. Data on outflows for Germany are available only since 2000. Between 2000 and 2008, the annual outflows of German medical doctors almost tripled (from 1097 to 3065), mostly to Switzerland, Austria, the United States and the United Kingdom. Some sources estimate much higher outflows. A rise in outflows cannot be confirmed for nurses in either country: numbers decreased in Austria and the German data are inconclusive.

The Italian data also suggest increasing outflows of medical doctors, as measured by Italian nationals registered in Germany and the United Kingdom. In the latter, the number of Italian general practitioners notably increased. This trend is also reflected for Italian nurses. Interestingly, while the United Kingdom is a major destination that absorbs high numbers of internationally trained health professionals it also loses increasing numbers of health professionals. However, the scale of outflows or outflow intentions is not comparable to that of inflows. Finland and Spain reported a declining trend in outflows and in outflow intentions (as well as important numbers of returnees), whereas time trends in Belgium and France remained inconclusive.

Both EU-12 and EU-15 countries are losing health professionals. But, unlike EU-12 countries, many EU-15 countries are simultaneously receiving health professionals.

Analysis in this section on quantifying mobility in Europe has been built on limited data, collected directly from the data sources in the respective countries and complemented by OECD data. Comparisons were made on a less than robust basis as the following section will argue.

2.3 *Methodological issues*

In the absence of any adequate commonly agreed definition of health professional mobility the readily available indicators of foreign nationality, foreign born and foreign trained have been used in this study. The figures illustrate how usage of these indicators differs between countries. For example, Austria and Poland use all three indicators for medical doctors (Fig.0.2) but have reported vast differences in the values: more than threefold for Austria and almost fivefold for Poland, depending on the indicator used. Comparison of the countries shows that not one of these indicators consistently estimates higher than another but without a good definition of health professional mobility it is not possible to judge their validity.

The case studies show variations in the availability of data on mobility – for example, a paucity of quantitative information in Romania, Serbia and Turkey but a relatively good evidence base in the United Kingdom. There are also large differences in the quality of data, in terms of coverage of the health professions, registration procedures, indicators used and periodicity.

Data on medical doctors and dentists were generally of better quality than those for nurses. Limited or no data on nurses were identified in Lithuania, Poland, Romania, Serbia and Slovenia. Nursing is not a registered profession in Austria and Germany but data from other sources are available. In several countries, nurses are grouped with other professions, for example: nurses and midwives in Germany and the United Kingdom; nurses and allied health professionals in Hungary.

Compulsory registration is not the practice in all countries. It does not cover all medical doctors in France and, although self-employed medical doctors and those in the private sector are registered in Poland, they are not included in public statistics concerning employment in a public sector. In Spain, registration is not mandatory in the public sector and covers only basic medical degrees. This may lead to an overestimate of mobility as it is assumed that almost all foreign medical doctors register. Reregistration procedures also influence data comparability. Whereas data in Austria cover *active* medical doctors, Belgium, France, Poland and the United Kingdom cover *total* registered health professionals. Germany, Hungary, Slovakia and Estonia provide information on both active and total numbers of registered medical doctors.

Analyses of time trends were only possible in a limited number of countries and good time-series data were rare or nonexistent in the vast majority of countries covered by the case studies. This was due to several reasons including simply the unavailability of data 10 or 20 years ago and changes over time concerning the coverage of data sources, registration and reregistration procedures; definitions used; or data holders (e.g. from government agencies to professional bodies).

3. Geographical patterns of mobility in Europe

The preceding section has focused on the magnitude of health professional mobility by analysing the reliance on foreign health professionals and the actual flows to and from countries. This section moves the analytical perspective towards a spatial focus, identifying the geographical patterns of health professional mobility in the EU. The three patterns analysed include mobility within and beyond the European free-movement area, mobility between neighbouring countries and the EU enlargements in 2004 and 2007. EU enlargements provide insight on the geographical patterns of mobility as they concern flows and the directions of flow. Given their importance as a policy issue, EU enlargements will be covered separately (section 4).

3.1 *Mobility within and beyond the European free-movement area*

The aim of this section is to identify regional clusters of health professional mobility in terms of the prevailing geographical sources of mobile health professionals. If policy responses to health professional mobility are envisaged it is important to know whether this is predominantly a global or a European phenomenon and whether it varies from country to country and from profession to profession.

For the analysis countries are organized according to three clusters: (i) the European free-movement area covering EU and EEA countries plus Switzerland; (ii) the wider Europe;[10] and (iii) the third countries[11]. A region is deemed to be dominant if it is the source of the larger part of the workforce. Estonia, Lithuania, Poland and Slovakia are excluded from the analysis since they have very low reliance on foreign health professionals. The analysis is based on both stock and flow data but is limited by inconsistencies in data reporting between the different case studies. For example, countries may be clustered either as EU or EEA countries or as EEA countries and Switzerland. However, the wider Europe of the World Health Organization (WHO) includes Israel, the central Asian republics and Kazakhstan which are not reflected in national data sources. In addition, the different data sources available in different countries produce slightly different figures, as reported for France and Italy. Data also may be presented as percentages or as absolute numbers and thus offer no possibility to calculate a common aggregate.

Austria, Belgium, France, Germany and Italy receive their foreign health professionals predominantly from the European free-movement area. The share of EU doctors among all medical doctors in Austria was 6.3% in 2008 compared to only 2.3% of foreign medical doctors from non-EU countries. In 2008, 10.5% of all medical doctors in Belgium were foreign nationals. The largest contingents were French (2.3%), Dutch (2.6%), German (0.8%), Italian (0.7%), Spanish (0.5%) and Romanian (0.5%). In France, 54% of all foreign medical doctors in 2005 were from EU countries; data from the French National Medical Council (CNOM) show an even higher share in 2010 (66%). In 2006, the majority (4488) of the 7616 newly registered nurses in France came from EU countries. Around 51% of Germany's foreign medical doctors are EU nationals. The proportion of foreign medical doctors in Italy has been estimated at around 4% with the major contingents coming from Germany (1276), Switzerland (869), Greece (851), the Islamic Republic of Iran (752), France (686), Venezuela (626), the United States (618), Argentina (584), Romania (555) and Albania (431). The share of foreign health professionals within the Italian

---

10 Countries of the WHO European Region outside the free-movement area.

11 All countries outside the WHO European Region

nursing workforce was around 11% in 2008. The largest groups were from the European free-movement area including Romania (25%), Poland (10.7%), Switzerland (7%), Germany (5.6%), France and Spain (around 3.5% each).

Slovenia is the only country in this study that receives the majority of its foreign health professionals from the wider Europe cluster. The stock of all active medical doctors in 2008 comprised 22.5% of foreign health professionals, primarily from Croatia, Bosnia and Herzegovina and Serbia. Some countries of the European free-movement area cluster (such as Germany, Austria, Finland) also receive considerable numbers of health professionals from wider Europe. In Germany, this is the source of around 20% of foreign medical doctors. The Russian Federation was the third most important source country in 2008, with 1685 registered medical doctors in the total stock. Croatia and Turkey are the main source countries for foreign nurses in Germany. Austria has also significant inflows of nurses from countries from the wider Europe. Health professionals from the former Yugoslavia amounted to 7% of the foreign workforce. Collectively, Finland receives more medical doctors from the European free-movement area but foreign medical doctors from the Russian Federation comprised the single most important group with around 70–80 new registrations per year in 2004–2008.

The United Kingdom and Spain receive their foreign health professionals predominantly from third countries. Spain recruits medical doctors from Latin America – 7706 of the 8282 foreign diplomas recognized in 2008 were from outside the EU.

Inflows to the United Kingdom have come largely from Commonwealth countries and 27% of all medical doctors in the United Kingdom come from outside the EEA. The most important source countries were India, Pakistan, South Africa, Nigeria and Australia but the trend has changed. Inflows of medical doctors from Asia reached a peak of 5366 in 2004 but had dropped to 1705 in 2008; the share of doctors from the European free-movement area countries rose from 6% in 1988 to 9% in 2008. There was a similar development in the inflows of nurses from Asia – these peaked at 7872 newly registered nurses in 2003 but had fallen to 1541 in 2008. These fluctuations are the consequences of the policy changes discussed in the section on policy, regulation, cross-border frameworks and general workforce measures.

Some countries that receive the majority of their health professionals from the European free-movement area also have close ties to third countries. In France, 36% (3659) of foreign medical doctors in 2009 came from Algeria, Morocco and Tunisia. Austria has small contingents of foreign health professionals from third countries – around 5% of foreign-trained medical doctors come from

Iran, 2% from Syria and 1% from Egypt. Between 2004 and 2006, 51 medical doctors with a diploma from the Congo and 93 with a diploma from Morocco undertook part of their specialization in Belgium. Nurses with Congolese and Lebanese diplomas also work in Belgium. In Germany, around 28% of foreign medical doctors come from third countries in Asia (4163), Africa (916), America (722), Australia and Oceania (17) and other countries (242).

3.2 *Mobility between neighbouring countries*

The second geographical pattern analysed in this section is mobility between neighbouring countries. Densely populated border regions, shared languages and cultural ties increase the likelihood of this. The analysis focuses on Austria-Germany, France-Belgium-Netherlands, Austria-Italy-Hungary-Slovenia-Slovakia and Finland-Sweden-Estonia-Russian Federation. Methodologically, the links were established in terms of the source country's importance in the destination country, for example as the single, second or third most important source country.

Neighbourhood movements are occurring throughout the EU. Box 0.2 focuses on some hot-spots with reciprocal or one-way flows.

4. Role of EU enlargements

This section examines the effects of the EU enlargements that added ten new Member States in 2004 and two in 2007. With a combined population of over 100 million citizens, these countries substantially extended the European labour market for health professionals. The portability of health professional qualifications was guaranteed by the European treaties establishing a free-movement area. This facilitated the mutual and, in most cases, automatic recognition of diplomas for medical doctors, nurses, dentists, midwives and pharmacists although some EU-15 countries set up labour market restrictions covering transitional phases.[12] Enlargement also added to the economic diversity of the EU and markedly lower salary levels in the accession countries provided new strong incentives to seek work elsewhere.

This section deals with four topics central to the analysis of European enlargement: (i) magnitude of outflows from EU-12 countries; (ii) magnitude of inflows to EU-15 (iii) pre-accession flows from eastern Europe; and (iv) the changing nature of mobility; followed by a short summary .

---

12 Labour market restrictions for EU-8 nationals still apply in Austria, Germany, Malta and Switzerland. Romanianand Bulgaria n nationals are subject to restrictions in Austria, Belgium, France, Germany, Iceland, Ireland, Italy, Liechtenstein, Luxembourg, Malta, Netherlands, Norway and the United Kingdom.

Box 0.2 *Hot-spots for mobility between neighbouring countries*

Austria-Germany

Relatively intense and roughly balanced two-way flows. In 2008:

→ 1802 Austrian-national medical doctors were registered in the German Federal Physician's Chamber

← 1453 German-national doctors were registered in the Austrian Medical Chamber

Each country is the other's most important destination for medical doctors. Yearly inflow data for 2008 and 2007 confirm close migratory ties.

France-Belgium-Netherlands

Reciprocal flows where linguistic proximity exists. The Netherlands recognize Belgian medicine, dentistry and nursing diplomas without systematically requesting conformity certificates.

→ 1576 Belgian nationals were registered with the French Medical Order in 2009 (16% of foreign medical workforce in France)

← 1163 French-national medical doctors registered in Belgium in 2008

← 1152 foreign nursing diplomas recognized in Belgium in 2004–2008, 40% were French

→ 81 nurses with Belgian diplomas registered in the Netherlands in 2006–2008

← 253 Dutch nursing diplomas recognized by Belgian authorities in 2004–2008

France and the Netherlands are main destinations for Belgian medical doctors, nurses and dentists.

Austria and neighbours

One-way flows to Austria:

→ Top destination country for nurses from Slovenia and Slovakia, 41% (728) of conformity certificates requested by Slovak nurses in 2004–2007 stated "Austria"

→ Among the top three destinations for medical doctors from Slovenia, Italy (particularly South Tyrol) and Hungary (to a lesser extent)

Finland-Sweden-Estonia-Russian Federation

Finland and Sweden: two-way flows of medical doctors and nurses

Finland: Estonia and the Russian Federation are main source countries for medical doctors – declared destination of 74% of recognition certificates issued to medical doctors and of 61% issued to nurses in Estonia.

Estonia: foreign medical doctors come mostly from the Russian Federation and Ukraine, followed by Finland and Latvia. Russian-speaking foreign medical doctors who do not move on (e.g. to Finland) often work in north-east Estonia where the population speaks Russian.

In most countries, the only data source available to estimate outflows is intention-to-leave data. In some countries, studies were conducted to explore health professionals' willingness to leave the country. Intention-to-leave data emanate from the EU's mutual recognition of diplomas that requires certificates of diploma recognition or of good standing. These documents are issued by the competent authorities at the request of the health professional seeking recognition of qualification in another EU country.

4.1 *Magnitude of outflows from EU-12 countries*

The magnitude of outflows of health professionals measured on the basis of intention-to-leave data was not as large as anticipated before accession (see Table 0.3). In those countries with data available, outflows have rarely exceeded 3% of the domestic workforce – in 2005 diploma recognition certificates issued represented approximately 3% of all registered Polish medical doctors, a maximum of 1% of the Slovenian workforce, approximately 2% of the Estonian active medical workforce after 2004 (but 6.5% at the height of mobility in 2004) and around 3% of medical doctors who actually left Romania in 2007. However, it is not only the EU-12 countries that lose health professionals and comparison with EU-15 data helps to qualify the magnitude of outflows.

Table 0.3 *Yearly outflows/outflow intentions of medical doctors from selected 2004 and 2007 EU Member States*

Country	Indicator	2004[h]	2005	2006	2007	2008	2009
Estonia	**Intention to leave**[a] (% among active workforce)	283 (6.5%)	79 (1.8%)	87 (2.0%)	75 (1.7%)	79 (1.8%)	106 (2.4%)
Hungary	**Intention to leave**[b] (% among active workforce)	906 (2.7%)	889 (2.7%)	721 (2.2%)	695 (2.1%)	803 (2.4%)	887 (n/a)
Lithuania	**Intention to leave**[c] (% among active workforce)	357 (2.7%)	186 (1.4%)	-	-	-	132 (0.9%)
Poland	**Intention to leave**[d]	n/a	3579[i]	1535[i]	1123[i]	901[i]	n/a
Slovakia	**Intention to leave**[e]	442	594	376	267	250	217
Romania	**Intention to leave**[f] (% among active workforce)	-	-	-	4990 (10.2%)	2683[k]	n/a
	Emigration study[g] (% among active workforce)	-	-	-	1421 (3%)	n/a	n/a

Sources: [a] Certificates of recognition of diplomas issued (HCB); [b] Applications for certification – all applicants, whether residing in Hungary or elsewhere (OHAAP); [c] Certificates of good standing issued to medical doctors (Lithuanian Ministry of Health); [d] Certificates issued in Poland (GUS 2006a–2009a and 2006b–2009b); [e] Certificates issued (Ministry of Health of the Slovak Republic), [f] Applications for diploma verifications (Ministry of Health of Romania), [g] Study on emigration among all practising medical doctors (Dragomiristeanu et al. 2008). *Notes*: [h] May–December only; [i] as of 30 June (numbers for 2005 may be cumulative); [j] as of 31 December; [k] covers 2008 and January to May 2009.

For Germany, for example, a study conducted to determine the outflow in 2008 showed that this amounted to 1% of active medical doctors.

Estonia, Poland, Slovakia and Romania faced initial strong outflows in the years of accession followed by a drop; Hungary faced initial strong outflows in the year of accession followed by more contained development. The highest numbers of mutual recognition of diploma certificates were issued in the year of accession or the next year, followed by a decreasing tendency. In Estonia, the numbers of certificates of recognition peaked in 2004 with 283 for medical diplomas, 118 for nursing diplomas and 29 for dental diplomas. Numbers dropped considerably in the following years, between three- and four-fold, but increased again slightly in 2009. There were similar patterns for Poland and Slovakia in 2005.[13] Following EU enlargement, medical doctors and dentists appear to have had greater increases in mobility than nurses. However, it may be that the real scale of nurses' migratory flows has been considerably underestimated due to the lack of good quality data in several countries including Poland, Romania and Slovakia. Intention-to-leave data from Romania indicate continuing high outflows of medical doctors; more than 300 certificates per month were issued to Romanian medical doctors in 2010. However, Romania provides a good example that intention-to-leave data must be interpreted with care as the reported outflow (based on intention-to-leave data) of 4990 medical doctors in 2007 contrasts sharply with the findings of a separate study that concluded that 1421 medical doctors actually left the country. Still, the scale of these yearly outflows is a matter of concern, particularly because the most economically deprived region in the north east of the country was most affected by outflows.

There are two possible explanations for the high number of intentions to leave in 2004 or 2005 in Estonia, Hungary, Slovakia and Poland and 2007 in Romania. Firstly, it may be that interest to leave these countries was greatest in the year of accession. Secondly, these numbers may reflect a culmination of both *prospective* and *retrospective* applications – including not only health professionals residing in the country and wishing to leave but also health professionals already living abroad but requesting recognition retrospectively, as demonstrated by the Hungarian case study.

4.2 Magnitude of inflows in EU-15 countries

The numbers of newly registered EU-12 medical doctors, nurses and dentists in destination countries such as Austria, Belgium, Finland, France and Italy increased modestly around 2004 and 2007. France experienced marked increases in the numbers of Romanian registered medical doctors – from 174 in 2007 to 1160 in January 2009. Spain and the United Kingdom reported

13 Numbers in 2005 may be of a cumulative nature.

Table 0.4 *Medical doctors, nurses and midwives from EU-12 countries newly registered in the United Kingdom, 2003–2008*

	2003	2004	2005	2006	2007	2008
Medical doctors	175	1 172	1 792	1 251	1 039	970
Nurses and midwives	84	87	305	848	958	932

Sources: GMC unpublished data 2009, NMC unpublished data 2009.

important inflows of medical doctors from Poland and Romania partly linked to the active roles of recruitment agencies targeting these countries.

For Austria, inflows for nurses seem to follow the accession. No nurses from future enlargement countries applied for diploma validation in 2003 but the number increased from 0 to 159 in 2004 to 278 in 2008. Similarly, the United Kingdom has become one of the major destination countries, attracting an increasing number of medical doctors from Poland but also from Hungary, Romania, Slovakia or Lithuania. Nurses from EU-12 countries are also clearly visible in the statistics (see Table 0.4). The United Kingdom, Ireland and Scandinavian countries were the main destination countries for Lithuanian nurses.

4.3 *Pre-accession flows from eastern Europe*

Health professional mobility across the European region existed well before the EU expanded, influenced by geopolitical contexts, labour markets and economic circumstances. A first wave of labour migration from east to west emerged after 1991 as the dissolution of the former USSR triggered outflows of health professionals from newly independent states to western European countries, Canada and the United States. Cumbersome and costly registration and licensing requirements in destination countries hampered mobility, however. The case studies show that the east-to-west mobility of health professionals predates the 2004 and 2007 expansions. EU enlargement thus reinforced existing patterns by facilitating freedom of movement.

4.4 *Changing nature of mobility*

Mobility has changed not only in terms of intensity and directions but also qualitatively, through diversification of the types of mobility. There is evidence of short-term mobility since the EU expanded, for instance weekend work, short-term contracts of several weeks/months and increasingly mobility to the home-care and long-term care sectors.

Outflows of health professionals from Estonia can be characterized not only as temporary but also (in several cases) as remarkably short-term. The Estonian shift system allocates specific working days and therefore some health professionals choose to provide services on weekdays in Finland, Sweden or Norway and return to work in Estonia at weekends. Following EU enlargement, there has been an emerging phenomenon of extremely short-term mobility from eastern Europe to the United Kingdom. Taking advantage of EU regulations on free movement, the so-called "Easyjet" phenomenon emerged – dentists and general practitioners supplement their main incomes in their home countries by using budget airlines to fly to the United Kingdom in order to provide services for a few weeks, months or just weekends. Inflows from Romania to Belgium also suggest that mobility is to some extent of a temporary nature. Generally, these are doctors without specialist or general practitioner diplomas who move temporarily either to undertake part of their specialization in Belgium or to cover on-call duties. The increasingly short-term nature of mobility is also demonstrated by the short-term (several weeks/ months) contracts that health-care facilities issue to Polish, Romanian or Slovakian health professionals working abroad.

Diversion of mobility is another example of the changing nature of mobility following EU enlargement. This is seen particularly in the numbers of nurses being shifted towards the long-term care sector. In Germany and Austria, anecdotal evidence shows that nurses work as caregivers or home-helps, often in illegal or unregulated areas. This may be due to labour market restrictions and to higher demand for care workers. Estimates in both countries suggest substantial increases in eastern European nurses and informal care workers.

4.5 Summary

Contrary to estimates and expectations raised by media and stakeholder groups, the 2004 and 2007 EU enlargements led neither to a "swamping" of the EU-15 countries nor to a massive brain drain of health professionals from the then accession states (EU-12). Enlargement did considerably increase existing flows from eastern and central EU Member States towards the western EU. Outflows were particularly visible in Estonia, Hungary, Poland, Slovakia and Romania although numbers often decreased slightly following initial high peaks. Yet although the scale of outflows did not reach the expected dimensions, many countries lost a considerable number of health professionals around the years of accession.

There are three possible reasons why EU enlargement did not produce the predicted dramatic effect on the mobility of health professionals, aside from the labour market restrictions applied in several EU-15 Member States in the transition periods. First, predictions were often based on the intention/interest to move which is certainly higher than actual migration. Second, workforce policies on salaries and working conditions in some eastern European countries may have helped to retain health professionals by reducing incentives to migrate. In Estonia, Poland and Lithuania there is evidence that health professionals may be returning due to policy changes that have triggered salary increases or improved working conditions. Salary negotiations with trade unions in Estonia and Poland produced increased remuneration levels, coinciding with fewer health professionals applying for recognition of diploma in subsequent years. Third, EU enlargements received much public and media attention which likely contributed to excessively high expectations (or fears) related to intra-EU mobility.

5. Motivational factors

Motivations, personal drivers and pull and push factors for migration have been widely described in the literature. The research in the 17 countries has added to existing evidence on the reasons why individual health professionals have moved in the first decade of 21st century Europe. Timing and geopolitical context are relevant since the EU enlargements in 2004 and 2007 have facilitated mobility between health systems with widely different levels of organization, technical development and remuneration, bringing new opportunities and incentives to the fore.

Authors were asked for the specific motivational factors within their country based on surveys, qualitative interviews, focus groups, grey literature and expert observations. Widespread interest in the topic is indicated by the use of surveys in several countries and most notably in the EU countries that joined in 2004 and 2007. Surveys among medical doctors and/or nurses were reported in Estonia, Lithuania, Hungary, Poland, Romania and Slovakia as well as in Germany and Turkey. Secondary sources were used for other countries.

A common finding in all chapters is the role of income. Pecuniary motivations have varying prominence across Europe and over time but were identified in all 17 countries and found to be key motivations in Estonia, Poland, Romania, Serbia and Slovakia. For example, wage differentials motivate Romanian health professionals to work in countries in which they can earn up to four times more. In addition, they encourage movements of French nurses in border regions to neighbouring Germany and Switzerland; Slovak health professionals to neighbouring Austria; Serbian health professionals to Slovenia; and Belgian Dutch-speaking nurses to the neighbouring Netherlands (while continuing to live in Belgium). A degree of interdependence can be seen between migration intentions and income levels in source countries. Fewer requests for diploma recognition certificates have been noted in Estonia, Poland and Slovakia at approximately the same time as the wages of health professionals were increased.[14] Also, outflows of medical doctors dropped in Spain in the

---

14 It should be mentioned that health professionals may make strategic use of requests for certificates – inflating numbers in order to exert pressure on governments during collective salary negotiations.

mid and late 2000s when salary levels rose. However, incentives can change rapidly. Stark salary and staff cuts in Romania in 2010 saw rising numbers of certificate requests from medical doctors and nurses; Estonian figures for 2009 show a similar situation. The current global financial crisis may re-intensify motivations for migration or may slow them if fewer job opportunities are present in destination countries. While there are no concrete data, income-related incentives to migrate and the perception of better opportunities can be expected to change considerably in the new economic environment.

The other most cited motivation is working conditions – covering elements such as the working environment, terms of employment, work relations and access to good infrastructures. Better working hours is a motivation for Austrian medical doctors to go to Germany; German medical doctors declare workloads and administrative burdens as motivations to migrate (or leave the health sector); and limited control over work as well as an effort-reward imbalance influence German nurses to migrate or leave. In the 1990s, job insecurity and temporary contracts drove Spanish health professionals to seek work in Portugal, France and the United Kingdom. Belgian nurses working in the Netherlands cite that country's less hierarchical working relations between nurses and doctors as a motivation. Turkish health professionals and Slovak medical doctors mentioned access to infrastructures and medical equipment as a reason to migrate (to technically more advanced health systems).

The possibilities of professional and career advancement were among the key motivations of Finnish medical doctors working abroad (second to family ties) and of Belgian nurses working in the Netherlands. Austrian junior doctors are attracted to Germany by the absence of waiting times for training places and by high-quality education in modern hospitals. Non-EU medical students are attracted to France by good access to research teams and technical equipment and Romanian medical doctors move to Belgium to specialize in fields for which there are no facilities in Romania. Arguably the most extreme lack of domestic opportunities is when health professionals are faced with unemployment in their own country. Oversupply of medical doctors in Italy and of medical doctors, nurses, dentists and pharmacists in Serbia are equally as strong motivations for migration today as unemployment was for Spanish medical doctors in the 1990s.

Social status also counts among motivations to migrate and, perhaps surprisingly, is mentioned with high frequency. Low social recognition or low esteem is felt by German and Polish nurses and throughout health professionals in Hungary, Romania and the Slovak Republic.

Dissatisfaction with wages, working conditions and/or social recognition are all expressions of health professionals' general perception of their current position in the health system in which they work. Incomplete health reforms, unrealized goals and/or a disappointed health workforce were noted to be among the reasons why health professionals leave Lithuania, Hungary, Romania and Slovakia. Time spent abroad and work experience in another health system also added to the aspirations of younger Hungarian and Romanian medical doctors. Surveys of Hungarian junior medical doctors show that they perceive target countries to be better in five out of six dimensions (social prestige, research opportunities, professional opportunities, working conditions and living circumstances). EU enlargement may have contributed to this by raising the expectations of health professionals in the EU-12 Member States.

The perception of better earnings and/or better opportunities motivates health professionals to move. The findings from the case-studies generally confirm existing knowledge about health professionals' motivations for migrating but add new insights on motivations in the EU-12 Member States.

6. Impacts on health system performance

A key rationale for the present volume was to understand how health professional mobility impacts on health system performance. In the context of this book, impact can be defined as an effect or consequence relevant to the health system caused directly or indirectly by health professional mobility. Health systems can be defined in terms of their goals and functions as set out in the WHO's *World Health Report 2000*. The WHO model reports the goals of health systems to be improving the health of the population; meeting the non-medical expectations of patients and citizens; and protecting against the financial consequences of ill health. The achievement of these goals and thus the performance of health systems is dependent on four functions of the health system: (i) service delivery (contributes to goal achievement by providing individual and collective services including, prevention, health promotion, diagnostics and curative treatment); (ii) resource creation (provides the infrastructure including buildings and technologies and produces the staff necessary); (iii) financing (collects and pools money to purchase health services); and (iv) stewardship (contributes to health by planning, regulating and providing information and intelligence).

The impact of health professional mobility will be analysed in terms of the four functions in order to identify whether and at what level mobility has repercussions for health systems. Impacts are developments which can be particularly hard to capture. One reason is the time lag between noticing and measuring a phenomenon. Another is the difficulty of establishing cause and effect, for example – how can a change in care delivery patterns be attributed to the inflows or outflows of health professionals? It may also take time before any effect trickles through and becomes visible. Moreover, impacts likely go un(der) reported as few resources are dedicated to monitoring health professional mobility. Finally, when mobility is associated with expectations, impacts may appear smaller if expected to be greater.

6.1 *Service delivery*

Service delivery contributes to health improvement by providing individual and collective services organized into primary, secondary and tertiary care and ensuring the quality of, and access to, services. The quantity, appropriateness and quality of services delivered will depend on the geographical distribution, skill mix and size of the health workforce. In turn, the health workforce is affected by health professionals entering or leaving the system.

In many countries, health professional mobility impacts on underserved areas. Some 15% of medical doctors in the Balearics and Canary Islands are of foreign origin and thus important in improving service delivery in Spanish remote areas. In France, non-EU medical doctors help to fill gaps in public hospitals especially in smaller cities, in positions with greater night-time responsibilities and in areas with socioeconomic problems. While shortages in sensitive specialties remain, foreign medical doctors are making noteworthy contributions in psychiatry, paediatrics and anaesthetics. Service provision in less affluent and sparsely populated regions in eastern Germany is increasingly dependent on foreign medical doctors. Similarly, a small number of medical doctors from Russia and Ukraine provide services to the Russian-speaking population in north-eastern Estonia. Foreign health professionals can also compensate for overall or specific workforce shortages as evidenced by the thousands of foreign medical doctors, nurses and carers who have increased service capacity in public health systems (or in the informal care sector) in the United Kingdom, Spain, Germany, Austria and Italy. In Belgium, foreign medical doctors with basic training compensate for what hospitals perceive to be a lack of interns and perform mainly on-call duties.

Of course, source countries have different perceptions of health professional mobility. In Hungary, experts argue that outflows could be threatening the sustainability of the health system even in the short run. The economically deprived regions in north-east Romania have the country's lowest coverage of medical doctors in rural areas and are disproportionately affected by the emigration of both medical doctors and nurses. Impacts are not necessarily related to the volumes of flows. In such cases the departure of even a few specialist doctors can produce a substantial effect on service delivery, as mentioned in Hungary, Estonia and Lithuania. Moreover certain specialties appear to be in demand across Europe. In Poland, the specialties with the highest number of vacancies are those with the highest proportion of medical doctors holding the certificates required for migration within the EU (issued to 19% of anaesthetists and 13% of specialists in emergency medicine between 2004 and 2008). Similar worrying observations have been made in Lithuania. In Slovakia, the relationship between the numbers of certificates and the numbers of graduates per specialty illustrate how (for example) specialties such as anaesthetics, intensive medicine and surgery are vulnerable to outflows. In Belgium, the emigration of child and youth psychiatrists to the Netherlands has been reported as problematic considering the important shortages in Belgium in this profession. Evidence confirms how outmigration can exacerbate problems in service provision for source countries.

Questions concerning health professional mobility's impact on quality of care have attracted much attention. The case studies provide some insight in the absence of any specific studies or robust data with which to measure this impact. Anecdotal evidence suggests that foreign health professionals are more likely to work under difficult conditions such as late or heavy shifts (as in France and Belgium) or in unregulated circumstances when working illegally (for example in home care in Italy, Germany and Austria). Unfavourable working (and living) conditions may increase risks for both patients and providers. With regards to quality and mobility, professional organizations in the United Kingdom have voiced concerns over the actual equivalence of education and training; the lack of language tests within registration processes; the issue of continuing professional development; and poor information sharing between regulators to restrict "unsafe" individuals moving within Europe. Despite the absence of data, it is more than likely that mobility (indirectly) impacts on quality by (directly) affecting the skill mix of, shortages in, and geographical distribution of, a health workforce.

A different aspect concerns the non-medical dimension of care delivery. In Spain and Germany, a culturally diverse health workforce is more likely to respond to an increasingly culturally diverse population. Polish medical doctors fly to Irish cities to cater for the needs of the Polish diaspora during weekends. However, systems must invest in supporting foreign health professionals to integrate and become familiar with a country's practices, language and culture, as noted in both Germany and the United Kingdom.

6.2 Resource creation

Resource creation produces the manpower, skills and knowledge required by a health system. The education and training of the necessary health workforce forms an essential part of this but mobility can shrink or expand the pool of human resources, skills and knowledge as health professionals come and go. From the perspective of countries which train health professionals who then leave, outmigration means no return on investment and possible disruption of planning efforts. For countries importing foreign-trained staff, immigration represents an additional workforce free of charge but has the potential to produce reliance on foreign health professionals.

According to estimates, Serbia and Montenegro have spent US$ 9–12 billion educating and training medical specialists who have left the country. Long-term migration may undermine the return on Serbia's investment in education and training. Real but hidden financial losses are even higher in terms of lost profits and inadequate replacement of the departed experts. In an effort to offset such financial losses, programmes in Slovakia require compulsory postgraduate service or monetary compensation if graduates migrate. In other countries, foreign students may take up domestic training positions. Inflows of Dutch and French students to medical and health-related studies in Belgium disrupted health workforce planning efforts by bypassing the *numerus clausus* and because foreign students are likely to return home after graduation. The volume of foreign nursing students could also aggravate nursing shortages in Belgium and there are similar concerns about the influx of Germans taking up medical student posts in Austria. In Spain, 36% of candidates sitting the entrance exam for specialist medical training were of foreign origin, mainly from Latin America.

For destination countries, mobility can expand resources. The United Kingdom and Spain have benefited greatly from importing knowledge and skills – the former's case study notes the double benefit gained as foreign recruitment helped to free up senior staff and allow them to expand training. Conversely, a system that relies on inflows for resource creation can become dependent upon them (see Sections 2 and 8) and was noted as one of the risks of mobility during debates in the United Kingdom. Almost one quarter of medical doctors and dentists in Slovenia are foreign but the slow-down of inflows from other former Yugoslav federal states led to shortages and staffing problems in the 1990s and 2000s. Such reliance is a particular issue in the context of forecasted domestic shortages such as in Finland where foreign dentists represented almost half of all new dentist licences in 2006–2008 (134 foreign-trained/176 Finnish-trained) and foreign medical doctors obtaining a licence to practice represented a quarter of the new medical workforce in 2004–2008. In Spain, the number of foreign degrees in general medicine recognized (5383) was 40% higher than the number of medical students (3841) graduating from Spanish universities in 2007. In the United Kingdom, 42% of newly registered medical doctors and

14% of newly registered nurses and midwives in 2008 were foreign-trained. If reliance on foreign workforce grows as domestic shortages worsen, health systems will becoming increasingly susceptible to the directions and intensity of flows which remain hard to predict. Hence, domestic production of a health workforce seems a more sustainable (and responsible) approach to resource creation.

6.3 *Stewardship*

The stewardship function contributes to health through planning, regulation and the provision of information and intelligence. Policy responses to health professional mobility are addressed in section 8 but the effects of health professional mobility on decision-makers' ability to steer health systems are easily overlooked. Three interrelated aspects can be identified concerning information, planning and regulation.

Firstly, there is a lack of information about which health professionals are leaving and which are entering the system. Without the capacity to track movements comprehensively, authorities' ability to supervise (and react) is affected in Belgium, France, Germany, Hungary, Italy, Lithuania, Poland, Romania, Serbia, the Slovak Republic, Spain, Turkey and the United Kingdom (specifically on the outflows of returnees). This situation is worsened when considering the illegal health workforce which is not only invisible in official statistics but also constitutes crucial sources of care in countries such as Italy, Austria and Germany. The implication is that governments lose sight of the services delivered outside the regulated frameworks in the home and elderly care sectors. In Finland, more information is needed on the reasons for high unemployment among foreign health professionals in order to integrate this workforce in the system.

The lack of evidence on mobility and its unpredictable nature further hamper the planning function of health systems (see section 6.2) as workforce planning is not informed by the necessary data. Under the procedure of Directive 2005/36/EC on the recognition of professional qualifications, health professionals are not necessarily obliged to inform public authorities when entering or leaving a country. Moreover, the mutability of flows makes it difficult to factor them into planning and within projections (see section 8).

Mobility as enshrined in the *acquis communautaire* impacts on stewardship by undermining EU Member States' ability to regulate. Governments have no legal instruments with which to limit or steer inflows and outflows between their own countries and other EU Member States. The United Kingdom faced this situation in 2006 when measures to rein in global migration could not be applied to EU citizens. Hungary has also had to adapt interventions on emigration to meet the EU prerogatives of free movement and, as part of the EU accession process. Turkey is debating radical reforms to its restrictive labour laws which currently conflict with EU principles of labour mobility.

6.4 *Financing*

Financing a health system involves collecting and pooling revenues in order to purchase health services. Payment of health providers is a sub-function of purchasing services.

There have been few reported impacts on the financing function of health systems, with the exception of the payment conditions for medical doctors. Regardless of the limited evidence, health professional mobility is bound to have important impacts on payments systems as demonstrated by income's prominence as both a motivational factor (section 5) and a retention strategy (section 8).

For an important destination country such as Spain, foreign medical inflows from Latin America served to keep salary levels in the public sector fiscally sustainable as the pool of providers grew. Conversely, countries of origin facing the threat of emigration are driven to consider increasing salaries in the same way as the Lithuanian government and Polish independent health-care providers seeking to retain medical doctors. But such measures may not be sustainable in the long term and raise questions about redistribution within the system. Salary increases are dependent on a favourable economic situation and it is doubtful whether incentives can be maintained in the context of a financial crisis. While there is no evidence on how the financial downturn has impacted on health professional mobility, it will surely have repercussions in both sending and receiving countries (see also Section 5 on motivations).

7. Workforce context and relevance of health professional mobility

Health professional mobility raises important policy questions on how to assess whether there is a need to intervene. The extent of the need for policy and regulatory intervention (see section 8) is dependent on the impacts of health professional mobility (see section 6) and on its relevance vis-à-vis other domestic workforce issues. It is necessary to understand the workforce context in which mobility takes place in order to decide whether it is a priority for policy action, either independently or as part of larger workforce policies.

Authors were asked to qualitatively assess the relevance of health professional mobility in comparison to domestic workforce issues including the maldistribution of health workers over the territory, workforce shortages, attrition, the demographic transition and problems with the training pipeline. Based on the findings presented here, it is suggested that countries should be classified according to the domestic relevance of health professional mobility (see below).

Territorial maldistribution of the health workforce is endemic in virtually all 17 countries and causes severe policy concerns in under-supplied and underserved areas. In Romania, 98 rural localities had no family doctor in 2005. The remote areas of northern and eastern Finland have the most severe lack of general practitioners and important specialties are missing in some districts, usually in the least privileged regions. Maldistribution of specialists is reported for Spain, Turkey, Romania and Estonia. Serious maldistribution can occur even in situations of oversupply such as in Serbia where medical doctors are facing outmigration or unemployment. Germany shows disparities with oversupply in urban areas such as Munich, Hamburg and Berlin but considerable shortages in sparsely populated areas in the less prosperous eastern *Länder*. In France, maldistribution causes greater problems than shortages.

Many case studies have reported shortages in the health workforce. In Finland this has affected primary health care and 36% of public-sector general practitioner posts were not permanently filled in 2007. Estonia has reported a limited shortage for family medicine, anaesthetics, psychiatry, pathology and gynaecology. But this situation is heterogeneous as countries such as Belgium report an oversupply in most specialties. For nurses, Hungary is facing shortages and vacant positions in Budapest. Italy has also reported a substantial shortage of nurses that is particularly manifest in the south. France has less critical shortages of nurses in regions (such as the Paris suburbs) or in some specialties. Shortages of nurses in Belgium are found to be more acute in urban areas such as Antwerp or Brussels and in nursing homes more than in hospitals. Some case studies (such as Austria) have stressed a lack of home-care nurses although this was not the focus of this research.

Attrition is an issue in some countries but good data are widely missing. Estonia is the clearest example of a country in which attrition is deemed more important than outmigration. Part of the observed decline in workforce numbers in Poland since the 1990s can be attributed to medical doctors and nurses moving into alternative careers. In Hungary, 6000 health workers were made redundant following health policy reform and budget cuts. The attempt to retain and redistribute them to underserved areas proved unsuccessful and they were lost to the system.

Ageing of the workforce is a concern across countries and already firmly on the political agenda, as reported in the French case study. Data from Slovakia illustrate the speed and extent of demographic transition. Between 2004 and 2007, the 50+ age group grew from 41% to 45% for medical doctors and 54% to 61% for dentists; the proportion of nurses aged 40+ increased from 49% to 53%. Longer training periods mean that specialists in most countries have a particularly high average age. The Spanish case study reports that the average age in most traditional specialties is 50 or over. In Lithuania, 47% of all otolaryngologists and 30% of gynaecologists are aged over 60 and in Estonia the mean age of internists, neurologists, gynaecologists, oncologists and pathologists ranges from 54 to 56 years. In Belgium, an early retirement scheme means that nurses aged 60 years and older comprise less than 1% of the total nursing workforce.

In some countries, projections indicate that retirement from the health workforce will outpace the replacement of health professionals. In Italy, 13 400 nurses were due to retire from the system in 2010 but only 8500 graduated with a nursing degree in the 2008–2009 academic year. The trend of workforce ageing and increasing retirement rates in the United Kingdom is set against recruitment that is failing to replenish workforce losses, particularly those of general practitioners.

In a situation of shortages, attrition and the fast pace of retirement, some countries are facing severe difficulties in producing and training sufficient numbers of health professionals. France is facing an underproduction of medical doctors due to the *numerus clausus* introduced as a cost-containment measure; until recently, Germany reported decreasing graduate numbers; and Slovakia has reported insufficient outputs of graduates particularly nurses, midwives, physiotherapists, radiological assistants and paramedics. Hungary has experienced a decline in outputs from medical education since 1988 and seen serious bottlenecks in supply caused by reductions in some nurse training capacities. In addition, student intakes are dwindling in some countries as the health professions have become less attractive. The Romanian case study reported that the number of applicants to the medical universities decreased from 7 to 8 to only 0.9 candidates per place over a period of 10 years. Unfilled specialist training places are being reported not only in Romania but also in Turkey, for medical doctors in France, nurses in Hungary and for some specialties in Austria.

Based on the case-study findings, countries have been classified according to the domestic relevance of mobility. Assessment of relevance is a subjective exercise and a matter of political prioritization but such a classification serves to illustrate the varying levels of relevance in Europe and commonalities between groups of countries. Sending and receiving countries clearly have different reasons for such an assessment but can still be classified by the degree of relevance. Countries can be identified within three gradations of relevance.

1. High relevance – health professional mobility makes a major contribution to the size and characteristics of the health workforce, either because immigration is significant in both absolute (inflows) and relative (reliance) terms or because the country has considerable outflows of health professionals: Austria, Hungary, Romania, Slovakia, Slovenia, Spain and the United Kingdom.

2. Medium relevance – varies by health profession/region but, for example, includes countries in which there are considerable inflows for at least one health profession and/or reliance on a foreign workforce hovers around 5%; inflows and outflows that are likely to be broadly balanced; or outflows are visible but not considered to be a fundamental problem for the health system: Belgium, Finland, Germany, Italy, Poland and Serbia.

3. Lower relevance – other workforce issues such as overall shortages, geographical maldistribution or attrition are reported to be more problematic and/or attracting more political attention; and mobility overall is not seen as a major cause for concern: Estonia, France, Lithuania and Turkey.

8. Policy and regulatory interventions

This section will show four policy and regulatory interventions: international and domestic recruitment policies, workforce planning, cross-border frameworks and general workforce measures.

8.1 *International and domestic recruitment policies*

Recruitment policies determine the source, whether domestic or international, of health professionals entering the health system. International recruitment policies aim to attract foreign-trained health professionals either to meet shortfalls or to complement the skills and competencies of the existing workforce. Self-sufficiency policies are explicit policies that strive to meet a country's demand for health personnel. A secondary orientation is to reduce the reliance on foreign health professionals in the workforce stock.

Recruitment policies have been developed by the United Kingdom, Slovakia and Slovenia. The United Kingdom adopted an international recruitment policy in 1998 to fill gaps in the National Health Service (NHS) but moved stepwise to a self-sufficiency policy in 2006 and 2008. The period of 1998–

2006 was characterized by the British government's workforce expansion targets within its plan of NHS investment. Unable to increase domestic training in the required timescale, the United Kingdom started a high-profile international recruitment policy leading to a large openness to immigration across many health professions. This policy development was also reflected in a steep rise in yearly inflow data in that period. In 2006, policy-makers recognized that the domestic training expansion was coming on stream. Subsequently, a set of restrictions for international recruitment were introduced from 2006–2008 and further tightened from 2008 onwards.

Domestic recruitment policies or explicit self-sufficiency policies have been in introduced in Slovakia and Slovenia. Slovakia adopted a self-sufficiency policy in 2006, aiming to give health professionals better remuneration and improved social appreciation and social status. The policy included amendments to the labour code and remuneration act, a proposed system of social appreciation, amended minimum training standards, improved transparency on the work of ethical committees, improved and expanded health professional training, motivational measures and improved continuous medical education. This policy was a reaction to the substantial loss of health professionals that resulted in the formerly self-sufficient Slovakia becoming a source country following the opening of the borders in 1989 and the 2004 EU enlargement. Slovenia moved towards a self-sufficiency policy following an unsuccessful attempt to recruit internationally between 2000 and 2004. The political motivations that led to these self-sufficiency policies differ widely in the reported examples. Austria has a self-sufficiency policy at country level but planning decisions are taken by federal states and the country still has a relatively high intake of internationally recruited health professionals. Self-sufficiency is a very important policy orientation that still has no common definition apart from its use as a converse to international recruitment.

8.2 *Workforce planning*

Workforce planning is the continuous process of aligning the numbers, skills and competencies of health professionals with the aims, priorities, needs and demands of the health system. To this end workforce monitoring, analyses and forecasts are conducted using a variety of methodologies. Workforce planning aims to guide the development of educational and training contents and capacities.

A growing interest in workforce planning and the application of sophisticated forecasting methodologies is documented by the case studies from Belgium, Estonia, Finland, Lithuania, Spain and the United Kingdom. Some countries have no nationwide planning but use procedures at regional level, as in Austria;

others disperse planning across different institutions and levels, as in Germany. Workforce planning may extend beyond the health system, as in Finland which introduced a comprehensive system including other sectors to cover competing labour market demands. Yet very often, planning decisions are taken in an ad hoc manner or there is a serious disconnect between workforce planning and the development of training capacities, as reported from Serbia and Romania. Most workforce planners struggle with health professional mobility as it is a factor of uncertainty and an issue of technical debate. Even when countries have workforce planning mechanisms, serious methodological problems arise from the lack of data that makes it difficult to factor in the loss of health professionals. Lithuania has conducted studies on health professional mobility to address this uncertainty and factor outflows into workforce planning.

8.3 *Cross-border frameworks*

Cross-border frameworks are used to steer and manage health professional mobility. They can be unilateral, bilateral or multilateral and may be led by national governments or local health- care institutions.

There are many cross-border frameworks for steering and managing health professional mobility but uptake varies widely within and between countries, with a strong focus on bilateral agreements, staff exchange and educational support (Table 0.5). Austria and the United Kingdom use many of these instruments but most countries use only a few types of cross-border frameworks, although they may use them frequently. For example, France has three different kinds of bilateral agreements (*conventions d'établissements, accord de réciprocité,* and *convention médicale transfrontalière*) with at least 10 countries, the majority of which are in northern or sub-Saharan Africa.

In 2001 the United Kingdom introduced a code of conduct for international recruitment aiming to prevent recruitment from countries with workforce shortages. A regional code was introduced in Scotland. The effectiveness of such codes is the subject of scientific debate. The United Kingdom's case study reports that further specifications and implementation measures were required before the code showed some effects. A national code was reported for Austria too even though planning and recruitment takes place at regional and local levels; the effects of this code were not reported (see Table 0.5).

Bilateral agreements are the most commonly used cross-border framework. Most country case studies do not cover these in depth but at least four types of bilateral agreements can be distinguished. First, agreements that limit or exclude recruitment from countries with workforce shortages, as used in the United Kingdom in support of the international code. The Italian case study

Table 0.5 *Cross-border frameworks for steering and managing health professional mobility*

	International code	Bilateral agreement	Twinning	Staff exchange	Education support	Compensation	Training for export
Austria	X		X	X	X		X
Belgium		X			X		
Estonia		(X)					
Finland		X					
France		X					
Germany		X					
Hungary		X					X
Italy		X	X		X		
Lithuania							
Poland				X			
Romania				X			
Serbia		X					
Slovakia				X			
Slovenia		X					
Spain		X					
Turkey					X		
United Kingdom	X	X	X	X			

Note: (X) informal agreement only.

also reported on the implementation of a code to reduce immigration from third countries but it is not clear whether this applies only to health professionals. Second, those that aim to facilitate health professional mobility by establishing systems for mutual recognition of diplomas, such as the agreement established between Belgium and South Africa and those established as part of the free trade agreements in Nordic countries in the 1950s. France has agreements with countries in north and central Africa, Monaco and Switzerland and has entered bilateral agreements on the establishment of health professionals (these include Monaco on the basis of its special relation to France). Third, those that foster active recruitment, such as the bilateral agreement between Germany and Croatia concerning nurses. Between 2001 and 2005, the United Kingdom concluded bilateral agreements with Spain, Germany, Austria and Italy on the active recruitment of medical doctors. Fourth, bilateral agreements such as those that allowed temporary opening of the labour markets to accession countries until enlargement was finalized and full mobility established. Country case studies report agreements between Hungary and Norway and between the United Kingdom and Poland.

Policy changes can lead to the removal of bilateral agreements, as was the case for the United Kingdom agreements on reciprocal recognition of pharmacists from Australia and New Zealand. Slovenia has agreements inherited from the former Yugoslav Republic that are being phased out or becoming irrelevant. Informal bilateral agreements between professional bodies assume similar functions in some cases as shown by the examples between Tyrol in Austria and South Tyrol in Italy, or between Finland and Estonia.

Twinning aims to support the development of modern institutions in the beneficiary country. Some twinning activities have been reported from the United Kingdom, Italy and Austria, led by the Royal College of Physicians, the International Training Academy for Health Professionals and EU-funded projects.

An abundance of initiatives focus on staff exchange and educational support but it is often difficult to distinguish between them because the same activity can cover both cross-border frameworks. These initiatives tend to be used more at regional or local level rather than nationally and often by professional bodies or health-care organizations. There are several examples in Belgium. In 1990, a Belgian university signed an agreement allowing Romanian third- or fourth-year medical students at a Romanian university to spend one to three years of their specialization in one its hospitals. By 2009, some 450 Romanian interns had taken part in the programme. A university hospital in Liège has signed an agreement with a Vietnamese hospital and a university in Brussels runs a scholarship programme for medical doctors.

The Italian-led SkyNurse project has involved 180 candidates in a fourteen-month training programme that includes three months of distance learning between classrooms in Padua and the partners' institutes in Bucharest and Pitesti. Other examples were reported for leading institutions from Austria, Turkey and the United Kingdom.

Country case-study authors were also asked to report on compensation schemes. These aim to mitigate the loss of investment in human resources in source countries but, while discussed in the international literature, no compensation schemes were found.

Training for international recruitment takes place in Europe but the examples are not straightforward and do not necessarily involve high-level or governmental involvement. No intentional training for international recruitment was reported but the oversupply situation in Serbia is de facto training for unemployment. Hungarian medical universities train foreign nationals for the European job market and have offered programmes in German since 1983 and in English since 1987. These courses are increasingly popular mainly among students from the Middle East, Nordic countries, Germany and the United States. Romanian doctors are offered the opportunity to undertake part of their specialist training in France. It is expected that most students will return to their countries on completion of their training.

8.4 *General workforce measures*

General workforce measures included in this study are those that facilitate retention and avoid attrition of health professionals and, to this end, aim to improve working conditions and the working environment. While not necessarily implemented with the primary aim to manage health professional mobility, they have had a distinct effect. The following paragraphs summarize the findings on the four policy and regulatory interventions.

A large number of general workforce measures have been implemented. Salary increases for health professionals, especially doctors, were reported in Lithuania, Poland and Slovakia and (locally) for Hungary. The memorandum on salary levels signed between the Lithuanian ministry of health and the medical associations in 2005 was a particularly important measure. Increasing salaries (20% annually for medical doctors and nurses during 2005-2008) is likely to have had positive effects on high dropout rates from medical studies, attrition to other better paid professions and on emigration rates.

There are also reports of improvements to staff working conditions; modernization of the infrastructure of health-care facilities, including the introduction of up-to-date medical technologies; incentives for practice in under-supplied and underserved areas; and flexible retirement policies adapted to the consequences of workforce ageing and the potential migration of health professionals. Finland is planning measures to recruit unemployed immigrant health professionals into the health sector. The Slovak and Lithuanian case studies also reported using funding from European structural funds for modernization of the health system. Poland, Slovenia, the United Kingdom and Slovakia all reported increased training capacities or increased intakes of health professionals. For example, Slovenia has opened a new medical faculty and new nursing schools. Many of these interventions were developed and implemented to address general workforce issues and challenges. Only some are direct responses to health professional mobility but all these activities are highly relevant for responding to this issue.

Overall, there are substantial variations in the levels of activity concerning policy and regulatory interventions. The United Kingdom is the only country that is responding to health professional mobility by developing activities in all four areas covered. Countries that are developing a variety of activities include Austria, Belgium, Slovenia and Slovakia. Poland, Romania and Hungary have been less active.

9. Summary of results

The case studies show the diversity within Europe, with large intercountry variations in terms of flows, impacts, motivations, relevance and responses.

Reliance on foreign health professionals is characterized by large differences across Europe and indications of an east-west asymmetry. Reliance levels gradually decrease towards the eastern part of Europe (ranging between <1% and 2% for both professions in most 2004 and 2007 accession countries). Reliance on foreign medical doctors is negligible in Turkey, Estonia and Slovakia (0.02–0.7%); relatively low in Poland, Hungary, Italy and France (>5%); moderate in Germany (5.2%) and Finland (6.2%); high in Belgium, Portugal, Spain, Austria, Canada, Norway and Sweden; and very high in Switzerland, Slovenia, Ireland and the United Kingdom (22.5%–36.8%). Fewer countries provide data on foreign nurses yet evidence shows lower reliance than for medical doctors. At 1.3%, Hungary shows the highest reliance on foreign nurses among the EU-12 countries but this is in sharp contrast with Ireland (47%). Reliance on foreign nurses is negligible in Turkey and Slovakia; relatively low in Spain, Hungary, France, Finland, Sweden, Germany, the United States, Portugal and Belgium; moderate in Canada and Italy; high in the United Kingdom and Austria (10–20%); and very high in Ireland. Analysis of the reliance on foreign dentists is limited by the lack of data and no conclusions could be drawn across Europe.

Flow analysis quantifies the numbers of health professionals leaving and entering a country. Despite differences in the availability and quality of data for medical doctors, nurses and dentists, the evidence suggests that foreign **inflows** for all three professions in 2008 rate higher in absolute and relative terms in the EU-15 than in the EU-12. For most EU-15 countries the growth of inflows of foreign medical doctors and nurses appears to have peaked and have been followed by lower inflows. Austria, Finland, France, Germany, Hungary, Lithuania, Poland, Slovenia, Spain and the United Kingdom provided data on inflows of newly registered foreign medical doctors. These show that, in absolute numbers, the largest inflows were reported in Spain (8282), the United Kingdom (5022) and Germany (1583); the lowest were in Lithuania (11). Data on inflows of foreign nurses were available in Austria, Belgium, Finland, France, Hungary, Italy and the United Kingdom. The highest numbers were in Italy (9168) and the United Kingdom (3724); the smallest reported number was in Finland (97). Austria, Belgium, Finland, Hungary, Poland, Slovenia and Spain provide data on inflows of foreign dentists. These show the highest absolute numbers in Spain (421) and Austria (100) and the lowest in Hungary (18).

The case studies show that mobility has also increased over time in terms of **outflows** although substantial data limitations on emigration imply that outflow data are rather approximate. Outflows and/or outflow intentions increased substantially in Estonia, Hungary, Poland, Romania, Slovakia and Slovenia at the time of EU enlargements. This was also true in Austria, Germany, Italy and the United Kingdom. Health workforce losses are occurring in EU-12 and EU-15 countries but it appears that many EU-15 countries are concomitantly receiving health professionals although poor data do not allow firm conclusions to be drawn.

Three geographical patterns can be identified in the case-studies: (i) mobility within the European free-movement area; (ii) neighbourhood movements; and (iii) the EU enlargements of 2004 and 2007.

In terms of the **geographical source** of mobile health professionals, Austria, Belgium, France, Germany and Italy receive their foreign health professionals predominantly from the European free-movement area with (at least) 50% of the foreign medical workforce from EU countries. In Italy, this also holds true for nurses. Slovenia is the only country receiving foreign health professionals predominantly from the wider Europe – 22.5% of all active medical doctors in 2008 were primarily from Croatia, Bosnia and Herzegovina and Serbia. The United Kingdom and Spain receive their foreign health professionals predominantly from third countries, the former from the Commonwealth and the latter from Latin America (for medical doctors) although the trend is slowing in the United Kingdom.

Mobility between neighbouring countries occurs across Europe as either reciprocal or one-way flows. This occurs mainly in densely populated border regions and is facilitated by shared languages and cultures. Prime examples include France-Belgium-Netherlands, Austria-Germany, Austria-Italy-Hungary-Slovenia-Slovakia and Finland-Sweden-Estonia-Russian Federation.

Although health professionals were already moving from eastern to western European countries, the **EU enlargements** opened the borders for health professionals from ten new Member States in 2004 and two in 2007. These had significant influence on migratory flows although the magnitude of outflows of health professionals (measured by intention to leave) was not as large as anticipated. In countries with data available, outflows rarely exceeded 3% of the domestic workforce.

Estonia, Hungary, Poland, Slovakia and Romania faced initial strong outflows followed by a slow-down or more contained development. The highest numbers of mutual recognition of diploma certificates were issued in the year of accession or the following year. In Estonia, the number of certificates issued peaked in 2004 with 283 for medical doctors, 118 for nurses and 29 for dentists. Numbers dropped in the following years but increased slightly in 2009. Hungary showed the highest numbers in 2004; and Poland[15] and Slovakia in 2005. High outflow intentions among Romanian medical doctors seem to be continuing – certificates were issued to more than 300 per month in 2010, although the data have to be interpreted with care. The mobility of medical doctors and dentists appears to have increased on a higher scale than for nurses after EU enlargement although the real scale of flows may be underestimated due to the lack of good-quality data on nurses (including those in Poland, Romania and Slovakia).

The net winners of EU enlargements have been predominantly those in the EU-15. The numbers of newly registered EU-12 medical doctors, nurses and dentists increased modestly in destination countries such as Austria, Belgium, Finland, France and Italy around 2004–2007. France experienced a higher increase in the number of Romanian medical doctors, from 174 in 2007 to 1160 registered doctors in January 2009. In Austria, nursing inflows seem to follow enlargement as no nurses from future enlargement countries had applied for diploma validation in 2000 but 278 did so in 2008. Spain and the United Kingdom reported important inflows of medical doctors from Poland and Romania, partly linked to the active roles of recruitment agencies targeting these countries.

---

15 Numbers for 2005 may be cumulative.

Contrary to estimates and expectations the 2004 and 2007 EU enlargements did not lead to "swamping" in the EU-15 countries or to massive brain drains of health professionals from the then accession states (EU-12). Enlargement did considerably reinforce pre-existing flows from eastern and central EU Member States towards western parts of the EU. Labour market restrictions in several EU-15 Member States in the transition periods and better salaries and working conditions in some eastern European countries may help to explain why mobility was less than expected.

In terms of the **motivational factors** which influence health professionals in their decision on whether to migrate, the case-studies confirm existing knowledge and add new insights from the EU-12 Member States. Key findings are the importance of income-related incentives in all 17 countries studied, good working conditions and the perception of better earnings and/or better opportunities.

The case-studies show how health professional mobility's **impacts on health systems** are seldom immediately or easily discernible and rarely produce visible effects on health outcomes. Information was of a qualitative, unsystematic and often anecdotal nature from a limited number of countries but the reported observations confirm the stark differences between sending and receiving countries in terms of the impacts. The evidence suggests that health professional mobility affects service delivery by alleviating or worsening pre-existing workforce issues of skill mix, shortages and geographical distribution. It also affects resource creation by cancelling returns on investment and disrupting planning efforts in countries which educate and train workforces for international recruitment (but involving savings for destination countries) and by the potential to induce reliance on a foreign workforce. Stewardship is affected as countries lack information about health professionals leaving and entering the system, which in turn hampers workforce planning. Countries are also restricted in their ability to regulate mobility within the EU free-movement area. Financing may be affected in terms of payment of providers. Mobility appears to have helped to keep salary levels under control in at least one destination country but has probably contributed to salary increases in source countries. Overall, the impacts of outflows often exacerbate pre-existing challenges in the health systems of source countries and are not necessarily related to the volumes of flows.

To understand health professional mobility's role in broader contexts and to identify the need for policy interventions, qualitative material was collected to assess its **relevance** in comparison to domestic workforce issues such as the maldistribution of health workers, workforce shortages, attrition, demographic transition and problems with the training pipeline. Geographical maldistribution of the health workforce is endemic in virtually all 17 countries in terms of under-supplied and underserved areas. Workforce shortages were reported among public-sector general practitioner posts in Finland; for family medicine, anaesthetics, psychiatry, pathology and gynaecology in Estonia; and among nurses in Hungary and Italy. France and Belgium reported some nursing shortages especially in urban areas. Good data on attrition are widely missing but in Estonia this is reported to more problematic than outmigration and has contributed to an observed decline in workforce numbers in Poland. Ageing of the workforce is a major concern across countries as projections show that retirement from the health workforce will outpace the replacement of health professionals in some places. This is exacerbated as educational systems are facing severe difficulties producing and training sufficient numbers of health professionals in countries such Hungary, Germany, France, Romania and Turkey. Based on these findings, countries have been ranked according to the relative importance of health professional mobility: high relevance for seven countries (Austria, Hungary, Romania, Slovakia, Slovenia, Spain, United Kingdom); of some relevance in six (Belgium, Finland, Germany, Italy, Poland, Serbia) and of relatively lower relevance in four (Estonia, France, Lithuania, Turkey).

Four different types of **policy and regulatory interventions** were identified in the case studies: (i) international and domestic recruitment policies; (ii) workforce planning; (iii) cross-border frameworks; and (iv) general workforce measures. Recruitment policies have been developed by the United Kingdom, Slovakia and Slovenia. Growing interest in workforce planning and the application of sophisticated forecasting methodologies is documented by the case studies from Belgium, Estonia, Finland, Lithuania, Spain and the United Kingdom. A host of cross-border frameworks have been established to steer and manage health professional mobility but the uptake of these instruments varies widely, with a strong focus on bilateral agreements (11 countries), staff exchanges (7 countries) and educational support (4 countries).

Overall activity levels concerning policy and regulatory interventions vary substantially. Some countries have unfolded a range of interventions; others have been rather inactive although no less affected by health professional mobility. The United Kingdom is the only country that is responding to health professional mobility by developing activities in all four areas covered. Countries that are developing a variety of activities include Austria, Belgium, Slovenia and Slovakia. Poland, Romania and Hungary have been less active.

Conclusions

Irene A Glinos, Matthias Wismar, Claudia B Maier, Willy Palm, Josep Figueras

1. Introduction

This study aims to enhance our understanding of health professional mobility in today's Europe. The endeavour comprises two distinct but closely connected parts. The first is to understand mobility in terms of the evidence on its extent and directions; the second is to understand mobility in terms of its impact, policy relevance and implications.

While information on health professional mobility is available for some countries, the general level of evidence across Europe is largely insufficient in quantity and/or inadequate in quality. These gaps have become manifest as mobility has started to attract policy interest. Without evidence on the extent and directions of migratory flows, decision-makers cannot know how their country is affected; without evidence on the implications of mobility and its relative weight in the context of domestic workforce priorities, they cannot know whether to address it.

The research underlying this book aims at addressing the glaring knowledge gaps. For the first time, evidence has been gathered from a large pool of countries in a systematic, standardized way that ensures intercountry comparability. In addition, authors have gone beyond numbers to grasp the impact and relevance of health professional mobility and assess the policy interventions applied in their country.

The present chapter concludes the research included in this volume. It first presents the reader with the mobility highlights of the 17 country case-studies. Based on this evidence, six key observations on health professional mobility are formulated to bring out the most policy-relevant dimensions of the research. The third section discusses the changing and uncertain context of mobility in the future while the fourth draws on the observations and changing context to explain the potential policy implications of mobility. The chapter closes with some brief reflections.

2. Mobility highlights from 17 countries

This section presents a summary of each of the 17 country case-studies, outlining the main features of mobility in order to highlight the individual and common challenges presented by health professional mobility. This provides a useful reminder of the uniqueness and diversity of the countries that provide the evidence base for this study, serving as the basis for discussion of the key observations and policy implications. The European Union (EU) Member States are ordered according to whether accession occurred before or after 2004, followed by Serbia and Turkey – countries that have applied for EU membership.

Austria (Chapter 1) is both a destination and a source for health professionals from neighbouring countries. The strongest connection exists with Germany and this mobility is two-way. Inflow and outflow volumes are roughly balanced for medical doctors and dentists but for nurses are characterized by a one-way inflow over years. Health professional mobility is of high significance for the home-care sector. High numbers of nurses from eastern Europe have been recruited to work in home care, often on an illegal basis. This remains an issue of public and political debate.

There are reciprocal flows of health professionals between **Belgium** (Chapter 2) and neighbouring countries with languages in common. Inflows from more distant countries such as Romania and Lebanon are also visible as foreign medical doctors with basic training and nurses are being recruited to alleviate domestic shortages. In particular inflows of foreign-trained dentists and medical doctors with basic training represent important shares of new registrations (19.3% and 25.3% respectively in 2008) while outflows are strongest for Belgian-trained specialists moving to France.

Over the last 20 years, **Finland** (Chapter 3) has changed from a source country to one with a mixed mobility profile. Outflows of health professionals have decreased and become comparable to inflows. Foreign medical doctors and dentists represent important shares of all new arrivals in the workforce. This signals that the Finnish system could become dependent on the inflows of foreign health professionals from abroad. In the context of a changing policy environment and health workforce shortages since 2006, recruitment programmes for foreign health professionals have gained more attention as a measure for tackling workforce shortages.

Evidence suggests that **France** (Chapter 4) is a destination country, especially for foreign medical doctors. These are mainly from neighbouring EU countries, followed by French-speaking countries of north and sub-Saharan Africa. Inflows have increased with EU enlargements (considerable numbers of Romanian doctors have migrated to France since 2007) but at lower levels than expected. Nationally, health professional mobility is of limited impact but the foreign workforce is important locally – in hospitals with shortages and in certain specialties.

Germany (Chapter 5) is both a destination and a source country. Around 5-6% of all registered medical doctors and dentists and 3.4% of all nurses and midwives[1] are of foreign nationality. Federal states and hospitals in eastern Germany are compensating for the shortage of medical doctors by recruiting from abroad. Foreign nurses from eastern European countries are increasingly working as self-employed or illegally, mainly as home-care workers for elderly people. At the same time, a rising number of German health professionals are leaving the country to work abroad, attracted by better working conditions and higher pay.

Health professional mobility to and from **Italy** (Chapter 6) is shaped by distortions in the domestic health workforce. Oversupply of medical doctors has led to outflows while structural nursing shortages have led Italy to recruit from abroad. One in ten nurses is of foreign origin, mainly from Europe (Romania and Poland) and also from Latin America (Peru). The elderly-care and home-care sectors rely heavily on foreign carers who nevertheless remain undocumented. Legislation partly reflects the needs of the system by easing entry requirements for nurses and seeking to regularize care workers.

Inflows and outflows of health professionals have increased substantially in **Spain** (Chapter 7) over the last decade. Responding to workforce shortages, medical doctors from Latin America have immigrated to work as general medical doctors and to train as specialists. Spanish doctors and nurses did show high outflows to other EU Member States but these have been declining since the mid 2000s. In 2007, foreign nationals comprised about 12.5% of all medical doctors but only about 1% of nurses. The importance of foreign inflows not only to the medical workforce (8282 foreign degrees recognized in 2008 alone)[2] but also to the nursing, dentistry and pharmacy professions suggests a degree of dependency on immigration.

Historically, the **United Kingdom** (Chapter 8) has been a major destination country for health professionals, predominantly from India, Pakistan, Nigeria and South Africa as well as Australia and New Zealand. More than a third of medical doctors and every tenth nurse are internationally trained. Old colonial ties and English as a common language have influenced migration patterns. This is also true for the EU enlargements but on a lower overall scale.

---

1 Subject to social insurance contributions.

2 Foreign degrees in general medicine recognized in Spain, equivalent to 213% of all diplomas delivered in Spain in that year.

The British government's policy of massive expansion in the National Health Service (NHS) workforce in the late 1990s instigated a period of active international recruitment on an unprecedented scale. The policy was reversed in 2006 and more restrictive immigration rules were introduced as earlier expansion in domestic training numbers came on stream.

Predominantly a source country, **Estonia** (Chapter 9) continues to lose health professionals not only to Finland but also to the United Kingdom, Sweden, Germany and Norway. Since EU accession in 2004, outflows (intentions) appear to have been of moderate scale (about 70–130 certificates issued yearly since 2005[3] to medical doctors and nurses and 20–40 to dentists). Constant increases in salaries since 2005 may have contributed to making working abroad less attractive. Mobility appears to be less significant than other domestic workforce issues such as ageing of the workforce or attrition. However, the active recruitment practices of Scandinavian (especially Finnish) health-care institutions may pose a threat in the near future.

Inflow and outflow data show **Hungary** (Chapter 10) to be mainly a source country. In 2008, 803 medical doctors showed intentions to leave[4] but there were only 45 newly registered foreign medical doctors. The magnitude and character of emigrating health professionals is a key health workforce challenge. Since EU accession, mainly medical doctors and dentists (intend to) leave. Around 2–3% of all medical doctors and dentists and around 0.2% of nurses have outflow intentions but the effect of migration is worsened by the age profile, specialties and skill-mix of leavers. There are indications that, in combination with other health workforce issues, outflows pose a risk to the sustainability of the Hungarian health system. Despite this, there has been little policy action.

Lithuania (Chapter 11) is best defined as a source country but outflows of health professionals have not been as important as anticipated prior to EU accession. Whereas 2.7% (357) of medical doctors and 3.6% (81) of dentists showed intentions to work abroad during the first year of EU enlargement,[5] numbers fell to 0.9% (132) of medical doctors and 3.1% (72) of dentists in 2009. Nurses had fewer intentions to leave the country (around 0.5–1% of the workforce). However, health professional mobility and its potential consequences for the health system have attracted political attention and workforce-planning processes have been initiated at national, regional and local levels. Ongoing reforms have focused on improving working conditions and it is likely that the 2005–2008 salary increases played a role in retaining health professionals.

---

3 With the exception of 2004. This is a clear outlier as 283 mutual recognition of diploma certificates were issued to medical doctors in that year.

4 By requesting recognition of diploma certificates.

5 Measured by the number of recognition of diploma certificates issued.

Poland's (Chapter 12) accession to the EU in 2004 led to an escalation of health professionals leaving the country, especially medical doctors and dentists. Mobility is a noticeable phenomenon but currently is not seen to pose a significant threat to the health system although it has been suggested that there is a link to the increasing number of vacancies in the Polish health sector. Emigration has slowed and health professionals have been returning since 2007, the year that salary levels were increased. Poland also attracts some inflows of foreign health professionals, mainly from the Ukraine, but these have been insignificant in comparison to outflows.

Outflows from **Romania** (Chapter 13) have been triggered by EU accession and the economic downturn. In 2007, the scale of emigration was high as 1421 medical doctors (around 3% of all practising medical doctors in Romania) left in that year alone. This affected one of the most economically deprived areas (North-East Region) more than other regions. Overall the phenomenon was not as dramatic as expected and showed no signs of jeopardizing the health system. By the end of 2009 the economic downturn had begun to impact on the health workforce, staffing levels and salaries. These developments combined with the emigration of health professionals to become a critical concern. An effective health workforce strategy has been lacking and some of the retention measures in rural areas have not proved effective.

Slovakia (Chapter 14) is a source country, losing considerable numbers of qualified health professionals to other EU countries. The opening of borders in 1989 and EU accession in 2004 affected a formerly self-sufficient system. Between 2004 and 2007[6] a total of 1377 medical doctors, 1780 nurses, 109 dental doctors, 164 pharmacists and 194 physiotherapists requested mutual recognition of diploma certificates to work abroad. The country now faces challenges from staff shortages, underproduction of health professionals and a looming demographic trend. Measures such as better data collection and retention strategies aimed at regaining self-sufficiency are a key priority.

Slovenia (Chapter 15) has been an attractive destination for medical doctors and dentists from the countries of the former Yugoslavia. In 2008, more than 20% of all active medical doctors and dentists were foreign-trained. Shortages of health professionals and consequent opportunities for foreign graduates may have triggered considerable inflows, as did the expanding health sector. There have been attempts to make Slovenia self-sufficient – training capacity was expanded by opening an additional medical faculty and four additional nursing schools. It is too early to comment on the effect of these measures.

The political, social and economic situation in **Serbia** (Chapter 16) has influenced health professional mobility since the 1960s. It is estimated that a total of 10 000 Serbian health professionals have moved to work abroad

6 1 May 2004–30 April 2007.

since 1960. Germany and Switzerland were the most popular destinations but neighbouring countries (predominantly Slovenia) are becoming more popular through their association with the EU, geographical proximity, similar languages and cultures and established social networks. Aside from Serbia's political and economic situation, health professional outflows are due to higher salaries and oversupply of medical doctors. They are also related to broader health system and workforce challenges such as working conditions and limited career development opportunities.

Turkey (Chapter 17) is characterized by one-way flows of health professionals as restrictive labour laws pose serious difficulties for individuals of foreign descent seeking to live and work there. However, foreign recruitment is beginning to be seen as a possible remedy to the problems caused by insufficient planning, a problematic skill-mix, unbalanced specializations, underproduction and the maldistribution of professionals. These considerations and a view to potential EU accession have led the current government to try to ease labour laws but this is a highly controversial policy option in Turkey.

3. Mobility matters: key observations

Health professional mobility is clearly a phenomenon that cannot be ignored by policy-makers, health workforce planners, managers or researchers. Some important observations can be derived from the evidence presented in this volume and this section will present six key observations formulated to highlight the most policy-relevant dimensions concerning the significant but diverse magnitude of mobility; the lower than expected effects of EU enlargements; worsening east-west asymmetries; money as a driver for mobility; the subtle but significant impacts of mobility; and the limited data available.

3.1 *Magnitude of mobility: significant but diverse*

The magnitude of health professional mobility is important in a number of countries in terms of reliance on the foreign workforce and of inflows. Reliance shows the share of foreign health professionals within a country's health workforce in a given year. As a share of total new entrants to the system, inflows show how migrants contribute to replenishing the workforce. There is considerable diversity in the magnitude of mobility across countries as well as within countries for different health professions.

Important reliance on foreign health professionals has been noted for the following countries. Foreign[7] medical doctors amount to at least one in every

---

7 Foreign born, foreign trained or foreign national.

ten medical doctors in Belgium, Portugal, Spain, Austria, Norway, Sweden, Switzerland, Slovenia, Ireland and the United Kingdom. Foreign-trained medical doctors comprised 36.8% of all medical doctors in the United Kingdom in 2008. Overall, reliance on foreign nurses seems less pronounced but does exceed 10% of the nursing workforce in Italy, the United Kingdom, Austria and Ireland. One in every two nurses in Ireland is foreign-trained. All other countries in the study show low (around 5%) to negligible (<1%) reliance on the foreign health workforce.

The magnitude of flows also shows the importance of mobility. In Europe, flows have been increasing since the major geopolitical changes that began in the late 1980s. The limited number of time series data that are available indicate fluctuating inflows – increasing, decreasing or stable depending on the country. Increases in outflows are suggested in more countries (see observation 3.2). In 2008, the proportion of foreign inflows within all new entrants[8] to the health workforce was particularly high for foreign medical doctors in the United Kingdom (42.6%), Belgium[9] (25.3%) and Austria (13.5%); for foreign nurses in Italy (28%), the United Kingdom (14.7%) and Belgium (13.5%); and for foreign dentists in Austria (40.8%), the United Kingdom (33.7%), Belgium (19.3%) and Hungary (9.7%). In Finland, 43.2% of newly licensed dentists in the period from 2006 to 2008 were foreign trained. Much lower shares were reported in Poland (around 3% for foreign medical doctors and dentists) and in Hungary (4.7% for foreign medical doctors and 2.4% for foreign nurses). Data were not available for other countries.

3.2 *Effects of EU enlargement: less than expected*

The EU enlargements in 2004 and 2007 added 12 new countries to the free-movement area. Health professionals from eastern Europe joined the mobile workforce in Europe and mobility became a more diverse phenomenon. The enlargements were associated with high expectations. Outflow intentions in Estonia, Hungary, Lithuania, Poland, Romania and Slovakia increased considerably at the time of accession but were lower than anticipated. In many countries, annual outflow intentions hovered at around 3% of all health professionals but showed some peaks – reaching 6.5% of all medical doctors in Estonia in the first eight months of 2004, for example. In most countries these outflow intentions subsequently decreased (between three and four times) but remained at higher overall levels than before enlargement. In Hungary, the outflow intentions of medical doctors have remained stable at around 2.5% per year. By contrast, outflow intentions have remained low (<1%) in Slovenia.

---

8 Newly registered or newly licensed depending on country and profession.

9 In Belgium, these were medical doctors with basic medical diplomas (as opposed to general practitioner or specialist diplomas).

Poland is an example of a country in which health professionals are reversing outflows by returning. Generally, outflows from the EU-12 have been lower than expected but are still higher than outflows from the EU-15.

It is important to note that intention-to-leave data are used as a proxy in the absence of data on actual outflows. However, these tend to overestimate emigration. Studies in Romania and Estonia showed that actual departures were two to three times lower than outflow intentions. Peaks such as the one recorded in Estonia in 2004 may be explained by retrospective applications for diploma certification from health professionals who migrated before accession.

Overall, the EU enlargements have led to increases in flows between EU countries but it is probably too soon to draw conclusions on the effects of EU enlargement. More recent (2009 or 2010) data from Estonia, Hungary and Romania point to a new surge in outflows, presumably related to the global economic downturn.

3.3 *East-west asymmetries worsened*

The analysis also reveals noticeable asymmetries between EU-12 and EU-15 countries. Flows are predominantly in one direction, from east to west and most destination countries are in the EU-15 (cf. observation 3.1). All European countries are subject to outflows but most EU-15 countries show simultaneous inflows, unlike most EU-12 countries. EU-15 countries thus have more possibilities to fill vacant positions with foreign health professionals.

These differences may signal the persisting importance of geopolitical contexts and economic incentives. Lower income levels (see observation 3.4), working conditions and standards of living as well as unfinished health reforms in some EU-12 countries all add to the perception of less promising perspectives. The lower inflows of foreign medical doctors and nurses as well as the lower levels of reliance on foreign health professionals in the EU-12 reflect and reinforce these asymmetries.

It should not be forgotten that outflows from eastern Europe started well before accession, following the political transitions that took place in various parts of the region. For example, high numbers of health professionals from Bosnia and Herzegovina, Croatia and Serbia in Germany's workforce stock in 2003 point to decades of outmigration from the former Yugoslav Republic. In some ways, it may still be too early to draw conclusions on the effects of enlargements. Less than 10 years have passed and the right to free movement acquired with EU membership will continue to facilitate mobility even decades from now. For the moment, mobility data show persisting differences between the EU-12 and the EU-15, albeit with variations within both groups.

3.4 *Money: a main driver for mobility*

Unsurprisingly, many of the country case-studies show that money motivates mobility. This may seem obvious when an Estonian medical doctor can earn six times more in Finland and a Romanian general practitioner can earn ten times more in France. Income is the most cited factor in deciding whether or not to migrate, and influences leavers, returnees and those who remain. In Lithuania, annual salary increases of 20% for medical doctors and nurses in 2005–2008 likely helped to reverse high dropout rates from medical studies as well as attrition and emigration. In Poland, better remuneration is reported to have diminished outflows and motivated returns. In Slovenia, increases in salaries arguably contributed to a smaller than expected loss of health professionals. Conversely, a 25% cut in the salary of health professionals in Romania may have contributed to higher outflow numbers in 2009. It remains to be seen how the global economic downturn will affect flows as mobility is dependent on what opportunities are (perceived to be) available in source and destination countries.

Money is an important motivator but only one among many factors that determine job satisfaction and willingness to stay or look for alternative options at home or abroad. The other most often mentioned motivation in the country case-studies is working conditions. This includes the working environment, terms of employment, work relations and access to infrastructures. Low social recognition and/or low esteem were also mentioned relatively frequently. Incomplete health reforms, unrealized objectives and disappointment among the workforce were mentioned in four EU-12 countries (Lithuania, Hungary, Romania and Slovakia).

3.5 *Subtle but significant impacts on the performance of health systems*

One aim of this study was to assess mobility's impact on health systems. The perceived effects on shortages, training new workforces and financing sustainability have received much public attention in several countries. In spite of intense debates, there is surprisingly little evidence on this subject and there appear to have been no systematic studies. The country case-studies address this gap by including some qualitative analysis based on expert interviews and authors' observations.

The case studies indicate how mobility contributes to shortages concerning the size, skill-mix and geographical distribution of the health workforce. Inflows to destination countries help to compensate for inadequate workforce planning and to improve access. Foreign medical doctors, nurses, dentists and/or carers increase service capacity in the United Kingdom, Spain, Austria and Italy. Shortages in the less affluent eastern parts of Germany are increasingly filled by foreign medical doctors –their numbers tripled between 2000 and 2008. In France, medical doctors from non-EU countries fill gaps in public hospitals especially in socioeconomically disadvantaged areas.

There may be many reasons for shortages in source countries and it is hard to prove that emigration is the cause. However, several case-studies mention that outflows can worsen service delivery. Losses become a particular problem if they involve large numbers, rare skills or occur in already undersupplied areas. Slovakia lost a reported 3243 health professionals between January 2005 and December 2006 but the real numbers are likely to be substantially higher. In Romania, rural areas with the lowest coverage of medical doctors report some of the highest emigration rates among medical doctors and nurses. Impacts are not always related to the size of flows. Hungary, Estonia and Lithuania noted that the departure of even a few specialists can upset service provision. Certain specialties appear to be more vulnerable. In Poland, most vacant posts concern anaesthetists and emergency doctors – specialists that show greatest intention to leave. In Belgium, the emigration of child psychiatrists has been reported as problematic given important shortages in the profession.

It is also important to recognize the accumulated effect of mobility. For instance, an annual outflow of 3% of total medical doctors may not appear to be significant but will leave a major mark on the size of the workforce if it continues over years. This implies that some impacts may take time to appear.

Training and financing are closely related in the mobility context. Mobility has implications for training due to the huge cost and time needed to educate and train health professionals. Several countries report (extremely) high foreign inflows in at least one health profession (cf. observation 3.1). In 2008, Spain recognized 8282 foreign degrees in general medicine – more than double the number of medical graduates produced that year. Whether or not this is a conscious strategy, the importation of health professionals expands knowledge and skills but at lower costs. As noted in the United Kingdom, foreign recruitment has the added benefit of freeing up senior staff to train a new workforce. Yet, while foreign inflows are substantial in many countries (observation 3.1), they may come at the expense of reliance on a foreign workforce.

Conversely, Serbia and Montenegro have spent an estimated US$ 9–12 billion educating and training medical specialists who have since left the country. This undermines returns on investment and possibly the necessary skill-mix of the country. Mobility of foreign students affects the availability of training positions and foreign students are less likely to stay in a host country following graduation. Health workforce planning in Belgium is affected as inflows of Dutch and French students bypass the *numerus clausus* that applies to domestic students of medical and health-related studies. There are similar concerns about the influx of Germans taking up medical student posts in Austria.

In addition to the financial consequences of gaining or losing health professionals, there is also evidence that mobility can impact on salary levels. Spain has reported that foreign inflows helped to keep salaries at sustainable levels within a context of high demand for health services. On the other hand, the Lithuanian government and Polish independent health-care providers increased salaries in order to retain medical doctors. Such incentives raise questions about long-term sustainability and redistribution within the system.

Impacts are subtle in the sense that they are often indirect, hard to discern and non-immediate. They may be insignificant at country-level but substantial at regional or hospital level. As mentioned, the analysis of impacts is also hampered by the difficulty of establishing causal effects. Moreover, the relative importance of mobility will depend on the domestic workforce issues facing planners and policy-makers in individual countries. These include shortages, unbalanced skill-mixes, geographical maldistribution, workforce and population ageing, attrition and/or underproduction of new health professionals. Within this context, mobility can be considered to be of high relevance in seven countries of this study (Austria, Hungary, Romania, Slovakia, Slovenia, Spain, United Kingdom), of medium relevance in six (Belgium, Finland, Germany, Italy, Poland, Serbia) and of lower relevance in comparison to other concerns in four (Estonia, France, Lithuania, Turkey).

3.6 *Data are still limited*

In 13 of the 17 country case-studies (Belgium, France, Germany, Hungary, Italy, Lithuania, Poland, Romania, Serbia, Slovakia, Spain, Turkey, United Kingdom) there was reported to be insufficient availability of updated and comprehensive data on migration. Decision-makers do not know exactly who is entering and who is leaving their systems and therefore it is harder to assess the implications for the workforce and for health system performance.

There are several aspects to the issue of data limitations. First, the absence of a proper definition of health professional mobility means that three indicators (foreign trained, foreign born, foreign national) are used to capture mobility. Limitations in the validity of each indicator and their unsystematic use across Europe make it difficult to assess the scale and character of mobility. Countries such as Austria, Poland and Slovenia collect more than one indicator and show data values that differ significantly. With careful interpretation these variations can provide a richer picture of mobility but they also raise questions about the validity of comparisons between indicators. Moreover, the inaccuracy of general stock indicators (for example, on licensed/active or full-time/part-time health professionals) makes it difficult to assess how mobility contributes to the health workforce. Data sources are also not able to capture certain types of mobility that may be on the rise in the EU such as returning migrants, short-term mobility, weekend work and dual practice, commuting and training periods abroad.

Second, most countries find it very difficult to provide time-series data, thereby hampering the ability to understand mobility trends and monitor fluctuations. Changes in professional definitions, new collection methods and new data holders also led to discontinuity of data in EU-12 countries.

Third, data on nurses suffer from greater limitations and inaccuracies than data for medical doctors in most countries. Even where data are available the professions and qualifications included vary widely between countries.

Finally, no country appears to have accurate outflow data. Intention-to-leave data are used to gauge emigration but, although an important signal, their validity is disputed. Health professionals may choose to leave without conformity certificates as they are not required by all employers; they may apply for certification retrospectively; or may apply but never leave. A study in Romania showed that only a third of medical doctors who requested certificates in 2007 actually emigrated; in Slovakia there is evidence that equivalence confirmations are severe underestimates of real outflows. Moreover, intention to leave may be susceptible to manipulation as health professionals can use requests for conformity certificates to pressurize governments and fuel political debate. Countries can address this information gap by searching the registries of destination countries but this remains a cumbersome and little used procedure. Such studies have been carried out in Lithuania, Germany and Belgium.

4. Mobility in a changing context

Mobility has become an increasingly important issue and its significance is bound to be reinforced by a series of contextual factors and uncertainties that will only increase. While we cannot predict how mobility will evolve, it is certain that this will be affected by the changing context in which it takes place. Five dimensions related to health system challenges, workforce shortages, Europeanization, reliance on foreign workforce, and ethical considerations will be examined in terms of their future meaning for health professional mobility.

Health systems face a series of current and future challenges caused by the changes in demography, technology and the economic environment. Planners and decision-makers cannot be sure that their systems have the required numbers of health professionals and adequate skills to respond to the demographic transition. In some countries, ageing of the workforce means that the rate of retirement is already outpacing the replacement of the workforce. Population ageing will require new skills as service provision is reoriented towards chronic, palliative and long-term care. In parallel, technological and medical progress will continue to make new treatment methods available which are bound to add to pressures on health expenditure. The economic outlook is uncertain yet it is clear that the current financial crisis impacts on public budgets. Political decisions determine whether health spending is cut (announced in the Baltic countries, Slovenia, Spain and the United Kingdom, for example) or protected (announced in Austria, France and Sweden, for example) but the financial crisis will clearly be an additional challenge for health systems.

Within this changing context, future health workforce shortages are bound to worsen. On one hand, there is a shrinking supply of candidates entering training and, on the other, demand for health services is rising. Different public employers, different sectors and different countries are increasingly competing for the same workforce and skills. The European Commission[10] forecasts that the EU will face a shortage of 1 million health professionals by 2020 if existing workforce problems are not addressed. In the United States, projections show that there could be a shortage of 159 300 full-time equivalent medical doctors by 2025 (AAMC 2008) and almost a million nurses by 2020 (Aiken & Cheung 2008). This will have implications since the United States is a major destination country for European health professionals.

Europeanization is defined as the process of increasing economic, political, social, cultural (etc) integration within Europe. This will contribute to mobility in three ways. First, the phasing out of transition periods for the countries which joined the EU in 2004 and 2007 means that any remaining labour market restrictions will be lifted. Second, future enlargements are planned. Croatia, Iceland, Macedonia, Montenegro and Turkey are official candidate states; Albania and Serbia have applied for membership; Bosnia and Herzegovina has concluded an association agreement and is preparing an application; and Kosovo is beginning negotiations for an agreement. Third, the increases in mobility arising from the sheer number of EU Member States will decrease national governments' ability to steer mobility as no unjustified restrictions may limit the freedom of movement within the EU.

---

10 The forecast on health professional shortages in the EU was presented by the European Commission during a policy dialogue in Leuven, Belgium in April 2010. An explanatory note detailing the methods and results was circulated later (Ref. Ares(2010)740064 - 25/10/2010).

Reliance on the foreign health workforce is bound to become an increasingly unsustainable approach to tackle workforce shortages. International competition for the health workforce will intensify and systems will become more susceptible to changes in the directions and volumes of flows if reliance on foreign inflows grows as a result of shortages. Mobility patterns are already hard to predict but are increasingly dependent on decisions taken in other countries. Finally, international recruitment may be a faster and cheaper solution for problems such as domestic underproduction, inadequate skill-mix or geographical maldistribution but it does not resolve the underlying causes of workforce problems and foreign health professionals may not fill the "right gaps".

Finally, ethical considerations are likely to evolve in tandem with mobility. In 2010, WHO Member States adopted the WHO Global Code of Practice on the International Recruitment of Health Personnel. The Code provides guidance on ethical aspects of recruitment but workforce shortages may drive countries to choose between insufficient health services for their own populations or recruitment from third countries facing even more severe shortages. Moreover, freedom of movement is an EU citizen's right and it is undeniably progress that this will extend to an increasing number of Member States. This gives rise to the question – what is the difference between recruiting from third countries and recruiting from less economically advantaged EU countries? The 2004 and 2007 enlargements have made the EU more diverse, as reflected in the World Bank and International Monetary Fund country classifications. Most EU-12 countries are considered to be emerging and developing countries and large salary differentials are apparent between the EU-12 and EU-15 (cf. observation 3.4). Future EU enlargements will add to this diversity and to ethical considerations.

5. Policy implications

In this section we discuss policy implications deriving from the key observations on health professional mobility and the changing context. Good information is the basis for all further action, therefore policy implications on data, intelligence and evidence will be presented first. These will be followed by a second set of implications focusing on workforce strategies as these appear to be of great importance for addressing mobility. A third set of policy implications will be presented for workforce planning and finally, implications for internationals frameworks will be discussed.

5.1 *Data, intelligence and evidence*

Any response to health professional mobility requires a sound evidence base as good-quality and timely data are essential for effective actions. Three main areas have emerged: (i) the need for better quality data on actual mobility; (ii) information on the workforce overall; and (iii) intelligence to evaluate the effectiveness of workforce strategies.

There is a clear need for better data to improve the measurement of mobility spanning from inflows to reliance on foreign health professionals and outflows. Data on the mobility of medical doctors are available in most countries but data for nurses are not, despite the fact that nurses are numerically the largest group of health workers. This health profession will become even more crucial for effective service delivery given future trends on population ageing, increases in chronic conditions and other contextual factors. But any performance measurement will require a sufficient evidence base on the profession including information on mobility. Data on outflows are non-existent in most countries and proxy measures[11] are used instead. Similarly, there is a lack of information on returnees. One option is to improve the information base by conducting specific surveys. A second is to collect personalized data on mobile health professionals although this involves several methodological challenges such as data protection issues. A third option is to trace health professionals in destination country registries, an action that can be undertaken by individual countries. A fourth, albeit ambitious, option would be collaboration between registries across Europe, forming a joint mechanism to relay relevant data to the sending countries.

The second policy implication relates to monitoring the workforce as information on mobility needs to be contextualized with data on the general workforce. There is scope for improved EU-wide intelligence on workforce policies and the training pipeline in Member States in order to anticipate European shortages and changes in recruitment policies. Some countries are very highly reliant on foreign health professionals and hence decisions made in other countries. Other countries are vulnerable to outflows and will need to know the context in which they operate. Intelligence on workforce policies and the training pipeline can also reduce uncertainties concerning forecasted shortages. However, this action can only be achieved as a joint measure and would require collaboration between the European Commission and the Member States.

The third policy implication is the need for investment in research to evaluate workforce strategies and measure their effectiveness. Countries have implemented a variety of measures (such as raising salary levels, improving

---

11

working conditions, increasing education and training capacities) but their effects on the mobility of health professionals have not been evaluated. Evaluation studies can therefore help to identify which workforce measures or bundle of measures are the right choice.

5.2 *Strengthening workforce strategies*

The need to improve countries' workforce strategies is a central policy implication of this research. This can build on strengthening retention, raising the domestic supply of health professionals and optimizing skills and their use within health systems.

Retention can be optimized by focusing on working conditions and the working environment. Measures include salary increases, improvement of infrastructures, introducing up-to-date technologies, facilitating part-time work and providing models for older health workers. These can reduce exits from the workforce due to emigration or attrition and increase the appeal of the health professions.

Another strategy is to raise the domestic supply of health professionals. This would require measures to expand the capacities of faculties and schools and to increase the number of training facilities and specialist training slots. This strategy can be closely connected to self-sufficiency policies which aim to meet a country's demand for health personnel by training its own health professionals for retention in the domestic health workforce. This can reduce unsustainable reliance on foreign inflows and the risks associated with important outflows.

Workforce strategies can also aim to optimize skills and their use within countries and health systems. One aspect of this is to achieve effective employment of foreign health professionals already in the country. This would require measures to attract foreign health professionals not working in the health sector; fast track recognition of non-EU qualifications; provide additional training or induction periods; and to deliver programmes enabling foreign health professionals to integrate within the system and society.

5.3 *Workforce planning*

The need to improve health workforce planning in countries is another policy implication based on the research included in this volume. Assessment of health workforce needs, the use of mobility data and a joint European workforce planning framework are three strategies that contribute to more effective health workforce planning.

Workforce needs assessment broadens the perspective of workforce forecasting and planning. It takes into account issues of recruiting, educating, distributing, retaining, motivating and managing the health workforce. Workforce needs assessment therefore goes beyond forecasting the numbers and the skills needed. It is sensitive to the potential loss of health professionals to other sectors and other countries that may be precipitated by changes in these factors. This also implies the need to improve understanding of the motivations of the health workforce, including monetary and non-monetary aspects.

The use of mobility data will improve the accuracy of forecasting since it allows losses that would have been unacknowledged to be factored in. It can also improve monitoring of the assumptions about retention in the assessment of health workforce needs.

A common European workforce planning framework would aim to maintain a European health workforce that can rely largely on health workers trained in Europe. To this end a European workforce planning framework would facilitate exchange on data sources and forecasting methodologies, reduce uncertainties about Member States' forecasts and workforce policies and provide transparency on the planning of the numbers and skill-mix in the health workforce.

5.4 *International frameworks*

International frameworks can contribute to managing health professional mobility by introducing strategies to improve the use of codes for international recruitment, the use of bilateral agreements and to facilitate local and organizational cross-border collaboration.

Codes on the international recruitment of health personnel discourage recruitment in countries facing workforce shortages. The research included in this volume indicates that three strategies can improve the use of these codes. First, a monitoring of inflows is necessary to understand whether or not the code is respected and effective. Second, accountability frameworks need to be introduced to support the code by ensuring that the public administration, public health-care providers and publicly contracted providers comply with the code. Scrutiny or sanctions need to be considered for cases of non-compliance. Third, strengthened workforce strategies support these codes by improving the retention and supply of health workers and thus moderating the need for international recruitment.

If used appropriately, bilateral agreements are flexible instruments that can help to manage health professional mobility and complement workforce policies. For example, they can be used to limit or exclude international recruitment from third countries; to establish systems for mutual recognition of diplomas with countries outside the free-movement area; or to foster active recruitment on a permanent or temporary basis.

International frameworks can be used by professional organizations, health-care providers or teaching hospitals and can address local workforce and mobility issues through forms of cross-border collaboration. These include twinning, staff exchange and educational support and are widely used throughout Europe.

6. Final reflections

The increasing importance of mobility, the changing context in which it takes place and the resulting policy implications combine with the EU legislative framework on freedom of movement to create a setting in which joint perspectives are needed to address health professional mobility as part of wider workforce strategies. Together, the European Commission and the EU Member States have initiated a policy debate on the future of the European workforce for health, publishing a Green Paper and launching a public consultation process. Member States have shown persisting interest in moving the topic up the EU agenda. Council conclusions on this issue were adopted under the Belgium Presidency in 2010 and the focus is continuing under the Hungarian Presidency in 2011.

We hope the 17 case-studies that follow will contribute to awareness and debates on the subject of health professional mobility in Europe.

References

AAMC (2008). *The complexities of physician supply and demand: projections through 2025.* Washington DC, Association of American Medical Colleges Center for Workforce Studies.

Aiken LH, Cheung R (2008). *Nurse workforce challenges in the United States: implications for policy.* Paris, Organisation for Economic Co-operation and Development (OECD Health Working Papers No. 35).

Part II

Case studies from countries that joined the EU before 2004

Positioned between old and new EU Member States: Austria as source and destination country for health professional mobility

Guido Offermanns, Eva Maria Malle, Mirela Jusic

1. Introduction

In Austria, there is a long tradition of health professionals crossing borders. Characterized as both a destination and a source country, most exchange occurs with neighbour countries. The strongest connection is between Austria and Germany and, interestingly, mobility is in both directions. European Union (EU) enlargement did not lead to the dramatic rise of inflows forecast by many experts but has reinforced the existing importance of the Czech Republic and Slovakia.

Mobility patterns in Austria differ according to health professions. For medical doctors and dentists mobility is characterized by a rough equilibrium between inflows and outflows, but nurses show a constant one-way inflow over years. Due to the mostly outbalanced flows, health workforce migration is of low to medium significance for Austria´s health system. The exception is the home-care sector as the majority of mobile or home care is currently performed by foreign nurses. The demand for these nurses has led to the emergence of an underground economy in recent years, mainly due to restrictions and the fact that foreign nurses provide mobile health care that official care services cannot cover (NÖGUS 2006). A high number of nurses from eastern Europe have been privately contracted to work in home care on an illegal basis (Georg 2007); amounting to about 40 000 illegal nurses (ÖGKV 2006). The Foreign Labour Act of Austria was amended for home-care nurses but could not resolve the problem entirely and this remains an issue of public and political debate. Overall, Austria lacks an explicit and coherent human workforce policy and policy responses on mobility are short-term reactions to acute problems. However, several regional and local level initiatives such as staff exchange and cross-border education programmes have flourished over the recent past.

This case study will give an overview of health professional mobility in Austria, with a focus on the neighbouring states with which most movements occur. Initially, it will describe the mobility profile with the aim of quantifying the scale of migration and time trends in Austria. The next section will cover how migration impacts on the Austrian health system and its relevance for other workforce issues in the country. This will be followed by discussion of the barriers and hurdles that hinder mobility as well as the factors that define Austria as an attractive destination country. The last section covers workforce and migration policies, regulatory measures and interventions and their relevance to mobility.

Limitations of the study

Austria faces a lack of relevant data on the mobility of health professionals, particularly foreign nurses. Furthermore, existing data are scattered throughout different institutions and data holders such as medical associations, the Austrian Federal Ministry of Health (*Bundesministerium für Gesundheit* – BMG), Austrian Association of Midwives (*Österreichisches Hebammengremium* – ÖHG) and the Public Employment Service Austria (*Arbeitsmarktservice Österreich* – AMS). This complicates data comparability and accessibility. Finally, health professional mobility has not been prioritized in past political discussions and so data on foreign health professionals were neither collected nor evaluated systematically.

2. Mobility profile of Austria

The long tradition of cross-border recruitment of health professionals and shortages of nurses in hospitals has led to a high share of foreign health professionals in the Austrian health-care system. Since 2003 the share of medical doctors of foreign nationality registered in the Austrian Medical Chamber (*Österreichische Ärztekammer* – ÖÄK) has constantly increased. There have been inflows of nurses since the 1960s when numerous nurses from the former Yugoslavia moved to Austria. Exchange programmes with countries such as the former Czechoslovakia and the Philippines also facilitated mobility (Biffl 2006, Lenhart & Österle 2007).

It is hard to obtain detailed documentation or proper studies about the full dimensions of the migration of health professionals – mainly because there is a lack of data on foreign nurses in Austria and different data sources on medical doctors show a diverging picture. The history of health professional mobility in Austria is an indication that a high percentage of staff in the Austrian health-care system has a migration background. However, it is particularly difficult to find this data because most data sources provide only information on citizenship, not the country of birth.

The last population census[1] from 2001 gives an idea of the dimension of mobility in Austria. Based on this data, a 2006 study published by the Austrian Institute of Economic Research *(Österreichisches Institut für Wirtschaftsforschung* – WIFO provides a record of foreign-born health professionals. Other data sources show foreign health professional numbers ranging between about 8% and 14% according to the indicators used. It should be noted that the foreign-born indicator includes health professionals who already possess Austrian citizenship; foreign nationals may include those who have foreign citizenship (Biffl 2006).

The 2001 census data show that more than 14% of the Austrian health workforce were foreign born. The shares vary between professions – unskilled workers show the highest proportion (25.1%), followed by nurses (14.5%), medical doctors (14.2%) and employees in public administration (9.4%) (Biffl 2006). The largest proportion of the foreign-born health workforce living and working in Austria came from the former Yugoslavia excluding Slovenia (30%), other EU-15 countries (23%), EU-10 countries (18%) and Asia (13%) (Biffl 2006). The development of data on newly registered health professionals in recent years shows that mobility occurs mostly between Austria and its neighbouring countries, with the strongest relationship between Austria and Germany. New EU countries such as the Czech Republic and Slovakia are also very important in recent developments of cross-border mobility, whereas the mobility of non-EU country nationals has slowed.

The following section describes and analyses in detail the existing data on the stock and flows of health professionals to and from Austria. The analysis focuses on medical doctors, nurses, midwives and dentists. These four groups are defined as either foreign nationals or foreign trained.

---

1 Austrian census takes place every 10 years.

2.1 *Medical doctors*

The number of active medical doctors is increasing steadily. The absence of a language barrier can explain why most staff exchanges take place between Austria and Germany. Also, the 2004 EU accessions induced a rise of medical doctors from eastern European countries. Different data sources show different migration figures (Table 1.1) – for example, the 2001 population census shows 14.2% of foreign-born active medical doctors while the number of foreign-national medical doctors registered with the ÖÄK reached about 8% in 2003. These differences may be attributed to several factors, including the different years. The indicators chosen are also significant and likely explain a substantial part of the differences as "foreign born" includes foreign health professionals who had already taken Austrian citizenship. Conversely, data from the Organisation for Economic Co-operation and Development (OECD) show a much smaller proportion of foreign-trained medical doctors in 2005. The authors believe that the number constitutes an underestimate of the actual magnitude of mobility. This may be explained not only by the indicator used but also because junior doctor[2] numbers are not included in OECD data but are included in ÖÄK data.

Table 1.1 *Foreign medical doctors in Austria, from different data sources and indicators*

Indicator					
Foreign born	**Foreign national**	**Foreign trained**	**Year**	**Data sources**	**Comments**
14.2% (active medical doctors)			2001	Census[a]	Includes foreign-born medical doctors who took Austrian citizenship
	8.8% (3 322 of 37 734 active medical doctors), all registered (including turnus doctors)		2008	ÖÄK[b]	Indicates medical doctors with foreign nationality (citizenship)
		3.3% (964 of 29 164 active medical doctors), only graduate medical doctors	2005	OECD[c]	Eventual underestimate of phenomenon due to different indicators; assumption that junior doctors are not included

Sources: [a] Biffl 2006; [b] ÖÄK unpublished data 2009; [c] Dumond et al. 2008.

---

2 In Austria doctors must complete three years of in-service training (turnus) after their medical degree. This is a legal precondition for working as a medical doctor. Specialist training takes (at least) another four years and general practice training take (at least) another three years.

The following section will describe the inflows and outflows of medical doctors on the basis of registry data from the ÖÄK.

Medical doctor inflows

In order to practise in Austria, medical doctors must be registered on the ÖÄK official registry – the *Ärzteliste*. They must inform the ÖÄK about every change in their employment as only active medical doctors can remain on the list. The inflows of medical doctors who migrated to Austria are therefore best illustrated by data on new registrations. These show short-term variations in the registration of foreign medical doctors and so trends over the last five years can be observed easily. Table 1.2 shows time trends in the number and percentages of newly registered active medical doctors according to nationality.

The share of foreign medical doctors peaked at 17.9% (269) in 2004 and at 17.7% (276) in 2007 and slowed to 13.5% (230) in 2008. Most were nationals of EU-15 countries, principally Germany and Italy (Fig. 1.1). Interestingly, the number of EU-10 nationals (including Romania and Bulgaria) among foreign newly registered medical doctors has increased since 2004 whereas the inflows from non-EU countries hold steady.

Fig. 1.1 *Newly registered German, Italian and other foreign-national medical doctors 2000 and 2003–2008*

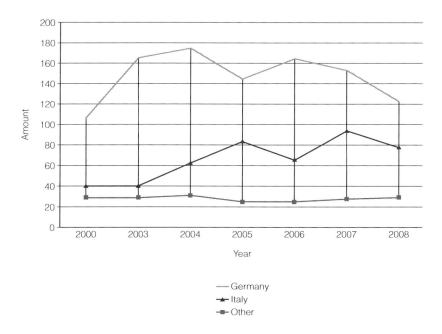

Source: ÖÄK unpublished data 2009.

Table 1.2 *Newly registered native and foreign medical doctors in Austria, by nationality, 2000 and 2003–2008*

Country	2000		2003		2004		2005		2006		2007		2008	
	N	%	N	%	N	%	N	%	N	%	N	%	N	%
EU-15[a]	149	11.6	210	14.3	210	13.9	177	11.7	195	12.2	197	12.6	167	9.8
EU-10	5	0.4	4	0.3	38	2.5	55	3.6	47	3	56	3.6	44	2.6
Romania & Bulgaria	1	0.1	2	0.1	2	0.1	2	0.1	1	0.1	6	0.4	3	0.2
Non-EU	20	1.6	20	1.4	19	1.3	19	1.3	13	0.8	17	1.1	16	0.9
Total foreign doctors	**175**	**13.6**	**236**	**16**	**269**	**17.9**	**253**	**16.8**	**256**	**16.1**	**276**	**17.7**	**230**	**13.5**
Austria	1 114	86.4	1 237	84	1 237	82.1	1 256	83.2	1 337	83.9	1 285	82.3	1 475	86.5
Total newly registered doctors	**1 289**		**1 473**		**1 506**		**1 509**		**1 593**		**1 561**		**1 705**	

Source: ÖÄK unpublished data 2009. Note: [a] excluding Austria.

Fig. 1.2 *Newly registered foreign-national medical doctors in Austria*

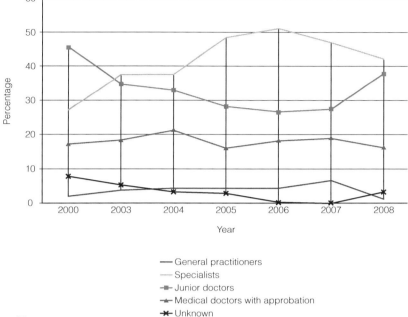

Source: ÖÄK unpublished data 2009.

More than half of the newly registered foreign medical doctors are of German nationality (Fig. 1.1). An arrangement between Austria and South Tyrol explains the high numbers of Italian doctors; the increase in other nationals can be attributed to EU enlargement in 2004.

Among these newly registered foreign-national medical doctors, by 2008 the proportion of specialists had increased to 42% whereas the proportion of junior doctors had decreased to 38%. There is a small, but increasing, proportion of general practitioners and medical doctors with approbation[3] until 2007 but in 2008 the proportions decline again (Fig. 1.2).

Foreign medical doctors in Austria

The stock of foreign-national medical doctors increased slightly but steadily from 8.1% in 2003 to 8.8% in 2008 and mostly comprises nationals of EU-15 countries, including a high proportion of German medical doctors. Among the EU-10 countries, numbers from Romania and Bulgaria climbed slightly, whereas those from non-EU countries decreased (Table 1.3).

In 2008, German nationals represent the highest share of foreign medical doctors (44%; 1453). Nationals from Iran (5%; 178), Syria (2%; 54) and Egypt (1%; 41) reflect the high share of non-EU countries. The break-up of Yugoslavia and

---

3 In Austria, approbation is awarded after in-service training. Other EU countries award approbation at the end of the medical degree or after a postdoctoral education lasting 3–24 months (Ärztekammer für Tirol 2009).

Table 1.3 Native and foreign-national medical doctors (stock) in Austria, 2003–2008

Country	2003		2004		2005		2006		2007		2008	
	N	%	N	%	N	%	N	%	N	%	N	%
EU-15	1 398	4.2	1 456	4.3	1 609	4.7	1 820	5	1 837	5	1 933	5.1
EU-10 (joined 2004)	286	0.9	283	0.8	304	0.9	386	1.1	394	1.1	444	1.2
Romania & Bulgaria (joined 2007)	92	0.3	89	0.3	88	0.3	86	0.2	85	0.2	93	0.2
Non-EU	906	2.7	903	2.7	890	2.6	875	2.4	867	2.3	852	2.3
Total foreign doctors	**2 682**	**8.1**	**2 731**	**8.1**	**2 891**	**8.4**	**3 167**	**8.6**	**3 183**	**8.6**	**3 322**	**8.8**
Austria	30 441	91.9	30 826	91.9	31 704	91.6	33 589	91.4	33 720	91.4	34 412	91.2
Total medical doctors	**33 123**		**33 557**		**34 595**		**36 756**		**36 903**		**37 734**	

Source: ÖÄK unpublished data 2009.

Czechoslovakia led to a rise of migration to Austria and explains why nationals from these countries comprise the highest share (7%; 215) among non-EU countries (see Table 1.11 for more details).

The next section compares stock data of inflows and outflows in order to analyse the risk of losing Austrian medical doctors to Germany.

Medical doctor outflows

As mentioned, the most significant movements of medical doctors occur between Austria and Germany and among emigrating Austrian medical doctors the highest percentage moves to Germany. The German Federal Chamber of Physicians shows 260 working Austrian medical doctors registered in Germany in 1988, increasing to 958 in 2003 and 1613 by 2007 (stock data).

In 2003, 989 German medical doctors were working in Austria. This number increased to 1376 in 2007 and 1453 in 2008 (see Table 1.11 for more details). Comparison of these data from the German Federal Chamber of Physicians and the ÖÄK shows mobility between Austria and Germany to be quite balanced. The absence of language barriers supports a flourishing exchange between these countries.

A service provider that supports health professional mobility reports the preferred destination countries of Austrian medical doctors to be not only Germany but also Switzerland, Sweden, Norway and Denmark. Young doctors prefer Australia or New Zealand (Going International 2009).

2.2 Nurses

In Austria, nurses are perceived to be one of the health professions with the highest numbers of movements. However, the relevant data are particularly scarce and of low quality as nurses are not registered in the same way as medical doctors, dentists and midwives. Statistik Austria (2010) shows that 57 367 nurses worked in hospitals in 2000 and numbers increased steadily to reach 62 657 in 2008. The 2001 census data show a high proportion of foreign-born nurses working in hospitals (25.1%). Regrettably there are no data that are more relevant to the stock of foreign nurses in Austria.

Nurse inflows

The 2004 EU enlargement had a clear effect on the inflow of foreign nurses to Austria. The total number from EU-10 countries increased substantially between 2004 and 2006 before decreasing, ranging between 18.1% and 37.9%. Table 1.4 provides the data on diploma validation but it should be noted that it includes no information about whether or not these nurses are still working in Austria.

Table 1.4 Foreign-trained nurses applying for diploma validation in Austria, 2003–2008

Training country	2003		2004		2005		2006		2007		2008	
	N	%	N	%	N	%	N	%	N	%	N	%
EU-15	415	97	708	80.6	990	69.4	859	61.4	572	72.8	481	62.2
EU-10	0	0	159	18.1	429	30.1	530	37.9	207	26.3	235	30.4
Romania & Bulgaria	0	0	0	0	0	0	2	0.1	4	0.5	43	5.6
Non-EU	13	3	12	1.4	8	0.6	9	0.6	3	0.4	14	1.8
Total	**428**		**879**		**1 427**		**1 400**		**786**		**773**	

Source: BMG unpublished data 2009.

Table 1.5 Foreign-national nurses from eastern European and non-EU countries* applying for work permits, 2003–2008

Country	2003		2004		2005		2006		2007		2008	
	N	%	N	%	N	%	N	%	N	%	N	%
EU-10	381	44	782	69	985	78	1 142	82	1 031	80.1	630	77.9
Romania & Bulgaria	31	4	26	2	21	2	23	2	67	5.2	68	8.4
Non-EU	461	53	330	29	249	20	232	17	190	14.8	111	13.7
Total	**873**		**1 138**		**1 255**		**1 397**		**1 288**		**809**	

Source: AMS unpublished data 2009. * Worldwide.

Austria's neighbouring countries play the most important role in nurse mobility. Germany is the main source country of foreign-educated nurses as the absence of language barriers enables them to validate their diplomas much more easily than nurses from non-German-speaking countries. Slovakia is the second most important source country, firstly because of geographical proximity and secondly because of the potential to commute.

Table 1.5 shows the numbers of nurses from eastern European countries (foreign nationality) who applied for work permits and are still working in Austria. Transitional arrangements are in place for nationals from the Member States that joined the EU in 2004 and 2007. These fall under the Foreign Labour Act[4] which prescribes a work permit issued by the AMS as a precondition to start employment in Austria (AMS 2009).

Fig. 1.3 shows the source countries of foreign-nationality nurses who applied for work permits between 2003 and 2008. Slovakia is the main source country, followed by Hungary, Poland and the Czech Republic. The proportion

Fig. 1.3 *Source countries of foreign-national nurses applying for work permits in Austria, 2003–2008*

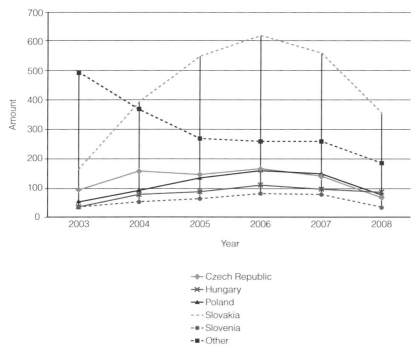

Source: AMS unpublished data 2009.

4 Nationals of non-EEA countries (excluding Switzerland) and new EU countries (excluding Malta and Cyprus) need a work permit to start employment in Austria (AMS 2009).

of Slovakian nurses increased constantly until 2006 – after which numbers decreased. This can be explained in part by the fact that home-care nurses have been exempted from the Foreign Labour Act since 2006 and no longer need work permits (for a detailed explanation see sections 4 and 7).

Nurse outflows

Austrian nurses prefer Germany as a destination country. The number of active Austrian nurses working in Germany decreased from 1100 nurses in 2003 to about 1000 nurses in 2008. Switzerland is another destination country but no data or studies are available on Austrian nurses in that country.

2.3 Midwives

Midwives show less mobility from and to Austria. Overall, Table 1.6 shows only a small number of newly registered foreign-national midwives between 2003 and 2008.

Generally, new registrations increased slightly until 2006 and then started to decrease. Again, the highest share of foreign midwives comes from Germany.

At 33 years, the average age of midwives in Austria is relatively young in comparison to other countries. A small number of Austrian midwives are interested in working abroad and, as the emigration age of Austrian midwives lies between 20 and 30 years, they are therefore in the prime of their careers (see Table 1.16 for more details). Italy and Germany are the target emigration and working countries.

2.4 Dentists

Dentist inflows

Dentists must be registered by the *Austrian Dental Association (Österreichische Zahnärztekammer)*. Table 1.7 shows the numbers of newly registered dentists with native or foreign nationality from 2003 to 2007.

The constant growth in the total numbers of this profession is clearly visible. Similarly, the number of newly registered dentists from EU-15 countries more than doubled between 2003 and 2007. Comparison of the total number of newly registered professionals (foreign and national) in 2003 and 2007 reveals a large increase in the proportion of dentists of foreign nationality. Hence, a high proportion of dentists in Austria are foreign nationals.

Table 1.8 shows all dentists working in hospitals or in private practice, classified by nationality. There is a slight increase in the total number of registered dentists

Table 1.6 *Newly registered foreign midwives in Austria, by nationality, 2003–2008*

Country	2003		2004		2005		2006		2007		2008	
	N	%	N	%	N	%	N	%	N	%	N	%
EU-15	2	100	13	76.5	14	82.4	15	75	8	61.5	12	63.2
EU-10	0	0	4	23.5	3	17.6	4	20	3	22.1	3	15.8
Romania & Bulgaria	0	0	0	0	0	0	0	0	0	0	2	10.5
Non-EU	0	0	0	0	0	0	1	5	2	15.4	2	10.5
Total	**2**		**17**		**17**		**20**		**13**		**19**	

Source: ÖHG unpublished data 2009.

Table 1.7 *Newly registered native and foreign dentists in Austria, by nationality, 2003–2007*

Country	2003		2004		2005		2006		2007	
	N	%	N	%	N	%	N	%	N	%
EU-15	18	13.3	26	13.9	38	20.7	46	22.6	42	17.1
EU-10	6	4.4	24	12.8	13	7.1	27	13.2	16	6.5
Romania & Bulgaria	7	5.2	10	5.4	4	2.2	12	5.9	17	6.9
Non-EU	8	5.9	12	6.4	15	8.2	15	7.4	25	10.2
Total foreign dentists	**39**	**28.9**	**72**	**38.6**	**70**	**38**	**100**	**49**	**100**	**40.8**
Austria	96	71.1	115	61.6	114	62	104	51	145	59.2
Total dentists	**135**		**187**		**184**		**204**		**245**	

Source: Österreichische Zahnärztekammer unpublished data 2009.

Table 1.8 *Registered dentists (stock) in Austria, by nationality, 2005–2007*

Country	2005		2006		2007	
	N	%	N	%	N	%
EU-15	207	5.7	255	6.6	302	7.3
EU-10	203	5.6	231	6	243	5.9
Romania & Bulgaria	87	2.4	96	2.5	120	2.9
Non-EU	168	4.6	187	4.9	217	5.2
Total foreign dentists	**665**	**18.3**	**769**	**19.9**	**882**	**21.3**
Austria	2 970	81.7	3 090	80.1	3 264	78.7
Total dentists	**3 635**		**3 859**		**4 146**	

Source: Österreichische Zahnärztekammer unpublished data 2009.

between 2005 (3635) and 2007 (4146). In 2005, there were 665 foreign-national dentists – 497 EU, Romanian and Bulgarian nationals and 168 non-EU nationals. By 2007 numbers had increased to 882 – 665 EU, Romanian and Bulgarian nationals and 217 non-EU nationals (see Table 1.15 for more details on individual countries).

3. Vignettes on health professional mobility

From Austria to Germany: experiences of a junior doctor

Raffaela decided to move abroad after graduating from Vienna University in 2002 as limited training posts for junior doctors were available in Austria. Specializing in paediatrics, she has been working in a paediatric intensive care ward and neonatal unit for almost a year in a 538-bed district hospital in Stade, close to Hamburg. She describes her experiences below (Hammerl 2007).

There is a lot of discussion about the working conditions in the German health-care system, not only for doctors but for the entire hospital staff, including changes in the general regulations. Aiming to abandon 24-hour shifts and more, most departments are working in shorter shifts now which increases the number of training posts needed by approx 40%. Most contracts do not include after-hours payment, but it is possible to take compensatory leave. There is a high workload as there are less doctors working during daytime than previously. Dealing with bureaucratic matters, such as medical letters, can seem quite frustrating at times for someone used to less paperwork in Austria. In contrast to Austria, junior doctors are given a lot of responsibility early on in their career in Germany, which is important. Senior support is very helpful and a lot of emphasis is put on teaching (Hammerl 2007).

> ### *From the Philippines to Austria: experiences of a qualified nurse*
>
> Zenaida moved to Austria mainly because she can earn much more money. As a nurse with a diploma she would earn only €200 in her homeland; in Austria she earns between €1500 and €1800. The nursing profession is not the job of her dreams, she chose it for economic reasons. Her goal was to emigrate easily and to ensure the financial support of her family in the Philippines. She obtained a work permit easily, learned German and started to work at the hospital at Schwarzach in Salzburg. She describes how very hard it was to migrate, especially leaving her family, but the prospect of improving her life prevailed over personal matters. Now her sister has also moved to Austria to work as a nurse and does not regret her decision (Rainer 2008).

4. Dynamics of enlargement

Migration to Austria boomed at the beginning of the 1990s as the flourishing economic situation led to a rapid growth of immigrants, especially from the countries of the former Yugoslavia and traditional sources of guest-workers such as Turkey (Fassmann 2007). The migration of health professionals increased In line with overall labour force migration. Data from the 2001 Austrian census reveal that a high proportion (around 30%) of foreign-born health professionals came from the former Yugoslavia, excluding Slovenia (Biffl 2006).

The 2004 EU enlargement was very important for Austria as it shifted into a more centralized geographical position. The border regions towards the Czech Republic and Slovakia were most affected by economic and structural changes. They also influenced the Austrian health system and economic development, such as the labour market and patient mobility. National health policy-makers, planners and service providers are faced with blurred boundaries that were once clearly defined. This is due to international politics, the law of the European Court of Justice, cost pressures and also financiers' and patients' awareness of these costs (NÖGUS 2006, Wieland & Burger 2006). Various regions in Austria and the neighbouring states are now working together to improve the quality of health care. Cross-border education and cooperation have great potential and increasingly are attracting attention to these areas (Rosenmöller et al. 2006).

Enlargement has not caused the dramatic rise in health professional mobility to Austria predicted by many experts. Nevertheless, there has been a visible surge in the numbers of health professionals, particularly nurses. In 2000, there were only 5 registrations for medical doctors who were EU-10 nationals; this number increased to 55 in 2006 with a reversing trend afterwards (Table 1.2).

The 2004 EU enlargement had a clear effect on the nursing profession, as shown by the number of diploma validations. In 2004, there were applications from 159 foreign-trained nurses from EU-10 Member States. Numbers rose almost fourfold to 530 in 2006, constituting 37.9% of all validations of nursing diplomas in that year (Table 1.4). However, numbers then fell to 235 (30.4%) in 2008.

In summary, the rising trend in the numbers of foreign medical doctors and nurses in the Austrian labour market after the 2004 EU enlargement stabilized and inflows were far from dramatic. Unlike some EU countries that completely opened their labour markets for the 2004 accession countries, Austria extended the transitional arrangements for two additional years until April 2011 (Die Presse 2009). It was argued that unrestricted opening could disturb the Austrian labour market in view of the 2008/2009 financial and economic crisis (WEKA 2009).

5. Impacts on the Austrian health system

Health professional mobility and its subsequent impacts on the Austrian health system are not yet central themes of political or public discussion. Austria does not suffer from a significant loss of health professionals and therefore there are rather few impacts on the Austrian health system in general. However, the subgroup of illegal nurses illustrates one important area of health professional mobility that has impacted on policies, health service delivery and financing in the Austrian health system.

Foreign nurses have increasingly met the rising shortage of service supply in home care and offer a low-cost form of 24-hour home care, which is illegal under the Austrian Employment Act. This supply cannot be replaced as it covers an existing demand that is not met by state services or by legal private affordable care-support services (NÖGUS 2006). In practice, thousands of elderly people in need of care cannot afford to pay licensed professionals and instead privately engage the services of illegal workers from abroad, mostly from eastern European countries and new Member States. These care workers work as geriatric nurses but often lack the relevant qualifications. Usually, they perform many specialized activities such as providing medication and physical care, as well as providing housekeeping services, general physical care and company for their charges (Georg 2007).

Elderly people in need of care are entitled to claim a statutory nursing allowance of up to €1536 per month, depending on the extent of their needs (Georg 2007), but often this is not sufficient to meet the costs of licensed nurses. Some patients may require 24-hour stand-by care which proves very costly. Many of the illegal nurses live in the same households as their patients and receive some form of allowance rather than regular pay (Georg 2007). Restrictions on new EU countries also propelled the rapid growth of this underground economy (NÖGUS 2006). Policy-makers were forced to step in and various political measures relating to the legalization of illegal nurses were taken in 2006.

Illegal nurses impact on long-term-care service delivery, existing policies and financing and may cause a domino effect because they also influence the health system objectives of responsiveness, fair financial distribution and health. Since accession, nurses moving to Austria from Slovakia and the Czech Republic have tended to have lower qualifications. More highly qualified nurses from these countries prefer other destination countries which have labour markets completely open to all EU countries. It is also important to consider that foreign nursing staff in 24-hour home care generally used to work for people with little need of specialized care but a high need for general support in everyday life. Now they mainly provide long-term care for people with demanding health-care needs (Schmid & Prochazkova 2006).

There are concerns that opening the market completely in 2011 will lead to dramatic losses of home-care staff to the domestic hospitals. These effects are likely to influence the responsiveness and the expectations of people in need of long-term care. Legal or social political solutions to current problems would lead to a dramatic rise in costs. These would have to be borne by private households or increasing use of public resources and could affect the financial distribution of health-care expenditures (Schmid & Prochazkova 2006).

6. Relevance of cross-border health professional mobility

Austria is not affected by significant losses of qualified health professionals to other countries, inflows and outflows are roughly balanced, therefore other human resource issues are currently of higher importance. For example, the training of sufficient medical doctors and the upcoming retirement of the baby-boom generation of medical doctors constitute workforce challenges with higher significance than mobility. Another major problem is the number of illegal nurses providing services in the home-care sector, although it is unclear how long this situation will persist.

A study by the Austrian Federal Institute for Health Care (*Österreichisches Bundesinstitut für Gesundheit* – ÖBIG) in 2006 predicted that until 2012 there will be no lack of medical doctors unless around 30% of graduates emigrate. Between 750 and 1000 medical doctors must be trained each year in order to safeguard supply until 2025. Currently, the medical universities offer 1500 places per year and it is predicted that between 1300 and 1600 students will graduate annually until 2011 (ORF 2007). The strict numerus clausus in Germany has caused many students to migrate to Austria in order to circumvent the restrictions (Medtest-Team 2009). There were concerns that a large number of foreign students could cause a lack of medical doctors in Austria if they returned to their home country after graduation (Schwarz 2008). Therefore, in February 2006 the Austrian National Council (*Nationalrat*) decided to implement quotas for medical degrees to ensure that 75% of the places at universities should be filled by home students (Schwarz 2008).

Moreover, although Austria does not face an overall lack of medical doctors, there is a lack of specialists in anaesthesia, pathology, paediatrics, operative dentistry and psychiatry. This already causes problems in some hospitals (Gallob 2008). The lack of home-care nurses, primarily in 24-hour care, is a human resource issue that has attained considerable attention in the past. Nurses from central and eastern Europe (CEE) countries continue to fill the demand (Ausweger 2009) but it is questionable whether this is the best option to secure the provision of home-care services. Researchers from the Department of Sociology at the University of Vienna showed that shortages of nursing staff in Austria could be ascribed to a shortage of training places and too few applicants for nursing.

Drop-outs are another problem that affects the supply of adequate health and nursing staff – high pressure and a lack of career options can lead to early exit from the profession (Krajic et al. 2003). Attrition takes place after about 20 years of work, on average, and results in a nursing staff that is generally relatively young. Most graduate nurses fall within the 25–39 age group but non-qualified nurses are characterized through different age patterns. Medical doctors have a different age structure as most of those practising are aged between 45 and 55 and therefore due to retire in the next one or two decades. Thus, in around 15 years there is the possibility of a severe lack of medical doctors which would undermine service provision in health care (ORF Steiermark 2009).

7. Factors influencing health professional mobility

Different individual decisions influence whether to stay or leave Austria and several structures that influence mobility motivation, nationally and elsewhere, have been investigated in order to understand why Austrians leave or stay. The aim was to identify the factors which encourage individuals to emigrate or to return to their country of origin.

7.1 *Instigating factors*

Mobility willingness manifests itself in personal advantages, such as improvements in the quality of life, salary, living standards, job security, employment conditions and occupational perspectives such as career opportunities. The primary motivation for migrating to Austria, especially for health professionals from eastern European and new EU countries (such as Czech Republic or Slovakia), results from Austria's position as a neighbouring country. Secondly, Austria offers both better pay for the same work and higher living standards (NÖGUS 2006). Nationals of new EU Member States are also attracted by job security, better conditions of employment and occupational perspectives, such as career and promotion prospects. In CEE countries health care is characterized by dramatic changes that influence conditions of employment, such as radical reductions in the numbers of beds (derStandard. at 2009a). Lachmayr (2009) interviewed 407 assistant medical technician[5] students and alumni in Austria. The study shows the most relevant issues for mobility to be health insurance, unemployment and retirement insurance. Interviewees also considered topics such as verification of diplomas, labour law and labour market questions to be important.

7.2 *Activating factors*

The highest percentage of emigrating Austrian health-care staff moves to Germany. An enquiry by the international department of the ÖÄK shows that arguments for moving to Germany include the absence of language barriers, excellent education in modern hospitals, regulated working hours, higher pay for assistant medical doctors (in comparison to Austria) and no wait for training places. In particular, given the limited number of places available in Austria, the absence of waiting times for education is becoming more and more attractive for junior doctors (ORF 2008).

7.3 *Facilitating factors*

As mentioned, the terms of the labour market and labour laws are very important factors in the choice of destination country. The open labour market within the EU motivates health professionals to move, primarily to Germany due to the common language. Junior doctors at Innsbruck Medical University also prefer countries such as the United Kingdom, Australia, the United States of America and the Scandinavian countries (ORF Tirol 2009).

---

5 Medical technicians are active in three divisions: (i) laboratory; (ii) radiology; and (iii) physiotherapy. Requirement to work is completion of training at one of the medical-technical academies or one of the colleges for medico-technical occupations.

7.4 *Mitigating factors*

Austria presents certain barriers to health professionals, such as the regulation that those from new EU Member States must apply for a work permit from the AMS. These regulations also deter staff because other countries have open labour markets. Austrian medical doctors who seek to emigrate are hindered by the different terms for awarding the licence of medicine (approbation) in different European countries. In Austria, the licence of medicine is granted after the three years in-service training. Other EU countries award the licence at the end of the medical degree or after a postdoctoral course lasting 3 to 24 months. In many cases Austrian medical doctors are unable to train as specialists in countries where the licence of medicine is a precondition (Ärztekammer für Tirol 2009).

8. Policy, regulation and interventions

8.1 *Policies and policy development on health professional mobility*

Austria does not have an explicit and coherent labour migration policy for the health-care sector and those seeking employment in the health sector face the same regulations as all other labour migrants. Several specific policies regulated health professional mobility in the past. However, these interventions were not part of a larger immigration policy but rather were short-term reactions to current and acute problems of the health sector (Schütz 2006).

Austria has a long history of recruiting personnel from abroad. Shortages of qualified nursing staff in the early 1970s and 1990s led hospital associations or single hospitals to recruit foreign health professionals. The City of Vienna recruited unmarried Philippine women to fill vacancies in hospitals and the ambulatory system – about 560 Philippine nurses were recruited between 1973 and 1982 (Schütz 2006). Employment contracts were issued for a minimum duration of three years and qualifications were legally recognized after a nurse had attended a German language course. The City of Vienna continued recruitment in the 1980s and 1990s through exchange programmes with countries such as the former Czechoslovakia, former Yugoslavia and the Philippines. The Missionary Sisters of the Queen of the Apostles also provided mobility by recruiting Indian sisters to work in Catholic hospitals in Austria in the 1970s. However, quotas for immigration and family reunification were introduced in 1993. Immigration slowed, especially for those organizations that had relied on recruiting high numbers of health professionals from the Philippines and India. Traditional recruitment for the health-care sector has been restricted further for these countries (Schütz 2006).

The restrictions on active recruitment from countries such as the Philippines and India further emphasized the role of Austria's neighbours in the mobility of health professionals. In recent years, recruitment from countries such as Germany, Slovakia and the Czech Republic has been particularly important. The placement of home-care staff from the Czech Republic and Slovakia is organized through job agencies. Founded as associations in all three countries, these agencies first attracted attention in the mid 1990s and numbers have increased to about 37 organizations (Schmid & Prochazkova 2006).

The transitional arrangements for the 2004 EU accessions have limited and disrupted the important recruitment of health professionals from Slovakia and the Czech Republic. Health professionals from the EU-15 countries and Switzerland are allowed unlimited access to the employment market in Austria; those from the 2004 and 2007 EU accessions and non European Economic Area (EEA)[6] states must apply to the AMS for a work permit in order to commence employment in hospitals. The Foreign Labour Act forms the legal basis of this regulation (AMS 2009). The additional attraction of legally and socially secured working conditions leads many qualified health professionals from new Member States to migrate to EU countries that have no labour market restrictions (NÖGUS 2006). Pressure from the provincial governments that bear political responsibility for long-term care institutions, and are therefore most affected by the lack of qualified personnel, has led to the introduction of a few exceptions for migrants from EU-10 countries. This group is now exempt from the *Bundeshöchstzahl*, the federal quota that determines the maximum share of third-country national employees and unemployed persons within the total labour supply (Schütz 2006).

As mentioned in the previous section, the transitional arrangements also led to the rapid growth of an underground economy in foreign nurses providing home care. Policy-makers decided to open the labour market for home-care nursing staff from new EU Member States in 2006. These nurses no longer fall under the Foreign Labour Act and can work in Austria without a work permit (NÖGUS 2006). A legal ordinance was introduced in order to tackle the problem of illegal nurses and to ensure affordable care. This will be discussed in the section on domestic interventions.

Austria has a small number of country-level instruments for steering and managing health professional mobility (Table 1.9). As mentioned, the Foreign Labour Act regulates migration to Austria. Also, the quota regulation for medical universities represents a country-level self-sufficiency instrument to ensure that enough Austrian medical doctors will receive training.

---

6 Austria, Belgium, Bulgaria, Cyprus, Czech Republic, Denmark, Estonia, Finland, France, Germany, Greece, Hungary, Iceland, Ireland, Italy, Latvia, Lichtenstein, Lithuania, Luxembourg, Malta, the Netherlands, Norway, Poland, Portugal, Romania, Slovakia, Slovenia, Spain, Sweden and the United Kingdom.

Table 1.9 *Country-level instruments for steering and managing health professional mobility*

Instrument/tool	Foreign health professionals
Country-level fast-tracking of health worker immigration	In general same regulations as for all other labour migrants, no preferential status or priority treatment
	Nursing staff, solely home-care providers from new EU countries (joined since 2004), is excluded from the Foreign Labour Act
	Health professionals from new EU Member States are exempted from the federal quota
Country-level recruitment code	Foreign Labour Act regulates immigration from new EU and non-EEA countries
Country-level self-sufficiency policy	Quota regulation for medical universities to ensure sufficient numbers of medical doctors or graduates

8.2 Workforce planning and development

The provision of health care in Austria is a federal matter in terms of legislation and execution. Competence for health does not lie exclusively with the BMG as responsibilities are also assumed by other federal ministries, provinces and municipalities and the social security institutions, as self-administrated public corporations. The BMG has no federal sub-authorities in the public health sector so health administration is executed by provincial and municipal administrations. Each provincial government has its own department with responsibility for health. In addition, each *Bezirksverwaltungsbehörde* (district administrative authority) has a health department. The ÖBIG is responsible for research and planning in the health sector, established as a separate legal entity under the aegis of the BMG (ÖBIG 2009, Schütz 2006).

The ÖBIG and the BMG jointly develop the Austrian Structural Plan for Health (*Österreichischer Strukturplan Gesundheit* – ÖSG) that sets out the planning of service provision for the Austrian health-care sector, including workforce planning. The ÖSG describes the framework for detailed planning at a regional level – especially for the Regional Structural Plan for Health (*Regionaler Strukturplan Gesundheit* – RSG), which is then created by the nine provinces and the health-care regions. The numbers of foreign health professionals are not part of the personnel planning (BMG 2010).

8.3 Cross-border regulatory frameworks and interventions

Mutual recognition of diplomas in the European Community

Medical doctors with EEA or Swiss nationality who wish to practise in Austria must provide proof of their diplomas in compliance with EU regulations, certifying appropriate training (licence or approbation) in the host country.

They also require a certificate from the competent authority of their homeland to confirm that this training complies with EU law or the successful completion of medical studies in Austria. Medical studies completed in a non-EEA country must also be inspected for their equivalency with Austrian standards by one of the medical universities in Austria (ÖAK 2009a).

Diplomas acquired in the new EU Member States are recognized under the same conditions as those acquired in the EU-15. Medical doctors holding a recognized diploma have the right to freely set up practice in Austria. However, nationals of Bulgaria, the Czech Republic, Estonia, Hungary, Latvia, Lithuania, Poland, Romania, Slovakia and Slovenia must obtain a work permit from the AMS in order to work in a hospital (ÖAK 2009a).

Nurses wishing to practise in Austria require a job entitlement. Qualifications acquired outside Austria must be verified by the appropriate public authorities; both employees without verification and their employers are liable to prosecution. Nurses apply for either nostrification (verification) or licence to work. Nostrification verifies foreign diplomas from non-EU Member States; licence to work is based on EU Directive 2005/36/EC on the mutual recognition of diplomas. This covers nationals of EU Member States, EFTA countries, Switzerland and those from non-EU countries who hold permanent residence permits (*Daueraufenthalt-EG*). The BMG is responsible for job entitlements of nursing staff from EEA countries or those from non-EEA countries who hold permanent residence permits. Other non-EEA country members apply to the federal state governments for verification of their diplomas. Midwives are regulated by the ÖHG (BMG 2009).

Bilateral agreements

Austria is characterized more by informal agreements than by official bilateral agreements. For example, the ÖAK responded to a shortage of medical doctors in eastern Germany by concluding informal agreements with the German provinces of Thüringen, Mecklenburg-Vorpommern, Brandenburg, Sachsen und Sachsen-Anhalt. These arrangements enable young Austrian medical doctors to work in 1 of 250 German hospitals (ÖAK 2008).

The two medical chambers of South Tyrol in Italy and Tyrol in Austria demonstrate a special model of cross-border collaboration. The Südtirol Enquête was established in 1987 in order to ensure that medical doctors from South Tyrol can be trained in South Tyrolean hospitals in accordance with Austrian law and receive the Austrian licence to practise medicine (approbation). Thus, Austrian medical training is secured for South Tyrolean graduates and Austrian medical doctors gain training possibilities in South Tyrol (Ärztekammer für Tirol 2007).

The Sanicademia and the Healthregio project are examples of bilateral agreements between Austria and its neighbouring regions. The Healthregio project (Regional Network for the Improvement of Healthcare Services) is implemented under INTERREG III A, the external border programmes of the EU. It aims to optimize the structure of health-care provision in the border regions of Austria, the Czech Republic, Slovakia and Hungary, thereby developing a quality location for health-care services in central Europe in the long term. The project priorities are the mobility of patients and health professionals; education and skills development for health professionals; legislative changes and need for progress in national systems; and comparable statistical data on the region (Healthregio 2004).

Sanicademia, the International Academy for Health Professionals, was established in 2006 as an interdisciplinary centre for education and further training of health professionals, to support the mobility of health professionals and to ensure high-quality cross-border education. The academy is the result of a long-term cooperation between the Friuli Venezia Giulia, Veneto and Carinthia regions. Sanicademia coordinates training and education programmes and promotes the worldwide exchange of experiences and knowledge, planning and participating in projects involving cooperation at interregional and international levels (Sanicademia 2009). Currently, Austria-Slovenia and Austria-Italy are collaborating in a cross-border cooperation project – INTERREG IV runs from 2007 until 2013 and deals with health professional mobility in the region. The project covers the harmonization of the training initiatives offered to health professionals. In this context it aims to compare the quality management systems of countries and regions and to organize thematic seminars and language courses; foster the mutual recognition of specialized training; and collect information for the exchange of personnel (Sanicademia 2009).

Cross-border education and exchange programmes encourage health professional mobility and are innovative ways to improve health care collaboratively. These models are becoming more and more popular in other regions in Austria and the neighbouring states (Sanicademia 2009).

Third-country health professionals

The Foreign Labour Act requires health professionals from third countries to obtain a work permit and a residence title for specific purposes before commencing work in Austria (AMS 2009).

Until the medical law was amended in 2009, every medical doctor from a third country had to apply for diploma verification at one of the three medical universities in Austria. Following the amendment, third-country medical doctors who acquire their diploma in an EEA country and work there for at least three years are no longer required to apply for verification at a university (ÖAK 2009b). The federal state governments verify the diplomas of third-country nurses.

Specific interventions and managerial tools

Austria uses both formal and more informal collaborations with neighbouring countries and regions to facilitate staff exchanges and cross-border education. In the recent past more and more models of collaboration have become important, aiming to ensure integrated service delivery and cross-border knowledge transfers (Busse et al. 2007, Offermanns 2008).

Austria uses several instruments to manage and steer health professional mobility (see Table 1.10). The majority of foreign home-care staff from the Czech Republic and Slovakia is placed in Austria by recruitment agencies founded as associations in all three countries (Schmid & Prochazkova 2006). Going International supports health professional mobility by searching for the best accredited and certified courses at regional, national and international levels. It also helps foreign and Austrian health professionals with the migration process (Going International 2009).

8.4 *Domestic interventions*

As mentioned, several specific interventions regulated health professional mobility in the past. These were not part of a larger immigration policy, but were rather short-term reactions to acute problems in the health sector.

Table 1.10 *Cross-border instruments and tools for steering and managing health professional mobility*

Instrument/tool	Description
Twinning	Arrangements with Germany and Italy ensure staff exchanges and staff support
	Slovakian and Czech Republic job agencies facilitate recruitment of nursing staff
Staff exchange	Agreement with South Tyrol (Italy) provides many staff exchanges
	Sanicademia in Carinthia works with Friuli Venezia Giulia (Italy) and Slovenia
	Healthregio project facilitates cooperation between Lower Austria region and Czech Republic, Hungary and Slovakia
	Going International founded to support mobility of health professionals
Educational support and cross-border projects	Sanicademia and Healthregio support cross-border education
	Austrian medical universities cooperate with other medical universities
	Going International focuses especially on education abroad

Interventions to tackle the high number of illegal nurses in the home-care sector have been introduced. In 2006, a legal ordinance changed the Foreign Labour Act to allow home-care staff from new EU countries to enter the Austrian labour market more easily. Other political changes were introduced in 2007, most notably – the Hausbetreuungsgesetz, a legal ordinance for home care that regulates labour legislation. This prescribes two models of foreign nurse recruitment: (i) employment as a self-employed person with a trade licence to provide personal care; and (ii) employment as an employee (Wirtschaft.Info. Service 2008). The *Pflegegeldgesetz*, the law relating to the allowance for nursing care, has also been changed in order to guarantee higher subsidies (derStandard. at 2009b).

The government introduced a deadline in order to motivate employers of illegal nurses – the Pflegeamnestie guaranteed that those who registered their employment as illegal nurses with the Social Insurance Department by 31 December 2007 would bear no legal consequences. The deadline was extended to 30 June 2008 following political and public discussions (Medical Tribune 2008). Since June 2008, the fine for illegal work has ranged between €730 and €2180 and the back payments of social insurance contributions and taxes have been especially high. In May 2008, 5000 registrations were counted but an estimated 35 000 cases were not accounted for (Gewinn 2008).

8.5 *Political force field of regulating and managing health professional mobility*

In 2006, the first prosecutions of illegal nurses in Austria made the topic a central theme of public debate and therefore an important theme for political parties during the general election. Political parties and social partners agreed on the need to introduce general regulations but offered different proposals (Rudda & Marschitz 2007). Subsequent political interventions, such as the changes to the Foreign Labour Act and the illegal workers' amnesty, led to further intensive public and political discussions.

Public opinion is still divided on the consequences of the reforms. Austria's labour restrictions led to losses of qualified health professionals as citizens of the new EU Member States in 2004 and 2007 chose to move to countries with open labour markets. However, the end of transitional arrangements could threaten the home-care sector if hospitals become more attractive to current home-care staff, inducing a significant lack of home-care staff in the ambulatory sector (NÖGUS 2006).

9. Conclusion

Austria benefits from its role as an attractive destination country for foreign health professionals in the EU, but also constitutes an important source country. The traditional two-way exchange of health professionals between Austria and Germany, particularly medical doctors and dentists, is significant for both countries. In particular, provinces in eastern Germany actively recruit Austrian medical doctors to balance their significant loss of medical doctors to western Germany and other countries. The strong tie between the countries is based not only on the common border and common language but also on agreements and exchange programmes between the countries, which may reinforce mobility further.

Currently, there is no shortage of nursing staff in Austria but staffing is tight in both inpatient and outpatient settings (Schmid & Prochazkova 2006). It is likely that any shortages in the near future would be covered quickly by professionals from countries with a weaker economic performance. Different wage levels, proximity, social security provisions and better living standards attract nurses from the Czech Republic and Slovakia, in spite of labour market restrictions. Such migration is important for Austria, especially for mobile health care – in which foreign professionals are particularly important (NÖGUS 2006). Therefore, it is important for Austria to retain its status as an attractive destination country for qualified nurses. The removal of mobile health professionals from the Foreign Employment Act was an important first step. However, there is a fear that the open access to the whole Austrian labour market gained by the disappearance of the transitional arrangements will reduce the availability of mobile health professionals from various EU countries who are currently employed in low-paid and highly stressful jobs (Schmid & Prochazkova 2006).

The EU enlargement has facilitated cooperation and integration in Austria's border regions, regardless of national differences. Existing bilateral projects and agreements, such as the activities of Sanicademia, INTERREG or the Healthregio projects, constitute important steps to ensure a balance of mobility between Austria and its neighbouring states. Countries involved in such interregional projects can benefit from cross-border knowledge transfers and working together to improve their health systems.

References

AMS (2009). *Aufenthalt, Niederlassung und Arbeitspapiere.* Vienna, Arbeitsmarkt Service Österreich (http://www.ams.or.at/sfu/14185_1274.html, accessed 10 June 2009).

Ausweger P (2009). Personalentwicklung im Gesundheitsbereich: Das sagen die Experten. *Informationen für Mitarbeiter und Mitarbeiterinnen der OÖ Ordensspitäler*, Issue 2 (http://www.ooe-ordensspitaeler.at/position/Pos.Gesundheit2. Ausgabe09.pdf, accessed 28 June 2009).

Ärztekammer für Tirol (2007). *Abkommen der Ärztekammern Tirol und Südtirol.* Innsbruck (http://www.aektirol.at/aerztekammer/aktuelles/ details/10056. aspx, accessed 14 September 2009).

Ärztekammer für Tirol (2009). *Approbation.* Innsbruck (http://www.aektirol.at/ inhalte/ 10243.aspx, accessed 14 September 2009).

Biffl G (2006). Teilstudie 16: Alternde Dienstleistungsgesellschaft. In: Aiginger K et al. *WIFO-Weißbuch: Mehr Beschäftigung durch Wachstum auf Basis von Innovation und Qualifikation.* Vienna, WIFO-Gutachtenserie.

BMG (2009). *Anerkennung.* Vienna, Bundesministerium für Gesundheit (http:// www.bmg.gv.at/cms/site/thema.html?channel=CH0941, accessed 9 June 2009).

BMG (2010). *Österreichischer Strukturplan Gesundheit 2010.* Vienna Bundesministerium für Gesundheit (http://www.bmg.gv.at/cms/site/standard. ht ml?channel=CH0716&doc=CMS1136983382893, accessed 13 December 2010).

Busse R et al. (2006). *Mapping health services access: national and cross-border issues (HealthACCESS).* Brussels European Health Management Association (http://ec.europa.eu/health/ph_projects/2003/action1/docs/2003_1_22_frep_en.pdf, accessed 16 December 2010).

derStandard.at (2009a). *Auswandern ist aufwändig.* Vienna (http://www. derstandard.at/fs/   1233309236290/Bedarf-an-Pflege-steigt-Auswandern-istaufwaendig?sap=2& _pid=12297550, accessed 10 June 2009).

derStandard.at (2009b). *Fast 22.000 angemeldete Selbstständige.* Vienna (http://derstandard.at/1256744270119/24-Stunden-Pflege-Fast-22000-angemeldete-Selbststaendige, accessed 2 December 2009).

Die Presse (2009). Arbeitsmarkt: EU billigt Verlängerung der Übergangsfrist. *Die Presse*, 8 June 2009 (http://diepresse.com/home/politik/eu/485681/index.do, accessed 4 September 2009).

Dumond J-C et al. (2008). *International mobility of health professionals and health workforce management in Canada: myths and reality.* Paris, Organisation for Economic Co-operation and Development (OECD Health Working Paper No. 40). Fassmann H (2007). *Österreichischer Migrations- und Integrationsbericht 2001–2006.* Drava, Klagenfurt-Celovec.

Gallob R (2008). Ärztemangel. *Consilium,* 6:14–15 (http://cms.arztnoe.at/cms/dokumente/1002950_100317/e8ed921f/AngAerzte_Consilium_0608.pdf, accessed 29 June 2009).

Georg A (2007). *Temporary work permits issued to illegal foreign care workers.* EUROnline (http://www.eurofound.europa.eu/eiro/2007/01/articles/at0701019i.htm, accessed 16 September 2009).

Gewinn (2008). Neue 24-Stunden-Pflege: Anmeldung bis Ende Juni! *Gewinn*, 6:60.

Going International (2009). *Wissensmanagement für Bildung und Karriere, Personalberatung und Vermittlung.* Vienna (http://www.going-international.at/de / aboutus/, accessed 17 September 2009).

Hammerl R (2007). *Working in Germany.* Vienna (http://www.goinginternational. org/ deutsch/jobs/eb_14.pdf, accessed 15 September 2009).

Healthregio (2004). *Abstract.* Vienna (http://www.healthregio.net/healthregio. htm, accessed 14 December 2010).

Krajic K et al. (2003). *Pflegenotstand in Österreich?* Vienna (http://lbimgs-archiv. lbg.ac.at/present/19112003.pdf, accessed 20 November 2009).

Lachmayr N (2009). Gesundheitsberufe in Bewegung: Mobilität im Medizinisch technischen Assistenzbereich. *Qualitas*, 1:14–17 (http://neu.oeibf. at/db/calimero/ tools/proxy.php?id=13159, accessed 10 June 2009).

Lenhart M, Österle A (2007). Migration von Pflegekräften: Österreichische und Europäische Trends und Perspektiven. *Österreichische Pflegezeitschrift*, 12:8–11 (http://www.oegkv.at/fileadmin/docs/OEPZ_2007/12/lenhart_oesterle.pdf, accessed 10 June 2009).

Medical Tribune (2008). Pflegeamnestie ausgelaufen. *Medical Tribune*, 40(28) (http://www.medical-tribune.at/dynasite.cfm?dsmid=93068&dspaid=708621, accessed 15 September 2009).

Medtest-Team (2009). *Zugang zum Medizinstudium in Österreich, Schweiz und Deutschland.* (http://www.eignungstest.ch/nc_oesterreich_medizinstudium.php #Austria, accessed 9 June 2009).

NÖGUS (2006). *Konsultation zu Gemeinschaftsmaßnahmen im Bereich der Gesundheitsdienstleistungen.* St. Pölten, Stellungnahme des Niederösterreichischen Gesundheits- und Sozialfonds (http://ec.europa.eu/health/ph_overview/co_operation/ mobility/docs/health_services_co166.pdf, accessed 10 June 2009).

ÖÄK (2008). *Ärztekammer schließt Freundschaftsabkommen mit Sachsen Anhalt.* Vienna, Österreichische Ärztekammer (http://www.aerztekammer.at/index.

php?id= 00000000020080901135107&aid=xhtml&id=00000000020080901135 107&type=module&noedit=true, accessed 13 September 2009).

ÖÄK (2009a). *Information for EEA citizens.* Vienna, Österreichische Ärztekammer (http://www.aerztekammer.at/pdf/ Infoblatt_EWR_E.pdf, accessed 9 June 2009).

ÖÄK (2009b). *ÄG-Novelle Zusammenfassung.* Vienna, Österreichische Ärztekammer (http://www.aekooe.or.at/cms/uploads/media/12 _aerztegesetz_ novelle_2009.pdf, accessed 7 September 2009).

ÖBIG (2009). *Österreichischer Strukturplan Gesundheit 2008.* Vienna, Österreichisches Bundesinstitut für Gesundheit (http://www.bmg.gv.at/cms/ site/ attachments/1/0/1/CH0716/CMS1136983382893/oesg_2008_-_gesamt.pdf, accessed 21 September 2009).

Offermanns G (2008). Behandlung ohne Ländergrenzen – Europäische Patienten werden mobil! *Soziale Sicherheit,* 61:148–154.

ÖGKV (2006). *Politische Lösungen für illegale "Pflegekräfte" sind mehr als fraglich!* Vienna, Österreichischer Gesundheits- und Krankenpflegeverband (http://www. oegkv.at/index.php?id=2594, accessed 16 September 2009).

ORF (2007). *Studie: Mittelfristig kein Ärztemangel zu erwarten.* Vienna, Österreichischer Rundfunk. (http://science.orf.at/science/news/147042, accessed 30 July 2009).

ORF (2008). *Immer mehr Ärzte gehen nach Deutschland.* Vienna, Österreichischer Rundfunk (http://oesterreich.orf.at/stories/271726/, accessed 10 June 2009).

ORF Steiermark (2009). *Experten prognostizieren Ärztemangel.* Graz Österreichischer Rundfunk Steiermark (http://steiermark.orf.at/stories/349262/, accessed 30 July 2009).

ORF Tirol (2009). *Deutsche werben um Ärzte aus Österreich.* Innsbruck, Österreichischer Rundfunk Tirol (http://tirol.orf.at/stories/348751/, accessed 10 June 2009).

Rainer J (2008). *Migration-Übersichtsfacharbeit.* Saalfelden, HTL Saalfelden (http://www.htlsaalfelden.at/Migration/4b/1_Uebersichtsarbeit.pdf, accessed 21 November 2009).

Rosenmöller M et al. (eds.) (2006). *Patient mobility in the European Union. Learning from experience.* Copenhagen, WHO Regional Office for Europe on behalf of the European Observatory on Health Systems and Policies.

Rudda J, Marschitz W (2007). *Reform der Pflegevorsorge in Österreich.* Vienna (http://www.sozialversicherung.at/mediaDB/MMDB116408_Rudda_ Pflegevorsorge-Artikel.pdf, accessed 14 September 2009).

Sanicademia (2009). *Crossborder health education.* Villach (http://www.sanicademia. at/projekte/interreg-iv-a-projekt-crossborder-health-education, accessed 4 December 2009).

Schmid T, Prochazkova L (2006). Pflege und Betreuung im Spannungsfeld zwischen Nötigem, Wünschenswertem und Finanzierbarem. *Soziale Sicherheit Online*, November 2006 (http://www.hauptverband.at/portal27/portal/esvportal/channel_ content/cmsWindow?action=2&p_menuid=63491&p_tabid=2&p_pubid=126199, accessed 8 September 2009).

Schütz B (2006). *Second Small Scale Study II: Managed migration and the labour market – the health sector. Austrian Report.* Vienna, International Organization for Migration.

Schwarz V (2008). Alarm in der Anatomie: Die Deutschen kommen! *Integration im Fokus*, 4:18–20 (http://www.integrationsfonds.at/de/wissen/integration_im_fokus/ integration_im_fokus_ausgabe_42008/oesterreich/alarm_in_der_anatomie/, accessed 10 June 2009).

Statistik Austria (2010). *Personalstand in den Krankenanstalten Österreichs seit 1980.* Vienna (http://www.statistik.at/web_de/statistiken/gesundheit/gesundheitsversorgung/personal_im_gesundheitswesen/022348.html, accessed 13 December 2010).

WEKA (2009). *Verlängerung der Übergangsregelungen für neue EU-BürgerInnen.* Vienna, Arbeitsrecht Online (http://www.weka.at/arbeitsrecht/kollektives-arbeitsrecht/news/alle/verlaengerung-der-uebergangsregelungen-fuer-neue-eu-buergerinnen/21969/?l=1, accessed 6 November 2009).

Wieland M, Burger R (2006). *"Healthregio" – regional network for the improvement of healthcare services.* (http://www.healthregio.net/bilder/AbstractGM.pdf, accessed 10 November 2009).

Wirtschaft.Info.Service (2008). *Neuregelungen bei 24h Betreuung.* Krems, Wirtschaftstreuhand-Steuerberatung GmbH & Co KG (http://infodienst.astoria.at/index.php?id=66, accessed 4 September 2009).

Annex

Table 1.11 *Foreign-national medical doctors in Austria, 2003–2008 (stock data)*

Country	2003	2004	2005	2006	2007	2008	2003	2004	2005	2006	2007	2008
Germany	989	1047	1173	1348	1376	1453	36.9%	38.3%	40.6%	42.6%	43.2%	43.7%
Italy	246	249	272	304	295	305	9.2%	9.1%	9.4%	9.6%	9.3%	9.2%
Iran	204	202	195	190	184	178	7.6%	7.4%	6.7%	6.0%	5.8%	5.4%
former Czechoslovakia	169	167	161	159	157	151	6.3%	6.1%	5.6%	5.0%	4.9%	4.5%
Poland	155	154	148	151	149	147	5.8%	5.6%	5.1%	4.8%	4.7%	4.4%
Hungary	87	86	96	130	130	156	3.2%	3.1%	3.3%	4.1%	4.1%	4.7%
former Yugoslavia	69	67	63	62	63	64	2.6%	2.5%	2.2%	2.0%	2.0%	1.9%
Greece	50	49	49	47	47	54	1.9%	1.8%	1.7%	1.5%	1.5%	1.6%
Syrian Arab Republic	58	58	57	56	58	54	2.2%	2.1%	2.0%	1.8%	1.8%	1.6%
Egypt	46	45	43	42	41	41	1.7%	1.6%	1.5%	1.3%	1.3%	1.2%
Others	609	607	634	678	683	719	22.7%	22.2%	21.9%	21.4%	21.5%	21.6%
Total foreign medical doctors	**2 682**	**2 731**	**2 891**	**3 167**	**3 183**	**3 322**						

Source: ÖÄK 2009a.

Table 1.12 *Foreign-trained nurses in Austria: diploma validation applications, 2003–2008*

Country of training	2003	2004	2005	2006	2007	2008
Czech Republic	93	158	145	165	141	67
Hungary	37	80	90	111	97	86
Poland	54	92	134	160	150	77
Slovakia	163	394	551	619	560	357
Slovenia	31	55	65	83	79	36
Other	495	359	270	259	261	186
TOTAL	**873**	**1138**	**1255**	**1397**	**1288**	**809**

Source: BMG 2009.

Table 1.13 *Nurses from eastern European countries: applications for work permits in Austria, 2003–2008*

Country	2003	2004	2005	2006	2007	2008
Czech Republic	93	158	145	165	141	67
Hungary	37	80	90	111	97	86
Poland	54	92	134	160	150	77
Slovakia	163	394	551	619	560	357
Slovenia	31	55	65	83	79	36
Other	495	359	270	259	261	186
TOTAL	**873**	**1138**	**1255**	**1397**	**1288**	**809**

Source: AMS 2009.

Table 1.14 *Newly registered dentists in Austria, by nationality, 2003–2007*

	2003	2004	2005	2006	2007
Austria	**96**	**115**	**114**	**104**	**145**
EU countries:					
Belgium			1		
Bulgaria		2		2	5
Czech Republic		5	2	3	3
Finland				1	
France	1				
Germany	16	21	34	42	36
Greece	1	1		1	2
Hungary	1	9	4	12	6
Italy		3	1	1	3
Latvia		1			1
Lithuania				1	
Netherlands			1		
Poland	4	7	2	7	4
Romania	7	8	4	10	12
Slovakia	1		2	3	
Slovenia		2	3	1	2
Spain					1
Sweden			1	1	
United Kingdom		1			
Total EU countries	**31**	**60**	**55**	**85**	**75**
Total non-EU countries	**8**	**12**	**15**	**15**	**25**
Total inflows foreign nationality	**39**	**72**	**70**	**99**	**100**

Source: Österreichische Zahnärztekammer unpublished data 2009.

Table 1.15 *Practising dentists in Austria, by nationality, 2005–2007*

	2005	2006	2007
Austria	**2970**	**3090**	**3264**
EU countries:			
Belgium	1	1	1
Bulgaria	10	12	17
Czech Republic	55	58	57
Denmark	1	1	1
Finland		1	1
France	1	1	1
Germany	171	216	256
Greece	6	7	9
Hungary	51	62	69
Italy	14	14	18
Latvia	1	1	2
Lithuania		1	1
Luxembourg	2	2	2
Netherlands	5	5	5
Poland	61	69	72
Romania	77	84	103
Slovakia	23	27	27
Slovenia	12	13	15
Spain	1	1	2
Sweden	2	3	3
United Kingdom	3	3	3
Total EU countries	**497**	**582**	**665**
Non-EU countries:			
Bosnia and Herzegovina	18	19	25
Croatia	31	34	36
Iran	19	21	26
Serbia	18	18	21
Syrian Arab Republic	12	13	17
Other	70	82	92
Total non-EU countries	**168**	**187**	**217**
Total foreign-national dentists practising in Austria	**665**	**769**	**882**

Source: Österreichische Zahnärztekammer unpublished data 2009.

Table 1.16 .*Newly registered midwives in Austria, by nationality, 2003–2008*

	2003	2004	2005	2006	2007	2008
A – foreign nationality						
Mean age	37	32	36	31	31	34
Country:						
Bulgaria						2
Czech Republic		0		0		
Finland			1			
France				1		1
Germany	2		9	13	5	10
Hungary		0				
Iceland					1	
Iran				1		2
Italy		0	4	0	3	1
Poland		2	1	3	3	2
Serbia					1	
Slovakia		2	1	1	0	0
Slovenia			1			
Turkey						1
United Kingdom	0			1		
B – Austrian citizen, foreign born						
Mean age		35	39	27	30	
Cape Verde			1			
Germany			0		1	
Iran (Islamic Republic of)		1				
Iraq				0	1	
Japan				1		
Philippines			1			
Poland		1				
Slovakia				0		
Spain			1			
Turkey				1		
C – Austrian born, foreign trained						
Mean age for all years						30
Finland			1			
Germany	1		2	2	2	1
Total inflows midwives (new registered)	**3**	**19**	**23**	**24**	**17**	**20**

Source: ÖHG unpublished data 2009.

Table 1.17 *Practising foreign-national, foreign-born and foreign-trained midwives in Austria, by country, 2008*

A – foreign citizenship		F – Austrian citizenship, foreign-born	
Bosnia and Herzegovina	3	Bosnia and Herzegovina	2
Bulgaria	3	Bulgaria	3
Switzerland	4	Switzerland	2
Chile	1	Côte d'Ivoire	1
Czech Republic	15	Cape Verde	1
Germany	83	Czech Republic	6
Finland	1	Germany	11
France	4	Spain	1
Greece	1	Hungary	3
Croatia	4	Iran	8
Hungary	3	Italy	1
Iran	4	Japan	1
Iceland	1	Philippines	30
Italy	9	Poland	30
Netherlands	2	Romania	1
Philippines	2	Serbia	1
Poland	31	Slovakia	9
Serbia	1	Turkey	2
Slovenia	4	former Yugoslavia	6
Slovakia	12	South Africa	1
Turkey	3	**G – Austrian born, foreign trained**	
United Kingdom	2	Germany	8
		Finland	1
Total		**322**	

Source: ÖHG unpublished data 2009.

Table 1.18 *Outflows of midwives from Austria, 2003–2008*

	2003	2004	2005	2006	2007	2008
Mean age	between 20 and 30					
H-applying for diploma verification to work in EU Member State						
Germany						1
Hungary			1			
Ireland					1	
Italy			5		1	1
Slovakia				1		
Sweden			1			
United Kingdom		1	1	1	1	
I-applying for visas to emigrate						
Australia					1	1
Ghana					1	
Luxembourg		1				
New Zealand						1
United Republic of Tanzania						1
J-emigrated midwives *						
Total outflow	**0**	**2**	**8**	**2**	**5**	**5**

* no reliable data; includes cross-border work, development assistance, etc.
Source: ÖHG unpublished data 2009.

Chapter 2

Of permeable borders: Belgium as both source and host country

Anna Safuta, Rita Baeten

1. Introduction

This chapter aims to capture the crucial aspects of health professional mobility between Belgium and the rest of the world. Most of the observed flows occur to and from neighbouring countries (France, the Netherlands, Germany) but research for this study also shows that Belgium is a recent host to migration from less obvious source countries – Romania (for medical doctors with basic training[1] and nurses), and Lebanon (nurses). Foreign nurses and medical doctors with basic training are often recruited to alleviate shortages in nursing staff and to compensate for the reduction in the number of Belgian doctors in training resulting from the introduction of a quota (see section 6.3). Evidence suggests that professionals from Romania and Lebanon who have migrated to Belgium are employed mainly in French-speaking hospitals. This indicates that language is an important facilitating factor for health professional migration. The prevalent facilitating factors for migration from neighbouring countries include shared language and cultural proximity.

Inflows and outflows are almost negligible for general practitioners; moderate for nurses and dentists; and more significant for medical doctors with basic training and for specialists. Inflows have increased for all professions in recent years, due to emigration not only from neighbouring countries but also from Romania and Lebanon.

---

1 As defined in the Directive on the recognition of professional qualifications (European Parliament and Council of the European Union 2005).

Limitations of the study

The statistical data analysed in this chapter have been retrieved and in some cases created specifically by the Belgian public authorities responsible for providing recognition or equivalence certificates and licences to practise to medical professionals with foreign diplomas. These data provide a relatively accurate account of the inflows since 2003; older data are either incomplete or unavailable.

In the absence of data, outflows have been estimated from applications for conformity certificates that certify compliance with the Directive on the recognition of professional qualifications (European Parliament and Council of the European Union 2005). These statistics provide a relatively accurate indication of outflows to some countries. However, not all destination countries systematically request these certificates from migrating health professionals and so actual outflows may be underestimated. Data interpretation is complicated further by the high proportion of foreign students who study in Belgium as the outflows of medical doctors and nurses include a proportion of these students returning to their home countries after graduation. For this reason, statistics on foreign inflows have also been collected from the two main destination countries – France and the Netherlands.

This chapter will first present Belgium's mobility profile in terms of medical doctors, nurses and dentists leaving or entering the country. This is followed by a brief discussion of the role of EU enlargement. The impact and relevance of health professional mobility are analysed in the wider context of the Belgian health-care system and its workforce. The final section is an explanation of the policy context and measures/interventions aimed at managing health professional mobility.

2. Mobility profile of Belgium

Belgium is both a source and a destination country. Cross-border flows are numerically relatively important in the investigated health professions and the most important exchanges have been found with neighbouring countries. Recently, inflows seem to have increased in all professions. Anecdotal evidence suggests that Belgium is also a transit country for some medical doctors – having completed basic medical training in their home countries they undertake one or two years of specialization in Belgium before returning home or moving elsewhere (see section 5).

2.1 *Outflows*

Holders of a Belgian medical, dentistry or nursing diploma who intend to practise in another EU Member State must apply for a conformity certificate that assures compliance with the directive on the recognition of professional qualifications (European Parliament and Council of the European Union 2005). Health professional outflows are estimated from the numbers of conformity certificates requested, from data supplied by the International Mobility Cell for the Health Professions of the Belgian Federal Public Service (FPS) Health, Food chain safety and Environment. This information is supplemented by inflow data from France (Le Breton-Lerouvillois 2007 & 2009) and the Netherlands (Ministry of Health, Welfare and Sport unpublished data 2009).

The data on conformity certificates should be interpreted with caution. Applicants do not always know or declare their destination – 10% of nurses and general practitioners, 11% of doctors with basic medical training, 14% of specialists and 22% of dentists did not. In addition, professionals may request these certificates but never leave Belgium to practise abroad, or may go to another country than that declared. Some countries (such as the Netherlands) recognize Belgian diplomas without systematically requesting a conformity certificate; other countries (such as France) request a conformity certificate from every foreign-trained health professional who intends to migrate. Aggregated conformity certificate statistics show that France and the Netherlands are the two most frequently declared destinations.

The outflow data take no account of the nationality of the person requesting the conformity certificate and thus do not distinguish between Belgian nationals and foreign nationals with a Belgian diploma. Also, the data do not distinguish foreign nationals who have studied in Belgium and are applying for conformity certificates before returning to their home countries after graduation. Finally, the outflow statistics include a very small number of requests that were declined (less than 2% according to the competent civil servant). Data on the delivery of conformity certificates were available only for the last three years (2006–2008), making it difficult to analyse trends over time. These data do not show any clear decreasing or increasing tendencies.

France is the destination of a large share of Belgium-trained migrating health professionals – specified by 57% (394) of specialists requesting conformity certificates (Table 2.1). It is assumed that these migrating professionals include many French nationals who studied in Belgium (Roberfroid et al. 2008). However, data collected by the French Medical Chamber (CNOM) also show important outflows of Belgian-national medical doctors moving to France (Le Breton-Lerouvillois 2007 & 2009). In early 2009, a total of 1576 Belgian

Table 2.1 *Annual outflows of specialists with Belgian diplomas estimated from number of conformity certificate requests, 2006–2008*

Declared destination country	2006	2007	2008	Total per destination country	%
France	142	180	72	394	57.27
Germany	2	2	5	9	1.31
Luxembourg	0	1	2	3	0.44
Netherlands	19	18	1	38	5.52
United Kingdom	22	35	16	73	10.61
Unknown	38	45	18	101	14.68
Other EU-15[a]	**7**	**10**	**7**	**24**	**3.49**
EU-12[b]	**0**	**0**	**0**	**0**	**0.00**
Non-EU	**9**	**31**	**6**	**46**	**6.68**
Total per year	**239**	**322**	**127**	**688**	**100**

Source: FPS Health, Food chain safety and Environment unpublished data 2009. *Notes*: [a] Austria, Denmark, Greece, Ireland, Italy, Spain, Sweden; [b] Bulgaria, Czech Republic, Cyprus, Estonia, Hungary, Latvia, Lithuania, Malta, Poland, Romania, Slovakia, Slovenia.

nationals were registered with the CNOM, 16.37% of all foreign medical doctors registered in France (Le Breton-Lerouvillois 2007). In 2007, Belgians accounted for 30% to 40% of all foreigners practising certain specialities in France.[2] The Paris region and the regions bordering Belgium and Germany had the highest numbers of foreign medical doctors.

Belgian data on outflows of medical doctors and dentists show that the United Kingdom is the second most popular stated destination.

It should be noted that the Belgian data on conformity certificate requests underestimate actual outflows as the Dutch authorities do not systematically request conformity certificates from the holders of Belgian medicine, dentistry and nursing diplomas. Therefore, the Belgian data have been supplemented by Dutch Ministry of Health, Welfare and Sport statistics on the number of health professionals with Belgian diplomas newly registered in the Netherlands in 2006–2008 (Fig. 2.1). These data allow a more accurate picture of outflows to the Netherlands since it is compulsory for medical doctors, dentists and nurses to register with the Dutch authorities.

---

2 Radiotherapy, physical medicine and rehabilitation, nuclear medicine, occupational medicine, orthopaedic surgery and traumatology, urological surgery, vascular surgery; 11 of the 17 foreign neuro-psychiatrists practising in France were Belgians (Le Breton-Lerouvillois 2007).

Dutch data show 373 doctors with basic training, general practitioners and specialists holding Belgian medical diplomas and newly registered in the Netherlands between 2006 and 2008. The majority of those migrating doctors are likely Dutch nationals who studied medicine in the northern, Dutch-speaking part of Belgium (see section 6.3). During the same period, 81 nurses and 69 dentists with Belgian diplomas registered in the Netherlands (Fig. 2.1).

Dutch data suggest that outflows to the Netherlands by medical doctors, nurses and dentists with Belgian diplomas are numerically important and of a similar size to the outflows to France estimated from the Belgian data on conformity certificates.

Fig. 2.1 *Annual outflows to the Netherlands of health professionals with Belgian diplomas, comparison of Belgian and Dutch data, 2006–2008*

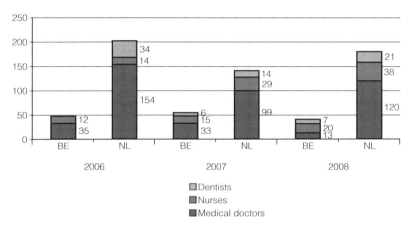

BE: Number of conformity certificates requested by Belgian doctors with basic training, general practitioners, specialists, nurses and dentists who declared Netherlands as destination (*Source*: FPS Health, Food chain safety and Environment unpublished data 2009).

NL: Number of newly registered medical doctors, nurses and dentists holding Belgian diplomas in the Netherlands (*Source*: Dutch Ministry of Health, Welfare and Sport unpublished data 2009).

The data on conformity certificate requests show that the emigrating specialists with Belgian diplomas represent a very high percentage of the total number of newly registered specialists in Belgium per year. Between 2006 and 2008, 3100 foreign- trained and Belgium-trained specialists registered in Belgium (Table 2.4), while 688 specialists with Belgian diplomas requested conformity certificates (Table 2.1). This suggests that nearly 2 of every 10 specialists who enter the Belgian health labour market emigrate.

2.2 Inflows

Health workforce data in Belgium are held at both federal and community level. Inflows of foreign-trained health professionals to Belgium have been estimated from three different sources – (i) International Mobility Cell for the Health Professions' data on European Economic Area (EEA) diplomas recognized between 2001 and 2008; (ii) French Community statistics on non-EEA diplomas and EEA diplomas not conforming with the EC directive[3], declared equivalent between 2003 and 2008; and (iii) the Federal Database of Health Care Professionals (*Cadastre des professionels de soins de santé*) (the register) on the number of registered general practitioners and specialists and on the number of medical doctors, nurses and dentists newly licensed to practise (see section 8.2). Theoretically, the number of newly licensed medical doctors with foreign diplomas should coincide with the sum of equivalences and recognitions granted (although there might be a time lag) but this is not the case with the data provided. However, recognition data are more reliable than register statistics.[4]

Medical doctors with no general practice or specialist training

Inflow data provided by the International Mobility Cell for the Health Professions show that 1704 foreign basic medical diplomas were recognized or declared equivalent in Belgium between 2001 and 2008 (FPS Health, Food chain safety and Environment unpublished data 2009). These were mostly French (355) and Dutch (313). Before EU accession, no Romanian diplomas were declared equivalent. In 2007, Romania became the third most frequent country of origin (267 recognitions) overtaking both Germany (213 recognitions) and Italy (187) which were the third and fourth source countries until 2006. The sharp increase in recognitions noticeable from 2007 (Fig. 2.2) is thus mostly attributable to inflows from Romania.

Belgian data on recognized foreign basic medical training include doctors with foreign general practitioner or specialist diplomas who might have further registered as a general practitioner or a specialist. Indeed, in Belgium, recognition of a foreign general practitioner or specialist diploma implies recognition of the applicant's basic medical training.

The proportion of foreign-trained newly licensed doctors with only basic training has been increasing since 2005 and in 2008 reached just over 25%

---

3 Only French Community (sub-national) data on EEA diplomas not in conformity with the EC directive were used as the Flemish Community data lacked precision. The 2003–2008 data on equivalences of dentistry, bachelor-level nursing and basic medical diplomas and the 2007 & 2008 data on equivalences of secondary-level nursing diplomas were analysed. Information on non-EEA diplomas was obtained from French Community data (2003–2008 for basic medicine, bachelor nursing and dentistry diplomas; 2007 and 2008 for secondary-level nursing diplomas) and 2004–2008 statistics on practice permits from the International Mobility Cell for the Health Professions.

4 Phone interview with the competent civil servant, Brussels, July 2009.

of all newly licensed medical doctors with basic training (Table 2.2). A major part of this significant increase can be explained by the increase in Romanian diploma recognitions mentioned above.

Table 2.2 *Estimated numbers of foreign-trained medical doctors with basic training licensed in Belgium per year, 2005–2008*

	2005	2006	2007	2008
A: Foreign-trained newly licensed medical doctors with basic training	199	258	417	459
B: Foreign-trained newly registered general practitioners and specialists	75	110	105	148
C=(A-B): Foreign-trained doctors not registered as general practitioners or specialists[a]	124	148	312	311
D: Total of newly licensed doctors with basic training	1 082	1 005	1 157	1 228
E=C/Dx100 : % of foreign-trained within total newly registered medical doctors with basic training	11.5%	14.7%	27.0%	25.3%

Source: FPS Health, Food chain safety and Environment unpublished data 2009. *Note*: [a] Category covers medical doctors who either have no general practitioner or specialist training or who did not register as general practitioners or specialists in Belgium.

Yearly inflows of Romanian doctors with basic medical training were comparable before Romania's accession to the EU, but based on a different legal provision limiting their stay in Belgium (see section 8.3). In 2004–2006, some 682 medical doctors with third-country diplomas (mostly from Romania, Morocco and the Congo) arrived to do part of their specialization in Belgium on the basis of this specific legal provision (Table 2.3).

Table 2.3 *Medical doctors with non-EEA diplomas undertaking part of their specializations in Belgium under Royal Decree No. 78*

Country of diploma	2004	2005	2006	Total per country
Congo	18	15	18	51
Morocco	27	40	26	93
Romania	51	114	113	278
Other	92	81	87	260
Total per year	**188**	**250**	**244**	**682**

Source: FOD Volksgezondheid 2007c.

General practitioners and specialists

Table 2.4 shows the number of general practitioners and specialists with a foreign diploma newly registered in Belgium between 2005 and 2008 – non-Belgian diplomas were held by about 3%–8% of newly registered general practitioners and about 8%–12% of newly registered specialists.

Table 2.4 *General practitioners and specialists in Belgium, 2005–2008*

	2005	2006	2007	2008
Foreign-trained newly registered general practitioners	11	14	7	17
Total newly registered general practitioners	259	281	238	218
Percentage of foreign-trained general practitioners	4.2%	5%	2.9%	7.8%
Foreign-trained newly registered specialists	64	96	98	131
Total newly registered specialists	821	1056	973	1071
Percentage of foreign-trained specialists	7.8%	9.1%	10.1%	12.2%

Source: FPS Health, Food chain safety and Environment unpublished data 2009.

The data on EEA diploma recognitions lead to similar conclusions to those drawn from the registration data – general practitioner inflows to Belgium appear to be rather insignificant and specialists migrate in larger numbers. A total of 91 general practitioner diplomas were recognized between January 2001 and December 2008. Of these, 38 were French. Surprisingly, the United Kingdom (15 diplomas) and Spain (10 diplomas) were the second and third country of origin for general practitioners. The neighbouring Netherlands had only five recognitions. During the same period, Belgium recognized 348 specialist diplomas from within the EEA, mostly German (83), Dutch (68), French (55), Italian (40) or Romanian (34).

Over time, there has been a steady increase in the share of foreign nationals in the medical workforce. In 2003, foreign nationals counted for only 8% of all registered medical doctors. However, these data should be interpreted with caution as they include foreign nationals who lived and studied in Belgium before enrolling in medicine in the country. Organisation for Economic Co-operation and Development (OECD) data for 2008 show that 2989 medical doctors (6.7% of the total Belgian medical workforce) were foreign-trained (OECD 2008). Stock data from the national database show that 10.5% of the 51 171 registered medical doctors in 2008 were not Belgian nationals – 2.3% were French, 2.6% Dutch, 0.8% German, 0.7% Italian, 0.5% Spanish and 0.5% Romanian.

Inflow charts show a steady increase in recognitions of all types of foreign medical diplomas. The sharp increase in specialist diploma recognitions in 2006 is mainly attributable to intensified inflows from France and the Netherlands (Fig. 2.2).

Fig. 2.2 *EEA medical diplomas recognized in Belgium, 2001–2008*

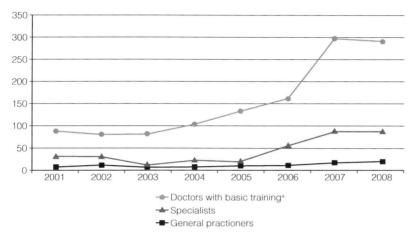

Source: FPS Health, Food chain safety and Environment unpublished data 2009. *Note*: [a] Values calculated by subtracting the number of recognized EEA general practitioner and specialist diplomas from the annual total of EEA basic medical training recognitions.

Nurses

Register, recognition and equivalence data suggest important inflows of foreign-trained nurses relative to total inflows to the profession. Register data for 2005–2008 show that the proportion of foreign-trained nurses within all newly licensed nurses varied between 5.8% and 13.5%, with a tendency to increase (Table 2.5).

Table 2.5 *Newly licensed nurses in Belgium, 2005–2008*

	2005	2006	2007	2008
Foreign-trained newly licensed nurses	205	268	330	565
Total of newly licensed nurses	3549	3798	4078	4170
Percentage of foreign-trained nurses	5.8%	7.1%	8.1%	13.5%

Source: FPS Health, Food chain safety and Environment unpublished data 2009.

Stock data show that 4.4% of the total of 175 111 registered nurses in 2008 were foreign nationals, mainly of French (2.5%), Italian (0.5%) and Dutch (0.4%) nationality (FPS Health, Food chain safety and Environment unpublished data 2009). Again, these data include second generation immigrants who studied in Belgium. This is illustrated by the high proportion of Italians as Belgium has had a sizeable Italian population since the 1960s. OECD data for that same year show a share of only 1.5% of foreign nationals in the nursing population (OECD 2008). However, there are good reasons to question the OECD data as the Belgian authorities stressed that nursing stock data with an acceptable degree of reliability could be provided only for the last trimester of 2009. Prior to this, the database for nurses included those who were no longer active in the workforce.

Recognition data show that 40.5% of the 1152 foreign nursing diplomas recognized between 2004 and 2008 were French, mostly of post-secondary level. Dutch nursing diplomas ranked second with 253 recognized diplomas balanced roughly between secondary and post-secondary level. German diplomas were the third most important group with 111 exclusively secondary level diplomas.

For all the medical professions discussed in this chapter, community data demonstrate that non-EEA and EEA diplomas that do not conform to the EC directive are seldom declared equivalent. The noticeable exceptions are 153 Romanian secondary level nursing diplomas that the French Community declared equivalent in 2007–2008 (94% of all secondary level nursing diplomas declared equivalent during that period)[5] and the 93 Lebanese post-secondary nursing diplomas declared equivalent in 2008 (80% of all post-secondary nursing diplomas declared equivalent by the French Community in that year). The competent civil servant reports that the majority of the 169 diplomas declared equivalent between January and August 2009 were also Lebanese.[6]

Federal level data for 2008 on diplomas first declared equivalent by Community authorities (Table 2.6) do not reflect the 93 Lebanese nursing diplomas declared equivalent by the French Community in that year. This is probably due to a time lag between the granting of equivalences and subsequent processing of the application. The 153 secondary level nursing diplomas from Romania that the French Community declared equivalent between 2007 and 2008 also do not figure because the federal data do not take account of diplomas that fall beyond the scope of the EC directive (Table 2.6).

Federal data show that 59 of the 175 nurses with a non-EEA diploma granted a Royal Decree of Exercise between 2004 and 2008 had a Congolese diploma (Table 2.6). Moreover, the increase in recognitions noticeable from 2006 onwards is almost exclusively attributable to an increase in post-secondary diploma recognitions.

---

5 The French Community could provide data on nurses for 2007 and 2008 only; no statistics were received from the Flemish Community. This made it difficult to evaluate the inflows of EEA diplomas within the scope of the directive as these data are not covered by the FPS Health, Food chain safety and Environment statistics.

6 Phone conversation with civil servant from the Foreign University Diplomas Equivalences Unit, Ministry of the French Community of Belgium, 1 September 2009.

Table 2.6 *Foreign nursing diplomas recognized or declared equivalent in Belgium*[a]

Country issuing diploma	2004	2005	2006	2007	2008	Total per country
France	79	66	93	96	133	467
Germany	37	18	14	28	14	111
Luxembourg	0	0	0	2	2	4
Netherlands	43	74	48	46	42	253
United Kingdom	6	3	2	3	3	17
Other EU-15	**10**	**13**	**20**	**15**	**16**	**74**
Romania	0	0	0	12	10	22
Other EU-12	**2**	**1**	**4**	**7**	**14**	**28**
Congo	1	5	16	14	23	59
Lebanon	0	6	1	7	35	49
Other non EU-27	**24**	**12**	**13**	**9**	**9**	**67**
Total per year	**202**	**198**	**211**	**239**	**301**	**1 151**

Source: FPS Health, Food chain safety and Environment unpublished data 2009. *Note*: [a] Does not include EEA diplomas that do not conform to the EC directive but have been declared equivalent.

Dentists

Recognition statistics from the FPS Health, Food chain safety and Environment show that 181 foreign EEA dentistry diplomas were recognized between 2001 and 2008. Register data for 2005–2008 show the percentage of foreign-trained workforce among newly licensed dentists varied between 9.6% and 19.3%, with considerable fluctuations over the period (Table 2.7).

Table 2.7 *Newly licensed dentists in Belgium, 2005–2008*

	2005	2006	2007	2008
Foreign-trained newly licensed dentists	11	28	21	37
Total newly licensed dentists	114	189	151	192
Percentage of foreign-trained dentists	9.6%	14.8%	13.9%	19.3%

Source: FPS Health, Food chain safety and Environment unpublished data 2009.

Stock data show that 6.1% of the 9 489 registered dentists in 2008 were not Belgian nationals – 2.3% were French, 0.8% Dutch and 0.5% Italian.

Summary

Federal data show that inflows of medical doctors, dentists and nurses have been increasing since 2001 (Fig. 2.3). Among medical doctors, this increase is less pronounced for general practitioners than it is for those with basic training and specialists (Fig. 2.2).

Fig. 2.3 *EEA diplomas for medicine, nursing and dentistry recognized in Belgium, 2001–2008*

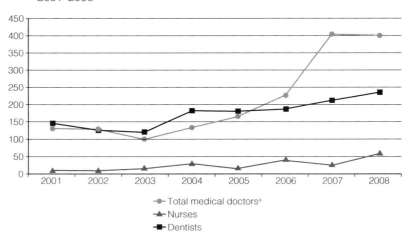

Source: FPS Health, Food chain safety and Environment unpublished data 2009. *Note*: ª Values calculated by summing up recognized EEA medical doctor diplomas (see Fig. 2.2).

Stock data show a steady increase of foreign nationals in the total registered workforce for all these health professionals.

3. Vignettes of health professional mobility

Belgian health professional commuting to Holland

HD is a 55 year old Belgian living in Belgium and commuting daily to Maastricht. At 18, he started a work-integrated learning programme in nursing at the University Hospital of Maastricht (azM). In continuous employment, he gained permanent status after a year. He graduated in 1975 and, while working in the same hospital, successively obtained post-secondary level diplomas as an operating theatre assistant (1976–1979), in management (1981–1982 and 1985–1986) and in law (1990–1997).

Since 1985, his duties have not included any contact with patients. His career developed both vertically and horizontally, in the following order – nurse, theatre assistant, deputy chief of theatres, chief coordinator of surgical care, administrator, manager, chief of the staff services department, education and labour market adviser.

He chose Maastricht because the employment structure seemed less hierarchical and less formal than that in the Belgian nursing schools he visited. Maastricht is very close to the Belgian border and therefore there was no need for him to move to the Netherlands. He is very satisfied with his choice of Maastricht and emphasizes that any Belgian nurse who takes up employment in the Netherlands, especially at azM, has no interest in being employed in Belgium.

Immigrant doctor with plans to move on

AM is a 28 year old Romanian who graduated in medicine in Romania and started a five-year specialization in internal medicine (neurology) at the Romanian University in Iaşi. After 18 months, he applied unsuccessfully for the exchange programme between his university and the Université catholique de Louvain (UCL) in Belgium. He signed a contract with a private agency that found him a position as assistant in a small rural hospital in Belgium on a contract running from 1 October 2008 to 30 September 2009. He is the sole intern on the neurology unit and also works regularly as an on-call medical doctor in internal medicine. He lives within the hospital premises.

AM chose to move to Belgium in order to work in centres of expertise that do not exist in Romania. He plans to stay in Belgium for another year. His internship tutor has promised to find him a place in another hospital as he cannot stay in his current hospital. He would like to finish his specialization in Belgium or France. His private life will determine whether he establishes himself permanently in Romania after his specialization but he would like to work in France.

---

4. Dynamics of enlargement

Romanian nurses and doctors with basic medical training (and specialists to a much smaller extent) appear to be the most numerous among the health professionals from the twelve new European Member States who moved to Belgium to work. This can be partially explained by the activity of private companies recruiting Romanian nurses and specializing doctors to work as assistants in Belgian hospitals (see section 8.3). As illustrated by Table 2.3, Romanian medical doctors with basic medical training were migrating to Belgium even before Romania's accession to the EU.

Belgium applied legal restrictions on immigration from the ten new central and eastern European Member States until 1 May 2009 (Government of Belgium 2004). This was later extended until 31 December 2011 for Romanian and Bulgarian citizens (Government of Belgium 2008c), who therefore still need work permits in order to work in Belgium. Attribution of working permits has been facilitated since 1 May 2006 for specific shortage professions in the Belgian labour market (Government of Belgium 2006a), including almost all the nursing professions (Government of Belgium 2006b).

Since the first day of accession there have been no limitations on self-employment. Foreign candidates for self-employment receive a five-month residence permit to start up their activity. Those who are successful are granted an open-ended residence permit. Since most doctors and dentists in Belgium are self-employed, even in hospital settings, this applies to most immigrant doctors and dentists. Specializing medical doctors have a *sui generis* status – they receive a fee but are neither employees nor self-employed.

5. Impact of health professional mobility

Health professional inflows and outflows are numerically relatively important but no impacts or potential impacts on the Belgian health system have been reported.

Foreign candidate specialists are not counted in the quotas limiting candidate specialists' and general practitioners' access to further training (see section 6.3). This has been the subject of debate as it could thwart Belgian health workforce planning policies (Roberfroid et al. 2008). Between 2004 and 2007, 7.4% of all applications for training plans in Belgium were submitted by holders of foreign medical diplomas (SPF Santé publique 2007). However, it is difficult to estimate the proportion of foreign-trained doctors with basic training who will remain in Belgium on completion of their specialist or general practitioner training (Roberfroid et al. 2008).

Furthermore, it is not possible to assess the long-term effects of the important recent inflows of Romanian doctors with basic training as outflow data show only conformity certificates delivered to holders of Belgian diplomas. It is not known how many of the recognized medical doctors with foreign basic training settle permanently in the country and how many leave (except those who start a specialization).[7] It can be assumed that at least some of these foreign-trained medical doctors return home, for example to finish their specializations. This has been confirmed during interviews with Romanian doctors and within Belgian institutions that host Romanian doctors with basic medical training.[8] If these doctors decide to establish themselves permanently in their home countries after undertaking part of their specialization in Belgium, such temporary migration could be considered positive for both the Belgian and their home health-care systems. This situation is too recent for an in-depth analysis to draw far-reaching conclusions. Indeed, Romanian doctors were undertaking part of their specialization in Belgium before their country's EU accession and the situation could now evolve as they are offered the possibility of staying to practise.

---

7 Between 2004 and 2007, only 241 graduates with a foreign medical diploma started general practitioner or specialist training in Belgium (SPF Santé publique 2007). A total of 925 foreign basic medical diplomas were recognized during the same period but only 234 of these were further recognized as general practitioner or specialist diplomas. Hence, approximately 450 holders of a foreign basic medical diploma neither applied for recognition of a foreign general practitioner or specialist diploma nor started a specialization in Belgium (at least during those years).

8 Interviews with Romanian doctors with basic training who specialize in Belgium; e-mail interview with a Belgian professor in charge of an exchange programme between a Belgian university and a Romanian medical school aimed at Romanian specializing doctors, 13 July 2009; phone interview with a Belgian specialist working in a rural hospital in southern Belgium, 14 July 2009.

Some Dutch care institutions situated on the border with Belgium employ important numbers of Belgian nurses from the Flemish province of Limburg[9] but institutions in this Belgian (rural) province seem to have fewer problems with nurse recruitment than those in larger cities (Jacobs 2007). The emigration of child and youth psychiatrists to the Netherlands has been reported as a problem (De Morgen 2007). Indeed, these professions have major shortages in Belgium and are on the list of specializations for which a minimum of candidates has to be filled each year (Government of Belgium 2008a). By contrast, it is suggested that the outflows of specialists to France result from an oversupply in most specialties in Belgium, particularly in the French Community (Anrys 2009).

The significant numbers of foreign residents in Belgian training institutions (see section 6.3) could impede the training of home students in shortage professions in Belgium, particularly nurses.

6. Relevance of cross-border health professional mobility

6.1 *Inflows and outflows*

The Belgian health workforce is characterized by oversupply in most professions, including dentists, specialists and physiotherapists. There are difficulties in the recruitment of nurses, especially in urban centres, and shortages of general practitioners are expected in the coming years. Attrition rates seem to be important in both nursing and general practice medicine. Furthermore, there is a reduction of the available labour volume as the health workforce is ageing and undergoing feminization. The professional mobility of general practitioners is negligible and thus has little impact on the available workforce. Inflows and outflows of nurses are more important – recent active recruitment of nurses from Romania and Lebanon aims at alleviating existing shortages.

6.2 *Distributional issues influencing composition of the health workforce*

Oversupply in most specializations has led to the introduction of a quota that limits access to general practitioner, specialist and dentistry training (see section 6.3). However, general practitioner density has decreased in a short period of time and shortages are expected in the coming years, especially in the Dutch-speaking north of the country (Roberfroid et al. 2008). A federal programme offers financial incentives to general practitioners willing to settle in sparsely populated areas or in urban positive action zones (NIHDI 2010).

---

9 Interview with a Belgian nurse working in the azM, Maastricht, 2 July 2009.

Regional variations in the density of practising general practitioners (9.8–14.4 per 10 000 inhabitants) are even more marked among specialists (8.4–24.0 per 10 000 inhabitants). Given the discrepancies in general practitioner and specialist coverage between the better-served French-speaking south and the medically less well-served Dutch-speaking north, it is likely that the quota system will see lower numbers of French-speaking medical graduates being able to specialize or to train as general practitioners (Roberfroid et al. 2008).

Shortages of nurses are found to be more acute in urban areas such as Antwerp or Brussels and in nursing homes more than in hospitals (Geets 2008). It is argued that increasing the involvement of auxiliary nurses by redefining the functions of nurses and auxiliary nurses and changing nursing home regulations could have a smoothing effect on the shortages (Geets 2008, Jacobs 2007).

6.3 *Factors within the system influencing size and composition of the health workforce*

Educational system

Oversupply led Belgium to introduce the *numerus clausus* system in order to limit the number of graduates with access to the practice of medicine and dentistry (see section 8.2). Quotas set the maximum number of graduates allowed to start general practitioner, specialist and dentistry training each year. For 2008–2011, the quota allows 757 medical graduates to pursue general practitioner or specialist training (Government of Belgium 2008a). The number of dentistry graduates allowed to practise was limited to 140 per year until 2010 (Government of Belgium 2008b).

In the Flemish Community, almost 10% of those who passed the entrance examination for medical/dentistry studies in 2007 had Dutch nationality (Janssen 2007).[10] Similarly, during the 2007–2008 academic year around 7% of medical and 19.5% of dentistry students in the French Community were French nationals with a non-Belgian secondary education diploma (Cref 2008, FOD Volksgezondheid 2007a).

The number of students with foreign basic medical diplomas who submit training plans in Belgium increases every year in both the French and the Flemish communities. In 2007, foreign-trained graduates started medical internships amounting to 10% of all internships initiated that year, in comparison to only 6.6% of all training plans submitted in Belgium between 2004 and 2006 (SPF Santé publique 2007). Holders of foreign diplomas are not subject to the *numerus clausus* and thus not included in the federal quotas (FOD Volksgezondheid 2007b).

---

10 The number of Dutch medicine and dentistry students in Flemish universities decreased by one third between 1996 and 2005, presumably due to the introduction of the quota system in Belgium (Nuffic 2007).

Foreign students apply almost exclusively for specialization rather than general practitioner training (SPF Santé publique 2007).

There are no restrictions in access to nursing training which can be studied at secondary level or at post-secondary/bachelor level. During the 2007–2008 academic year, 16% of all enrolled post-secondary nursing students and 40% of all enrolled secondary level nursing students in the French Community were not registered as Belgian residents (Service statistique de l'ETNIC unpublished data 2009). French nationals accounted for 95% and 98% respectively of those non-resident students (Service statistique de l'ETNIC unpublished data 2009). It is likely that most of the French nationals who study in Belgium without being officially registered as residents practise in France after graduation.

Quotas limit the number of physiotherapists registered with the statutory health insurance system, but only for outpatient practice. The number of physiotherapists working in nursing homes and hospitals is not subject to limitations.[11] Unlike doctors, candidate physiotherapists with a recognized or equivalent foreign diploma are included in the physiotherapists' quota.

Similar to the situation for nurses, there are extremely high proportions of French-national physiotherapy and paramedical students in the French Community. In 2006, 74.4% of physiotherapy students in higher education institutions and 78.1% of those studying physiotherapy at the university were students officially residing abroad, mainly in France. The same was true for 68.2% of podiatry, 59.5% of speech therapy and 63.2% of midwifery students (Simonet 2006a). This is due to the educational quotas in France (Simonet 2006a & 2006b) and relatively low registration fees in Belgium (France 3.fr 2009). In 2006, this caused the French Community to introduce a 30% quota for non-residents enrolling for the first time on certain medical and paramedical curricula in a higher education institution within its territory (Ministère de la Communauté française 2006, Simonet 2006a). The introduction of this quota has been justified by evoking possible shortages in some professions (Simonet 2006a & 2006b).

The impact on the education budget produced by such significant numbers of non-resident foreigners studying in Belgium probably also played a role in the introduction of these limits. The European Commission challenged the quota measure in an infringement procedure. This was subsequently suspended as the Commission accepted that, without an appropriate safeguard measure, the French Community would not be able to maintain a sufficient level of territorial coverage and quality in its public health-care system (Europa 2007). In case C-73/08, the European Court of Justice ruled that such legislation is

---

11 Interview with Henk Vandenbroele, civil servant from the FPS Health, Food chain safety and Environment, Brussels, November 2009.

precluded by the Treaties "unless the referring court … finds that it is justified in the light of the objective of protection of public health" (Court of Justice of the European Union 2010).

Demographics

The medical and dental professions are ageing rapidly. In 2005, 47.7% of practising general practitioners and 46.2% of practising specialists were aged over 50 years. Activity levels (expressed as the number of patient contacts per year) decrease gradually from 50 years onwards for general practitioners and from 60 years onwards for specialists (Roberfroid et al. 2008). The 42–56 age group is heavily overrepresented among active dentists. Many dentists stop practising from the age of 55 onwards and activity levels decrease among those who remain active (Gobert et al. 2007). Most medical doctors and dentists are self-employed and therefore have no legal retirement age.

Women comprise 30% of the current medical workforce and 60% of new graduates (Roberfroid et al. 2008). Among female doctors over 30, both general practitioners and specialists have significantly lower activity levels than their male counterparts. Women comprise 43% of active dentists and the majority of newly qualified dentists. The activity rate of female dentists is about 75% of that of their male peers (Gobert et al. 2007). The gender ratio of immigrating medical doctors appears close to one and they are markedly younger than the average age of domestic medical doctors (FOD Volksgezondheid 2009). The ageing and feminization of the medical workforce could reinforce the expected shortages of general practitioners. No such problems are forecasted for the other medical professionals discussed in this chapter, given their current oversupply.

Nursing is considered to be a heavy profession and therefore most nurses have the right to take early retirement from the age of 58. This results in nurses over 60 years comprising less than 1% of the total nursing workforce (Pacolet & Merckx 2006c). Furthermore, nurses aged 45 years or more have the right to reduce their working hours progressively by up to 15%.

As of 31 December 2008, the Federal Database of Health Care Professionals shows that 87% of the holders of a licence to practise nursing are women, with a median age of 44 years. Nurses have high attrition rates, especially those aged 50 and over (Geets 2008). The fact that the profession is highly feminized impacts strongly on labour volume as reduced working time, career breaks, parental leaves etc. are more common among female professionals (Pacolet & Merckx 2006d). It is estimated that nurses work an average of 75% of a full-time working schedule (Pacolet & Merckx 2006d).

Health professionals leaving or returning to the profession

Only 53.3% of registered general practitioners practise medicine and only an estimated 5 500 (43%) of these work full time as general practitioners (Meeus 2009). Between 65.4% and 87.4% of registered specialists work full time but activity levels vary between specialities. Other registered medical doctors work in non-curative sectors (Roberfroid et al. 2008). The number of practising general practitioners decreased from 12 531 to 11 626 between 2002 and 2005, possibly the result of significant professional attrition rates. Suggested factors include long working schedules and/or low earnings (Roberfroid et al. 2008).

6.4 *What does cross-border mobility mean for Belgium?*

While migration flows in some health professions are not negligible, most appear to be the initiative of individuals looking for opportunities elsewhere.

Intentional recruitment of foreign-trained health professionals by Belgian hospitals has been observed for nurses and for medical doctors with basic training (see section 8.3). There are no elements to assert that the Belgian health system has any dependency on migratory flows and no indication of any negative effects from the workforce lost from emigration.

7. Factors influencing health professional mobility

7.1 *Facilitating factors*

Language and geographical proximity appear as the crucial facilitating factors for any group of health professionals. In the case of outflows from Belgium, there is no language barrier for Dutch-speaking professionals migrating to the Netherlands or for French-speaking professionals willing to practise in France. The relatively important inflows of Romanian professionals are facilitated because Romanian is a Romance language[12] and the country has traditional ties with the *Francophonie*. The latter is also true for Lebanon. The recent important inflow of Lebanese nurses with a post-secondary diploma, apparent in the French Community equivalence statistics, comprises graduates of a French-speaking nursing bachelor course organized in Lebanon (Geets 2008). It is suggested that French-speaking hospitals in Brussels turned to Lebanese nurses after Romanian nurses experienced language difficulties (Metro 2008).

7.2 *Activating factors*

Standard activating factors include perceived opportunities of personal

---

12 Rocour 2006a and interviews with Romanian specializing doctors working in Belgian hospitals.

development; competence diversification; and horizontal and vertical career opportunities that can be linked either to national differences in work styles or to particularities of the destination institution (Van Den Heuvel et al. 2007). Partner-like and less formal relations between nurses and doctors are commonly cited as activating factors for Belgian nurses seeking employment in the Netherlands (Nursing voor verpleegkundigen 2006).[13] Employers also appeal to potential employees by offering in-service training opportunities[14] or work in specialized care units (and thus learning opportunities and higher incomes). Romanian doctors specializing in Belgium underscore that Belgian hospitals provide specialized care for which there are no expertise centres in Romania (e.g. treatment of the neurovegetative state).[15]

Income and pension differentials remain among the key activating factors for Belgian nurses migrating to the Netherlands.[16] However, Belgian health professionals working in the Netherlands often choose to live in Belgium and commute, whether for family reasons, lower housing prices or specific social benefits.[17] Although it was not mentioned during the interviews, it is likely that financial motives are also significant for Romanian doctors coming to Belgium, particularly those recruited by private companies.[18]

7.3 *Instigating factors*

The surplus of specialists is cited as the main instigating factor encouraging Belgian specialists (mainly from the French Community) to migrate to France (Anrys 2009). Significant variation in the activity levels of specialists (Roberfroid et al. 2008) does suggest oversupply and this would impact on income as specialists are generally self-employed.

Literature cites potential instigating and activating factors for Belgian-trained general practitioners considering migration to the Netherlands – the past shortage of general practitioners in the Netherlands and the simultaneous surplus observed in Belgium (Van Den Heuvel et al. 2007); financial motivations; differences in both status and working conditions; and work style or, more generally, cultural differences. Despite these potential instigating/activating factors, and efforts to attract Flemish general practitioners to the

---

13 Interview with Belgian nurse working in azM, Maastricht, 2 July 2009.

14 In-service training allows nurses with a secondary level certificate to obtain a bachelor diploma in nursing or to specialize. BBL (*Beroeps Begeleidende Leerweg*) programmes combine three or four days of practical employment with one or two days of paid theoretical courses per week, allowing the student to acquire a diploma mainly through experience.

15 Interview with Romanian medical doctor with basic training working in Belgium, July 2009

16 Interview with Belgian nurse working in the azM, Maastricht, 2 July 2009.

17 Interview with Belgian nurse working in the azM, Maastricht, 2 July 2009.

18 Recruitment companies often promise Romanian candidates that they will be able to top up their income by working as on call physician as often as possible. Interview with Romanian doctor with basic training working in Belgium, July 2009.

Netherlands (Van Den Heuvel et al. 2007), inflow data from the Dutch authorities show that surprisingly few Belgian general practitioners migrated to the Netherlands (Ministry of Health, Welfare and Sport unpublished data 2009). This could indicate potential mitigating factors. General practitioners tend to be more embedded in the local community and this could explain the important difference between the low outflows of general practitioners and the much higher outflows of specialists (see section 2.1).

8. Policy, regulation and interventions

8.1 *Policies and policy development on health professional mobility*

No public policy at federal or regional level that specifically aims at encouraging or discouraging health professional migration has been reported.

8.2 *Workforce planning and development*

Belgium has had explicit health workforce planning policies since 1996, when the Committee for Medical Supply Planning (*Commission de planification médicale*) was established to advise the federal authorities on a quota system (Government of Belgium 1967). The committee comprises representatives of the public authorities, relevant health professions, experts and other stakeholders. Following the committee's advice, in 1997 a quota for training places was introduced at federal level for medical doctors and further extended to dentists and physiotherapists (see section 6.3). The committee's remit also covers nursing, midwifery and speech therapy.

A specific register to centralize data on health-care professionals was set up in 2003 in order to provide the Committee for Medical Supply Planning with necessary information on the current medical workforce (Government of Belgium 1967). The Federal Database of Health Care Professionals gathers information on professionals of all regulated health professions.

A mathematical model is used to forecast future supplies of medical doctors, dentists, physiotherapists and nurses (FOD Volksgezondheid 2009). This is intended to support the Committee for Medical Supply Planning in assessing the needs and sustainability of the system in order to determine health workforce planning policies. This stock-flow model should take account of the numbers, gender and age of foreign-trained health-care professionals migrating to Belgium as well as the outflows of Belgium-trained graduates. However, the outflows have not been included in simulations to date as the Belgian authorities lack complete data on emigration (FOD Volksgezondheid 2009).

8.3 *Cross-border regulatory frameworks and interventions*

Mutual recognition of diplomas in the European Community

Chapter 4 of the Belgian law on the exercise of the health professions specifies the means by which the EC mutual recognition directive was implemented in May 2005 (Government of Belgium 1967). The provisions of this chapter are extended to third-country nationals with qualifications that conform with the directive. Professional qualifications that fall under the scope of the directive must be recognized by the Health Minister. Authorities can ask for a document certifying that the candidate's qualifications are in compliance (a conformity certificate) and this is a systematic requirement for professionals from new Member States.[19] Professions that are recognized automatically are granted recognition when the authenticity and conformity of the documents have been verified, up to three months after the complete file has been introduced. For nurses, the recognition distinguishes between secondary level and post-secondary level diplomas.[20]

The Belgian system distinguishes between nurses with secondary-level education,[21] nurses with post-secondary/bachelor-level education[22] and assistant nurses.[23] All three diplomas meet the criteria for nursing diplomas listed in the EC directive and holders of these three types of diplomas are granted the same conformity certificates. Belgian law allows all three categories of nurses to perform the same functions, with two exceptions: (i) nursing assistants are not allowed to undertake work delegated by a doctor; and (ii) only nurses with post-secondary level diplomas can specialize. There are also de facto differences as hospitals generally prefer to hire nurses with bachelor-level diplomas and nursing homes are staffed predominantly by nurses with secondary-level diplomas.

For diplomas that fall outside the automatic recognition procedure, the FPS Health, Food chain safety and Environment additionally enquires whether the applicant complies with all the conditions on professional training and experience stipulated in the EC directive and defined in a Belgian Ministerial Decree. The FPS Health, Food chain safety and Environment have one month (two in exceptional cases) to inform the applicant about the results of the verification procedure. The professionals meeting the requirements are granted recognition within four months. Specialist and specialist nursing diplomas that do

---

19 Interview with competent civil servant, FPS Health, Food chain safety and Environment, Brussels, 7 July 2009.

20 Competent civil servant said that authorities make this distinction because Belgian employers want to know whether a foreign diploma corresponds to secondary or post-secondary level. Further, if no distinction was made, employers would recruit all foreign-trained candidates as if they held secondary-level diplomas and pay them (less) accordingly.

21 Infirmières brevetées/gebrevetterde verpleegkundigen.

22 Infirmières graduées/gegradueerde verpleegkundigen.

23 Aides-soignantes/verpleegassistenten.

not fall under the automatic recognition procedure must be recognized by the competent recognition commission (comprising representatives of the relevant profession).

As foreseen by the EC directive, EU nationals who are legally established in other EEA countries can provide health services in Belgium on a temporary and occasional basis without the recognition, licence to practice and registration. However, they are required to apply for provisional licences to practise. Before the first provision of care, these professionals must give written notice informing the FPS Health, Food chain safety and Environment of their intentions and provide information on their professional liability insurance. In practice, it appears that some health professionals do not apply for this provisional licence to practise.[24]

Fig. 2.4 *Recognition or equivalence route for medical doctors, dentists or nurses with EEA nationality*

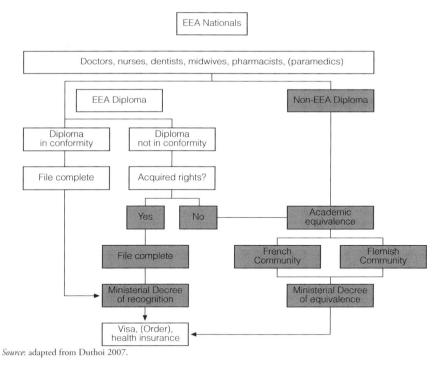

Source: adapted from Duthoi 2007.

Bilateral agreements

A bilateral agreement signed with South Africa in 1965 establishes a system of mutual recognition of basic medical diplomas and has been in use for 40 years (Government of Belgium 1970).

---

24 Interview with the competent civil servant, FPS Health, Food chain safety and Environment, Brussels, 7 July 2009·

Third-country health professionals

A qualification that does not conform to the EC directive must be declared equivalent by the French or the Flemish Community. Furthermore, third-country nationals with a non-EU diploma must obtain a Royal Decree before applying for a licence to practise and registering with the competent order. Applications from doctors, dentists and pharmacists are also submitted to the competent Royal Academy.

Doctors and nurses are granted equivalences only for the basic medical/nursing diploma. In addition, specializations must be recognized by the competent federal recognition commission. In practice, such recognitions are very rare.[25]

Belgian law allows foreign-trained non-EEA medical graduates to undertake part of their specialization in Belgium. This is conditional upon a signed declaration of their commitment to return to their country of origin on completion of the assigned training period (Government of Belgium 1967).

Fig. 2.5 *Recognition or equivalence route for medical doctors, dentists or nurses with non-EEA nationality*

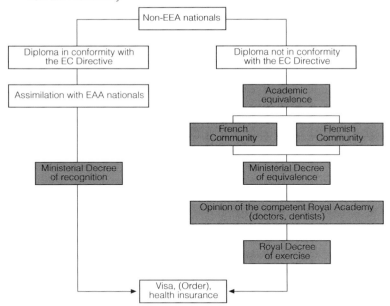

Source: adapted from Duthoi 2007.

Specific interventions and managerial tools

Some hospitals recruit nursing staff by setting up exchange programmes with foreign schools or by using the services of liaison or temporary work agencies that recruit abroad. Several Brussels hospitals have used this method to hire

25 Interview with competent civil servant, FPS Health, Food chain safety and Environment, Brussels, 7 July 2009.

Romanian or Lebanese nurses (Metro 2008). In 2005 the University Hospital of Antwerp (UZA) hosted several Polish nursing students and, more recently, nurses from the Philippines (Vandaag.be 2009). Such private companies provide Belgian hospitals not only with nurses but also with specializing foreign medical doctors who are willing to work as assistants in Belgium (Anrys 2009, Geets 2008).[26]

Private companies not only recruit in the country of origin but often also arrange travel, accommodation and administrative requirements (such as residence permit, diploma recognition/equivalence) for their recruits. Hospitals that have hosted or recruited foreign-trained nurses evaluate these experiences overall as positive or mixed, mentioning communication difficulties due to insufficient command of their hospital's working language (Metro 2008).

An HR manager at the azM reports that the hospital would not survive without recruiting nurses from Belgium – situated near the border it employs 400 Belgian nurses (in a total of 1100). Hence, the azM collaborates closely with the Flemish Public Employment and Vocational Training Service (VDAB) and publishes recruitment adverts in the Dutch-speaking Belgian local, national and specialized press.[27]

Certain Belgian hospitals recruit foreign doctors with basic training for less attractive tasks, mainly on-call duties (Geets 2008). Often, these duties are funded from the pooled income of a hospital's medical doctors who therefore tend to prefer the lower cost of trainee doctors. Some hospitals claim that they are not assigned enough Belgium-trained interns following the introduction of the quota system as the *numerus clausus* limits the number of doctors eligible to specialize (Rocour 2005) (see section 8.4).

In 1990, the French-speaking UCL and the Romanian University of Medicine and Pharmacy (UMF) "Gr. T. Popa" Iaşi signed an agreement allowing Romanian doctors with basic training to spend one year (potentially extendable to two years) of their specialization in one of UCL's hospitals. Each year, this agreement brings around 70 third or fourth year Romanian medical students to Belgium. By 2009, some 450 Romanian interns had taken part in the programme.[28] Before Romania's accession to the EU, participants could undertake part of their specialization in Belgium, under the responsibility of a qualified doctor, without obtaining equivalence of their diploma and a licence to practise (see section 8.3).[29] Some other hospitals signed similar cooperation agreements with foreign training institutions. For example, a university hospital in Liège signed such

---

26 Phone interview with specialist working in a rural hospital in southern Belgium, 14 July 2009.

27 Interview with Belgian nurse working in the azM, Maastricht, 2 July 2009.

28 Interview with Philippe Meert, Brussels, 13 July 2009.

29 The legal basis for such practices was art. 49 ter, Royal Decree No.78.

an agreement with a Vietnamese hospital (Janssens 2006) and the French-speaking University of Brussels runs the Fonds de Soutien à la Formation Médicale (FOSFOM) scholarship programme.[30]

8.4 *Political force field of regulating and managing health professional mobility*

Professional associations in Belgium generally disapprove of the recruitment of foreign nurses and medical interns, rejecting hospitals' shortage arguments (Vandaag.be 2009). They argue that migrant professionals accept less favourable working conditions (Rocour 2006a & 2006b) that could potentially lead to social dumping. Hospitals experimenting with the recruitment of foreign professionals are much less sceptical and declare that they are well aware of the short-term character of such solutions (Rocour 2006a).[31]

Simultaneously with the decision to lift transition periods for the citizens of the eastern European Member States that joined the EU in 2004, the Belgian federal Minister for Migration and Asylum Policy evoked migration as a way of alleviating nurses' shortages, probably in order to make the opening of the Belgian labour market more acceptable to the public (Turtelboom 2009).

Belgian medical associations cite the numerically significant outflows of specialists to France as an illustration of the oversupply of specialists in Belgium, especially in the French Community. These are used to refute arguments for an increase in the training places allowed by the quota system or even to push for stricter quotas (Anrys 2009). Several parliamentary questions have linked the recently increasing foreign inflows of medical doctors with basic training and the quotas preventing numerous graduates with a Belgian diploma from pursuing a specialization (Brotchi 2008, Van Ermen 2009). Thus, the issue of foreign inflows is used to regenerate debate on the quota system.

The linguistic capacities of the Romanian nurses and doctors with basic training recruited by bilingual hospitals in Brussels have also been the subject of parliamentary debate. At both federal and regional level, Flemish Members of Parliament have criticized the fact that these professionals are unable to speak Dutch (Vanackere 2006, Van Linter 2006). The debate on professional mobility has thus become part of the Belgo-Belgian discussion. The generally insufficient Dutch language skills of health professionals (whether Belgian or foreign) working in Brussels' bilingual hospitals has long been a very sensitive political issue (Gatz et al. 2005).

---

30 http://www.ulb.ac.be/facs/medecine/fosfom/, accessed 15 July 2009.

31 See section on specific interventions and managerial tools.

9. Conclusion

Based on the figures obtained for this study, it can be can be concluded that migration flows to and from Belgium are numerically significant in most health professions. However, mobility does not constitute a health workforce planning issue for the moment. The most important flows are observed to and from neighbouring countries, in particular France and the Netherlands. Inflows of foreign-trained health professionals in 2005–2008 represented 5% of all new general practitioner registrations; 10% of new specialist registrations; 9% of newly licensed nurses; 15% of newly licensed dentists and a remarkable 20% of newly registered medical doctors with basic training. Outflows of specialists with Belgian diplomas, especially to France, are seriously exceeding inflows of specialists with foreign diplomas. This may be explained by an oversupply of specialists in the French Community. Stock data for 2008 show that 10.5% of medical doctors, 4.4% of nurses and 6.1% of dentists registered in Belgium were foreign nationals.

Inflows appear to be increasing in all professions over recent years, mainly due to migration from neighbouring countries and from Romania. The increase in inflows from Romania is attributable mainly to the migration of medical doctors with basic training. The national quota system means that hospitals receive fewer specializing Belgian medical doctors and try to compensate for this by hiring foreign-trained doctors with basic training. It is too early to assess the stability of these inflows. Hospitals (mainly French-speaking) recruit foreign-trained nurses to alleviate shortages in nursing staff. Recent inflows of Lebanese and Romanian nurses recorded by the French Community have been noticeably higher than in previous years but still appear negligible when estimated as a proportion of the average yearly number of nurses newly licensed to practise in Belgium.

The significant number of foreign (especially French) nursing students could aggravate the shortages in nursing staff, since most of these students are likely to return to their home countries after graduation. The high proportion of foreign students in Belgian medical and paramedical facilities calls for attention to the potential negative consequences for health workforce planning policies in their countries of origin if students choose to study in Belgium in order to avoid domestic enrolment quotas. Furthermore, foreign candidates are not counted in the Belgian quotas that limit candidate specialists' access to further training. This could have a negative impact on Belgian health workforce planning policies.

Overall, migration flows seem rather natural as Belgium is a country with generally high levels of individual and professional mobility – a country with permeable borders.[32] However, recent developments indicate that this requires close monitoring.

References

Anrys H (2009). *Numerus clausus. Le nombre de spécialistes qui quittent la Belgique correspond à un manque de postes.* Official note for the ABSyM-BVAS, Belgian Association of Medical Trade Unions, 16 January 2009.

Brotchi J (2008). Oral question No. 4-224 to the Federal Minister for Social Affairs and Public Health, Laurette Onkelinx. *Annales* No. 4-25. Brussels, Belgian Senate, 17 April 2008 (http://www.senate.be/www/?MIval=/publications/viewPubDoc&TID =67110623&LANG=fr, accessed 20 December 2010).

Cref (2008). *Annuaire statistique 2008* (http://www.cref.be/Annuaire_2008.htm, accessed 20 December 2010).

Court of Justice of the European Union (2010). Nicholas Bressol and others, Céline Chaverot and others v. Gouvernement de la Communauté francaise. Case C-73/08 (http://eur-lex.europa.eu/LexUriServ/LexUriServ.do?uri=CELEX:62008J0073:EN: NOT, accessed 14 February 2011).

De Morgen (2007). Nederlanders lokken Belgische psychiaters met belastingvoordeel [The Dutch attract Belgian pyschiatrists with fiscal advantages]. *De Morgen,* 5 March 2007.

Duthoi I (2007). Application des directives européennes pour la reconnaissance des diplômes des professionnels de la santé. *Human Resources in Health Care Symposium, Brussels, 10 March 2007.*

Europa (2007). Access to higher education: the Commission suspends its infringement cases against Austria and Belgium. *Europa,* Press release 28 November 2007 (http://europa.eu/rapid/pressReleasesAction.do? reference=IP/07/1788&format=HTML&aged=1&language=EN&guiLanguage=en, accessed 22 November 2010).

European Parliament and Council of the European Union (2005). Directive 2005/36/EC of the European Parliament and of the Council of 7 September 2005 on the recognition of professional qualifications. *Official Journal of the European Union*, 255(48):22–142.

Eurostat (2010). Population of foreign citizens in the EU27 in 2009: Foreign citizens made up 6.4% of the EU27 population. *Eurostat,* Press release

---

32 In 2008, Belgium's total population included 9.1% of foreigners, 6.2% of whom were citizens of other EU Member States (Eurostat 2010).

7 September 2010 (http://epp.eurostat.ec.europa.eu/cache/ITY_PUBLIC/3-07092010-AP/EN/3-07092010-AP-EN.PDF, accessed 20 December 2010).

FOD Volksgezondheid (2007a). *De planning van het medisch aanbod in België: tandartsen, Statusrapport 2006* [*Medical supply planning in Belgium: dentists*]. Brussels, FOD Volksgezondheid, Veiligheid van de Voedselketen en Leefmilieu, Directoraat-generaal Basisgezondheidszorg en Crisisbeheer [Federal Public Service Health, Food chain safety and Environment, Directorate-general Basic Healthcare and Crisis Management].

FOD Volksgezondheid (2007b). Planning van het medisch aanbod in België: artsen. Statusrapport 2006 [*Medical supply planning in Belgium: doctors*]. Brussels, FOD Volksgezondheid, Veiligheid van de Voedselketen en Leefmilieu, Directoraat-generaal Basisgezondheidszorg en Crisisbeheer [Federal Public Service Health, Food chain safety and Environment, Directorate-general Basic Healthcare and Crisis Management].

FOD Volksgezondheid (2007c). *Rapport betreffende het aantal gevallen artikel 49ter van het Koninklijk Besluit nr. 78 voor de jaren 2004–2006* [*Report on the application of article 49 of RD No. 78 in 2004–2006*]. Brussels, FOD Volksgezondheid, Veiligheid van de Voedselketen en Leefmilieu, Directoraat-generaal Basisgezondheidszorg en Crisisbeheer [Federal Public Service Health, Food chain safety and Environment, Directorate-general Basic Healthcare and Crisis Management].

FOD Volksgezondheid (2009). *Basisscenario Rapport Artsen 2009* [*Simulation scenario: doctors 2009*]. Brussels, FOD Volksgezondheid, Veiligheid van de Voedselketen en Leefmilieu, Directoraat-generaal Basisgezondheidszorg en Crisisbeheer.

France 3.fr (2009). Des étudiants étrangers en Belgique. *France 3. Info Champagne-Ardenne*, 29 September 2009 (http://lorraine-champagne-ardenne.france3.fr/info/ champagne-ardenne/Des-%C3%A9tudiants-%C3%A9trangers-en-Belgique-57668564.html accessed 20 December 2010).

Gatz S et al. (2005). *Drie jaar Raad van Europa over Brusselse ziekenhuizen. Het Actieplan & Terugblik* [*Three years of Council of Europe on Brussels hospitals. The action plan and retrospection*]. [Memorandum] (http://www.gatz.be/documents / raadvaneuropa.pdf, accessed 22 December 2009).

Geets J (2008). *Medisch en verpleegkundig personeel met buitenlands diploma en/ of herkomst in België: een kwantitatieve en kwalitatieve verkenning* [*Medical and nursing workforce with a foreign diploma and/or of foreign origin: a quantitative and qualitative exploration*]. Antwerp, Steunpunt Gelijkekansenbeleid [Flemish Equal Chances Policy Support Point].

Gobert M et al. (2007). *Offre et besoins en soins dentaires: Perspectives d'avenir. Rapport de synthèse.* Louvain-la-Neuve, UCL-Ecole de santé publique, SESA-Socio-Economie de la Santé and KUL-HIVA.

Government of Belgium (1967). Arrêté royal n° 78 relatif à l'exercice des professions des soins de santé [Royal Decree No. 78 of 10 November 1967 on the practise of healthcare professions]. *Moniteur belge*, 14 November 1967.

Government of Belgium (1970). Accord du Cap entre le Gouvernement du Royaume de Belgique et le Gouvernement de la République d'Afrique du Sud du 25 mai 1965 relatif à l'admission réciproque de médecins à la pratique [Agreement concluded on 25 May 1965 in Cape Town between the Kingdom of Belgium and the Republic of South Africa, concerning the mutual recognition of medical doctors' right to practise medicine]. *Moniteur belge*, 11 July 1970.

Government of Belgium (2004). Arrêté royal modifiant, suite à l'adhésion de nouveaux Etats membres à l'Union européenne, l'arrêté royal du 9 juin 1999 portant exécution de la loi du 30 avril 1999 relative à l'occupation des travailleurs étrangers [Royal Decree of 12 April 2004 modifying, due to the accession of new Member States, the Royal Decree of 9 June 1999 executing the Law of 30 April 1999 on the professional activities of foreign workers]. *Moniteur belge*, 21 April 2004.

Government of Belgium (2006a). Arrêté royal modifiant l'arrêté royal du 9 juin 1999 portant exécution de la loi du 30 avril 1999 relative à l'occupation des travailleurs étrangers, en vue de la prolongation des mesures transitoires qui ont été introduites suite à l'adhésion de nouveaux Etats membres à l'Union européenne [Royal Decree of 24 April 2006 modifying the Royal Decree of 9 June 1999 executing the Law of 30 April 1999 on the professional activities of foreign workers, with a view to extend the transitional measures introduced with the accession of new Member States to the EU]. *Moniteur belge*, 28 April 2006.

Government of Belgium (2006b). Bericht over de vaststelling van de lijst van beroepen voor versoepelde procedure van arbeidskaarten in het Vlaamse Gewest ter uitvoering van het koninklijk besluit van 21 april 2006 tot wijziging van het koninklijk besluit van 9 juni 1999 houdende uitvoering van de wet van 30 april 1999 betreffende de tewerkstelling van buitenlandse werknemers, naar aanleiding van de verlenging van de overgangsbepalingen die werden ingevoerd bij de toetreding van nieuwe lidstaten tot de Europese Unie [Message on the definition of the list of professions for relaxed procedure for work permits in the Flemish Region, in execution of the RD of 21 April 2006 modifying the RD of 9 June 1999 concerning the execution law of 30 April 1999 on the professional activities of foreign workers, with a view to extend the transitional measures introduced with the accession of new Member States to the EU]. *Moniteur belge*, 18 May 2006.

Government of Belgium (2008a). Arrêté royal relatif à la planification de l'offre médicale [Royal Decree of 12 June 2008 on medical workforce planning]. *Moniteur belge*, 18 June 2008.

Government of Belgium (2008b). Arrêté royal portant modification de l'arrêté royal du 25 avril 2007 relatif à la planification de l'offre de l'art dentaire [Royal Decree of 28 November 2008 on dentistry workforce planning]. *Moniteur belge*, 12 December 2008.

Government of Belgium (2008c). Arrêté royal modifiant l'arrêté royal du 9 juin 1999 portant exécution de la loi du 30 avril 1999 relative à l'occupation des travailleurs étrangers en vue de la prolongation des mesures transitoires qui ont été introduites suite à l'adhésion de la Bulgarie et de la Roumanie à l'Union européenne [Royal Decree of 18 December 2008 modifying the Royal Decree of 9 June 1999 executing the Law of 30 April 1999 on the professional activities of foreign workers, with a view to extend the transitional measures introduced with the accession of Romania and Bulgaria to the EU, *Moniteur belge*, 30 December 2008].

Jacobs M (2007). *Impact van de vergrijzing op het tekort aan verpleegkundigen. Arbeidsmigratie: een oplossing?* [*Impact of the ageing population on the shortage of nurses. Labour migration: a solution?*] [Master's thesis]. Antwerp, Universiteit Antwerpen, Faculteit Politieke & Sociale Wetenschappen.

Janssen PJ (2007). Vlaanderens toelatingsexamen arts-tandarts [Flanders' entry examination for candidate medicine and dentistry students]. *Tijdschrift voor geneeskunde* [*Medicine Periodical*], 62(22):1579–1581.

Janssens P (2006). Trois questions à Michel Meurisse. Accords bilatéraux avec Ho Chi Minh Ville (HCMV) au Vietnam. *Le 15e jour du mois*, No. 152 (http://www2.ulg.ac.be/le15jour/Archives/152/troisquestions.shtml, accessed 22 November 2010

Le Breton-Lerouvillois G (2007). *Les médecins de nationalité européenne et extra-européenne en France*. Paris, Conseil national de l'Ordre des Médecins.

Le Breton-Lerouvillois G (2009). *Atlas de la démographie médicale en France: Situation au 1er janvier 2009*. Paris, Conseil national de l'Ordre des Médecins.

Meeus P (2009). Optimalisering van het kadaster: wat kunnen we wel of niet verwachten van de informatie die beschikbaar is bij het RIZIV omtrent activiteit? [Optimalization of the medical register: what can we expect from the NIHDI activity information?]. Presentation at the symposium: Towards an Evidence-based Workforce Planning in Health Care? Brussels, 25 April 2009.

Metro (2008). Les infirmières étrangères, une solution? *Metro*, 2 February 2008 (http://www.vandaag.be/binnenland/20015_zna-trekt-verpleegkundigen-aan-uit-de-filipijnen.html#, accessed 8 December 2009).

Ministère de la Communauté française (2006). Décret régulant le nombre d'étudiants dans certains cursus de premier cycle de l'enseignement supérieur. Moniteur belge [Belgian official journal], 6 July 2006.

NIHDI (2010). *Impulseo I - Financement pour l'installation des médecins généralistes.* Brussels, National Institute for Health and Disability Insurance (http://www.riziv.be/care/fr/doctors/specific-information/impulseo/index_ impulseoI.htm, accessed 20 December 2010).

Nuffic (2007). *Vlaanderen in trek bij Nederlandse student* [*Flanders attracting Dutch students*]. The Hague, Nederlandse organisatie voor internationale samenwerking in het hoger onderwijs [Netherlands Organization for International Cooperation in Higher Education (http://www.nuffic.nl/nederlandse-organisaties/nieuws-evenementen/nieuws-archief/nieuws-archief-2007/juni/vlaanderen-in-trek-bij-nederlandse-student, accessed 20 December 2010).

Nursing voor verpleegkundigen (2006). Vlaamse verpleegkundigen vluchten naar Nederland [Flemish nurses flee to the Netherlands]. *Nursing voor verpleegkundigen* [*Nursing for nurses*], 9 June 2006 (http://www.nursing.nl/home/nieuw/157/vlaamse-verpleegkundigen-vluchten-naar-nederland, accessed 14 July 2009).

OECD (2008). *Share of foreign-trained or foreign nurses in selected OECD countries in 2008.* Paris, Organisation for Economic Co-operation and Development (http://www.oecd.org/dataoecd/8/0/44783714.xls, accessed 22 November 2010).

Pacolet J, Merckx S (2006c). *Het planningsmodel verpleegkunde en vroedkunde: vraag en aanbod* [*The planning model for nursing and midwifery: demand and supply*]. Brussels/Leuven/Louvain-la-Neuve, FOD Volksgezondheid, Veiligheid van de Voedselketen en Leefmilieu [Federal Public Service Health, Food chain safety and Environment], HIVA-K.U.Leuven and SESA-UCL..

Pacolet J, Merckx S (2006d). Manpowerplanning voor de verpleegkunde en vroedkunde in België: synthese [*Workforce planning in nursing and midwifery in Belgium: synthesis*]. Brussels/Leuven, FOD Volksgezondheid, Veiligheid van de Voedselketen en Leefmilieu [Federal Public Service Health, Food chain safety and Environment], HIVA-K.U.Leuven and SESA-UCL).

Roberfroid D et al. (2008). Het aanbod van artsen in België. Huidige toestand en toekomstige uitdagingen [*Physician workforce supply in Belgium: current situation and challenges*]. Brussels, Federaal Kenniscentrum voor de

Gezondheidszorg [Belgian Health Care Knowledge Centre](KCE Reports No.72A).

Rocour V (2005). Ces médecins venus d'ailleurs. *La Libre Belgique*, 15 February 2005 (http://www.lalibre.be/actu/belgique/article/206369/ces-medecins-venus-d-ailleurs.html, accessed 22 November 2010).

Rocour V (2006a). Des infirmières recrutées en Roumanie. *La Libre Belgique*, 28 April 2006 (http://www.lalibre.be/actu/belgique/article/283141/des-infirmieres-recrutees -en-roumanie.html, accessed 22 December 2009).

Rocour V (2006b). La Roumanie et son énorme réservoir de main-d'œuvre médicale. *La Libre Belgique*, 9 May 2006 (http://www.lalibre.be/actu/belgique/article/284787/la-roumanie-et-son-enorme-reservoir-de-main-d-oeuvre-medicale.html, accessed 22 December 2009).

Simonet M-D (2006a*). Avant-projet de décret régulant le nombre d'étudiants dans certaines filières: le Gouvernement poursuit la concertation.* Press release of the Minister for Higher Education of the Communauté française, 9 March 2006 (http://www.marie-do.be/ministrecommuniques2006-03-09.html, accessed 11 May 2009).

Simonet M-D (2006b). *Préserver un enseignement supérieur de qualité et de proximité pour les étudiants de la Communauté française: limitation à 30 % du nombre d'étudiants non-résidents.* Press release of the Minister for Higher Education of the Communauté française, 3 February 2006.

SPF Santé publique (2007). *Le nombre de plans de stage débutés au cours de la période 2004–2007.* Note à la Commission de planification – offre médicale. (Rapport annuel 2007, v. 1.0 FR).

Turtelboom A (2009). Economische migratie kan arbeidsdruk zorgsector helpen verlichten [Economic migration can help lift the pressure from the health sector workforce]. *De Morgen*, 8 June 2009.

Vanackere S (2006). Parliamentary question to the Flemish Minister for Employment, Education and Training Frank Vandenbroucke. Flemish Parliament, 3 May 2006 (Plenary noon meeting no. 41) (http://www.vlaamsparlement.be/Proteus5/ showJournaalLijn.action?id=449466&persId=2619, accessed 22 December 2009).

Vandaag.be (2009). ZNA trekt verpleegkundigen aan uit de Filipijnen [The ZNA attracts nurses from the Philippines]. *Vandaag.be*, 18 November 2009 (http://www.vandaag.be/binnenland/20015_zna-trekt-verpleegkundigen-aan-uit-de-filipijnen.html#, accessed 8 December 2009).

Van den Heuvel J et al. (2007). The migration of Flemish doctors to the Netherlands. *Eurohealth*, 13(3):12–16.

Van Ermen L (2009). Parliamentary question to the Federal Minister for Social Affairs and Public Health, Laurette Onkelinx. Belgian Senate, 12 February 2009 (http://www.senate.be/www/?MIval=/publications/viewPubDoc&TID=67113 198&LANG=fr, accessed 20 December 2010.

Van Linter G (2006). Parliamentary question to the Flemish Minister for Culture, Youth and Sport Bert Anciaux. Flemish Parliament, 3 May 2006 (Plenary noon meeting no. 41) (http://www.vlaamsparlement.be/Proteus5/showJournaalLijn.action? id=449466&persId=2619, accessed 20 December 2010).

Chapter 3

Cross-border mobility of health professionals in Finland

Hannamaria Kuusio, Meri Koivusalo, Marko Elovainio, Tarja Heponiemi,
Anna-Mari Aalto, Ilmo Keskimäki

1. Introduction

Traditionally, there has been little international mobility of health-care professionals in Finland. Inflows of foreign health professionals have been very small and Finland acted as a source country until the late 1990s, particularly for nurses who migrated in low numbers to other European (for example, Germany or the United Kingdom) and Nordic countries. However, there have been some changes in mobility patterns over the last 20 years. The country now has a mixed mobility profile as the outflows of health professionals have decreased and become comparable to the inflows. Moreover, foreign medical doctors and dentists represent important shares of all new arrivals to the medical workforce. This signals that the Finnish system could become dependent on the influx of health professionals from abroad – within a context of serious shortages, especially of general practitioners.

Migration policies in Finland have traditionally been formulated on humanitarian bases. However, in 2006 the government adopted a programme in which immigration was promoted in order to alleviate shortages in the Finnish labour market. The changing policy environment and labour shortages in the health-care sector have created new grounds for international recruitment of health professionals. Since 2006 the recruitment programmes for foreign health professionals have gained more attention as a measure for tackling workforce shortages in the health sector, especially in primary health care.

Since 2000, Finland has granted increasing numbers of licences to practise to health-care professionals of foreign origin, particularly medical doctors and dentists. However, not all who received a licence have migrated to Finland and not all of those who did migrate are employed in the health-care sector. Further studies are needed to examine the reasons for this and to develop effective practices to recruit and employ these health-care professionals who have the potential to become part of the active workforce.

The aim of this study is to assess the cross-border mobility patterns of medical doctors, nurses and dentists in Finland. The specific aims are to: (i) map the magnitude of professional mobility and identify critical data gaps and limitations; (ii) assess the contextual, health system and personal factors that influence professional mobility; and (iii) assess the impact of professional mobility. The overview of mobility among health professionals is based on a literature search, interviews and registers. Five Finnish national databases were searched.[1] In addition, senior experts on professional and workforce migration in government agencies were interviewed on the challenges and forthcoming actions regarding Finnish migration policies in the health sector. Data on the inflow and outflow of health professionals were obtained from the National Supervisory Authority for Welfare and Health (Valvira) and the employment statistics database maintained by Statistics Finland.

Limitations of the study

One limitation of this study concerns the datasets on health professional mobility that are available in Finland. Applications for residence permits in Finland do not include information on academic or vocational education. However, those wishing to practise in the health professions in Finland must apply for a licence from Valvira and this information was available to the study. The Valvira register on licensed health professionals covers all health professionals who have completed their vocational education outside Finland and then been granted a licence to practise in Finland. The register does not allow identification of the limited number of native Finns who have studied abroad and subsequently returned to work in Finland or those foreign licensed health professionals who have since left the country. Furthermore, the Valvira register covers only applications for licences and holds no information on those with a health-care education who do not apply for a licence to practise.

---

1 Using search terms for "mobility" or "immigration" or "emigration" AND "health care" AND "physician" or "registered nurse" or "dentist" or "public health nurse". Publication years ranged from 1990 to 2009.

2. Mobility profile of Finland

Traditionally Finland has been a source country for workforce migration. Nurses in particular have migrated from Finland to other Nordic countries such as Norway and Sweden. However, the direction of health professional mobility has changed and become more balanced over the last few years. Inflows of foreign-born health professionals have gradually increased (to some extent in line with the overall expansion of the health workforce) while outflows of Finnish-born health professionals have decreased. The country remains a source country, particularly for emigrating nurses, but has also become a destination for foreign medical doctors, nurses and dentists. In 2007, around 200 nurses and 50 medical doctors left the country; in 2008, 97 nurses and 135 medical doctors from abroad obtained a licence to practise in Finland. In 2006, foreign medical doctors, dentists and nurses represented between 2% and 7% of the total number of each profession in Finland, while around 5% of both medical doctors and nurses licensed in Finland worked abroad. The yearly inflows of medical doctors and dentists in particular represent important shares of total new arrivals to the medical workforce. This could indicate some dependency on migrating health professional

The term foreign-health professional is used to describe foreign-trained health professionals who have been granted a licence to practise their profession in Finland. They can be foreign nationals or foreign-born with Finnish nationality. Finnish nationality can be granted on the basis of application after living in Finland for at least five years.

2.1 *Inflows of health professionals*

While comparatively few health professionals have migrated to Finland, their relative importance in terms of new arrivals to the health workforce has been rising. Between 1980 and 2006, a total of 3499 foreign health professionals (1471 medical doctors, 228 dentists, 1800 nurses) obtained licences to practise in Finland (Statistics Finland unpublished data 2009). The number of foreign health professionals has remained small but has increased significantly over the last 20 years. In 1988, only one foreign medical doctor was licensed; 135 were licensed in 2008. Nine nurses and two dentists applied for licences in 1988; in 2008 the corresponding numbers were 97 and 20 (Valvira unpublished data 2009). In 2006, 6.8% (1517) of medical doctors, 4% (232) of dentists and 2.2% (1813) of nurses were foreign born,[2] held a Finnish licence to practise and lived in Finland (Fig. 3.1) (Statistics Finland unpublished data 2009). Recent statistics (OECD 2010) on health professional mobility give other numbers for

---

2 In 2006, total numbers were 22 191 medical doctors, 5989 dentists and 68 098 licensed nurses (Statistics Finland 2009).

Fig. 3.1 *Total accumulated numbers of foreign-born health professionals with licence to practise in Finland, 2000–2006*

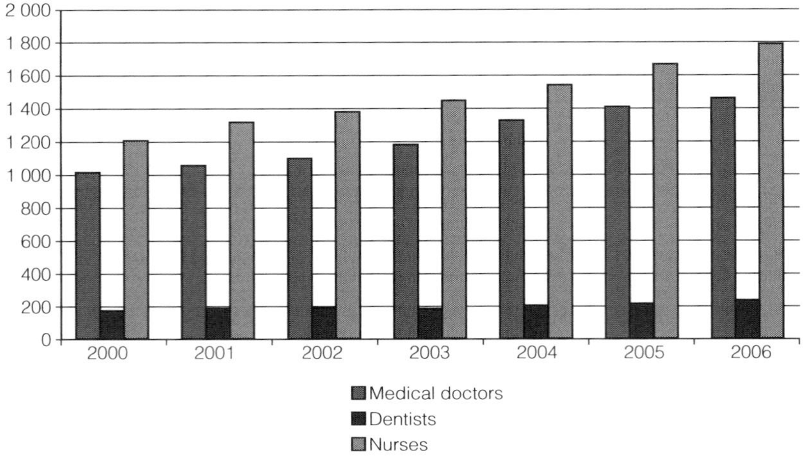

Source: Statistics Finland unpublished data 2009.

the foreign health workforce in Finland. However, these data are based on the Valvira registry data on numbers granted practising licences and include people of Finnish origin who studied abroad and foreign professionals who had already re-emigrated from Finland.

Dentists have comprised the most significant foreign inflows to the health workforce, representing almost half of all those with new licences in the profession. Licences were issued to 134 foreign-trained and 176 Finnish-trained dentists in 2006–2008 (Valvira unpublished data 2009). The number of newly licensed medical doctors of Finnish origin has been around 500 per year. In recent years, around 120 foreign medical doctors per year have obtained a licence to practise (Valvira unpublished data 2009), a quarter of the new medical workforce (Fig. 3.2). Foreign-trained nurses represent about 3% of new inflows to the nursing workforce – licences have been granted to about 75 foreign-trained and about 2500 Finnish-trained nurses per year (Valvira unpublished data 2009).

The majority of foreign health professionals have come from European Union (EU) or European Economic Area (EEA) countries or the Russian Federation. The latter is the most important source country for foreign medical doctors – around 70–80 per year in 2004–2008. Since 2006, Estonia has been a growing source country for all three professions. In 2006–2008, 266 medical doctors, 186 nurses and 53 dentists moved to Finland from Estonia (Valvira unpublished data 2009). Sweden and Germany are the third and fourth most important source countries.

Fig. 3.2 *Inflows based on numbers of newly licensed Finnish and foreign-born medical doctors and dentists in Finland, 2006–2008*

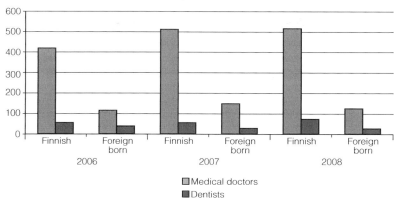

Source: Valvira unpublished data, 2009.

Foreign nurses migrating to Finland are predominantly female (81%); the mean age is 37 years for female and 34 for male nurses. Nearly one half of foreign medical doctors are female. Of 228 foreign dentists in Finland, 67% are female (Valvira unpublished data 2009).

2.2 *Outflows of health professionals*

About 4010 Finnish nurses and 840 Finnish medical doctors worked abroad in 2006 (Statistics Finland unpublished data 2009). These numbers correspond to 5.9% of the total number of licensed nurses (68 098) and 3.8% of all medical doctors (22 191). Outflows of health professionals have gradually decreased over the years – 595 nurses and 175 medical doctors emigrated in 2000 but only 215 nurses and 50 medical doctors left the country in 2007 (Fig. 3.3) (Statistics Finland unpublished data 2009). These numbers include foreign health professionals who have been granted a licence to practise as well as Finnish-born health professionals (Statistics Finland unpublished data 2009). The most attractive destination countries were Sweden and Norway for nurses and Sweden and the United States of America for medical doctors.

It is interesting to note that a proportion of the outflows of Finnish health professionals are temporary. A register-based follow-up of those who had emigrated found that about 40% of nurses, 40% of medical doctors and around 30% of dentists had returned to Finland within two years. The study was based on an exercise linking data from the licence registries of the three health professions with population data on place of residence (Ailasmaa 2010).

Fig. 3.3 *Yearly outflows of Finnish medical doctors and nurses, 2000–2007*

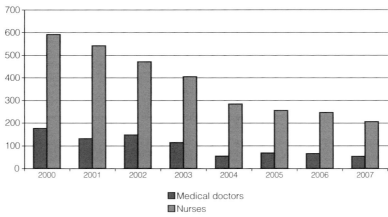

Source: Statistics Finland unpublished data, 2009.

3. Experiences of medical doctors moving to Finland

Interviews were carried out with ten medical doctors working in primary health care in order to map the experiences of health-care professionals who had migrated to Finland. Five of the interviewees came from the Russian Federation, four from EU/EEA countries and one from North Africa. They had been living in Finland for between 4 and 19 years, 14 years on average; the age range varied from 31 to 61 and the mean age was 45 years.

Factors such as higher pay, better working conditions, better careers and post-basic education are among the commonly known drivers for health workforce mobilization. However, only two of the medical doctors interviewed had moved to Finland for these reasons – family-related factors were the most important reason for migrating. This may be due to the fact that Finland has a large group of migrant medical doctors who trained in Russia, many of whom are Ingrian Finns[3] with relatives and family already living in Finland.

These foreign medical doctors found that the need to learn the Finnish language delayed the integration process. In addition, the licensing process was more complicated for non-EU/EEA nationals or those trained in non-EU/EEA countries. They were required to undertake additional studies and to pass the compulsory test for non-EU/EEA citizens before being granted a licence to practise as a medical doctor in Finland. Some non-EU interviewees had taken more than ten years to learn Finnish and pass the test. Meanwhile, they gained work experience in primary health care and fixed-term and part-time licences in hospitals. Some had also worked outside the health sector, in cleaning and commerce for example.

---

3 Ingrian Finns are considered to be of Finnish origin or to have other such close connections with Finland and can be granted a residence permit on this basis.

Most interviewees had experienced difficulty obtaining relevant information on the licensing process, language courses and jobs in Finland. The Internet and connections with doctors (migrant or Finnish) already working in Finnish health care were mentioned as the best sources of information. Moreover, references from Finnish colleagues were found to be helpful in acquiring employment.

The interviewees described their work in the Finnish primary health-care centres as multifaceted and challenging. Job descriptions for general practitioners are sometimes more wide-ranging than in their native countries. Everyone mentioned the need to work very long hours in order to complete all daily duties. They also found patient information systems to be complex because of the many different systems used, depending on the health-care centres and municipalities in which they worked. These are very common reasons for decreased job satisfaction among Finnish medical doctors too.

The foreign medical doctors underlined the challenge of acquiring the licence to practise and employment in Finland. However, those already employed are relatively well integrated into their work. The interviewees' career plans were similar to those of their Finnish colleagues – indicating their interest in moving from primary to specialized care.

4. Dynamics of enlargement

Cyprus, Malta and eight central and eastern Europe (CEE) countries joined the EU in May 2004 – the EU-10. As the latter included the Baltic countries and Poland, it was expected that the process would involve relative large labour force mobility to Finland. Consequently, Finland applied for a two-year transition period (ended 1 May 2006) for the free movement of labour from joining countries. This was not considered necessary for the countries involved in the 2007 enlargement (Bulgaria and Romania). Moreover, by that time the public debate had begun to anticipate labour force shortages.

The procedure to obtain a licence to practise as a health professional in Finland is easier for EU/EEA citizens than for those with qualifications from outside the EU/EEA areas. In spite of the free movement of labour and mutual recognition of qualifications, Finland has not been an attractive country for EU citizens, except for Estonians. Since 2006, Finland has received 11 health professionals from Poland and a total of 21 from Latvia and Lithuania (Valvira unpublished data 2009). However, no health professionals from Latvia or Lithuania had migrated to Finland before 2006.

The migration of Estonian health professionals to Finland has been facilitated by active recruitment, similar languages, geographical proximity and close ties between medical organizations. Between 2006 and 2008, Finland granted 505 licences to health professionals from Estonia, mostly medical doctors (266). Migration from Estonia to Finland was limited before implementation of the free movement policy for the new EU Member States (Valvira unpublished data 2009).

5. Impact of health professional mobility

International mobility of health professionals has been relatively small scale in Finland but the numbers of foreign-born health professionals have increased steadily over the last few years (see Fig. 3.1). There is virtually no research on the reasons for the increasing inflows of these migrants, or on their circumstances in Finland, and cross-border mobility's impact on the Finnish health-care sector remains poorly understood. It remains to be seen how the combination of active recruitment, free movement of labour and the new Government Migration Policy Programme (Government of Finland 2006) will influence health professional mobility and its impact on the health system in Finland.

6. Relevance of cross-border health professional mobility

In Finland, health care is among the sectors predicted to suffer from labour shortages in the near future. According to different scenarios, it has been estimated that health and social services will have 185 000–210 000 new posts in 2005–2020, corresponding to a need to recruit an annual average of 11 500–13 000 new employees (Ministry of Employment and the Economy 2007).

Unemployment among medical doctors, dentists and nurses was practically non-existent until the deep economic recession of the early 1990s when the government and municipalities cut their spending on public services and health and welfare programmes. However, unemployment rates among medical doctors dropped rapidly from a high of 700 in 1994 to virtually zero in 1998 (Kota unpublished data 2009) and had become a shortage of medical doctors by 2000.

Shortages in the health workforce can therefore be explained partly by the economic recession. Unemployment necessitated reductions in the yearly intake of medical schools from 1993. In recent decades the number of students admitted to medical schools has varied from around 350 to 640 students per year (Kota unpublished data 2009). Numbers have increased continually in all the medical faculties since the late 1990s but so far the measure has failed to alleviate the chronic lack of medical doctors seeking general practitioner positions.

The workforce shortage has hit primary health care in particular. In 2007, 36% of public-sector general practitioner posts were not permanently filled; 8% of the posts were managed by labour-leasing companies (Parmanne 2007). Medical doctors have been recruited actively through labour-leasing companies (Kokko 2007) in order to alleviate the chronic lack of health professionals, especially general practitioners. In practice, these are private employers that "rent" health personnel on a temporary basis to public sector health providers, particularly primary health centres. The health personnel are paid by the leasing companies.

The rural areas of the northern and eastern parts of Finland suffer from the most severe lack of general practitioners (Parmanne 2007). The problem is well-recognized but remains unresolved. At local levels, health-care management has suggested that migrant medical doctors should be recruited to the primary health centres in geographically remote areas that find it difficult to recruit native medical doctors. A few hospitals and primary health centres have recruited health professionals from abroad. International recruitment relies on private companies or health centres that recruit health professionals directly, especially from Estonia.

A relatively high number of licences are granted to foreign health professionals, especially medical doctors and dentists. However, there is a major problem with the large numbers who have been granted licences to practise but are not employed. Over 30% of the total foreign health professionals in Finland were not working in 2006 (Table 3.1) (Statistics Finland unpublished data 2009). Unemployment rates were 29% for foreign dentists and 4% for Finnish dentists. Similarly, unemployment rates for foreign medical doctors (24%) and foreign nurses (36%) were notably higher than those of their Finnish peers (2%) (Statistics Finland unpublished data 2009). The reasons behind this phenomenon are not known and further studies are needed to improve understanding and develop effective practices for recruiting non-employed health professionals into the active workforce.

The ageing population poses additional challenges for the Finnish health-care system and workforce. Over the next few decades the labour market will lose more people than it gains and it will become difficult to replace retiring health professionals in the near future. Moreover, working as a general practitioner in a primary health-care centre has lost much of its attractiveness as a career option among Finnish medical doctors during the past 15 years (Kankaanranta 2007). This may be due to developmental trends in public health care and the changes in general practice. The personal doctor system was introduced in Finland in the 1980s in order to improve access, continuity of care and cost savings (Vuorenkoski 2008). The system implies that a person is listed with one

Table 3.1 *Employment rate of health care professionals at working age in Finland. Finnish and foreign born medical doctors, dentists and nurses in 2000-2007.*

Years	Medical doctors					
	Finnish native			Foreign born		
	Employed		Total	Employed		Total
	N	%	N	N	%	N
2000	15 499	95.3	16 270	690	66.8	1033
2001	15 455	95.6	16 170	731	66.9	1092
2002	15 628	95.7	16 336	790	69.3	1140
2003	15 977	96.1	16 622	857	70.5	1215
2004	16 653	96.3	17 300	992	73.3	1354
2005	16 955	96.5	17 570	1078	75.1	1436
2006	17 160	96.0	17 871	1163	76.7	1517
2007	17 393	96.1	18 096	1283	77.4	1657
	Dentists					
2000	4476	96.5	4636	109	60.9	179
2001	4447	97.1	4581	121	63.4	191
2002	4390	97.0	4528	125	65.1	192
2003	4327	96.6	4478	132	66.0	200
2004	4309	97.2	4431	133	63.0	211
2005	4310	97.5	4419	157	69.5	226
2006	4242	97.4	4354	164	70.7	232
2007	4234	98.1	4318	189	75.0	252
	Nurses					
2000	44 791	84.6	52 960	625	51.1	1223
2001	47 054	87.2	53 967	684	51.4	1330
2002	48 721	88.8	54 844	762	54.4	1402
2003	49 476	89.9	55 009	832	56.4	1475
2004	50 250	90.5	55 500	909	57.6	1578
2005	50 880	91.4	55 680	1064	63.2	1684
2006	51 429	92.4	55 685	1164	64.2	1813
2007	52 195	92.9	56 172	1293	67.1	1926

Source: Employment Statistics Data, Statistics Finland

health centre general practitioner, usually on the grounds of place of residence. During the same period, the average length of hospital stays has become shorter and long-term care has shifted increasingly to primary health care. These developments have led to the diversification of tasks and an increasing workload for general practitioners.

7. Factors influencing health professional mobility

Health professional mobility is affected by factors such as motivation, opportunity and means. Health professionals may practise their professions in Finland only if their qualifications are recognized, a work permit is granted and jobs are available. They move if the destination country provides more attractive alternatives to their existing position.

A recent study on the mobility of Finnish medical doctors (Eskelinen et al 2007) found that the most important reasons to move overseas were social factors, such as family ties. Other activating factors were professional motives, such as improving professional competence and language skills. Low wages and high taxes in Finland were among the most important instigating factors.

Residence permit requirements and licensing rules can be facilitating or mitigating factors, depending on the applicant's country of origin and qualifications. The free movement of labour and recognition of qualification in EU and EEA countries have enhanced the opportunities of Finnish medical professionals wanting to work abroad and of foreign health professionals wanting to work in Finland. However, health professional mobility has remained relatively low between Finland and other European countries (Heikkilä & Pikkarainen 2008).

Non-EU residents face a more complicated process to obtain a licence to practise and this is likely to decrease willingness to work in Finland. However, recruitment of non-EU health personnel (from the Philippines and the Russian Federation, for example) is a new and rapidly growing phenomenon. It remains to be seen how this will affect the number of foreign health professionals migrating to Finland and how this may change the health-care system.

The geography of Finland and its language may pose additional challenges for foreign health professionals. The entire territory of Finland is north of 60° latitude and, as the northernmost country of the European continent, is relatively far away from many other European regions. Finnish differs from many other languages that are commonly studied and is widely believed to be difficult to learn. Also, other countries offer few options to study this language.

8. Policy, regulation and interventions

8.1 *Policies and policy development on health professional mobility*

The Finnish health-care system is regulated by 21 acts and several decrees. Act 559/1994 (Government of Finland 1994a) and Decree 564/1994 (Government of Finland 1994b) are the main national legislation on health professionals; both cover foreign health professionals' rights to practise in Finland. The main purpose of Act 559/1994 is to promote the safety of patients and to improve the quality of health-care services.

Since the early 1990s, Finland has had no explicit national-level planning system for the health-care infrastructure. However, the Ministry of Social Affairs and Health national plans for health and social care have been indicative and addressed mainly the objectives and activities of the services. Municipalities and hospital districts are responsible for concrete planning at municipal and local levels. At the national level, the National Institute for Health and Welfare (THL)[4] gathers information concerning infrastructure and provides this on a regular basis to municipalities and hospital districts for planning purposes. Private health care is planned solely by the provider companies. The Ministry of Social Affairs and Health and the THL gather information on health professional mobility including inflows and outflows of foreign and national health professionals. In addition, they monitor the regional variation of foreign professionals in the country.

The National Development Programme for Social Welfare and Health Care – the KASTE Programme – sets long-term strategic objectives for the social and health-care system. It also introduces measures to recruit unemployed migrants into the health sector. The current government has accepted this programme, coordinated by the Ministry of Social Affairs and Health, for its term of office from 2008 to 2011. The KASTE Programme also aims to ensure that there is sufficient staff and to develop the average occupational competence of health-care professionals through the creation of new forms of vocational adult education programmes. The focus of the education programmes should be the health professions that lack resources and have employment opportunities for migrants (Ministry of Social Affairs and Health 2008). The interim evaluation of the KASTE Programme (Ministry of Social Affairs and Health 2010) focused on the strategic appropriateness, launching and organization of the programme as well as the start-up of the funded projects. For this reason, as yet there are no specific data on its practical outcomes.

---

4 The National Research and Development Centre for Welfare and Health (STAKES) gathered information on the infrastructure until it merged with the National Public Health Institute (KTL) to form the THL on 1 January 2009.

The pathways by which foreign health professionals arrive in the Finnish labour market are not well-known. However, active measures for recruiting foreign health professionals have increased in Finland over the past few years. A private company has recruited nurses from the Philippines and the Continuing Education Centre at the University of Joensuu is planning a project for recruiting medical doctors from the Russian Federation. The THL's International Affairs Unit and Helsinki University Central Hospital have launched a pilot project to recruit nurses from other EU countries. The project aims to develop ethical recruitment among health-care personnel. The Government Migration Policy Programme issued in October 2006 also emphasizes active recruitment of a migrant labour force (Government of Finland 2006

The Ministry of Social Affairs and Health ensures that international recruitment in Finland adheres to the WHO global code of practice on the international recruitment of health personnel (WHO 2010).

8.2 *Mutual recognition of diplomas in the European Community*

Finland has implemented Directive 2005/36/EC (European Parliament and Council of the European Union 2005) on the recognition of professional qualifications. Health professionals must obtain licences from the Valvira in order to practise. The licensing procedure varies according to whether the applicant is an EU/EEA citizen and whether the applicant's qualifications were obtained within or outside the EU/EEA. Medical doctors who are not EU/EEA citizens must complete additional studies in Finland and pass an examination in Finnish in order to obtain a permit or licence. The examination consists of three parts: (i) basic knowledge of clinical medicine and health care; (ii) basic knowledge of the health-care system in Finland (including issues central to the practise of medicine in Finland); and (iii) clinical skills. A minimum of six months of hospital training must be completed before taking the test.

The same procedure applies for EU/EEA citizens who have qualified as medical doctors outside the EU/EEA. A medical doctor with a licence to practise from another EU Member State is not required to undertake additional education in Finland. Authorization is valid for a fixed period and may be restricted to a specific hospital or health-care centre. In principle, citizens of Finland or other EU/EEA Member States do not require language certificates. However, an employer (such as municipalities, health centres or hospitals) may require a certificate of language skills. The Act on the Status and Rights of Patients (Government of Finland 1992) gives patients consulting a health-care professional the right to use Finnish or Swedish, the official languages of Finland. The Language Act (Government of Finland 2003) ensures that those using health and social services are granted similar linguistic rights.

In addition, those wishing to practise a profession in Finland require a work permit. Citizens of EU/EEA countries can reside and work freely for a three-month period; those who wish to work for longer must register their intention to reside in Finland. Citizens of non-EU/EEA countries need a residence permit to live in Finland and a residence permit for employed persons if they wish to work. These permits are issued by the Finnish Immigration Service (Migri)[5] and are either temporary or continuous, depending on the basis on which they are granted. A residence permit for an employed person is normally granted for a certain professional field; the application process considers the needs of the labour market.

8.3 *Bilateral and multilateral trade agreements*

The mobility and mutual recognition of health professionals has been relatively open between the Nordic countries since the 1950s, enabled by a framework of agreements allowing broader mobility across countries. The first agreement on the common Nordic labour market was introduced in 1954 and amended in 1982 (Norden 1982). The agreement for particular health professionals (Norden 1993) was specified in 1993 and amended in 1998. These have been negotiated as part of a broader set of agreements and cooperation between the Nordic countries. It is likely that the existence of common labour markets has contributed to the mobility of health professionals, particularly when there have been large salary differences.

Multilateral and bilateral agreements in trade policies have had a limited impact on the mobility of health professionals in Finland. However, this is an area in which trading interests are now emerging more prominently within the country – as an alternative response to labour force costs and supply, and as part of global trade policies. This is due in part to the interests of countries exporting and trading health professionals and the engagement of global recruitment and employment agencies. Only a very limited number of health professionals have been actively recruited from countries such as the Philippines that are neither EU Member States nor neighbouring states. Multilateral, bilateral and regional trade negotiations already include (and likely will continue to develop) enhanced mobility of health professionals, including negotiations on mutual recognition of qualifications.

The General Agreement on Trade in Services (WTO 2005) governs multilateral trade in professional services. To date, this includes only nurses as a part of professional services. However, the European Commission is currently negotiating with several countries on bilateral or regional trade and investment agreements that also cover professional services. These are likely to influence

5 Directorate of Immigration (UVI) until 2008.

the legal framework that governs how Finland can limit, expand and regulate cross-border mobility of health professionals.

9. Conclusion

This report has assessed the cross-border mobility patterns of medical doctors, nurses and dentists in Finland. Over recent years, Finland has changed from a source country to one with a mixed profile of health professional mobility as increasing numbers of foreign medical doctors and dentists arrive and falling numbers of medical doctors and nurses leave. Foreign medical doctors and dentists represent important shares of the newly licensed medical workforce and signal a degree of dependence on foreign inflows. Reasons for these changes have not been clarified thoroughly but some tentative conclusions on contributing factors can be drawn. In May 2006, the free movement of labour was allowed between Finland and the EU-10 countries. This facilitated especially the movement of health professionals from Estonia to Finland. At the same time, the Government Migration Policy Programme was adopted to promote labour migration to Finland in order to alleviate workforce shortages.

The Finnish health sector suffers from important workforce shortages and it is estimated that the need for more qualified health professionals will only grow in the coming decades. The shortages can be explained partly by the economic recession that hit Finland in the early 1990s, leading to unemployment among medical doctors and cuts in the yearly intakes of medical schools. In addition, the ageing population poses challenges for the Finnish workforce.

Primary health care has lost much of its attractiveness as a career option for Finnish health professionals. All medical faculties have increased the number of student posts since 1999 but still there is a chronic lack of candidates seeking general practitioner posts. It has been suggested that migrant medical doctors should be recruited to primary health centres in geographically remote and underserved areas. However, one important bottleneck is the numerous foreign health professionals who are licensed in Finland but not employed in the health-care sector. The KASTE Programme has introduced measures to recruit unemployed migrants to work in the health sector. However, this is ongoing and no information is available to assess these actions.

The Ministry of Social Affairs and Health in Finland supports the draft of the WHO code of practice on the international recruitment of health personnel. In practice, international recruitment relies on private companies or health centres that recruit foreign health professionals directly.

The international migration of health professionals has been a growing feature in Finland since the early 2000s. However, little information is available on their integration into the health-care system, workplaces or the reasons behind their high non-employment rates. Further studies are needed on the obstacles faced by foreign health professionals, their career plans and intentions to stay in Finland. These will inform the development of effective policies and interventions to transform the large number of non-employed foreign medical doctors, dentists and nurses into an active workforce.

References

Ailasmaa R (2010). *Sosiaali- ja terveyspalveluiden ulkomaalainen henkilöstö ja suomalaiset ulkomailla. [Foreign health professionals abroad and Finnish health professionals working abroad]*. Helsinki, National Institute for Health and Welfare, Statistical Report 18/2010 (http://www.stakes.fi/tilastot/tilastotiedotteet/2010/Tr18_10.pdf, accessed 21 June 2010).

European Parliament and Council of the European Union (2005). Directive 2005/36/EC of the European Parliament and of the Council of 7 September 2005 on the recognition of professional qualifications. *Official Journal of the European Union*, 255(48):22–142.

Government of Finland (1992). *Act on the Status and Rights of Patients (785/1992)*. Helsinki, Ministry of Social Affairs and Health (http://www.finlex.fi/en/laki/kaannokset/ 1992/en19920785.pdf, accessed 10 January 2011).

Government of Finland (1994a). *Act on Health Care Professionals (559/1994)*. Helsinki, Ministry of Social Affairs and Health (http://www.psyli.fi/files/48/psyli-english-1.pdf, accessed 12 October 2009).

Government of Finland (1994b). *Decree on Health Care Professionals (564/1994)*. Helsinki, Ministry of Social Affairs and Health (http://www.finlex.fi/fi/laki/alkup/1994/ 19940564, accessed 14 December 2010).

Government of Finland (2003). *Language Act (423/2003)*. Helsinki, Ministry of Justice (http://www.finlex.fi/pdf/saadkaan/E0030423.PDF, accessed 12 October 2009).

Government of Finland (2006). *Government Migration Policy Programme. Government Resolution 19.10.2006*. Helsinki (http://www.mol.fi/mol/en/99_pdf/en/90_publications/ migration_programme2006.pdf, accessed 12 October 2009).

Eskelinen O et al. (2007). Suomalaiset lääkärit ulkomailla – Keitä he ovat, missä he ovat ja miksi he muuttavat? [Finnish doctors abroad – who are they, where are they and why do they move?] *Suomen Lääkärilehti*, 10/2007 vsk 62. (http://www.laakariliitto.fi/files/2007/ laakarit_ulkomailla.pdf, accessed 6 September 2009).

Heikkilä E, Pikkarainen M (2008). Väestön ja työvoiman kansainvälistyminen nyt ja tulevaisuudessa. [Internationalization of population and labour force from the present to the future]. Turku, Siirtolaisuusinstituutti [Institute of Migration].

Kankaanranta T et al. (2006). Factors associated with physicians' choice of working sector: a national longitudinal survey in Finland. *Applied Health Economics and Health Policy*, 5(2):125–136.

Kokko S (2007). Towards fragmentation of general practice and primary healthcare in Finland? *Scandinavian Journal of Primary Health Care*, 25(3):131–132.

Ministry of Employment and the Economy (2007). *Työvoima 2025. Täystyöllisyys, korkea tuottavuus, ja hyvät työpaikat hyvinvoinnin perustana työvoiman työikäisen väestön vähentyessä* [*Workforce report 2025. Full employment, high productivity and good jobs will provide the foundation for well-being as the working age population diminishes*] Helsinki (http://www.mol.fi/mol/fi/99_pdf/fi/06_tyoministerio/06_julkaisut/06_tutkimus/ tpt325.pdf, accessed 6 September 2009).

Ministry of Social Affairs and Health (2008). *KASTE - Sosiaali- ja terveydenhuollon kansallinen kehittämisohjelma. KASTE 2008–2011.* [*National Development Plan for Social and Health Care Services. Kaste Programme 2008–2011*]. Helsinki (http://pre20090115.stm.fi/hl1212563842632/passthru.pdf, accessed 6 September 2009).

Ministry of Social Affairs and Health (2010). *Evaluation of the National Programme for Social Welfare and Health Care (KASTE). First progress report.* Helsinki (Reports of the Ministry of Social Affairs and Health 2010:8).

Norden (1982). *Agreement concerning a common Nordic labour market.* (http://www.norden.org/en/about-nordic-co-operation/agreements/treaties-and-agreements/labour-market, accessed 14 December 2010).

Norden (1993). *Gemensam nordisk arbetsmarknad för viss hälso- och sjukvårdspersonal och veterinärer* [*Agreement concerning a common labour market for certain health and social care personnel and veterinarians*] (http://www.norden.org/en/about-nordic-co-operation/agreements/treaties-and-agreements/labour-market, accessed 14 December 2010).

OECD (2010). *International migration of health workers: improving international co-operation to address the global health workforce crisis.* (OECD Policy Brief). Paris (http://www.oecd.org/dataoecd/8/1/44783473.pdf, accessed 20 January, 2011).

Parmanne P (2007). *Terveyskeskusten lääkäritilanne [Physicians in health-care centres].* PowerPoint presentation (http://www.laakariliitto.fi/files/tklaakaritilanne07.ppt, accessed 3 June 2009.

Vuorenkoski L (2008). Finland: health system review. In: Mladovsky P, Mossialos E (eds.). *Health systems in transition.* Copenhagen, WHO Regional Office for Europe on behalf of the European Observatory on Health Systems and Policies.

WHO (2010). *WHO global code of practice on the international recruitment of health personnel.* Geneva, World Health Organization (http://www.who.int/hrh/migration/code/ WHO_global code_of_practice_EN.pdf, accessed 12 October 2010).

WTO(2005). *General agreement on trade in services (GATS).* Geneva, World Trade Organization (http://www.wto.org/english/tratop_e/serv_e/gatsintr_e.htm, accessed 12 October 2009).

Chapter 4

Nationally moderate, locally significant: France and health professional mobility from far and near

Marie-Laure Delamaire, François-Xavier Schweyer

1. Introduction

With the exception of foreign personnel in hospitals, the phenomenon of foreign mobility tends to be overestimated in France. Immigration of medical doctors has only a marginal impact and does not solve the difficulties of geographical maldistribution of physicians. The proportions of foreign dentists and nurses are even lower. Hence, France has no dependence on a foreign health workforce and, contrary to general opinion, there is no evidence that foreign doctors compensate for the lack of medical doctors in isolated rural areas. This widespread belief is probably due to the media's high-profile coverage of a few cases.

The French health sector is particularly affected by immigration policies through state regulation of health qualifications and the labour market. There is a great difference in the treatment of health professionals who are European Union (EU) citizens and those who are third-country nationals – the former have full authorization to practise but mobility of the latter is not encouraged, despite several longstanding state agreements with French-speaking countries.

Foreign medical labour is an important part of the health workforce in some public hospitals with recruiting difficulties. However, the numbers in public hospitals are likely to be underestimated due to lack of clarity on the status of foreign medical doctors. Reliable data on migratory flows of health professionals are rare and the reason why this complex subject is not perfectly understood. However, the key facts and issues are summarized below.

France appears to be a destination rather than a source country – the number of leavers is low but not all who leave are registered. Limited data on outflows make it difficult to obtain a complete picture of health professional mobility in France but the available evidence and estimates indicate that the country has a mixed mobility profile. Different occupational categories show different patterns, with more important flows of foreign medical doctors than of foreign nurses and dentists. Foreign medical doctors come mainly from neighbouring EU countries, followed by the French-speaking countries of north and sub-Saharan Africa. Inflows have increased as countries have gained accession to the EU (for example, noticeable numbers of Romanian doctors have migrated to France since 2007) but globally the inflows from the new EU Member States have been lower than expected. In general, health professional mobility has a limited impact at national level but can be more marked at local level, in hospitals with shortages and in certain specialties. This study has found that inflows and outflows of health professionals are affected by the same factors as those identified in the literature, such as wages, working conditions and the quality of training.

Sources and limitations of the study

The main sources for this study are shown in Table 4.1. There are fewer data on dentists and, to a certain extent, on nurses. The obligation to register with the National Medical Council (*Conseil National de l'Ordre des Médecins* – CNOM) when working outside the public sector means that there are better quality data on doctors in private practice than on those working in public hospitals. Moreover, the lack of clarity on the status of foreign medical doctors in public hospitals may explain the underestimation of the foreign medical workforce. Hence, the figures on Automatisation des Listes (ADELI) registration and on medical doctors at hospital level are not exhaustive. Also, the CNOM does not keep separate account of foreign-trained doctors who complete their degree in France and then adopt French nationality.

There is little information on outflows. The CNOM and the National Council of Dental Surgeons (*Ordre National des Chirurgiens-Dentistes* – ONCD) each maintain a specific list of French professionals who have left France but have authorization to practise on their return without any further procedure. Nevertheless, the national councils do not know whether or not these listed doctors and dentists actually practise abroad.

Table 4.1 *Main data sources and data holders on health professional mobility in France*

Source	Data holder	Comments
ADELI (lists of practising health professionals during latest year available)[a]	Sickness fund and DREES (see below)	Yearly series. Registration of medical doctors at hospital level incomplete
CNOM	Medical profession	Yearly series and thematic studies. Not all foreign-born doctors are included, immigration registration is not compulsory for all
DREES (*Direction de la Recherche, des Etudes, de l'Evaluation et des Statistiques*)	Ministry of Health	Yearly series and thematic studies
IRDES (*Institut de Recherche et Documentation en Economie de la Santé*)	Sickness Fund	Thematic studies
OECD (Organisation for Economic Co-operation and Development)	International organization	Thematic studies
ONCD	Dental profession	Yearly series. No reliable data on outflows
ONDPS (*Observatoire National de la Démographie des Professions de Santé*)	Ministry of Health	Annual report includes some data on foreigners

Note: [a] A project is underway to replace ADELI with a new national database (Répertoire partagé des professionels de santé – RPPS) in 2011.

The National Council of Nurses (*Ordre National des Infirmiers* – ONI) was created only in 2008 and data are not yet centralized at national level. The creation of this new national council may be seen as an official acknowledgment of the nursing profession and a means by which the state has introduced a new partner to improve regulation of the health system.

Another important source of information has been interviews with relevant institutions. The authors carried out interviews with representatives of the:

- ONCD – May 2009;
- CNOM – April and June 2009;
- HOPE (European Hospital and Healthcare Federation) – May 2009;
- OECD (Organisation for Economic Co-operation and Development) – June 2009;
- EHESP (*Ecole des Hautes Etudes en Santé Publique*, Rennes & Paris) – April and July 2009;
- ONDPS – March, April, June, September 2009;

- *Ministère de la Santé et des Sports* – April, May 2009 ;
- *Centre de sociologie et de démographie médicales* – April 2009.

2. Mobility profile of France

Health professional mobility is a rather less important phenomenon in France than in other European countries but is not the same in all occupational categories.

Important data limitations make it difficult to obtain a complete picture of health professional outflows. However, stock data show that the proportion of foreign-national medical doctors practising in France is rather low in comparison to countries such as Norway or the United Kingdom (see Chapter 8). The CNOM reported 10 165 registered EU and third-country nationals as at 1 January 2010, representing 4.75% of the total medical workforce (213 995). This compares to 8431 (or 4.5%) in 2008 (Kahn-Bensaude & Montane 2008). In 2006, 1.6% of the 478 483 nurses working in France were foreign – 3552 with French degrees; 4046 with foreign degrees (Table 4.4). 'n 2008, 2.5% of the total stock of 44 801 dentists were foreign (ONCD unpublished data 2008).

Most health professional mobility occurs between France and neighbouring countries – Belgium is the principal source of foreign-trained medical doctors; Spain and Belgium are equally important source countries for nurses. There are important flows of medical doctors from Germany and Italy and of nurses from Germany and the United Kingdom. Medical doctors from north Africa and, more recently, from Romania also play a role.

2.1 *Medical doctors*

Stocks and inflows

The stock of foreign-national medical doctors registered with the CNOM on 1 January 2010 was 10 165 or 4.7% of the medical workforce, a 20.6% increase over the last three years. Foreign medical doctors come mainly from neighbouring EU countries, followed by those of north and sub-Saharan Africa. In 2007, more than half (53%) of the foreign medical doctors were from the EU – Belgians (1125), Germans (732) and Italians (566) were the most numerous. However, by 1 January 2010 Romanians represented 15.4% of foreign medical doctors in regular work, Belgians 15.1%, Germans 9.6% and Italians 8.4%. Overall, the share of medical doctors from the EU had increased to 64% (CNOM 2010).

It is not just the nature of inflows from EU countries that have changed in recent years. Non-EU countries have also played significant roles in changing the structure of the stock of medical doctors. In 2005, there were 2275 doctors from north Africa, 490 from sub-Saharan Africa, 373 from the Middle East, 136 from Asia and 121 from South and North America (Cash & Ulmann 2008). CNOM data as at 1 January 2009 show that 47% of foreign medical doctors held a degree from outside the EU, mainly from north Africa (Algeria 10.3%, Morocco 7.8%, Tunisia 4.8% (CNOM 2009). However, inflows from the Maghreb[1] have been decreasing, falling from 45.6% of new registrants in 1999 to 12.1% in 2010 (CNOM 2010).

Inflows of foreign medical doctors have increased steadily over the years. Inflows from the EU have exceeded those from non-EU countries since the mid 1990s (Table 4.2) (Cash & Ulmann 2008). Growing feminization is also a clear trend even though 62% of the stock of foreign doctors practising regularly in 2009 were men (68% in 2008) (CNOM 2010, Kahn-Bensaude & Montane 2008).

The type of indicator is crucial when looking at migration data. For example, OECD data based on the CNOM registry indicate that there were 12 124 foreign-trained medical doctors in France in 2005, 5.8% of the medical workforce. The figures from Cash and Ullman (2008) are based on CNOM data but show that there were 7665 foreign-national medical doctors in 2005 (Table 4.2).

Table 4.2 *Foreign-national medical doctors from EU and third countries (stock), 1990–2010*

Doctors	1990	1995	2000	2005	2010[b]
EU	1 071	1 884	2 700	4 149	6 506
(%)	(43)	(56)	(50)	(54)	(64)
Non EU	1 402	1 452	2 674	3 516	3 659
Total	**2 473**	**3 336**	**5 374**	**7 665**	**10 165**

Sources: Cash & Ulmann 2008, [b] CNOM 2010.

The numbers of foreign-born doctors in France are significant, amounting to 33 879 (16.9%) of the 200 358 French doctors in 1999 (INSEE 1999). A CNOM interview revealed that a total of 18 000 foreign-born doctors held French citizenship in 2009. Among foreign-born doctors, 7.2% are locum doctors, 7.3% are away from the labour market and 5.4% have retired. Of the 80% who are working regularly as medical doctors, 33% work as general

---

1 Algeria, Tunisia and Morocco.

practitioners[2] (CNOM 2010). This compares to 39% in 2007 (Kahn-Bensaude et al. 2008). The number of foreign-born doctors is rather high as France has a long history of migration and a policy of naturalization.

Box 4.1 *Hidden mobility: foreign-trained French nationals and foreign nationals trained outside the EU*

In 2008, only 6700 (79%) of 8431 foreign medical doctors had a regular professional activity (Kahn-Bensaude & Montane 2008). However, the numbers of foreign-*national* medical doctors (8431 in 2008; 9631 in 2009) are underestimated because they exclude French nationals who obtained their degrees elsewhere (e.g. in Belgium). This partly explains the higher numbers of foreign-trained medical doctors (12 124 in 2005).

The CNOM registry also omits medical doctors trained in non-EU countries who work in public hospitals under the responsibility of another doctor and are not registered at the CNOM. These are examples of hidden statistics as databases do not cover these movements. This was also true for foreigners classified as medical trainees and working in public hospitals but some efforts have been made to regularize their professional status in recent years (Dumont & Zurn 2007). In 2010, the CNOM estimated that the 10 165 foreign doctors registered represented 94.5% of the total of foreign doctors, that is − 5.5% (559) were not subject to compulsory registration (CNOM 2010).

A Ministry of Health study shows that public hospitals employ 5000 doctors with non-EU medical degrees (ONDPS 2005). Another survey from ONDPS[3] shows that 6733 medical doctors do not have full authorization to work in France but work in hospital under the responsibility of a French doctor, 91% of these have the legal status of *Praticiens adjoints contractuels* (PAC) or trainee (AFS or AFSA).[4] Consequently, 9% (614) of these foreign doctors have a very vague status that is more or less illegal.

The CNOM estimates a total of 6750 foreign practitioners who trained outside the EU (Praticiens à diplômés Hors Union Européenne − PADHUE). Of these, 4420 are trainees (AFS/AFSA) and 2330 are PACs (Cash & Ulmann 2008). These include 2359 French nationals with foreign degrees. Indeed, CNOM data show 8000 foreign-trained medical doctors working in France in 2001, many with French nationality − 73% of doctors with a degree from outside the EU, 56% of PACs and 17% of EU-trained medical doctors (2572) (Couffinhal & Mousques 2001). These figures most likely include foreign-born doctors because the proportions are high in comparison to other sources. In the 2007−2008 academic year about 7% of medical students in Belgium were French nationals (see Chapter 2). In 2004, the CNOM counted 1582 medical doctors who had been trained in Belgium (OECD 2008) .

---

2 In France, general practice/family medicine has been recognized as a medical specialty since 2007.

3 Survey in hospitals conducted by the local authorities of the Ministry of Health for the ONDPS in 2006.

4 *Attestation de formation spécialisée* (Attestation of specialized training) and *Attestation de formation spécialisée approfondie* (Attestation of specialized training, higher level).

The OECD (2008) reports that migration has played a more important role in the structure of the global medical workforce over the past ten years than at any time since before the 1970s and the increase is particularly significant for France. The CNOM (2007) highlights the increased inflows of foreign medical doctors – a 24% (1875) increase in the stock of active foreign-national medical doctors in France between 2003 and 2006, reaching a total of 7966 by 1 January 2007. Table 4.3 shows some fluctuation in the numbers of new foreign enrolments such as the higher inflows in 2000 that resulted from significant immigration from Algeria. More recently, 1000 Romanian and 121 Bulgarian doctors registered between 1 January 2007 and 1 July 2008 (CNOM interview). They tended to have a younger profile and included a majority of women.

Table 4.3 *Annual inflows: newly registered foreign-national medical doctors in France, 1988–2006*

New enrolments with the CNOM	1988	1998	2000	2002	2003	2004	2005	2006
	88	364	621	528	481	558	384	452

Source: CNOM 2007.

The CNOM reports that 39% of foreign medical doctors work in general practice and 61% in other specialities. Foreign specialists tend to work in shortage specialties that lack a sufficient French medical workforce – 14% are in thoracic and cardiovascular surgery; 9% in gynaecology and obstetrics; and 8% in nephrology (CNOM 2007). There was a significant proportion of EU doctors in the surgery and anaesthetics specialty in 2001 (CNOM CREDES 2001). Today, foreign medical doctors constitute 9.5% of anaesthetists in France (CNOM 2009).

Outflows

There is a lack of quantitative knowledge on the outflows of domestically trained doctors and foreign returnees and movers (Cash & Ulmann 2008). The few data collected indicate that these numbers are marginal in France. In 2005, 6% of French medical doctors were trained abroad and were practising in another European country (Mullan 2007 cited in WHO 2007). However, interviews for this study indicated that informal agreements for student exchanges make it very difficult to establish the number of medical doctors who emigrate for training. The CNOM maintains a "special list" of registered medical doctors who practise abroad – for example, in the United States (128), Canada (98), Switzerland (90), Lebanon (39), United Kingdom (30) and Morocco (29). This list totalled 870 in 2009 but the figures are underestimates because doctors are not obliged to notify the CNOM about migration.

Data from other countries give some indication of outflows. In 2005, Belgium was home to 930 French-national medical doctors and 422 medical doctors in Canada had trained in France. In 2006, there were 649 French-national medical doctors in Italy (OECD 2008). In 2007, the United Kingdom had a total of 529 medical doctors who had trained in France (OECD 2008) and 583 French-trained medical doctors registered in the United Kingdom between 2003 and 2008 (see Chapter 8). There were 407 French-national medical doctors working in Germany in 2008 (see Chapter 5).

It is difficult to identify temporary moves as EU doctors on short-term contracts may be registered in their country of origin and not in France.[5] Universities operate traditional exchanges of medical trainees, based on informal and (less often) more formal agreements between hospitals.

2.2 Nurses

Stocks and inflows

In comparison to other European countries, France has low numbers of active foreign-national nurses with a French or a foreign degree – only 7616 (1.6%) of a total of 478 483 nurses in 2006, with the majority (4488) from the EU (Cash & Ulmann 2008). Table 4.4 shows that important numbers of foreign-national and foreign-trained nurses come from the border regions of neighbouring countries: Spain (1284), Belgium (1177), Germany (432) and the United Kingdom (421). Among the 7616 foreign-national nurses, 3552 have a French degree and 4046 have a foreign degree – 3743 from the EU and 303 from elsewhere (Cash & Ulmann 2008). Like doctors, a small number of French-national nurses have foreign degrees: 4281 from other EU countries and 559 from outside the EU (Cash & Ulmann 2008). Nevertheless, 23 308 (5.5%) of the 421 602 total nursing workforce were foreign-born and working in France in 1999 (Dumont & Zurn 2007).

Estimates of inflows show that authorizations to practise in France were issued to 490 EU/EEA nurses in 2005 and 439 in 2006 (Table 4.5). Information received from the Ministry of Health indicates that these figures are far from exhaustive and can be considered minimum numbers.

One likely source of inflows is the numerous French-national students who take nursing degrees in Belgium. In 2007–2008, 16% of all students enrolled in post-secondary nursing training and 40% of all students enrolled in secondary level nursing training in the French-speaking part of Belgium were from abroad. Within these foreign students, 95% and 98% respectively were French nationals (see Chapter 2).

---

5 Art. L4112-7 of the CSP 2011.

Table 4.4 *Nurses registered in France (stock) by nationality and origin of degree, 1 January 2006*

Nationality	French degree	Foreign degrees EU	Non-EU	Unknown	Total
Danish	6	43	0	0	49
Swedish	4	18	3	0	25
Finnish	16	11	0	0	27
German	64	363	4	1	432
Austrian	1	11	0	0	12
Italian	48	119	5	0	172
Belgian	79	1 093	4	1	1 177
British	21	388	12	0	421
Spanish	113	1 167	4	0	1 284
Dutch	17	165	6	0	188
Irish	7	101	2	0	110
Luxembourg	0	7	0	0	7
Portuguese	214	59	4	0	277
Other EU/ EEA[a]	109	89	104	5	307
EU nurses[b]	699	3 634	148	7	4 488
Non-EU	2 853	109	155	11	3 128
Total foreign nurses	3 552	3 743	303	18	7 616
French nurses	463 628	4 281	559	2 399	470 867
Total	**467 180**	**8 024**	**862**	**2 417**	**478 483**

Source: Cash & Ulmann 2008. *Note*: [a] European Economic Area, [b] excluding French nationals.

Table 4.5 *Authorizations to practise issued to foreign nurses and foreign-trained nurses by competent authority (DDASS)[a], 2005 and 2006*

Country in which degree was obtained	2005	2006
Germany	18	11
Belgium	338	355
Denmark	3	4
Spain	83	31
Italy	5	5
Netherlands	9	8
Poland	2	3
Portugal	5	5
United Kingdom	18	18
Switzerland	11	15
Total	**490**	**439**

Source: European Observatory on Health Systems and Policies unpublished data 2008.
Note: [a] Direction Départementale des Affaires Sanitaires et Socials. The figures are not exhaustive and give only an idea of flows. Table shows only countries in which more than five nurses obtained authorization.

> **Box 4.2** *A clear definition of the nurse statute in France*
>
> The French nurse statute is clear – only candidates who pass both the first-year competitive exam and the final (third-year) examinations can become *Infirmiers diplômés d'Etat* (IDEs). These nurses can then specialize in three fields: paediatrics, surgery wards and anaesthetics. The *Hôpital, Patients, Santé et Territoire* (HPST 2009) is a new law that classifies the IDE as a bachelor degree.

Outflows

As for medical doctors, it is difficult to capture information on nurse outflows on anything but the regional level. For example, 5.4% (903) of nurses from the Lorraine region are employed in neighbouring Luxembourg and 7% from Franche-Comté work in neighbouring Switzerland, with 3% of the latter commuting between France and Switzerland. Similar movements are visible between the border region of Alsace and Germany and Switzerland (ONDPS 2005, Recensement 1999). There is almost no evidence on the number of nurses who have returned to the country after practising abroad (returnees). However, there is evidence on certain returning immigrants – 5% of the 770 Spanish nurses who responded to the national recruitment drive returned to Spain in 2004–2005 (Polton et al. 2004).

National data from other countries also give some indication on outflows. Nurses with French nationality amounted to 2.4% of the foreign nurse workforce in Ireland and 9.4% of the 23% of foreign nurses working in Switzerland in 2001 (Simoens et al. 2005). In 2005, 831 French-national nurses were living in Belgium and 379 nurses who had trained in France were living in Canada (OECD 2008).

Nurses make few temporary moves although there are some exchange programmes for nurses with managerial responsibilities – under the Leonardo da Vinci programme of the European Commission, for example. There are also individual initiatives such as the agreement between Lille Regional University Hospital (CHRU) and a hospital in Poland which facilitated the temporary recruitment of 20 Polish nurses in 2004.

Until 2004, some foreign medical doctors applied to become candidates in nursing schools in order to qualify for practise as a nurse in French hospitals. Although this authorization was legally suppressed in 2006, foreign doctors may still apply for admission by submitting a file for consideration by the local health authorities. Those considered to have the relevant qualifications may be admitted to a nursing school and required to complete only part of the curriculum.

2.3 *Dentists*

Stocks and inflows

There are few foreign dentists in France – in 2007, only 1108 (2.5%) of the total dental workforce (44 392) held foreign nationality and were registered by the ONCD. Of this 1108, 698 are EU nationals (including 423 Belgians, 73 Germans, 50 Romanians, 37 British, 32 Polish) and 410 are from elsewhere (including 107 Algerians, 51 Lebanese, 38 Syrians). In 2007, 234 French dentists had a foreign degree. Nevertheless, the 130 foreign-national candidates who applied to work in France in 2007 represented more than double the increase in the *numerus clausus* for that year.[6] The state-determined *numerus clausus* sets the annual maximum number of students admitted following success in the annual competitive entrance exam.

Since the 1980s, there has been a rising trend in the numbers of EU-national dentists practising in France – 97 in 1988, 211 in 1993, 321 in 2000 (includes EEA nationals from 1994), 406 in 2003 and 474 in 2004. Proportionally, the increase is much higher for dentists from the EU than for third-country nationals whose proportion is decreasing somewhat. As with medical doctors, growing feminization of the workforce is also noticeable.

2.4 *Physiotherapists*

Finally, it should be noted that many French students who failed the competitive exam to enter a professional school of physiotherapy in France applied successfully to train in Belgium. According to an ONDPS interview, this significant inflow of students has induced the competent Belgian authorities to reduce the numbers of French candidates accepted since 2006.

3. Vignettes on health professional mobility[7]

Algerian medical doctor works and settles with long-term perspective

Dr G is an Algerian medical doctor who qualified in internal medicine in 1998. He has both French and Algerian nationality. On his first visit to France in 2002 he met a hospital consultant in charge of specialty training who agreed to take him as a trainee. Having returned to Algeria in order to obtain a trainee's visa and collect his family, he moved to France. He worked as a *faisant fonction d'interne* (FFI)[8] and then as a PAC in a small hospital. After three years he sat an exam to gain authorization for practice,

---

6 Box 4.6 in the annex explains the recognition of diplomas for dentists and nurses.

7 Interviews conducted May 2009 in hospitals in northern France, Brittany and Paris, respectively.

8 FFI is a medical trainee who works in a hospital but still has the status of student.

failed but passed a subsequent exam in 2006. He is required to practise for three years before applying for a job as a *praticien hospitalier* (PH) and hopes to become a medical doctor in 2012. The process of integration is long and difficult because of the precarious position, annual contracts and a gap between his status and that of French doctors. His principal motivations are the working environment and a good wage. His wife is also a medical doctor but she works as a nurse. Dr G does not plan to return to Algeria – he prefers public service and does not wish to practise in a private Algerian clinic.

Romanian internist with no career plan hesitates to stay in France

Miss T, a Romanian internist, taught in a public Romanian university until 2001 and then in a private university until 2009. She had good social status but was dissatisfied with the lack of means and autonomy within her job. During her medical training, she spent two years in the United States and six months in France. She decided to move to France for better work conditions and to improve her French. She searched online for jobs and applied successfully to become an internist in a hospital in a small town. This post offered her the chance to gain wider experience as it includes some work in geriatrics. She appreciates the welcoming medical team and the open attitude of patients. She has been working for a trial period and has had a very positive experience with no problems regarding official papers and registration. She hopes to obtain an annual contract but her family lives in Romania and so she is undecided about the future – whether to stay in France and become a PH (which could take at least seven years) or to return to her own country but leave the medical profession.

Spanish nurse with a two-year contract: temporary migrant

Nurse C is Spanish, 25 years old and has worked for three months in a hospital in a Paris suburb. She moved with a friend (also a nurse) after contacting a specialized Spanish agency via the Internet. The agency found the job and dealt with all the administrative paperwork. Nurse C paid for her diploma to be translated and her flight ticket and had to register with the local health authorities. She works in a medical ward every day and is learning French through an intensive training course that the hospital has organized for all Spanish health professionals. It helps that the chief nurse is a Spanish speaker. She experienced a warm welcome and is content with the professional recognition and her job. She does have two problems: (i) the language; and (ii) a two-year commitment that the agency arranged without her knowledge. She earns a high salary (€1400 per month). She is motivated by the opportunity to have her first professional employment (difficult to obtain in Spain) and the language training, both of which improve the chances of gaining a permanent job and becoming a civil servant in Spain. She does not plan to work longer in France.

4. Effects of EU enlargement: the Romanian case

Research shows that the immigration of labour from new Member States is less significant than anticipated (Borzeda et al. 2002, Cash & Ulmann 2008). Bui (2004a) reports that the French authorities were concerned about potentially important inflows following the first EU enlargement. This contrasts with the current situation in which the French authorities are concerned about a shortage of medical doctors, especially in rural areas. Immigration has continued to rise in the last few years but has been limited, despite wage inequalities between France and some eastern European countries. For instance, general practitioners in France earn ten times more than the €500 per month salaries of their counterparts in Romania. France has not imposed any specific restriction on workforce mobility from new Member States.

Immigration from Romania has increased considerably since the country's accession to the EU – there were 174 registered Romanian doctors in 2007, 819 in 2008 and 1160 as at 1 January 2009 (CNOM 2009). In 2009, Romanians represented 73% of medical doctors from the new EU countries registered by the CNOM. In the same year, Romanians were the most numerous group among female foreign doctors although Belgians remained the most numerous group among male foreign doctors.

Romanian culture has important Latin influences with an affinity to French culture and Romanians often speak French. Romanian doctors generally work on permanent contracts and in 2010 constituted the largest national group of medical doctors (15.4%), outnumbering those from neighbouring Belgium, Germany and Italy (CNOM 2010). Romanian doctors tend to be younger, with a high proportion of women (70% in 2009) and are employed mainly in the public sector. However, it should also be noted that some French medical students are currently studying in Romania (JIM 2009a).

The number of migrants from other accession countries remains small – a total of 432 in 2009, excluding Romanians; 121 Bulgarian medical doctors were registered in 2008 (CNOM 2009). It seems that being French-speaking plays an important role. Migration to France or to other western European countries has been limited to some extent by the reactions of some eastern European countries. For example, Lithuania has improved the working conditions of health professionals (Cash & Ulmann 2008).

5. Relative and contrasted impact of migration

France has been recruiting foreign health professionals for the last two decades to meet shortages not only of medical doctors but also of nurses and dentists.

However, the lack of staff depends on geographical areas and specialties and the current main workforce issues concern the maldistribution of the workforce within France. This is due to a lack of regulation and incentives for medical doctors (especially in primary care and certain other specialties) and a rapidly ageing workforce. Until the early 2000s, national policies caused an underproduction of medical doctors – the *numerus clausus*[9] was introduced to control growing health expenditures but failed to take account of the long-term effects (Bui et al. 2004b). Health professional demography is now firmly on the agenda of the French health authorities.

Research by the ONDPS shows that, in some cases, regional maldistribution of the workforce causes greater problems than real shortages of the three professions studied. France's large size contributes to the imbalances in the geographical distribution of health professionals. Health services in rural areas and socially disadvantaged suburbs are fragile, with a trend of desertification. These imbalances are increased as medical trainees tend to avoid specialties that are perceived to be more difficult or to involve great responsibilities.

Interviews with representatives of the CNOM, Ministry of Health, ONCD and ONDPS showed that foreign health professional mobility is not currently considered to be a key solution to demographic difficulties as the competent authorities are more concerned about the length of training that contributes to the foreseeable shortage of medical doctors. The French government does not think that foreign inflows can solve geographical imbalances in the health workforce as foreign doctors tend to prefer the same areas as their French peers (large cities and southern France). Available statistics show that the impact of migration is limited or marginal, even in rural areas. Furthermore, foreign doctors represent an average of only 3.5% of the entire specialist medical workforce and are dispersed across different specialties (CNOM 2007).

Non-EU medical doctors employed in public hospitals have helped to reduce the drastic decrease of young medical doctors in training – *internes*. Cash and Ulmann (2008) note that recruitment of foreigners to work as PACs is more important in small cities and priority is given to vacant positions in hospitals in which French doctors are more reluctant to work. It is also pointed out that PACs may carry greater medical responsibility during night duties and that there are more non-EU medical doctors with full authorization to practise in poor areas with socioeconomic problems. This contribution explains the good quality of service in shortage specialties (ONDPS 2005), in zones less favoured by their French peers and in demanding positions.

---

9 There are annual quotas for the concours (competitive exam) to become a medical doctor or a dentist (see explanation of *numerus clausus* in section 2.3).

Despite the non-negligible numbers of foreign specialist doctors (see section 2), the CNOM reports that foreign medical doctors do not redress deficits in shortage specialties, with the possible exception of anaesthesia. Stocks of foreign specialist doctors may be higher in a few sensitive specialities such as psychiatry or paediatrics (5.5% and 5.3%, respectively, on 1 January 2009) (CNOM 2009) but their proportions in comparison to French doctors remains relatively low – EU and non-EU doctors represent an average of 3.5% of medical specialties in 2007 (CNOM 2007). Anaesthetics is the exception as foreign doctors comprise 9.5% of the workforce and the high demand for doctors in this specialty.

Moreover, it is interesting to note the character of new inflows. Among medical doctors newly registered with the CNOM in 2007, 40% of specialist anaesthetists came from the EU and one in two of these were from Romania. In paediatrics, one in five new registrants were from the EU, also prevalently from Romania (50%).

The latest CNOM (2010) survey shows that 64% of foreign doctors are salaried and 29% work in private practice. The comparable proportions for French medical doctors are 42% and 47%, respectively. Primary care in France is essentially provided by doctors in private practice which may explain why immigration has had a negligible impact on the shortage of general practitioners in some areas, with the possible exception of the Centre region.

There are less critical shortages of nurses but this is still a key issue in some areas (such as the Paris suburbs) or in some specialties (such as surgery). Globally, the effect of nurse migration is marginal although Spanish recruitment in the mid 2000s had a noticeable impact. Spanish nurses were recruited in 2003 and have helped to limit immediate shortages of nurses in several French hospitals. An internal (unpublished) survey by the Direction de l'Hopitalisation et de l'Organisation des Soins showed rather good results in the short term although some interviewees were much less optimistic. The small proportion of foreign nurses within the total stock (1.6% in 2005) means that the impact of nurse migration is low overall, but greater near the French borders.

The ONCD asserts that the quality of services is guaranteed for foreign health professionals who have registered since 2003. The conditions for working in France became stricter after this date, requiring three years of post-graduate practice and a recognized degree.

6. Factors affecting flows of health professionals

The main factors governing inflows to France are geography, wages (confirmed by Buchan & Sochalski 2004) and having a native language similar to French. Migration from neighbouring countries is playing a key role near the French borders, with large inflows of Belgian, German and Italian medical doctors (Table 4.6) and of Belgian and Spanish nurses. France's border regions also show higher proportions of foreign-trained specialist doctors than elsewhere in the country (Table 4.6).

Table 4.6 *General medical doctors and specialists: numbers with degrees from practice regions and with foreign degrees*

Region	General practitioners		Specialist medical practitioners	
	Degree obtained in practice region	Foreign degree	Degree obtained in practice region	Foreign degree
Alsace	85.3	2.1	75.6	3.8
Aquitaine	71.5	1.5	67	1.6
Auvergne	66.8	1.4	59.1	1.6
Bourgogne	51.4	1.5	41.6	3.6
Bretagne	65.2	1	56.8	2.5
Centre	43.9	1.7	38.3	2.6
Champagne-Ardenne	61.1	2.8	46.6	6.9
Franche-Comté	73.0	1.3	61.1	3.1
Ile-de-France	84.2	3.5	80.5	3.9
Languedoc-Roussillon	63.8	2.4	57.9	2.9
Limousin	72.3	0.3	53.2	3.7
Lorraine	82.4	1.5	72.1	4.4
Midi-Pyrénées	70.5	1.9	67.4	2.2
Nord-Pas-de Calais	89.3	1.6	76.4	4.6
Basse-Normandie	60.8	1.1	47.5	2.1
Haute-Normandie	69.0	0.9	52.5	2.1
Pays de la Loire	59.6	1.0	54.9	1.7
Picardie	50.6	1.0	39.7	2.4
Poitou-Charentes	42.6	1.4	31.8	1.9
Provence-Alpes-Côte d'Azur	65.9	2.3	63.3	2.5
Rhône-Alpes	73.9	1.7	72.3	2.1

Source: DREES 2006 in Cash & Ulmann 2008.

Among activating factors, the most important criteria are both wages and quality of life. The vignettes (see section 3) confirm the findings of Borzeda et al's (2002) survey of Hungary, Poland and the Czech Republic. Economic environment is also a push factor – in 2003, nurses in Spain had less job security than nurses in France and therefore were interested in working in French hospitals.

Quality of care and the good reputation of the French health system are also incentives to move among medical doctors from third countries. Training and technical support are seen as activating factors. Medical students are particularly interested in joining French research teams that have high-quality training, medical teams and technical equipment. The interviews also indicated that political context is sometimes an issue – many Algerian men moved to France as a result of the difficult political situation in Algeria in 1999 and 2000.

French nurses are motivated to migrate to Switzerland or Germany where wages are higher (Cash & Ulmann 2008, ONDPS 2005). An ONCD interview confirmed that dentists also identify higher wages as an incentive to move abroad – especially to Luxembourg, Spain, Switzerland and Abu Dhabi in the United Arab Emirates.

Within facilitating factors, the recruitment policy led by the French Ministry of Health was a key factor in the retention of Spanish nurses. The French authorities have also signed conventions which facilitate migration with Algeria, Monaco, Morocco and Tunisia. At individual level, welcoming hospital staff and relatives or friends who have already settled in France also play a role. In addition, migration from Romania and Lebanon is facilitated by the existence of some initial medical or dental training courses taught in the French language.

Language is also a mitigating factor, a main barrier. Interviews with dentists and nurses have also highlighted cultural barriers. France is perceived to have a quite restrictive regulation for immigration and the complexity of the bureaucratic processes acts as another barrier. Furthermore, the French training system is less attractive than those of other countries – for example, foreign students who undertake training such as the AFS or AFSA do not get a degree.

Box 4.3 *Activating, facilitating and mitigating factors in health professional mobility*

Activating factors

Only assumptions can be made as there are insufficient data to draw clear conclusions. Interviews indicate that France has long had a reputation for a good quality of life but, among recent migrants, Polish and Lithuanian medical doctors mainly decided to live elsewhere.

Facilitating factors

French governments have signed conventions with non-EU countries (Algeria, Monaco, Morocco, Tunisia) that considerably facilitate migration.

Interviews at the Ministry of Health indicate that the recruitment policy was a key factor in the retention of the Spanish nursing staff.

Romania and Lebanon provide some initial medical training in French. The ONCD reports that this is also the case for dentists.

Mitigating factors

Language is definitely a key issue although it may be only what one foreign interviewee calls: "a temporary barrier". Interviews confirm the conclusions of some reports (e.g. Borzeda et al. 2002) that language is a main barrier. This is true at least initially.

Culture and way of life are other key issues. A CNOM interview reported that foreign medical doctors prefer to settle near large cities and the south of France, like their French colleagues. Similarly, young foreigners find it difficult to live in isolated areas such as the Picardie region. The CNOM reports that those who do move there tend not to stay.

Interviews with Spanish nurses and with dentists have also highlighted cultural barriers.

The French government has decided to cut new recruitment of Spanish nurses because of the lack of demand from French hospitals.

France seems to have a quite restrictive regulation for immigration in order to prevent brain drain. Moreover, there are major ethical issues. In hospitals, for instance, foreign doctors provide real support but can be paid substantially less. There are some exceptions – for example, foreign specialist anaesthetists can be very well paid for short periods of activity. It is also difficult to ascertain all the activities taking place within hospitals employing foreign-born medical doctors who do not have legal status; such practices often remain unknown.

Finally, it would not be fair to French students who fail their exams if foreigners were able to work in France without careful verification of their skills.

7. Policy, regulations and interventions

7.1 *Policies and policy development on health professional mobility*

During the 1990s, French hospitals recruited numerous non-EU medical doctors as trainees in order to counter the decreases in medical students caused by the introduction of the *numerus clausus*. This inflow was reduced by the CMU law in 1999 that introduced a new authorization process and a wave of regularizations but no clear policy. In parallel, EU doctors have had full authorization to practise since 1975. The 2006 law on selective immigration has encouraged general labour since 2007 with a list of 150 qualifying jobs for new EU countries and a list of 30 professions (in different fields). Unfortunately, the concrete effects of the 2006 law are not yet known in the health sector.

The health sector has specific immigration policies determined by the state's strict control of qualifications and entry to the labour market. Three conditions govern entitlement to practise as a medical doctor in France. Candidates must:

1. hold French or EU nationality or be a native of Andorra. Foreign medical doctors can also fall under the scope of an official bilateral agreement of the EEA or can be a national of Morocco, Tunisia or a country linked to France by a *convention d'établissement*;

2. have obtained a degree or certificate stipulated in Article L 4131-1 of the *Code de la santé publique* (CSP 2011);

3. have enrolled at the CNOM.

The CSP (2011) mentions two criteria – nationality and training place. The recognition of a foreign medical doctor's qualifications is the most important criterion used although some derogations can be obtained. However, it is clear that EU citizens have a very different recognition process in comparison to third-country nationals although both groups are required to meet the same administrative requirements for enrolment with the CNOM.

Directives on the mutual recognition of diplomas have given EU medical doctors full authorization to practise since 1975 (Council of the European Communities 1975a & 1975b, European Parliament and Council of the European Union 2005). The length of medical training has been harmonized to six years in the 27 Member States. In France, enrolment with the CNOM is compulsory for EU doctors, requiring each applicant to produce an attestation or other guarantees (such as proof of a foreign degree and a certificate of good conduct). France has also signed an agreement, *convention médicale transfrontalière*, with Monaco and Switzerland (Box 4.4).

Box 4.4 *Bilateral agreements*

France has *conventions d'établissements* with Morocco, Tunisia and Monaco. There are state agreements between France and several African countries – the Central African Republic, Chad, the Congo, Gabon, Mali and Togo. Medical doctors from the countries listed can practise in France if they have a French medical degree or one title mentioned in Article L431-1 of the CSP (2011).

An *accord de réciprocité* with Monaco (agreement of 14 December 1938) allows equal numbers (currently 14) of French and Monegasque doctors to work and settle in the host country. France has had agreements with other countries but only the Monaco accord is still active.

A *convention médicale transfrontalière* enables medical doctors who work next to the French border to practise on the other side of the border under specific conditions included in the contract. Two agreements have been signed – with Monaco and Switzerland, respectively.

Two special commissions are responsible for the recognition of dentistry diplomas obtained in the EU. Nurses trained in the EU need only to submit an application form issued by the local competent authority in the region in which they intend to work. Nurses with a specialization need additional authorization, depending on the content of their degree, and may be required to sit an exam or to retrain.

Policies and regulations covering third-country nationals

Mobility from non-EU countries is not encouraged and there is no real policy on this. An authorization of mobility can be given if a health professional has been offered a job in France (and therefore a recognition of qualification). France has bilateral agreements with Monaco, Morocco and Tunisia and state agreements with several countries in Africa (see Box 4.4). In practice, the policy is vague with room for flexibility: the state can issue derogations in some cases, including in public hospitals; some foreign health professionals work as medical doctors but are officially classified as students (FFIs). Since 19 July 2010, the *Centre National de Gestion* (CNG) has been responsible for administering the *concours* for foreign doctors who have: (i) EU degrees and non-EU nationality, or (ii) non-EU degrees and EU nationality. The Ministry of Health is still responsible for the attestation of degrees (confirming conformity with Directive 2005/36). Since the same date, attestations have replaced written examinations of the French language. Non-EU doctors seeking to become specialists must obtain approval from a commission comprising members with specializations in the candidate's chosen specialty.

Two statutes are currently in operation for third-country nationals. The first is the *Procédure d'Autorisation d'Exercice*[10] which makes a distinction between medical doctors from third countries who have already worked in France and those who have not. The second is a temporary statute that can be applied to junior or senior doctors who have experience in their home country. Usually, this requires them to sign a contract with a large hospital which conducts

10 Candidates must complete an application form in order to sit a national exam.

research or allows them to practise for a short period of one to five years.[11] In addition, a bill under process in 2010 would allow foreign doctors from non-EU countries to have their own practice in primary care on condition that they hold a French, EU or EEA medical degree. This law had not been adopted at the time of writing.

Non-EU nurses do not have mutual recognition and candidates are required to sit the usual *concours* of the French nursing schools. In practice, nursing school directors may issue derogations that allow candidates to be integrated directly into the second or third year of study. Moreover, the competent local authority, the DDASS, can authorize candidates to work as auxiliary nurses during the application procedure.

The precarious nature of their statutes led third-country medical doctors to establish a union in 2005 – the *Syndicat National des Praticiens a Diplôme Hors Union Européenne* (SNPADHUE). This was joined by two other unions to create the *Intersyndicale Nationale des Praticiens a Diplôme Hors Union Européenne* (INPADHUE) on 24 March 2007. This federation's objective is to obtain more equity in wages and working time and more clarity in an authorization regime that is perceived to be unfair and too selective (218 of 3800 applicants accepted in 2005). The health ministry was prompted to clarify their statute following a demonstration by non-EU doctors staged in Paris in 2008. Several successful measures were obtained in 2009 (JIM 2009b) with the support of the *Haute Autorité de Lutte contre les Discriminations et pour l'Egalité* (HALDE), the nondiscrimination authority.

7.2 *Workforce planning and development*

Workforce planning is implemented in France but data on foreign health professionals are only partially integrated even though immigration affects planning measures such as the *numerus clausus*. The Ministry of Health has responsibility for manpower planning, aiming to make it more effective and to ensure self-sufficiency in the number of medical doctors, nurses and dentists. Some models of projections do exist but the impact of migration has often been overestimated. The issue is sensitive, causes political debate and is widely reported in the media due to the French population's interest in the subject.

The French system is multilevel, combining a national framework with local and empirical initiatives. Some public hospitals recruit non-EU doctors on short-term contracts for which official authorization is not compulsory. Their contracts are renewed annually and such doctors are used to "*boucher les trous*".

---

11 More details are given in Box 4.6 in the annex.

Hospitals or local elected representatives pay private agencies to attract foreign health workers. Special programmes are scarce: the national agreement between the Spanish and French authorities signed in early 2000 is the only one observed, initiated by both local and national authorities. French hospitals were facing difficulties recruiting nurses and working to implement the 35-hour law. This led the French Federations of hospitals to cooperate with the Ministry of Health in order to recruit 770 Spanish nurses. Local hospital managers are required to give written guarantees (*chartes*) to smooth the arrival and integration of Spanish nurses and to help them in their work.

8. Conclusion

This research on health professional mobility to and from France has found that data on the migratory flows of health professionals are neither exhaustive nor always reliable. It is suggested that the ONDPS could improve the accuracy and usefulness of data by including foreigners more systematically within demographic studies as well as in information on outflows.

The available data show France to be a destination country with no evidence of important losses due to emigration in the three professions studied. Relatively modest numbers of foreign health professionals are working in France, foreign medical doctors being most concerned by mobility (foreign nationals represented 4.7% of medical doctors in 2010; 3.5% of specialists in 2007; 1.6% of nurses in 2006, and 2.5% of dentists in 2007). This remains true despite increasing inflows over the last few years (not least from countries such as Romania). Yet, the significant rate of naturalization tends to hide the phenomenon of migration and the several thousands of foreign doctors in training positions, mainly from non-EU countries, who do not appear in official registries.

Foreign medical doctors are more numerous in sensitive specialities but in comparison to French doctors their proportion remains small. Immigration of medical doctors has only a marginal impact in France and does not solve the difficulties of geographical maldistribution which is a characteristic of the French health system as there is no obligation but only incentives to establish in isolated areas. This comment is even more relevant for the dental and nursing professions that have even smaller proportions of foreigners. Hence, there is no dependency on a foreign health workforce in France.

Medical doctors and nurses within the health workforce in France have the freedom to apply for any available position in any hospital and independent medical doctors may choose where to practise. Nevertheless, foreign medical labour is important and provides real support in some hospitals that have recruiting difficulties. Foreign mobility partially compensates for the lack of regulation in the health workforce in France, specifically in hospitals. In 2009–2010, measures were taken to regulate the choice of specialty and training hospitals although this has not been enough to solve shortages in certain disadvantaged areas (such as rural and poorer suburbs) and in some specialties (such as obstetrics). Foreign medical labour provides important support in some hospitals that have recruiting difficulties and partially compensates for this lack of regulation.

There have been some attempts to improve the working conditions of foreign medical doctors arriving from third countries but regulations have not provided sufficient protection and there are unresolved ethical issues. There is a need for wider recognition of the qualifications of foreign doctors from non-EU countries and to consider additional training that will optimize their employment in the French system, especially in hospitals.

References

Borzeda A et al. (2002). *Elargissement de l'Union européenne: les professionnels de santé des pays candidates envisagent-ils de migrer ? Les cas hongrois, polonais et tchèque*. Paris, Délégations aux Affaires Européennes et International.

Buchan J (2006). Migration of health workers in Europe: policy problem or policy solution? In: Dubois C-A et al. (eds.). *Human resources for health in Europe*. Maidenhead, Open University Press (European Observatory on Health Systems and Policies Series).

Buchan J, Sochalski J (2004). The migration of nurses: trends and policies. *Bulletin of the World Health Organization*, 82(8):587–594.

Bui D-H-D (2004a). La démographie médicale en observation: dix chroniques des années charnières (1999–2004). *Cahiers de Sociologie et de Démographie Médicales*, 7(9):271–348.

Bui D-H-D et al. (2004b). Projection démographique de la profession médicale en France (2000–2050): quel numerus clausus pour quel avenir? *Cahiers de sociologie et de démographie médicale*, 44(1):101–148.

Cash R, Ulmann P (2008). *Projet OCDE sur la migration des professionnels de santé: le cas de la France*. Paris, Organisation de coopération et de développement économiques (OECD Health Working Papers No. 36).

CNOM (2007). *Les médecins de nationalité européenne et extra-européenne en France (inscrits au tableau de l'Ordre de Médecins)*. Paris, Conseil National de l'Ordre des Médecins (Etude No. 40-1).

CNOM (2009). *Atlas de la démographie médicale en France. Situation au 1er janvier 2009.* Paris, Conseil National de l'Ordre des Médecins.

CNOM (2010). *Les médecins de nationalité européenne et extra-européenne, Situation au 1er janvier 2010.* Paris, Conseil National de l'Ordre des Médecins.

CNOM/CREDES (2001). *La démographie médicale française: situation au 31 décembre 2001.* Paris Conseil National de l'Ordre des Médecins (Rapport CREDES).

Couffinhal A, Mousques J (2001). Les médecins diplômés hors de France: statuts et caractéristiques. *Questions d'économie de la santé*, 45:6.

Council of the European Communities (1975a). Council Directive 75/362/EEC of 16 June 1975 concerning the mutual recognition of diplomas, certificates and other evidence of formal qualifications in medicine, including measures to facilitate the effective exercise of the right of establishment and freedom to provide services. *Official Journal*, L 167, 30 June 1975, p. 1–13.

Council of the European Communities (1975b). Council Directive 75/363/EEC of 16 June 1975 concerning the coordination of provisions laid down by law, regulation or administrative action in respect of activities of doctors, *Official Journal*, L 167, 30 June 1975, p. 14–16.

CSP (2011). Code de la santé publique. *LegiFrance*, 18 February 2011 (http://www.legifrance.gouv.fr/affichCode.do?cidTexte= LEGITEXT000006072665&dateTexte=20110218, accessed 18 February 2011).

Dumont JC, Zurn P (2007). Immigrant health workers in OECD countries in the broader context of highly skilled migration. In: *International migration outlook 2007*. Paris, OECD publishing.

European Parliament and Council of the European Union (2005). Directive 2005/36/EC of the European Parliament and of the Council of 7 September 2005 on the recognition of professional qualifications. *Official Journal of the European Union*, 255(48):22–142.

HPST (2009) Loi n° 2009-879 21 juillet 2009 portant réforme de l'hôpital et relative aux patients, à la santé et aux territoires. *Legifrance*, 22 July 2009 (http://www.legifrance.gouv.fr/affichTexte.do;jsessionid=7629C7354363244707A2CD0BC8F24389.tpdjo11v_1?cidTexte=JORFTEXT000020879475&categorieLien=id, accessed 16 February 2011).

Jakoubovitch S (2009). *La formation aux professions de santé en 2008*. Direction de la Recherche, des Etudes, de l'Evaluation et des Statistiques (Document de travail, Série Statistiques, No. 139).

JIM (2009a). France/Roumanie: le chassé croisé des médecins et des étudiants. *Journal International de Medicine,* 13 February 2009 (http://www.jim.fr/en_direct/pro_ societe /e-doccs/00/01/9E/CB/document_actu_pro. phtml, accessed 28 January 2011).

JIM (2009b). Médecins étrangers: un pas historique pour les titulaires d'un diplôme français. *Journal International de Medicine,* 12 February 2009 (http://www.jim.fr/ en_ direct/pro_societe/e-docs/00/01/9E/B2/document_actu_pro. phtml, accessed 28 January 2011).

Kahn-Bensaude I, Montane F (2008). Zoom sur la démographie des médecins étrangers. *Bulletin de l'Ordre des Médecins*, 2008-002.

Kingma M (2005). Les migrations des professionnels de santé. *Cahier de sociologie et de démographie médicales*, 45(2–3):287–306.

OECD (2008). *The looming crisis in the health workforce, how can OECD countries respond?* Paris, Organisation de coopération et de développement économiques (http://www.oecd.org/dataoecd/43/43/41522822.xls, accessed 2 February 2011).

ONDPS (2005). *La nécessaire prise en compte des mouvements migratoires internationaux des professionnels de santé.* Paris, Observatoire National de la Démographie des Professions de Santé (Synthèse générale, rapport 2005).

Polton D et al. (2004). Infirmières. In: *Tome III – Analyse de trois professions sages-femmes, infirmières, manipulateurs d'électroradiologie médicale, Rapport 2004 de l'Observatoire national de la démographie des professions de santé.* Paris, Observatoire National de la Démographie des Professions de Santé.

Recensement (1999). *Recensement de la population française de mars 1999.* Paris, Institut national de la statistique et des études économiques (http://www.recensement-1999.insee.fr/RP99/rp99/page_accueil.paccueil, accessed 19 February 2011).

Schreiber A (2004). *La formation aux professions de santé en 2002 et 2003.* Direction de la Recherche, des Etudes, de l'Evaluation et des Statistiques (Document de travail, Série Statistiques No. 69).

Simoens S et al. (2005). *Tackling nurse shortages in OECD countries.* Paris, Organisation de coopération et de développement économiques (OECD Health Working Papers No. 19) (http://www.oecd.org/dataoecd/11/10/34571365. pdf, accessed 28 January 2011).

WHO (2007). Politiques relatives au personnel sanitaire dans la Région européenne. Résolution, *Comité regional de l'Europe, 57eme Session, Belgrade, 17–20 September 2007* (EUR/RC57/R1) (http://www.euro.who.int/__data/assets /pdf_file/ 0010/74557/RC57_fres01.pdf, accessed 4 February 2011).

Annex

Table 4.7 *Medical doctors in France by nationality and origin of degree, 1 January 2006*

Nationality	French degree	Foreign EU degree	Non-EU degree	Unknown	Total
Danish	2	7	0	0	9
Norwegian	3	0	2	0	5
Swedish	5	13	1	0	19
Finnish	7	3	0	0	10
Lithuanian	0	0	1	0	1
German	149	471	6	1	627
Austrian	2	15	2	0	19
Hungarian	0	0	3	1	4
Slovak	0	0	7	0	7
Polish	0	0	15	0	15
Greek	35	66	2	0	103
Italian	47	403	7	0	457
Belgian	55	965	4	0	1 024
British	23	50	1	1	75
Spanish	33	223	4	0	260
Dutch	12	41	1	0	54
Irish	0	17	0	0	17
Luxembourg	59	17	0	0	76
Portuguese	29	8	1	0	38
Maltese	0	0	1	0	1
Other EU	99	83	124	7	313
EU (excluding France)	560	2382	182	10	3134
Non-EU	2590	14	443	34	3081
Foreign medical doctors	**3150**	**2396**	**625**	**44**	**6215**
French	202 841	656	1703	296	205 496
Total	**205 991**	**3052**	**2328**	**340**	**211 711**

Source: Répertoire Adeli, corrected by DREES (Cash & Ulmann 2008).

Table 4.8 *Foreign-born, foreign-national and foreign-trained nurses applying for professional registration on completion of studies in France, 2003 and 2008*

	Total nursing workforce		Foreign nurses		Foreign nurses in total nursing workforce (%)	
	2003	**2008**	**2003**	**2008**	**2003**	**2008**
Institut de formation en soins infirmiers (IFSI) – initial three-year training	74 461	80 988	670	427	0.9	0.5
Ecole d'infirmiers anesthésistes (ISARs) – post-graduate school for nurse anaesthetists	1 134	1 149	2	1	0.2	0.1
Ecoles d'infirmiers de bloc opératoire (IBODE) – post-graduate school for theatre (surgical) nurses	729	504	14	4	1.9	0.8
Ecole de cadres de santé – post-graduate school for nurse-managers	1 780	2 056	6	1	0.3	0.05

Sources: Jakoubovitch 2009, Schreiber 2004. *Note*: The sources give no information on paediatric specialization.

Box 4.5 *International exchanges*

According to interviews, professors are exchanging medical students. This is creating a dynamic of research and contributing to increases in the pool of expertise. Foreign exchange students can be trained for a few years before returning to their countries – 4418 enrolled in AFS or AFSA courses for the 2004–2005 academic year (Cash & Ulmann 2008). Similarly, French medical trainees travel to countries such as the United States to complete their studies. Nevertheless, some of the foreign workforce is used in hospitals to limit immediate shortages of labour and to "*boucher les trous*".

French hospitals do not always offer good conditions of work although new statutes have brought some improvement in recent years. For instance, PACs are paid much less and have far less job security too. Moreover, some apply to become a FFI as a pretext to stay in France for many years. The figures indicate that France does not lose out from global exchange (inflows exceed outflows). This remains true even when France loses some very good doctors who decide to remain in their foreign host countries.

Little is known about exchanges for dentists. The situation is similar for nurses – very little evidence could be found and it seems that, globally, there are very few exchanges.

Box 4.6 *Recognition of diplomas in France*

Doctors

Two statutes currently apply to immigrating medical doctors and to foreign medical trainees and doctors who intend to stay in the country for only a short time.

1. Non-EU doctors work under the *Procédure d'Autorisation d'Exercice* which makes a distinction between candidates who have already worked in France and those who have not. This replaced the *Nouvelle Procédure d'Autorisation* which required candidates firstly to sit examinations in one or several specialties and, secondly, to have worked in a hospital for three years. Thirdly, a commission was required to give an opinion on their cases before the Ministry of Health could grant an authorization to practise. The Ministry of Health still sets an annual quota for authorizations.

2. Junior or senior doctors who wish to complete their studies in France may apply for temporary status (Law of 4 February 1995 and Decree of 20 April 1998). Candidates must provide proof of three to six years of practice in their home country and are required to sign a contract with a large hospital conducting high-level research in France – a *centre hospitalier universitaire*. They can also be allowed to practise for a short period (one to five years) before (usually) returning to their home countries.

It should also be noted that non-EU medical doctors seeking to become specialist doctors must be approved by a commission comprising members in that particular specialization. In 2001, the number of non-EU (??) medical doctors who managed to pass the exam was still low.

Past procedures

For EU citizens, Council Directive 93/16/EEC of 5 April 1993 aimed to facilitate the free movement of doctors and mutual recognition of diplomas, certificates and other qualifications. Repealed and replaced by Directive 2005/36/EC as of 20 October 2007.

Non-EU doctors with full authorization to practice (applied 1972–2003): French health ministry set annual quotas – between 40 and 100 until 1997 but increased between 1997 and 2001. Candidates were required to sit an exam; the last examination took place in 2001.

Non-EU doctors with a limited practice: PACs were medical doctors authorized to work only in hospitals. This statute was created in 1995 and replaced by the NPA. After 1999, PACs could sit the PH competitive exam in order to be integrated fully within the French system.

Those seeking to become a PAC had to have worked for at least three years in a public hospital or in a hospital which had close links with the public sector (Participant au service public hospitalier – PSPH) and were required to sit exams. PACs were enrolled with the CNOM. Before 1995, medical doctors from outside the EU or from the EEA could become *attachés associés, assistants généralistes* or *spécialistes associés*, working under the responsibility of a French doctor. The last PAC examination was held in 2002.

Dentists

Three commissions cover different categories of dentists.

1. Commission of foreigners (article R. 4111-2 of the CSP) – covers non-EU dentists required to sit an exam.

2. Hocsman (article R. 4111-14 and following of the CSP): covers EU dentists with non-EU degrees.

3. Dreessen: covers EU dentists with degrees obtained in home countries before accession to the EU.

Nurses

EU nurses are required only to submit a form to the local competent authority (Agence régionale de santé – ARS). However, nurses with a specialization may require further authorization if the content of their studies is very different from that of the French degree. This requires them to sit an exam or to undertake further training before a further assessment.

Non-EU nurses do not have mutual recognition and candidates are required to sit the usual examinations of the *concours* of French nursing schools. In a few cases, a nursing school principal may grant a derogation enabling a candidate to be integrated directly into the second or third year of studies. The DDASS may authorize candidates to work as auxiliaries whilst this procedure is in process.

Chapter 5

Germany: a destination and a source country Managing regional disparities in the health workforce by drawing upon foreign physicians

Diana Ognyanova, Reinhard Busse

1. Introduction

Germany is both a destination and a source country for migration in the health-care sector. A number of foreign health professionals have long had a presence within Germany's health services and nearly half of these hold European Union (EU) citizenship. However, the 2004 and 2007 EU enlargements have not produced the expected strong effect on the migration inflows of health professionals. Foreign-national health professionals still represent a relatively small percentage (about 6%) of the total health workforce in the country. This is lower than the percentage of foreign workers in the German labour market as a whole.

The decentralized and corporatist health-care system in Germany hampers active nationwide recruitment of health professionals. However, mainly in the less affluent and sparsely settled regions of eastern Germany, federal states and hospitals affected by a shortage of medical doctors are increasingly recruiting personnel from abroad. While the number of foreign nurses and midwives subject to social insurance contributions is declining, other forms of employment (self-employment, illegal employment) offer foreign nurses the possibility to work in Germany, mainly as home-care workers for elderly people. At the same time, a rising number of German health professionals are leaving the country to work abroad, attracted by better working conditions and higher pay. Regional disparities in the supply of health professionals, an ageing population and an ageing health workforce are causing health professionals trained abroad to become increasingly important for the provision of sufficient inpatient care, as well as home care for elderly people and those with disabilities.

Following a common template this case study assesses the magnitude and directions of the movements of health professionals to and from Germany and the effects of the eastern European expansion of the EU. Next it discusses the impacts of migration on the health system and its relevance in relation to other domestic workforce issues. Then it outlines the factors influencing health professionals' inflows and outflows. The last section of the study focuses on migration policies, workforce planning and domestic interventions affecting the mobility of health professionals.

Limitations of the study

Data on the mobility of health professionals to and from Germany have been collected from a number of different sources: the Federal Statistical Office, Federal Employment Agency, Federal Chamber of Physicians, Federal Association of Statutory Health Insurance Physicians and the Federal Chamber of Dentists. The most detailed data on immigration concern employees subject to social insurance contributions and therefore exclude a large number of self-employed practice-based health professionals, particularly medical doctors and dentists.

The data collected from registries in Germany mainly refer to the nationality of health professionals. Hence, those who were born and/or trained in Germany but who do not hold German citizenship appear in the statistics as foreign health professionals. Microcensus data were collected to overcome this shortcoming in the registry data by providing further relevant characteristics such as country of birth and country of training.[1]

Data on the annual outflows of health professionals from Germany are partially available. The regional chambers of physicians record the annual outflows of medical doctors from Germany; no corresponding data could be found on nurses and dentists. Data on the stock of German health professionals working abroad have been compiled only for medical doctors.

---

1 The microcensus is an annual random sample survey. With a sampling fraction of 1% of the population, it is the largest household sample survey in Germany. The microcensus sampling units are artificially delimited areas (sampling districts). The statistical units are all households living in the sampling districts (330 044) and all persons living in those households (691 361). The total number of foreign (-national/-born/-trained) health professionals is obtained through extrapolation and refers to active health professionals.

2. Mobility profile of Germany

Health care is one of the most important economic sectors in Germany, employing 4.6 million people (3.5 million full-time equivalents) or roughly 11% of the country's total workforce. Total health-care spending in 2008 amounted to €263 billion, 10.5% of the gross domestic product (GDP) (Federal Statistical Office 2010).

Foreign-national health professionals

Microcensus data from the Federal Statistical Office shows that the share of health professionals with foreign citizenship amounted to approximately 5% of all health professionals between 2003 and 2007 and increased to 6% in 2008. This included medical doctors, dentists, nurses and midwives, as well as nursing assistants. However, a significant percentage of all foreign-national health professionals are second or third generation migrants and have not migrated themselves. In 2008, roughly 15% of all health professionals with foreign citizenship were born in Germany and around 57% were estimated to have been trained in Germany (Federal Statistical Office unpublished data 2010).[2]

Between 2003 and 2008, the share of foreign nationals employed in the health-care sector and subject to social insurance contributions amounted to approximately 4.5% of the total number of employees – medical doctors, dentists, nurses, midwives and nursing assistants. This is lower than the percentage of foreign-national employees (subject to social insurance contributions) in the labour market as a whole, which averaged 6.8% in 2008 (Federal Employment Agency 2009).

Foreign-trained health professionals

Among all health professionals in Germany, the proportion of those (including both foreign and German nationals) who were trained outside Germany increased from roughly 3.7% in 2003 to 5.5% in 2008 (Federal Statistical Office unpublished data 2010).

Foreign-born health professionals

In 2008, roughly 13% of all health professionals working in Germany had been born outside the country (Federal Statistical Office unpublished data 2010). A study conducted by the Robert Koch Institute and based on the microcensus data for 2007 showed that 11.5% of all health professionals in the public health sector in Germany have personal experience of immigration. These include all persons who were born elsewhere but migrated to Germany, as long as they

---

2 Health professionals are categorized as foreign-trained if they obtained their degrees before moving to Germany (only the last year of entry to Germany is relevant). Hence, the number of health professionals trained abroad is an overestimation because it does not exclude those health professionals who were trained in Germany, subsequently lived (and presumably worked) abroad and then returned to Germany.

belong to one of three categories: (i) foreign citizen (4.5%); (ii) naturalized person – *Eingebürgerte* (4.6%); (iii) ethnic German – *Spätaussiedler* (2.4%) (Afentakis & Böhm 2009).[3]

Currently, there are no reliable data on the total number of German health professionals working abroad. Incomplete and partly outdated stock data are available for medical doctors only. Data compiled by the regional chambers of physicians show that the annual outflows of German and foreign medical doctors have increased since 2000.

2.1 *Medical doctors*

Germany is affected by international migration of physicians in both directions. Increasing numbers of foreign medical doctors are seeking employment in the country and a growing number of German medical doctors are leaving to work abroad.

The total number and the annual inflows of foreign-national medical doctors registered in Germany are recorded by the regional chambers of physicians. At the end of 2008 there were 21 784 medical doctors of foreign nationality in Germany, approximately 5.2% of the total number of registered medical doctors, and 18 105 active (practising) foreign medical doctors, around 5.7% of all active medical doctors in the country. The absolute numbers of registered and active foreign medical doctors have increased since 2000, as have their percentages among all registered and all active medical doctors in the country (Figs. 5.1 and 5.2).

Fig. 5.1 *Registered and active foreign-national medical doctors (stock) in Germany, 2000–2008*

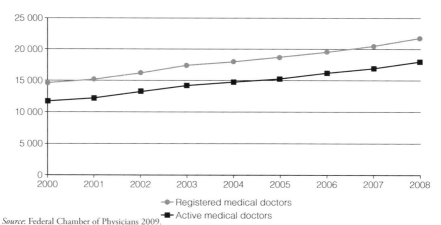

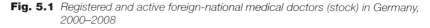
Registered medical doctors
Active medical doctors

Source: Federal Chamber of Physicians 2009.

---

3 The number of ethnic Germans is an underestimation as many appear under '"naturalized person". Between the mid 1980s and 2000, ethnic Germans were obliged to undergo naturalization and hence it is not possible to differentiate clearly between an ethnic German and a naturalized person.

Fig. 5.2 *Registered and active foreign-national medical doctors as percentages of all registered and all active medical doctors in Germany, 2000–2008*

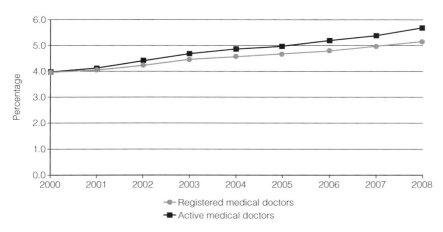

Source: Federal Chamber of Physicians 2009.

Microcensus data indicate that in 2008 approximately 11% of all foreign-national medical doctors were born in Germany and roughly 42% were trained in Germany. Hence, registry data based on nationality does not accurately reflect the migrant stocks and inflows of medical doctors in the country (Federal Statistical Office unpublished data 2010).

The main source countries for medical doctors (Table 5.1) are Austria (1802 registered medical doctors), Greece (1708), the Russian Federation/former USSR (1685), Poland (1428), the Islamic Republic of Iran (1092) and Romania (927) (Federal Chamber of Physicians 2009).

Until 2000, the total number of foreign-national medical doctors practising in Germany had been growing largely in line with the general development in the number of medical doctors. Immigration of foreign medical doctors began to increase in 2001 and peaked in 2003, as can be seen from the annual growth rate in the total number of registered foreign medical doctors. This was highest in 2002 (6.7%) and 2003 (7.2%) and decreased to 3.9% and 3.3% in 2004 and 2005 respectively. The annual inflow of foreign doctors demonstrates a similar pattern (Fig. 5.3).

One explanation for this is media hype of a looming shortage of medical doctors, induced by the physicians' organizations. This peaked in 2003, following a European Court of Justice ruling stipulating that on-call duty should be considered as working time. The physicians' shortage was traced to the poor working conditions and unattractive pay for medical doctors in Germany. However, one major reason for the perceived shortage was not mentioned

Table 5.1 *Registered foreign-national medical doctors in Germany, by nationality, 1988 and 2003–2008*

	1988	2003	2004	2005	2006	2007	2008
Total foreign medical doctors	9 376	17 318	17 991	18 582	19 513	20 434	21 784
EU	2 553	4 751	7 072	7 554	8 156	10 069	10 984
Austria	260	958	1 130	1 269	1 438	1 613	1 802
Belgium	263	235	224	222	228	231	239
Bulgaria	-	308	349	365	393	462	541
Cyprus	-	42	43	42	46	52	58
Czech Republic	351a	175	211	239	263	304	346
Denmark	59	66	63	59	62	61	59
Estonia	-	23	25	26	27	27	30
Finland	-	113	111	109	112	106	110
France	297	360	366	382	383	398	407
Greece	710	1 162	1 265	1 357	1 453	1 554	1 708
Hungary	169	248	252	271	305	359	430
Ireland	17	30	30	32	32	32	33
Italy	325	584	615	660	694	719	755
Latvia	-	37	40	40	37	43	41
Lithuania	-	37	49	48	51	61	69
Luxembourg	116	133	135	129	137	147	159
Malta	-	4	4	4	4	5	5
Netherlands	453	487	497	500	400	525	552
Poland	511	919	1 086	1 171	1 283	1 332	1 428
Portugal	-	52	62	68	73	74	77
Romania	283	635	660	692	718	824	927
Slovakia	-	155	255	297	375	454	503
Slovenia	-	11	18	22	24	28	31
Spain	149	295	320	326	338	356	369
Sweden	-	92	91	91	91	99	100
United Kingdom	141	184	181	190	200	203	205
Europe (excluding the EU)	-	7 060	5 342	5 471	5 639	4 557	4 740
Russia/former USSR	-	1696	1591	1572	1616	1624	1685
Africa	-	786	820	813	832	850	916
America	-	643	655	655	685	710	722
Asia	-	3 770	3 808	3 818	3 937	3 994	4 163
Iran	982	1316	1265	1201	1165	1106	1092
Australia and Oceania	-	12	17	15	15	17	17
Other	-	296	277	256	249	237	242

Source: Federal Chamber of Physicians 2009. *Note*: ᵃ Czechoslovakia.

Fig. 5.3 *Annual gross inflows of registered foreign-national medical doctors in Germany, 2000–2008*

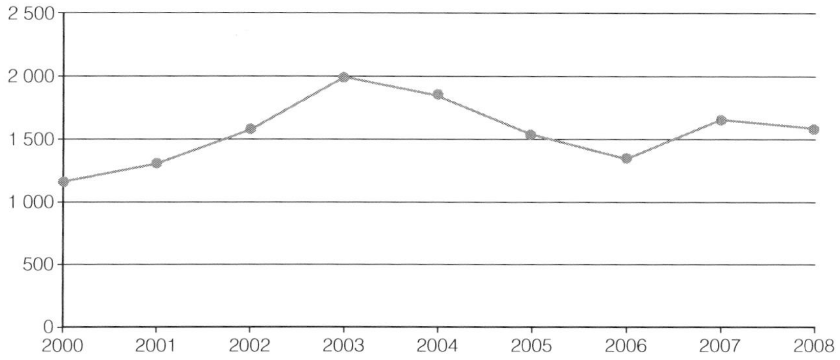

Source: Federal Chamber of Physicians 2009.

at that time – the decrease in the number of medical students in the winter semester of 1990/1991 (Hoesch 2009).

Box 5.1 *Statutory bodies and other organizations representing the interests of physicians*

Physicians' interests are well-organized and well-represented within Germany's health-care system. The regional chambers of physicians are responsible for secondary training, certification and continuing education and membership is a mandatory prerequisite to practise as a medical doctor. Within the Statutory Health Insurance (SHI) scheme, SHI-affiliated physicians' and dentists' associations represent the corporatist institutions on the provider side; the sickness funds and their associations operate on the purchasers' side. Furthermore, there are lobbying organizations such as the Hartmann Union and the Marburg Union. The former was established to defend the economic interests of physicians and has its main membership base in the outpatient sector; the latter was formed to defend the rights of hospital physicians (Busse & Riesberg 2004).

Immigration affects the whole country but the growth in the absolute number of foreign medical doctors and in their share among all medical doctors has been considerably higher in eastern Germany (Figs. 5.4 and 5.5). In the period from 2000 to 2008 the number of active foreign medical doctors in the states of the former West Germany rose by 40%, while the corresponding figure for the former East Germany was roughly 309%. Only 6% of all active foreign-national medical doctors in Germany were practising in eastern Germany in 2000 but this proportion had reached 15% by 2008. In particular the percentage of eastern European doctors among all medical doctors in eastern Germany is growing rapidly (Fig. 5.6).

Source: Kopetsch 2010.

Fig. 5.4 *Active foreign-national medical doctors in western and eastern Germany (stock), 2000–2008*

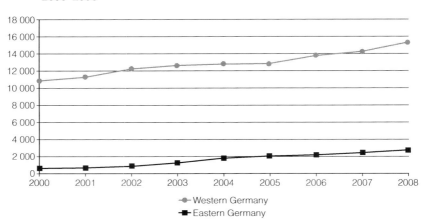

Fig. 5.5 *Active foreign-national medical doctors as percentages of all active medical doctors in western and eastern Germany, 2000–2008*

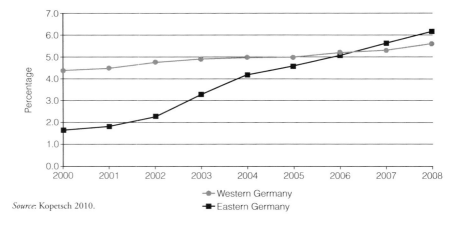

Source: Kopetsch 2010.

When immigration does occur, it is quite rare for foreign medical doctors to become self-employed. In 2008 only 3534 foreign medical doctors ran private practices – 2.8% of all practice-based medical doctors. The share of foreign medical doctors is considerably higher in the hospital sector – 13 207 (8.6%) of 153 799 medical doctors (Federal Chamber of Physicians 2009). Possible reasons for this imbalance are the legal framework and the high investment costs which discourage foreign medical doctors from opening a practice.

Data on the annual outflows of German medical doctors have been collected by the majority of regional chambers of physicians since 2000.[4] There are no data

---

4 Data from 14 regional chambers of physicians were supplemented by a projection for the missing data from three chambers.

Fig. 5.6 *Eastern European medical doctors as percentages of all medical doctors in western and eastern Germany, 2000–2008*

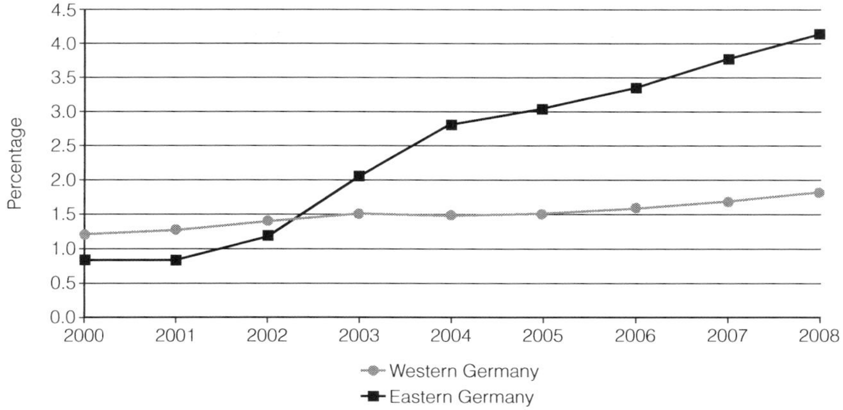

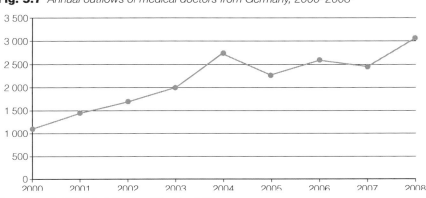

Source: Kopetsch 2010.

on the number of medical doctors who returned to Germany after practising abroad as return migration is not recorded.

Fig. 5.7 shows that the annual outflows of (German and foreign-national) medical doctors have increased since 2000. In 2008 a total of 3065 medical doctors who originally practised in Germany (approximately 1% of all active medical doctors) moved abroad, 67% of these held German nationality. Compared with the previous year, this represents a 26% increase in the total number of medical doctors leaving Germany and a 10% increase in the number of German medical doctors leaving the country (Fig. 5.8). The highest emigration rates in 2008 were recorded by the states of Hesse and Bremen (Kopetsch 2009b).

Fig. 5.7 *Annual outflows of medical doctors from Germany, 2000–2008[5]*

Source: Kopetsch 2007; Federal Chamber of Physicians 2009.

5 Based on the number of medical doctors who cancelled their registrations with regional chambers of physicians.

Fig. 5.8 *Annual outflows of German and foreign-national medical doctors from Germany, 2006–2008*

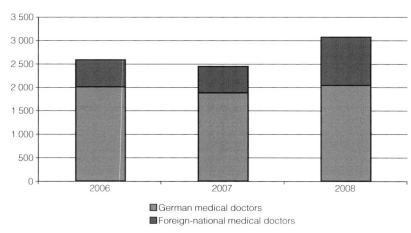

Source: Federal Chamber of Physicians 2009.

Data provided by the Federal Chamber of Physicians show that the most popular destination countries for all medical doctors who left Germany in 2008 were the German-speaking countries of Switzerland (729) and Austria (237), followed by the United States of America (168), the United Kingdom (95) and Sweden (86).[6] This ranking is unchanged from the previous year.

The total number of German medical doctors working abroad differs from source to source. A study conducted by the Federal Association of Statutory Health Insurance Physicians indicates approximately 17 000 physicians practising abroad, the majority based in Switzerland, followed by the United Kingdom, the United States and Austria (Kopetsch 2010).

2.2 Nurses and midwives

Aggregated data on foreign-national nurses and midwives were provided by the Federal Employment Agency. These record all employees subject to social insurance contributions and the majority of legally employed nurses fall under this category. No registry data are available as nurses and midwives are organized through voluntary membership of a variety of professional organizations and are not required to register with a particular organization or chambers. Nurse organizations have become part of an umbrella organization – the German Nursing Council (DPR) – which must (by law) be consulted on SHI decisions

---

6 Other destinations include the Netherlands (64), Spain (62), France (59), Greece (53), Poland (40), Norway (39), Denmark (36), Australia/Oceania (74). In 2008, the most popular destinations for German medical doctors were: Switzerland (626), the United States of America (144), Austria (81), the United Kingdom (74), Sweden (66), Netherlands (47), Spain (47), France (43), Norway (32) (Federal Chamber of Physicians 2009).

affecting nursing (Busse & Riesberg 2004). In practice, however, nurse organizations have considerably less influence and fewer resources than the strong physicians' organizations.

At present, there is no monitoring system for the number of nurses and their professional qualifications. Also, there is no system of workforce planning that considers future nursing needs (Weinbrenner & Busse 2006). Currently, there is a discussion on the introduction of a mandatory chamber of nurses. This should strengthen the position of the relatively weak and poorly organized nursing staff (Igl 2008).

Fig. 5.9 demonstrates that the number of foreign nurses and midwives subject to social insurance contributions has decreased since 2003.[7] The share of foreign nurses and midwives among all nurses and midwives subject to social insurance contributions decreased from 3.7% in 2003 to 3.4% in 2008. The number of nurses and midwives of foreign EU nationality shows only a slight decrease (3%) while there were more pronounced decreases in the numbers of nurses and midwives from Asia, Europe (excluding the EU) and Africa – at about 30%, 7% and 5% respectively. The share of nursing assistants decreased from 7.6% in 2003 to 7.0% in 2008 (Federal Employment Agency unpublished data 2009).[8]

Fig. 5.9 *Foreign-national nurses and midwives subject to social insurance contributions in Germany, 2003–2008*

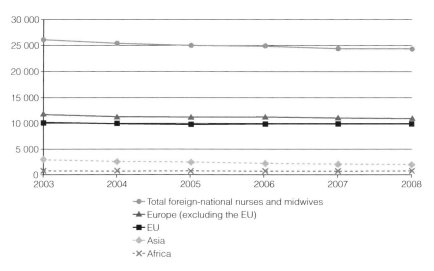

Source: Federal Employment Agency unpublished data 2009.

---

7 Reference date is 30 September for 2008 and 31 December for all other years.

8 Reference date is 31 December for all years.

There are several possible explanations for the decrease in the number of foreign-national nurses subject to social insurance contributions. Firstly, demand for foreign nurses often follows cyclical patterns linked to economic activity in the country – in times of economic upturn the nursing profession is considered less attractive than other employment opportunities and foreign nurses need to be recruited to fill the vacancies; in times of economic decline the nursing profession is regarded as a secure employment and recruitment of foreign nurses is less pronounced (Hoesch 2009). Hence, the recent financial crisis might have increased the attractiveness of the nursing profession.

Another possible explanation is a shift from dependant employment (subject to social insurance contributions) to other forms such as self-employment and illegal employment, concerning particularly elderly care. According to microcensus data the number of foreign-national nurses and midwives working in Germany decreased from 45 000 in 2003 to 42 000 in 2008, while the percentage of foreign-national nurses and midwives among all nurses and midwives remained stable at about 5%. However, the percentage of those foreign nurses who were trained outside Germany increased from 29% in 2003 to 43% in 2008.

Estimates of the number of nursing staff working illegally in the country, mostly as home nurses, differ from source to source (Spielberg 2009). A study conducted by the German Institute of Applied Research in Nursing mentions 100 000 home helps from eastern European countries, a considerable number of whom are estimated to have a nursing background (Neuhaus et al. 2009).

The main source countries for nurses and midwives subject to social insurance contributions are Croatia (3058), Turkey (2886), and Poland (2390), followed by Serbia/the former Federal Republic of Yugoslavia (1553), Bosnia and Herzegovina (1413) and Austria (989).[9] Data on the outflows of German nurses are not available but, according to German Nursing Association (DBfK) estimates, the annual outflow of nurses does not exceed 1000. The most important destination countries are Switzerland, Austria and the United Kingdom which offer better training opportunities, higher incomes and flatter hierarchies (Hoesch 2008).

2.3 Dentists

Data on foreign dentists practising in Germany are only partially available. Figures for 2007 compiled by the Federal Chamber of Dentists give a total of 1573 dentists with foreign EU nationality[10], around 2% of the total number of

---

9 Reference date is 30 September 2008.

10 Data for Schleswig-Holstein, Rheinland-Pfalz and Niedersachsen are missing.

Table 5.2 *Foreign-national nurses and midwives subject to social insurance contributions in Germany, by nationality, 2003–2008*

	2003	2004	2005	2006	2007	2008[a]
Total foreign nurses and midwives	26 364	25 452	25 115	24 977	24 489	24 387
EU	10 259	9 967	9 939	10 041	9 992	9 971
Austria	1 129	1 124	1 068	1033	992	989
Belgium	208	204	190	195	198	195
Bulgaria	249	220	219	221	233	237
Czech Republic	431	425	414	405	406	413
Denmark	117	112	104	108	100	94
Estonia	17	15	19	21	17	20
Finland	252	227	219	202	185	172
France	481	461	456	445	441	416
Greece	524	507	526	535	541	538
Hungary	291	282	282	292	308	310
Ireland	66	66	61	57	49	49
Italy	959	945	946	978	1 016	968
Latvia	35	34	36	39	37	40
Lithuania	62	73	86	92	96	102
Luxembourg	44	42	38	41	45	45
Netherlands	807	777	764	750	718	708
Poland	2 325	2 269	2 298	2 373	2 353	2 390
Portugal	524	511	521	546	530	544
Romania	593	568	574	576	591	606
Slovakia	139	134	147	162	173	180
Slovenia	194	195	198	214	219	221
Spain	411	390	401	396	392	393
Sweden	57	60	54	53	52	52
United Kingdom	340	323	315	304	297	286
Europe (excluding the EU)	11 776	11 519	11 369	11 306	11 055	11 013
Croatia	2446	2471	2581	2703	2963	3058
Turkey	3042	2930	2881	2901	2868	2886
Bosnia and Herzegovina	1107	1082	1115	1155	1359	1413
Serbia/former Federal Republic of Yugoslavia [b]	3483	3263	2978	2668	1844	1553
Africa	729	702	680	678	690	690
America	554	523	542	545	509	560
Asia	2 999	2 693	2 539	2 359	2 192	2 103
Australia and Oceania	47	48	46	48	51	50

Source: Federal Employment Agency unpublished data 2009. *Note*: [a] 2008 reference date is 30 September, [b] No clear classification to the succession countries of the former Federal Republic of Yugoslavia (1992–2003) was possible.

dentists in the country. Of these, 913 were working as practice-based dentists, 350 as assistants or employees in practices, 69 as civil servants or employees working as dentists but not in practices and 241 were non-active dentists. At the end of 2007, the main EU source countries were Greece (306), the Netherlands (300), Romania (157), Poland (124) and Sweden (120).

The Federal Employment Agency generated data on foreign dentists who are employed and subject to social insurance contributions. The statistics demonstrate an increase in the number of foreign-national dentists from 336 in 2003 to 490 in 2008,[11] split fairly evenly between citizens of EU Member States and of non-EU European countries. Microcensus data show that the number of dentists of foreign nationality in Germany hovered around 2000 (3% of all dentists) between 2003 and 2006 and increased to 3000 (5% of all dentists) in 2008.

3. Vignettes on health professional mobility[12]

Better prospects for eastern European doctors

Wiktor migrated from Bulgaria to Germany shortly after completing his medical studies in 2003. He was driven to leave not only by the poor pay but also by limited access to post-graduate training, the need to take additional work in order to cover his living expenses and the lack of prospects in an underfunded and poorly organized system.

Germany was an attractive destination as Wiktor had learned German at school and had friends already working in Germany. He was also in contact with an agency that placed eastern European doctors in German hospitals. This agency arranged an appointment with the head of a specialist department in a hospital in Mecklenburg-Western Pomerania. Wiktor was not attracted by the region and was apprehensive about the services offered by the agency, so decided to apply directly for some vacancies listed in the German Medical Journal. Having applied successfully to a hospital in Brandenburg, it took a few months to obtain a temporary professional work permit and a residence permit.

Wiktor has found it difficult to adapt to the German system. The language barrier, increasing amount of bureaucracy that doctors face, pace of work and frequent night shifts have often made him doubt his choice. Some of his colleagues have already moved on to other countries such as the United Kingdom.

---

11 Reference date is 30 September for 2008 and 31 December for all other years.
12 Based on information and interviews retrieved from the media, the names have been invented.

Back to Germany

Katja left Germany mainly because of the atmosphere in the hospital where she worked. After several years working for the British National Health Service, Katja returned to her native country to work as a hospital consultant in Berlin. With work experience in both countries, she has no doubts about the advantages of the British system:

Firstly you get excellent training in Britain, but there are other issues such as the flat hierarchy which means that when you have a good idea it doesn't matter how high up you are, people listen and take you seriously.

In Britain, the top level is more widely spread. Consultants are very independent and the system is fed sensibly. But in Germany, even the very senior doctors who are specialists in their own right have to bow down before the head doctor, who can make life miserable for anyone he chooses.

Germany has a higher physician density than the UK. This is a reason for both bad behaviour in the upper ranks of German hospitals and for slow career progress. In the UK, junior doctors are allowed to do many things because there are not as many doctors, whereas in Germany only the top people get to perform.

German doctors often mention their dissatisfaction when talking about their working conditions, not only with remuneration but also with hospital structures. Katja said:

Although the conditions in the UK seem enticing for young German graduates, there is no doubt that they would really like to see conditions at home improve, and hence not have to work abroad.

Growing need for elderly care

Anna is a 28-year-old nurse from Poland. An agency sent her to a small town in Rhineland-Palatinate to look after an 87-year-old woman who could not get around by herself and did not want to go into a nursing home. Anna is not the only one in this neighbourhood to offer cheap 24-hour care. The area is home to growing numbers of Poles, Romanians and Bulgarians caring for the elderly local population. Many do not stay long in Germany but they are replaced easily.

A growing number of agencies now provide home-help services from these eastern European countries. Many operate in a legal grey area, given Germany's restrictions on the free movement of labour within the EU. Carers can circumvent these regulations by registering as self-employed in their home country. This allows them to work in Germany if they prove that they are working for more than one client. Agencies tend to send a carer to various clients for limited periods. Other agencies offer eastern European professionals contracts with companies in their home countries that work with partner agencies in Germany. They are sent not only to private homes but also to understaffed hospitals and clinics.

> ### *Heading north*
>
> Miriam, a young German dentist, completed her internship at a dental practice and decided to pursue a career in Norway. Her time in the practice made her decide on Scandinavia as she did not like sacrificing quality for quantity. Her boss in Germany had pressurized her to complete procedures quickly as the next patient was already waiting – "Here in Norway I can take an entire hour for a filling, which means the quality is higher."
>
> Miriam is not alone among professionals in seeking her fortune, and future career, beyond Germany's border. The work pace and hours, as well as the higher pay, make the northern country an attractive destination to live and work, especially in comparison to Miriam's home region in eastern Germany. Patients sometimes have to drive 80 km to reach the nearest orthodontist in the states of Brandenburg, Saxony or Saxony-Anhalt. Few dentists will risk setting up a practice in such a sparsely settled region and few of those who wish to do so have the resources required to start a new practice.
>
> Another problem is emigration. The poor economy and lack of jobs have forced many to leave eastern Germany. Even if new dentists have the desire to open a practice there, they face the real danger that their patients will disappear.

4. Dynamics of enlargement

Against expectations, the migration of health professionals from eastern Europe to Germany did not increase considerably after the 2004 EU expansion. The number of foreign medical doctors from the new Member States has increased constantly since 2000 but the highest growth rate (around 21%) in the number of medical doctors from the EU-12 occurred in 2003, before EU enlargement (Fig. 5.10).

The total number of nurses and midwives coming from the new Member States (excluding Malta and Cyprus) and subject to social insurance contributions increased only slightly in the years after the 2004 EU enlargement (Fig. 5.11). However, it is estimated that there has been a higher increase in the number of nurses from the new EU Member States who are working in Germany as home helps or caregivers, mainly for elderly people and those with disabilities. Even though eastern European caregivers usually do not replace professional nursing services, they play an important role in facilitating care at home (Neuhaus et al. 2009).

Fig.5.10 *Registered foreign-national medical doctors from new and old EU Member States (stock) in Germany, 2000–2008[13]*

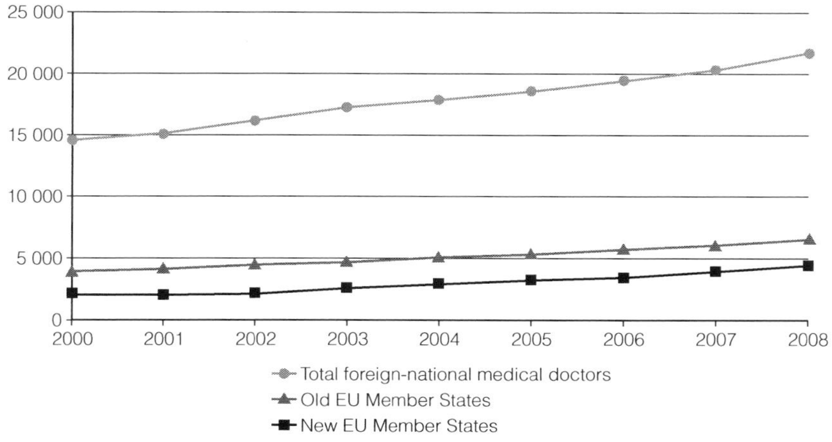

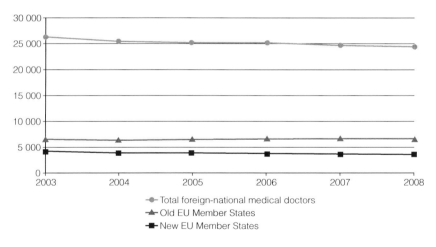

Source: Federal Chamber of Physicians 2009.

Fig. 5.11 *Foreign-national nurses and midwives subject to social insurance contributions from new and old EU Member States (stock) in Germany, 2003–2008[14]*

Source: Federal Employment Agency unpublished data 2009.

The number of dentists from the new EU Member States who were subject to social security contributions increased from 48 in 2003 to 72 in 2008.[15] However, there was a slight decrease in the years following the 2004 enlargement.

---

13 New EU Member States refers to the number of physicians from the EU-12 also before EU accession. No data were available for Cyprus, Estonia, Latvia, Lithuania, Malta and Slovenia for 2000 and 2001.

14 Including Bulgaria and Romania for all years. Missing data for Malta and Cyprus.

15 Missing data for Cyprus, Estonia, Latvia, Lithuania, Malta, Slovakia and Slovenia (<3).

In summary, the numbers of health professionals from the new Member States peaked before the 2004 EU expansion. This occurred at a time when demand was first diagnosed to be high (particularly for medical doctors) but the restrictive immigration policy for non-EU nationals still applied to these countries. Thus, it appears that high demand for foreign personnel and sufficiently large incentives to migrate (such as wage differentials, better working conditions) seem to have had a far greater effect than migration law in the country (Fellmer 2008).

Curiously, the increase in the number of medical doctors from the new EU Member States in Germany slowed after EU enlargement in 2004. This may be due in part to the fact that countries such as the United Kingdom did not limit the freedom of movement of labour. Moreover, as the prospect of higher wages was offered alongside this more immigration-friendly policy, many eastern European health professionals wishing to emigrate may have preferred the United Kingdom.

5. Impacts on the German health system

The scale of health professional migration to and from Germany is relatively limited in comparison to other major destination countries and therefore there has been little research on its impact on the country's health-care system. However, several studies indicate that the migration of health professionals has a growing effect on service provision. In particular, the provision of health services in eastern Germany is increasingly dependent on foreign medical doctors (Kopetsch 2009a).

The outflow of German medical doctors has a negative impact on the human resources and knowledge base in the health-care system. Conversely, the inflow of foreign medical doctors increases the pool of human resources and diversifies the knowledge, language and skills mix. As yet, migration has not had a pronounced impact on the general design, priority formulation and policy direction of the health system.

Furthermore, there are no sound studies on how health professional migration affects population health. The immigration of foreign medical doctors has increased the responsiveness of the health system by containing waiting times in less attractive regions in eastern Germany. Greater cultural and language variety among health professionals makes the system more responsive to the diversity in patients. However, a perceived reduction in responsiveness is caused by language differences and communication problems between foreign health professionals and German patients.

Integration programmes for structured training on the working procedures in German hospitals and for systematic improvement of the German language are rare. The often inadequate language skills of foreign health professionals are problematic, for both patients and colleagues. In the extreme, insufficient language skills might cause misdiagnoses (Flintrop 2009). As administrative tasks increasingly occupy health professionals, inadequate writing skills can lead to dissatisfaction among the foreign health professionals themselves and their German colleagues (Kopetsch 2009a).

6. Relevance of cross-border health professional mobility

The mobility profile of the country shows limited health professional migration to and from Germany. Health professionals of foreign nationality still represent a relatively small share (about 6%) of the total health workforce. However, foreign health professionals are becoming increasingly relevant – physicians for the provision of inpatient care in eastern Germany; nurses for the provision of home care for elderly people.

With a relatively high and rising density of physicians and nurses (OECD 2009), the German health-care system as a whole is not largely dependent on foreign-trained health professionals. However, Germany faces significant disparities in the provision of health-care personnel. An oversupply in and around big cities such as Munich, Hamburg and Berlin contrasts with considerable shortages in sparsely populated areas in the less prosperous eastern part of the country. This situation has been described as "shortage in the surplus" (Neubacher 2008).

According to directives, undersupply of SHI-authorized physicians in a particular planning area occurs when the actual number of physicians is less than 75% (for family physicians) or less than 50% (for all other specialties) of the determined optimal number of physicians. Under that definition, no serious undersupply could be established nationwide for any specialty. Nevertheless, regional maldistribution of medical doctors persists (Klose et al. 2007). In case of regional shortages the sickness funds can grant extra bonuses [*Sicherstellungszuschläge*] to attract physicians and ensure the financial viability of medical practices.

The Federal Association of Statutory Health Insurance Physicians reports that the medical health workforce in Germany is expected to face serious challenges from diminishing graduate numbers, feminization of the medical profession and an ageing medical staff (Kopetsch 2007). Between 1999 and 2008 the number of family doctors[16] in eastern Germany decreased by approximately

16 Including general practitioners and internists but excluding paediatricians.

10% as young doctors increasingly followed the higher pay and better working conditions offered in western Germany.

The *Hospital Barometer 2008* (Blum et al. 2008) reports that around two thirds (67%) of the hospitals surveyed had problems filling vacancies, compared to 28% in 2006. The situation in eastern Germany is of particular concern as nearly 81% of hospitals had vacant positions they could not fill, compared to 65% in western Germany. It was estimated that some 4000 vacancies could not be filled throughout the country, representing around 3% of all medical doctors working in the inpatient sector. This number has tripled since 2006 when the number of vacancies was estimated to be 1300 (Blum et al. 2008).

In summary, Germany has traditionally had a high physician-population ratio but it is likely that increasingly it will seek to recruit medical doctors from other parts of Europe in order to maintain current levels of supply. This may be temporary, until the distribution of human resources in the country has improved. Steps are already being taken to match the salaries of medical doctors in eastern Germany with those in western Germany. Given the lower costs of living in the eastern states this should provide an incentive for doctors to move there.

Data collected from the Federal Employment Agency suggest that the nursing system is growing less dependent on foreign-trained health professionals as the share of foreign-national nurses and midwives subject to social insurance contributions is declining. However, microcensus data suggest that the share of all foreign-national nurses and midwives has remained stable at around 5%.

Traditionally, recruitment of foreign nurses has played an important role in Germany, especially in times of recorded high demand. Bilateral agreements for the recruitment of nurses have been in place since the early 1970s – first to recruit nurses from the Republic of Korea, then with a number of eastern European countries. Currently, Germany has a bilateral agreement with Croatia, which provides the highest number of foreign nurses and midwives subject to social insurance contributions. With no monitoring system for nurses and no system of workforce planning that considers future nursing needs, recruitment of foreign nurses to Germany occurs on an ad-hoc basis, whenever a shortage is perceived (Hoesch 2009). The demand for nurses is expected to rise as a result of demographic changes and the declining appeal of the profession, especially in times of economic upturn. The health system's dependence on foreign-trained health personnel is already noticeable in areas such as elderly care and is likely to increase.

7. Factors influencing health professional mobility

7.1 *Inflows*

A significant instigating factor driving young foreign medical doctors to seek work in Germany is poor pay in their country of origin. In addition, limited training opportunities, chronic underfunding of the health system, shortages in medical equipment and medicine, corruption and strikes have led to dissatisfaction among the medical staff in some eastern European EU Member States. The main activating factors are therefore relatively high wage differentials, better working conditions and better training opportunities (Fellmer 2008).

Prospective migrants can be discouraged by the perceived costs of migration. These can include the monetary costs of the migration process – for transportation, finding relevant job vacancies, new accommodation and other such practicalities. Further deterrents are the loss of cultural and regional knowledge, the inability to receive the same wages as equally qualified citizens of the host country and possible hurdles that may hinder or prevent spouses wishing to work in their own professions (Fellmer 2008).

The legal framework regarding the migration of health professionals to Germany is often perceived as a deterrent factor. Legal possibilities to work in the country are still limited to some groups of migrants and the process of meeting the general work and occupational requirements is burdensome for many migrants, especially non-EU citizens.

It has become easier for citizens of the new EU Member States to enter and work in Germany since EU accession. One factor that facilitates the migration of health professionals is the mutual recognition of professional qualifications in the EU. Also, the growing numbers of agencies which specialize in recruiting nursing staff (mainly for elderly care) and medical doctors from eastern European countries are facilitating the information, job-seeking and application process.

The main instigating factors for nurses were found to be low pay and poor employment, economic, safety and working conditions. Facilitating factors were found to be easing of the migration regulations within EU countries, active recruitment and the mutual recognition of diplomas in the EU (Hasselhorn et al. 2005).

7.2 *Outflows*

A number of surveys have explored the reasons why German medical doctors leave the country. A survey conducted by Ramboll Management (2004) indicates three main instigating factors for either emigrating or ceasing to practise curative medicine altogether. Firstly, the level of remuneration –

medical doctors consider this to be inadequate for the services they provide. Secondly, the workload and the poor work-life balance. Thirdly, the increasing bureaucracy and administrative burden faced by medical practitioners. Further factors are the hierarchical structure and leadership style in German hospitals, as well as poor mentoring.[17]

German medical doctors willing to leave the country are attracted by a range of activating factors, including: systematic postgraduate training; better working conditions and pay; opportunities for professional development; and a relaxed working climate. A study by Janus et al. (2007) suggests that non-monetary factors are important determinants of physicians' job satisfaction, possibly more important than monetary incentives. Factor analysis revealed that decision-making and recognition, continuous education and job security, administrative tasks and collegial relationships were highly significant; specialized technology and patient contact were significant; but research and teaching and international exchange were not significant in contributing to physicians' job satisfaction (Janus et al. 2007).

The instigating determinants of nurses' decisions to leave their profession or move abroad include dissatisfaction with working conditions, the work content and work organization; low esteem; a marked effort-reward imbalance and perceived low pay (Hasselhorn et al. 2005).

8. Policy, regulation and interventions affecting health professional mobility

8.1 *Immigration law*

Immigration of health professionals to Germany is generally regulated by the provisions on the right of residence and work permit for foreign nationals. Medical doctors and other health professionals fall largely into the category of "qualified labour". There is no distinct national policy on health professional migration.

Non-EU citizens

Non-EU citizens wishing to take up qualified employment can obtain a temporarily restricted residence permit with approval by the Federal Employment Agency. This approval generally requires a labour market assessment which reviews (among other considerations) whether: (i) there are no negative consequences for the labour market; and (ii) access to the labour market is safeguarded for German and preferential non-German unemployed persons (such as citizens of EU Member States) (Derst et al. 2006).

---

17 The ranking differs slightly according to gender and career phase.

Migrants classed as "highly skilled persons" do not require Federal Employment Agency approval and hence no labour market assessment. This category includes: (i) academics with exceptional professional qualifications; (ii) lecturers and researchers in leading positions; (iii) specialists and executive employees with incomes over the contribution assessment ceiling for statutory pension insurance.

Residence and work permits for foreign nursing staff from certain non-EU/EEA countries are regulated with special procedures for recruitment. These involve a joint administrative procedure by the Federal Employment Agency and the labour administration of the country of origin. At present, Germany has a bilateral agreement of this type only with Croatia.

The Immigration Act of 2005 introduced a residence permit for self-employed persons, which might be applicable for setting up a medical practice. This regulation postulates a broader economic interest or a special regional need for the occupation, as well as a positive impact for the economy resulting from that type of occupational activity. As a rule, these requirements are met with an investment of at least €250 000 and guaranteed creation of at least five jobs. In the case of setting up a medical practice, the required amount of investment might be reduced and the assessment made on the basis of a potential special regional need for medical care (Derst et al. 2006).

Citizens from the new EU Member States

Citizens of the new EU Member States (excluding Malta and Cyprus) are subject to transition periods that restrict workers' freedom of movement. The transitional periods for those who joined the EU in 2004 will end in April 2011; for Bulgaria and Romania by December 2013 at the latest. Until these dates, these citizens need Federal Employment Agency approval (principally involving a labour market test) in order to take up employment.

Since 2009, citizens of the new EU Member States who hold a university degree do not require a labour market assessment in order to obtain a work permit to exercise a profession which corresponds to their qualifications. Their family members are also exempt from the labour market test. Hence, medical doctors from the new EU Member States can freely access the German labour market if they meet the occupational requirements described below.

Labour market assessment remains a prerequisite for nurses and midwives although the specific requirements, as well as the prospect of obtaining a work permit, differ from state to state. Within the framework of freedom of establishment and services, nurses from the new EU Member States can circumvent the labour market test and provide their services in Germany by registering as self-employed in their country of origin. However, this requires proof that they have more than one client. A second possibility is to sign a contract with a company in their home country which is entitled to send personnel to Germany. A number of agencies have sprung up to offer their services in facilitating this process in the elderly care arena.

Qualified workers from eastern Europe[18] aged between 18 and 40 years can take up temporary employment in Germany through the so-called guest worker procedure with the involvement of the Federal Employment Agency. This procedure allows them to work in Germany for up to 18 months and is intended to enhance their professional qualifications and language skills. It does not require a labour market test but has to comply with certain country quotas (Federal Employment Agency 2007). After a year of legal employment in Germany, EU citizens have the right to obtain a work permit of unlimited duration.

Legal occupational regulations

Fulfillment of the legal occupational requirements for practising medical and nursing professions in Germany is a prerequisite for obtaining a residence permit. A medical doctor wishing to practise medicine in Germany requires a medical licence [*Approbation*] or a temporary professional authorization [*Berufserlaubnis*]. The medical licence is issued by the responsible authorities in the federal states, following application and submission of the required qualification certificates. The medical licence entitles a medical doctor to practise medicine in hospitals, at institutes and other facilities as well as in his/her medical practice after completion of a specialist medical training. A medical licence is issued when the applicant is a German or an EU citizen.

Directive 2005/36/EC (European Parliament and Council of the European Union 2005) regulates the mutual recognition of professional qualifications. The educational qualifications of medical doctors whose education started after the date of EU accession are recognized as fully equal. The relevant authorities might request further specifications (such as confirmation of working experience) from health professionals whose education started before EU accession (European Commission 2007).

Non-EU medical doctors who are not eligible for a medical licence can apply for a temporary professional authorization [*Berufserlaubnis*] from the local health authority responsible for the administrative district in which they intend to practise. This requires applicants to certify that they have graduated as medical doctors or have the right to practise the medical profession in their countries of origin. The specific requirements differ from state to state.

---

18 Albania, Bulgaria, Croatia, the Czech Republic, Estonia, Hungary, Latvia, Lithuania, Poland, Romania, the Russian Federation, Slovakia and Slovenia.

The authorization to practise the medical profession is issued principally for the purpose of further education and for a period of four years. In certain cases, it is possible to extend this to up to seven years. The authorization is restricted to a specific position and foreign medical doctors are not allowed to work independently in their own medical practices, only as employees under supervision (Yamamura 2009).

Foreign nurses require vocational qualifications that are similar to the corresponding levels of qualification and legal vocational regulations in Germany. They also require sufficient knowledge of the German language as it is implicitly required for medical doctors and other medical staff. Council Directive 77/452/EEC (European Union 1977) regulates the mutual recognition of qualifications of nurses responsible for general care.

8.2 *Workforce planning and development*

Germany lacks a comprehensive national health workforce strategy that is implemented in a planned and systematic manner and takes account of the inflows and outflows of health professionals. There is also no explicit national self-sufficiency policy.

Workforce planning of health professionals follows different patterns for inpatient and outpatient care. SHI-authorized physicians are the major providers of outpatient care. Their planned numbers are determined by directives which classify all planning areas into one of ten groups (from large metropolitan areas to rural counties). These define the need for physicians per area group and per specialty according to the corresponding population-to-physician ratio in 1990 (Busse & Riesberg 2004).

The inpatient sector in Germany is characterized by a dual financing system – the states finance investment costs out of taxes; sickness funds or private insurers pay running (including personnel) costs within a system of diagnosis related groups (DRGs), except for psychiatric care and certain defined services (Busse & Riesberg 2004). This dual financing leads to inadequate dual planning – the number of hospitals and beds is planned at state level while workforce planning is left to individual hospitals.

The Health Care Structure Act of 1993 introduced workforce planning for nurses in order to overcome the perceived shortage. The nursing time standards resulted in the creation of almost 21 000 new nursing positions between 1993 and 1995. This surpassed the expectations of policy-makers who had anticipated an increase of 13 000 nursing positions during that period and therefore nursing time standards were abolished in 1997 (Weinbrenner & Busse 2006).

One major reason for inadequate workforce planning in Germany is the country's federal and corporatist system in which health-care goals are fixed and implemented within a complex set of institutional mechanisms acting at different levels. Purchasers and providers of health services work within a corporate framework that includes around 200 sickness funds, 17 regional physicians' associations, 18 regional dentists' associations and their corresponding federal associations. The corporatist nature of the system creates rigidities that make it difficult to introduce changes (Altenstetter & Busse 2005). In this highly fragmented environment, the state has only limited options to regulate the diverse aspects of the workforce (Weinbrenner & Busse 2006). As an example, the government is legally restricted from regulating workforce planning by directly controlling the number of students in medical schools. This led to overproduction of physicians in the post-war period (Mable & Marriott 2001).

Box 5.2 *Medical and nursing training in Germany*

Medical training

Medical training is a shared responsibility of the federal government, state governments and professional bodies. In general, the states are responsible for financing education. The annual intake of medical students is determined by the number of places available at medical schools. The annual total of accepted students for each medical school is based on the Physicians Approbation Ordinance [*Approbationsordnung*], which determines the scope and quality of medical training.

The Capacity Ordinance [*Kapazitätsverordnung*] translates these quality requirements into an administratively practicable formula. The higher the quality requirements, the fewer student places that are available, if the resources at medical universities remain the same. Physicians' organizations can indirectly influence the number of student places through the Physicians Approbation Ordinance, which is set by the Ministry of Health upon approval by the Federal Council. In 1989, the chambers of physicians pressed for a more detailed and complex ordinance in order to restrict the number of medical doctors. As a result, the intake of new students dropped by 22% in the winter semester of 1990/1991 (Schacher 1996).

Nursing training

Unlike medical training, nursing is not integrated in the German training system and is not a tertiary education. Training takes place in schools affiliated with hospitals; is not included in the state budget for science, research and higher education; and is financed by the health-care providers. For business management reasons, the number of nurses trained and the content of their training is often tailored to the needs of the specific hospital. This results in fluctuations in the annual number of trained nurses and discrepancies in the content of training. The number of training places dropped by 30% to 40% between 2000 and 2004 due to health reforms such as the transition to DRGs (Hoesch 2009).

8.3 *Domestic interventions*

National interventions to either recruit or retain health personnel are restricted. Recruitment or retention strategies are typically implemented at state or hospital level – for example, hospitals in eastern Germany are increasingly recruiting medical doctors from the new EU Member States. A number of private employment agencies specialize in recruiting health professionals from countries with lower salary levels. Such agencies recruit medical doctors in eastern Europe, predominantly for eastern German hospitals that are unable to recruit sufficient German medical doctors (Kopetsch 2009a).

The shortage of health personnel in eastern Germany has forced regional authorities to ease the bureaucratic hurdles concerning both the work permit and the legal occupational regulations. The number of medical treatment centres (*Medizinisches Versorgungszentrum* – MVZ) is increasing as they offer medical doctors the possibility of dependent employment in the outpatient sector, thereby circumventing the more restrictive regulations regarding self-employment of foreign physicians (Hoesch 2009).

In cooperation with the Otto Benecke Foundation, the state of Brandenburg in eastern Germany has started an initiative to retrain foreign-trained medical doctors who have not practised in Germany (mainly Jewish and ethnic German immigrants) and to prepare them for the verification of equivalency test (Nieland 2008).

In addition to foreign recruitment, some hospitals in the eastern states are trying to attract young medical doctors with offers of extra bonuses such as cheap loans, low rent and mortgages (Tuffs 2003). Furthermore, policy-makers are increasingly looking for innovative managerial solutions to overcome the German system's strong dependency on medical doctors by transferring tasks and responsibilities to nurses. For example, as part of the AGnES project[19] in the sparsely populated rural areas of Mecklenburg-Western Pomerania, district nurses rather than medical doctors are paying home visits to elderly patients (Hardenberg 2008). Their tasks include taking blood samples and checking that patients are taking the correct medicine. This successful project is now to be introduced nationwide.

8.4 *Political force field of regulating and managing immigration*

For many years Germany ignored the economic necessity of opening up for immigration and politicians contested even the idea of Germany being officially designated an immigration country. From the mid-1990s, experts warned

---

19 Community-based, e-health-assisted systemic support for primary care project.

vigorously that the country should make efforts to attract young and highly qualified migrants in order to stabilize the welfare system and ensure a sufficient pool of qualified workers.

The discussion was ongoing when negotiations for the accession of the eastern European countries started in 1998. The immediate question was whether eastern European workers should be granted full freedom of movement, including free access to the labour markets of the old EU Member States. Germany insisted on restricting this freedom.

During the accession process, experts and the media observed with alarm that Germany had a shortage of medical doctors in some regions. Facing the same problem, the British government took the opportunity to accept health professionals from the new Member States while Germany imposed transitional arrangements. However, as the demand for health personnel grows in some parts of the country and in some sectors, the migration of health professionals is perceived increasingly as a viable option to ensure the short- and medium-term provision of health care in the country.

9. Conclusion

Germany is affected by the international migration of health professionals in two ways. Firstly, a number of health professionals are leaving each year to work abroad. Secondly, rising numbers of foreign health professionals are working in the country. The mobility profile of the country shows that foreign-national health professionals still represent a relatively small share of the total health workforce in the country in comparison to other sectors of the economy and overall the German health system has a relatively low dependence on foreign-trained health professionals. However, foreign physicians are increasingly important for the provision of inpatient medical care in eastern Germany; as are foreign nurses for the provision of home care for elderly people. Rising demand for health personnel in certain sectors and regions of the country is likely to increase recruitment of foreign health professionals, at least for as long as they can fill gaps in the provision of health and long-term care and their incentives to migrate are sufficiently high.

References

Afentakis A, Böhm K (2009). *Beschäftigte im Gesundheitswesen. Gesundheitsberichterstattung des Bundes.* Berlin, Robert Koch Institut.

Altenstetter C, Busse R (2005). Health care reform in Germany: patchwork change within established governance structures. *Journal of Public Health Politics, Policy and Law*, 30(1–2):121–142.

Blum K et al. (2008). *Krankenhaus Barometer. Umfrage 2008*. Düsseldorf, Deutsches Krankenhausinstitute e.V.

Busse R, Riesberg A (2004). *Health-care systems in transition: Germany*. Copenhagen, WHO Regional Office for Europe on behalf of the European Observatory on Health Systems and Policies.

Derst P (2006). *Arbeitsmarktbeteiligung von Ausländern im Gesundheitssektor in Deutschland. Studie im Rahmen des Europäischen Migrationsnetzwerkes*. Nürnberg, Bundesamt für Migration und Flüchtlinge.

European Commission (2007). Mutual recognition of diplomas of the new Member States in the context of sectoral directives. Brussels (http://ec.europa.eu/internal_market/qualifications/docs/specific-sectors/overview_en.pdf, accessed 22 June 2009).

European Parliament and Council of the European Union (2005). Directive 2005/36/EC of the European Parliament and of the Council of 7 September 2005 on the recognition of professional qualifications. *Official Journal of the European Union*, 255(48):22–142.

Federal Employment Agency (2007). *Hinweise zur Vermittlung von Fachkräften aus osteuropäischen Ländern nach Deutschland (Gastarbeitnehmerverfahren)*. Nuremberg.

Federal Employment Agency (2009). *Statistik Beschäftigung*. Nuremberg (http://www.pub.arbeitsagentur.de/hst/services/statistik/detail/b.html?call=l, accessed 22 June 2009).

Federal Chamber of Physicians (2009). *Ärztestatistik*. Berlin (http://www.bundesaerztekammer.de/page.asp?his=0.3, accessed 22 June 2009).

Federal Statistical Office (2010). *Gesundheit – Personal 2008*. Wiesbaden.

Fellmer S (2008). Germany restricted the freedom of movement for Polish citizens – but does it matter? In: Across fading borders: the challenges of east-west migration in the EU. *EUMAP* [online] (http://www.soros.org/initiatives/media/articles_   publications/publications/across_20080429/fellmer.pdf, accessed 14 October 2010).

Flintrop J (2009). Integration Ausländischer Ärzte: Neben sprachlichen gibt es auch kulturelle Hürden. *Deutsches Ärzteblatt*, 106(10):438–439.

Hardenberg N (2008). Notruf aus der Provinz. *Süddeutsche Zeitung*, 64(7):3.

Hasselhorn H-M et al (2005). *Nurses Early Exit Study: NEXT Scientific Report*. Wuppertal (http://www.econbiz.de/archiv1/2008/53602_nurses_work_europe.pdf, accessed 18 October 2010).

Hoesch K (2008). Ärzte-Migration nach Großbritannien und Deutschland. In: Thränhardt D. (Hg.) *Entwicklung und Migration*. Jahrbuch Migration – Yearbook Migration 2006/2007. Berlin, Lit-Verlag.

Hoesch K (2009). *Was bewegt Mediziner. Die Migration von Ärzten und Gesundheitspersonal nach Deutschland und Großbritannien*. Berlin, Lit-Verlag.

Igl G (2008). *Rechtsgutachten zu Voraussetzungen und Anforderungen an die weitere rechtliche Regulierung der Pflegeberufe und ihre Tätigkeit*. Berlin, Deutscher Pflegerat.

Janus et al. (2007). German physicians "on strike" – shedding light on the roots of physician dissatisfaction. *Health Policy*, 82(3):357–365.

Klose J et al. (2007). *Daten zur Versorgungsdichte von Vertragsärzten*. Bonn, Wido Wissenschaftliches Institut der AOK.

Kopetsch T (2007). *Dem deutschen Gesundheitswesen gehen die Ärzte aus! Studie zur Altersstruktur- und Arztzahlentwicklung*. Berlin, Bundesärztekammer und Kassenärztliche Bundesvereinigung.

Kopetsch T (2009a). The migration of medical doctors to and from Germany. *Journal of Public Health*, 17(1):33–39.

Kopetsch T (2009b). Hohe Abwanderung ins Ausland – sehr geringe Arbeitslosigkeit. *Deutsches Ärzteblatt*, 106(16):757–760.

Kopetsch T (2010). *Dem deutschen Gesundheitswesen gehen die Ärzte aus! Studie zur Altersstruktur- und Arztzahlentwicklung*. Berlin, Bundesärztekammer und Kassenärztliche Bundesvereinigung.

Mable Al, Marriott J (2001). *Steady state: finding a sustainable balance point – international review of health workforce planning*. Ottawa, Health Human Resources Strategies Division Health Canada.

Neubacher A (2008). Mangel im Überfluss. *Der Spiegel*, 31 March 2008 (http://wissen.spiegel.de/wissen/image/show.html?did=56388070&aref=image036/2008/03/29/ROSP200801400340035.PDF&thumb=false, accessed 22 June 2009).

Neuhaus A et al. (2009). *Situation und Bedarfe von Familien mit mittel- und osteuropäischen Haushaltshilfen*. Köln, Deutsches Insitut für angewandte Pflegeforschung e.V.

Nieland W (2008). Meine Ärztin, die Russin. *Zeit Online*, 21 July 2008 (http://www.zeit.de/2008/30/C-Zugewanderte-Aerzte, accessed 22 June 2009).

OECD (2009). *OECD health data 2008*. Paris, Organisation for Economic Co-operation and Development (http://www.oecd.org/document/16/0,3343,en_2649 34631_2085200_1_1_1_1,00.html, accessed 22 June 2009).

Ramboll Management (2004). *Gutachten zum "Ausstieg aus der kurativen ärztlichen Berufstätigkeit in Deutschland."* Hamburg, Erstellt im Auftrage des BMGS.

Schacher M (1996). *Vorausschätzungen des Angebots an Absolventen der Humanmedizin und Auswirkungen auf den Bestand an Ärzten bis zum Jahr 2030*. Reihe: HIS Hochschulinformations-System Hochschulplanung 119. Hannover.

Spielberg P (2009). Zukunft der Gesundheitsberufe in Europa: Herausforderung Fachkräftemangel. *Deutsches Ärzteblatt,* 106(10):440-442. (http://www.aerzteblatt.de/v4/archiv/pdf.asp?id=63649, accessed 18 October 2010).

Tuffs A (2003). German doctors shun eastern states. *BMJ*, 327(7421):949.

Weinbrenner S, Busse R (2006). Germany. In: Rechel B et al. (eds.). *The health care workforce in Europe: learning from experience*. Copenhagen, WHO Regional Office for Europe on behalf of the European Observatory on Health Systems and Policies.

Yamamura S (2009). "Brain waste" ausländischer Ärztinnen und Ärzte in Deutschland. *Wirtschaftsdienst*, 89(3):196–201.

Oversupplying doctors but seeking carers: Italy's demographic challenges and health professional mobility

L Bertinato, E Boscolo, L Ciato

1. Introduction

The distorted supply of health professionals largely determines health professional mobility to and from Italy. Statistics from the Organisation for Economic Co-operation and Development (OECD) show that Italy has one of the highest ratios of medical doctors in the world – 4 medical doctors for every 1000 citizens. This compares to the OECD average of 3 doctors per 1000 (OECD 2008). Over-enrolment in medical studies has led to a surplus of medical doctors, although shortages are expected when the current cohort retires. In a context of oversupply, it is difficult for both foreign-trained and domestically trained foreign medical doctors to find stable employment in Italy. Consequently, medical doctors tend to leave, rather than enter, the country.

The nursing profession in Italy confronts entirely different but equally severe problems. There is estimated to be a structural shortage of over 70 000 nurses; insufficient numbers graduate from nursing schools and the replacement of the nursing workforce is not ensured. Traditionally given by families, care of the elderly is increasingly provided by (often illegal) migrant workers. General entry requirements to the country for nurses have been eased and currently one in ten registered nurses is of foreign origin, suggesting that Italy has become dependent on foreign inflows. However, health professionals from non-EU countries cannot hold permanent public sector positions and are thus disproportionally affected by less favourable working conditions. Recruitment of foreign nurses has been a necessary response to the changing needs of Italian society over the past five years, especially following the EU accession of eastern European countries in 2004 and 2007.

It is in this context of inefficient allocation of human resources for health that health professional mobility in Italy will be analysed. The categories considered in this study are medical doctors, nurses (general care) and care workers (*badanti*).

Data sources and limitations of the study

In June, July and August 2009, representatives of the following institutions were interviewed for this study: Department of Health and Social Affairs of the Veneto Region and the Office of Human Resources within this department; the Veneto branch of the National Board of Nursing (*Federazione Nazionale Collegi Infermieri* – IPASVI); Order of Medical Surgeons and Dentists (*Federazione Nazionale Ordini Medici Chirurghi e Odontoiatri* – FNOMCeO); National Institute of Statistics (*Istituto Nazionale di Statistica* – Istat); *Caritas Italiana*; National Institute for Social Security (*Istituto Nationale Previdenza Sociale* – INPS; Italian Workers Compensation Authority (*Istituto Nazionale per l'Assicurazione contro gli Infortuni sul Lavoro* – INAIL; and the National Council for Economics and Labour (*Consiglio Nazionale Economia e Lavoro* – CNEL). They confirmed the shortage or even absence of data at national level, exacerbated by the ongoing devolution of the public health system.

The Italian national health system is the responsibility of the 20 regions (Chaloff 2008). Law reforms in the 1990s paved the way for a process of political devolution (and fiscal federalism) aimed at investing local authorities (regions, provinces, municipalities and local health units) with greater authority in planning, funding, organizing and delivering services to citizens. In particular, the *Legge Bassanini* (Government of Italy 1997) was an important reform that has significantly extended the power transferred to regions via the principle of subsidiarity.[1] Each of the 20 regional services is composed of local health authorities/public enterprises (*unita locale socio sanitaria* – ULSS) and hospital public enterprises (*aziende ospedaliere* – AO).

The representatives of the ULSS in the Veneto Region who were surveyed[2] for this study maintained that the presence of foreign doctors and nurses in their

---

1 This aims to redefine and change the role of the public authorities in Italy and other European countries by redefining the relationships between central and local government (vertical direction) and among public and private actors (horizontal direction).

2 From February to June 2009, questionnaires were sent to all ULSS in the Veneto Region. ULSS 18, 4, 13 and 5; Azienda Ospedaliera di Padova and Azienda Ospedaliera di Verona responded.

institutions could only be inferred from the numbers of work permits granted. These *permessi di lavoro* are a mandatory requirement for foreign EU and non-EU professionals seeking to work within the Italian hospital network. However, there is no similar system to allow identification of foreign health professionals working outside hospital settings.

Those seeking to work as medical doctors and dental practitioners in Italy have a mandatory requirement to enrol with the relevant medical association at *provincial* level. These enrolments are another necessary source of data for this research. However, this also highlights the need for more comprehensive and reliable national data on the inflows and outflows of registered medical doctors (general medical doctors, specialist doctors, pharmacists) and dentists.

It can be difficult to establish whether foreign medical doctors have completed their training in Italy or in their home countries. The largest foreign medical doctors' association (*Associazione Medici di Origine Straniera* – AMSI) reports that 80% of its members have been trained in Italy (Chaloff 2008).

The IPASVI constantly monitors the flow of nurses. Readily available data in the systematic reports show greater inflows of nurses from new EU accession countries, mainly Romania and Poland. The Italian Ministry of Health provides data on foreign nursing and health sector qualifications by category and nationality but only for certain years.

Badanti working in the informal care sector are the most difficult category of foreign health professionals to measure.

Compilation of a detailed picture of trends at the national level would require consolidation of these data at various levels.

2. Mobility profile of Italy

The most recent estimates available show that foreign nurses have a strong presence in the country, comprising between 9.4% and 11% of the profession in 2008. There is some ambiguity over the proportion of foreign medical doctors, with estimates varying between 1% and 4%. However, these data do not include the invisible foreign workforce such as undocumented providers of elderly care and workers in the home-care sector (such as *badanti*) and there are no reliable data on the outflows of health professionals from Italy.

Given these limitations, Italy appears to have a mixed mobility profile. It is predominantly a destination country with higher levels of inflows for certain categories of health professionals such as nurses and care assistants (both legal and illegal), largely due to chronic nursing shortages which have shifted attention to recruitment from abroad. On the other hand, emigration mostly concerns medical doctors and medical/biomedical researchers.

2.1 Inflows

Stock and inflows of foreign nurses

IPASVI's systematic monitoring reports began in 2007. Before this time, nursing training schools were organized at regional level and each hospital ran its own school and managed its own personnel needs. Indeed, comprehensive national-level data on foreign nurses systematically recruited within the Italian health system through bilateral agreements between local authorities and universities are only available from 2008 onwards (interview with President of Collegio IPASVI Veneto).

The foreign nursing stock has increased remarkably over the past years. The IPASVI registries included 2612 foreign nurses in 2002 and 6730 in 2005 (2% of the workforce) (EMN 2009). By late 2008, the total number of foreign-registered nurses had risen to 34 043, 33 364 of whom were professional nurses. These represented 11% of the nursing workforce and just over half were from EU countries. The major source countries were Romania (8497; 25% of foreign professional registered nurses), Poland (3557; 10.7%), Switzerland (2386; 7%), Germany (1877; 5.6%) and Peru (1766; 5.3%) (EMN 2009). Albania, France, India and Spain respectively were the source countries of between 1100 and 1300 nurses, each nationality representing around 3.5% of foreign stocks. The proportion of nurses of European origin has remained constant at 70% of foreign stocks since 2002 but has risen from 12% to 16% for nurses from the American continent (302 in 2002; 5333 in 2008) (EMN 2009). According to OECD (2010) data, 33 364 foreign-national nurses in 2008 represented 9.4% of the nursing workforce. This suggests that the OECD used a larger nominator than that used in the EMN (2009) report.

Inflow data vary according to the source. Foreign nurses represented 28% of all new IPASVI registrations (9168) in 2008 (EMN 2009). The Ministry of Health web site shows that 7247 holders of diplomas from non-EU countries or newly acceded Member States were recognized to work as nurses between July 2000 and February 2011.[3] In 2005, the Ministry of Health recognized 4994 foreign nursing qualifications – 3864 from non-EU countries and 1130 from the EU and Switzerland. Foreign nurses were mostly from Romania (2420), Poland (1000), Peru (348), Albania (174), Serbia (155), India (127) and Bulgaria (121)[4] (Chaloff 2008). At least 2597 authorizations to enter Italy

---

3 The authors searched the Ministry of Health web site (http://www.salute.gov.it/professioniSanitarie/professioniSanitarie. jsp, accessed 28 February 2011) using search term "infermiere" under "Ricerca per nome o per professione".

4 Ministry of Health, Human Resources Directorate General 2006 cited in Chaloff 2008.

were issued in 2004 under the quota exemption for nurses, 50% of which were for nurses from Romania and 18% for nurses from Poland (Chaloff 2008).

The majority of foreign nurses have migrated to central and northern Italy (see section 5).

Stock and inflows of foreign medical doctors

The actual numbers and proportions of foreign medical doctors in Italy remain elusive. EMN (2009) reports that 14 548 foreign-born medical doctors were registered with the FNOMCeO in 2008–2009,[5] equivalent to around 4% of the medical workforce. Of these, 1276 were from Germany, 869 from Switzerland, 851 from Greece, 752 from the Islamic Republic of Iran, 686 from France, 626 from Venezuela, 618 from the United States, 584 from Argentina, 555 from Romania and 431 from Albania (EMN 2009). In 2004, 12 527 foreign-born medical doctors (3.4% of the total medical workforce) were registered with the FNOMCeO (Chaloff 2008). OECD (2010) data show slightly more – 14 747 foreign-national medical doctors in Italy in 2008, representing 3.7% of the medical workforce.

However, these data on foreign-born medical doctors should be contrasted with the results of an FNOMCeO census in 2006 which showed that 3525 of its members held foreign nationality (1562 EU nationals) (Chaloff 2008). Further differences arise when comparing the data on specific countries. For example, 575 medical doctors *born* in Venezuela were registered with the professional body in 2004 but only 23 medical doctors of Venezuelan *nationality* were registered in 2006. Similar differences are visible for many other countries including Argentina, Switzerland and the United States. This suggests that important numbers of foreign-born medical doctors are Italians born abroad or foreigners who have been naturalized after living for long periods in Italy (Chaloff 2008). If data on nationality are considered, the foreign share in the medical workforce drops to about 1%. Chaloff (2008) asserts that this is a more realistic number given the few opportunities for jobs and career advancement in the context of high unemployment among young medical doctors and budget cuts within the Italian health system.

The only inflow data that could be retrieved concern foreign-trained medical doctors. The Ministry of Health web site shows that 1310 holders of foreign (EU and non-EU) diplomas were recognized to work as medical doctors in Italy between April 2001 and January 2011.[6]

There is significant diversity in the provenance of medical doctors but most foreign medical doctors practising in Italy come from countries with significant

---

5 Report does not specify exact year.

6 The authors searched the Ministry of Health web site (http://www.salute.gov.it/professioniSanitarie/professioniSanitarie. jsp, accessed 28 February 2011) using search term "medico" under "Ricerca per nome o per professione".

Italian migrant communities. Hence, they do not face the language barrier that other foreign-trained doctors in Italy cite as one of the biggest obstacles to migration. The geographical distribution of foreign medical doctors shows that around 50% of foreign medical doctors practise in the north, 25% in the central regions and around 20% in the south. The remaining 2.7% are registered but are temporarily practising abroad (EMN 2009).

Inflows to the home-care and elderly care sectors: the badanti phenomenon

Sociodemographic change, an ageing population and the consequent increasing demand for assistance for elderly people are considered to be the main factors influencing international health professional mobility in Italy. The demand for *badanti* is estimated to be three times higher than the demand for nurses (Chaloff 2008). Surveys conducted in the Veneto Region show that 5% of people aged over 65 in 2005 were assisted by a *badante* (Osservatorio Regionale Immigrazione 2008).

Various sources show the importance of the foreign workforce in the home-care and elderly care sectors but it can be hard to establish a clear picture of this workforce. In 2008, the legal foreign workforce providing elderly care was estimated to be 500 000, 1% of the total Italian population. The Ministry of Labour reports that the home-care sector absorbed some 1.2 million people in 2007 including around 500 000 irregular workers, the vast majority being immigrants (Chaloff 2008). An INPS survey carried out in 2007 on a sample of 1003 foreign home-care workers of 66 different nationalities indicated that 29% were from NIS countries and 31% from eastern Europe (the remainder being from Asia, Latin America and Africa) (INPS 2009a). Unsurprisingly, women play an important role in this field in which low salaries and a lack of relevant experience or qualifications are common. For these reasons, the sector is also characterized by significant turnover with major outflows to the countries of origin.

In order to quantify the number of *badanti* it is necessary to differentiate this workforce from the traditional household workers registered with the INPS. The INPS reports that more than 250 000 foreign nationals worked as domestic workers in early 2009 (INPS 2009b). Official data do not show the real situation although the available information helps to underline important aspects such as an increasing number of foreign workers since 2002.

2.2 *Outflows*

National, regional and local medical associations (Di Marzio 2003) indicate that the United Kingdom and Germany are the main destination countries of an important share of Italian health professionals. These are mainly medical doctors (general practitioners and specialists) and medical researchers, trained in Italy. The main reasons for these outflows are the over-supply of these health professionals, poor career opportunities and inadequate working conditions in Italy as well as increasing demand for some medical specialties in destination countries (at least before the recent global financial crisis). Data on foreign-trained medical doctors in the United Kingdom show that 1692 new registrants with primary medical education from Italy registered with the General Medical Council between 2003 and 2008 (Chapter 8). Stock data from Germany and France do not suggest any important immigration of Italian health professionals. In Germany, the number of Italian-national medical doctors increased from 325 in 1988 to 755 in 2008 while the number of Italian nurses remained constant at around 950 over the twenty-year period (Chapter 5). In France, 566 Italian medical doctors were registered in 2007 (Chapter 4).

Driven by the lack of merit considerations and low salaries for health professionals, many Italian doctors have responded to the increasing demand for general practitioners in the United Kingdom since 2000. Reports indicate that psychiatrists and paediatric neuropsychiatrists were the Italian medical specialists most in demand in the United Kingdom (DoctorNews 2007).

The British press has highlighted the growing phenomenon of Italian general practitioners moving to the United Kingdom for brief periods in order to cover local shortages, even in emergencies. There are reports of Italian general practitioners taking a weekend's leave of absence to collaborate with a local health authority in exchange for substantial payments, especially in underserved areas such as the Scottish highlands, remote Welsh mountain villages and some densely populated urban areas (Camber 2010, Macrae & Pisa 2007). However, data on this phenomenon are anecdotal.

The wages and working conditions of nurses have deteriorated in Italy in the last decade. Although there is no evidence of systematic recruitment by other countries, recent data confirm the increasing outflow of qualified Italian nurses to countries that offer better salaries and more stable career opportunities (Chaloff 2008).

A number of information gaps should be kept in mind when examining outflows. Generally, these data need to be analysed very carefully. First, medical doctors and dentists working abroad can be commuters (from South Tyrol to Austria; or from Piedmont/Liguria Regions to France) living in Italy, rather than migrants. Second, data on Italian medical doctors and dentists with a foreign official address are not fully reliable in comparison to the data on doctors and dentists living in Italy. Legal addresses can be used purely for fiscal reasons and in such cases do not indicate the true home addresses.

3. Vignettes on health professional mobility[7]_

This 24 year old Italian registered nurse graduated in 2005. After a year working in a residential care home, she moved to Ireland to "improve her language competence and to gain more skills and experience in her profession." In order to enrol with the nursing board she was required to present her degree as well as a formal declaration from IPASVI confirming her participation in post-graduate nursing training activities. She has not decided whether she will remain in Ireland.

Arriving in Italy in 2009, this 42 year old Romanian nurse is currently working on the wards and in the operating theatre. Having gained recognition of her qualifications and nursing diploma, she enrolled in IPASVI. She migrated because she can earn more than in her home country and the economic stability she has in Italy helps her to take care of her husband and daughter in Romania.

Valentina is a 54 year old, Moldovan *badante*. She graduated as a physiotherapist in a university in her home country and worked as an official sports physiotherapist for the Olympic gymnastics team of the USSR. Following the dissolution of the USSR and the death of her husband, she lost her job and had no means of looking after her two children. An unofficial contact (newspaper advert) put her in touch with Italian families looking for home help for elderly residents in north east Italy. She initially travelled to Italy by bus on a tourist visa but obtained a work permit as a result of the 2002 regularization. She now works 40 hours per week as a live-in home help for an 86 year old woman in Padua.

Dr MW arrived in Italy in 1996 as a postgraduate medical researcher specializing in arterial hypertension. Having obtained a PhD at the Medical University of Gdansk, he had been invited to work as part of an *équipe* at the Department of Clinical Medicine at the University of Padua. This was facilitated through a bilateral agreement between the two medical faculties. In 2000, a grant from the American Medical Association enabled him to conduct two years of specialist research in

7 In October 2009 the authors interviewed the President of Collegio IPASVI; an employment agency for *badanti* in the Veneto Region and ULSS no. 5 concerning nurses, *badanti* and medical doctors respectively. These vignettes are all real-life experiences as reported by these interviewees.

hypertension at the University of Michigan in Ann Arbor. He has since married an Italian national, also a medical doctor. He is now 39 years old and works as a consultant medical doctor in various departments of the Veneto Region's hospital network. He also undertakes consultancy work in the private sector.

4. Impacts on the Italian health system

Foreign nurses and *badanti* bring extra capacity but such migration flows have only a partial impact on Italy's health system and on the shortage of nursing staff in hospital settings (EMN 2009). However, the composition of nursing staff in some hospitals suggests dependency on the foreign workforce (see section 5). Moreover, the significant (if uncertain) numbers of both legal and unofficial carers clearly indicate that the Italian system is dependent on migrants for the provision of home and elderly care.

Data indicate shortages of specialists in radiology, anaesthetics, paediatrics and emergency medicine (Chaloff 2008). For instance, the Italian press recently reported the high demand for psychiatrists and child psychiatrists in the United Kingdom and the resulting large outflows from Italy in the past four years (DoctorNews 2007).

5. Relevance of cross-border health professional mobility

5.1 *Demography and ageing*

Population forecasts suggest that people over 65 could comprise up to 26% of the total population by 2025 (Regione del Veneto undated). Demographic ageing and ageing of the health workforce contribute to the declining number of Italians entering the labour force, the increasing demand for health care and the difficulties of finding a health workforce that is sufficient for one of the greyest populations in the world. The Italian system has not adapted to meet the growing need for elderly care and, in the absence of appropriate measures (Chaloff 2008), the IPASVI considers the national nursing shortage to be at least 71 000 nurses (EMN 2009). The situation appears to be worsening – an estimated 13 400 nurses were due to retire from the system in 2010 (Silvestro 2010) but only 8500 graduated with a nursing degree in the 2008–2009 academic year (Binello 2010).

The chronic shortage of nurses has shifted attention to recruitment from abroad although this is hampered by high levels of bureaucracy and the lack of stability and career advancement within the public sector. There is a sharp contrast between the highly regulated nursing sector and the growing and diverse group of foreign *badanti* who generally work illegally but constitute a convenient and relatively affordable alternative to care homes or hospitalization. Definition of this workforce is further complicated by the multiplication of job titles in recent years including *assistenti socio sanitari* (ASS) and *operatori socio sanitari* (OSS) (Chaloff 2008).

In the Veneto region, the high prevalence of mononuclear families, decreasing birth rates, financial opportunities and the widespread ageing population have particularly contributed to increase the need for *badanti*. The majority of immigrants in this region work as *badanti* and represent the only alternative to hospitalization. This phenomenon is a consequence of many factors including the lack of residential homes for the elderly, the need for budget cutting and the psychological benefits gained when older people remain in their own environments. These have pushed many families towards the alternative private solution in the Veneto Region.

5.2 *Regional variations*

Nurse shortages are most severe in southern Italy – 5.7 nurses per 1000 population in comparison to the OECD average of 9 per 1000 in 2005 (OECD 2008). However, foreign health professionals are mainly present in the north. In 2008, there were 34 000 foreign nurses in Italy – 56% in the north, 25% in central Italy and just 11% in the south. Lombardy has a high concentration of private clinics that can hire foreign staff directly and one in three nurses is foreign. The proportion of foreign new nurses registering in Turin Province, rose from 14.5% in 2000 to 41% in 2007. This amounted to 2869 foreign nurses on the regional IPASVI register, 37% of whom were from non-EU countries (EMN 2009). Foreign nurses constitute up to 60% of the nursing staff in certain large hospitals in Turin. In the Trieste Maggiore Hospital on Italy's eastern border, 10% of nurses are foreign and come mainly from neighbouring Slovenia and other countries of the former Yugoslavia (Mellina et al. 2006).

5.3 *Public versus private sector*

There is greatest demand for foreign qualified nurses in private clinics, residential homes and institutes for people with disabilities or in need of support (Mellina et al. 2006). Nurses are free to choose whether to work in the public or the private sector but access to the public sector depends on the successful completion of highly competitive state examinations. This is not required in the private sector which therefore can be more flexible in response to its greater demand for nurses.

5.4 *Medical studies*

Italy faced over-enrolment of medical students from the 1970s to the early 1990s and the number of doctors increased by 40% between 1984 and 1994. A *numerus clausus* was introduced to cap this growth and the number of doctors rose by only 5.4% between 1994 and 1999 (Chaloff 2008). The number of students enrolling has reduced from 17 000 in 1980 to 5623 in 2006 (Chaloff 2008). Ministerial decrees set the total number of specialist doctors to be trained at 8848 in the 2009–2010 academic year (Ministry of Health 2010) and limited the number of graduate posts in medicine and surgery to 9527 in 2010–2011 (Ministry of Education, Universities and Research 2010). The Ministry of Health sets the numbers of training posts for each specialization and the Ministry of Education defines the total number and distribution of posts at Italian universities. Medicine has low attrition rates in comparison to other studies, with around 90% of enrolled students going on to graduate (Chaloff 2008).

5.5 *Nursing studies and shortages*

Students must complete three years of university education in order to obtain a degree in nursing. Nurses can practise in public and private hospitals and in rehabilitative settings, as employees or self-employed (EMN 2009). Enrolment numbers for nursing students increased from 10 700 in 2003 to 13 000 in 2006 and 9200 students graduated in 2006 (Chaloff 2008). Yet the demand for nursing training continues to exceed the supply of university places. There were 30 000 requests for a total of 14 849 student places in the 2008–2009 academic year, 28% of which were from foreign students (Binello 2010). There are also regional disparities in the distribution of these places – proportional to the population, fewer posts are allocated in the south (IPASVI 2005).

6. Factors influencing health professional mobility

In 2006, the Institute for Professional Training (IAL) Veneto conducted a survey of women from the Republic of Moldova. This study revealed that the main factors prompting migration of this workforce are generally linked to political instability, high rates of unemployment and poverty in the home countries. In most cases, these women had lost their jobs as a consequence of the dismantling of the public welfare system and had chosen to move to the Veneto Region to look for better living conditions and to fund their children's education (Osservatorio Regionale Immigrazione 2008).

The main obstacles that face foreign medical doctors moving to Italy include the risk of unemployment and job insecurity (both of which also encourage Italian medical doctors to emigrate), language barriers and a slow recognition process for non-EU medical degrees. Whilst the Ministry of Health certifies degrees within a year of a complete application being filed, it can take five years to compile the necessary documentation (Chaloff 2008). In a context of oversupply, there may also be a certain resistance to integrating foreign medical doctors in the health sector.

Factors influencing the brain drain of medical researchers include underfunding of research, poor career prospects, the absence of a meritocracy and inadequate infrastructures in some Italian universities. Moreover, the Italian public sector does not offer good job opportunities and staff budgets allocated to the 183 local health authorities were cut by 2% between 2004 and 2007 (Chaloff 2008). This has contributed to prospects that are already unpromising and thus to the outflow of medical doctors. The President of the FNOMCeO has suggested that part of the problem is the poor linkage between universities and the labour market which means that medical doctors are often in their mid 30s before they start working (with precarious contracts). The President of the Italian Society of Psychiatry (*Società Italiana Psichiatria* – SIP) has cited "ridiculous salaries" and punishing working conditions as reasons why young specialists leave the country (DoctorNews 2007). Indeed, the salaries of medical doctors in Italy are far from competitive with the remuneration levels in the international labour market.

7. Policy, regulation and interventions

7.1 *Entry requirements*

The Ministry of Health is the competent authority which issues certificates of conformity and of good standing at the request of an Italian-trained health professional's intended destination country. It also carries responsibility for recognizing the diplomas of foreign-trained health professionals, with recognition procedures differing according to profession, nationality and the country in which the qualifications were obtained. The Ministry of Health (2011) presents 14 distinct procedures. Generally, EU citizens who have qualified as medical doctors, medical specialists, nurses or pharmacists in an EU country are required to produce:

- a copy of the valid identity document;
- a copy of the relevant degree;

- a copy of the authorization to exercise the health profession (where applicable)

- an original certificate of conformity as stipulated by the relevant EU legislation on the mutual recognition of diplomas, issued by the competent authority of the country in which the degree was obtained

- an original certificate of good standing, dated no more than three months prior to submission of the recognition request.

Nurses are moreover required to submit documentation proving any postgraduate professional experience, as well as any additional specializations. The instructions for nurses include a reminder that Italian law forbids the exercise of a health profession prior to diploma recognition.

Third-country nationals who have obtained their diploma in an EU country or applicants who have qualified in a non-EU country (regardless of nationality) must also provide:

- a copy of the study programme for which recognition is requested, detailing the courses, years of study, accumulated hours (both theoretical and practical) and disciplines covered;

- an original declaration from the Italian diplomatic or consular authority in the country of qualification, testifying:

  - that the diploma is granted by the competent authority of the country;

  - that the access requirements for the study were fulfilled (basic schooling);

  - that the qualification enables the exercise of the relevant health profession in the country where obtained;

  - the number of years of the undergraduate degree;

  - the authenticity of the signature on the diploma and the compliance of the diploma itself;

  - the professional activities that the diploma gives the right to exercise in the issuing country.

- Certificate of the absence of any penal or professional impediments to the exercise of the relevant profession, issued by country of origin and/or the country of residence

- Certificate detailing any professional activities performed in the country of origin and/or the country of residence after obtaining the qualification in question.

Third-country nationals who obtain their diplomas in an EU country must also submit the original certificate of conformity issued by the competent authority of the country in which the degree was obtained. When a diploma has already been recognized by another EU Member State, all relevant documentation must also be submitted (Ministry of Health 2011).

Foreign health professionals wishing to exercise a health profession legally in Italy must also register with the relevant professional order and pass a written and oral Italian language exam (EMN 2009).

7.2 Migration policy

Foreign citizens are allowed to enter Italy for tourism, study and work purposes or for family reunions. A labour migration policy allows foreign (non-EU) workers with employment to enter the country, subject to annual quotas set by the Flux decree at ministerial level (EMN 2009). Following the EU accessions in 2004 and 2007, entry regulations for foreign health professionals from a number of the eastern European Member States have been eased.

The regulations[8] that enable third-country nationals to reside and work as health professionals in Italy also allow non-EU citizens to become members of professional orders, granting an exemption from the requirement of citizenship. The Ministry of Health's circular of 12 April 2000 defines the procedures for the recognition of health professional qualifications obtained outside the EU and the procedures for obtaining authorization to practise these professions (Mellina et al. 2006).

Nationality is an important determinant of the employment perspectives of foreign health professionals. Only Italian and EU citizens can take part in public competitions for positions in public institutions, therefore third-country nationals are left with the less favourable options of employment on shorter-term contracts (for example, recruited by cooperatives or interim work agencies) or of working in the private sector (Chaloff 2008, EMN 2009). This situation applies particularly to foreign nurses and carers. However, this discrimination based on nationality has been challenged on various occasions. In 2001, a regional administrative court (TAR) ruled in favour of a Moroccan nurse who had graduated in Italy but was excluded from a competition in Liguria. More recently, courts such as the Tribunal of Milan (n.2454 of 27 May 2008) and the Tribunal of Genoa (n.3749 of 3 June 2007) have ruled in favour of opening permanent employment positions in Italian hospitals to third-country nationals (EMN 2009).

---

8 Legislative Decree 286/98 – Consolidation Act on Immigration Regulations (*Testo unico delle disposizioni sull'immigrazione*) and Presidential Decree 394/99 – Implementation Regulations (*Regolamento di attuazione*).

Driven by the critical nursing shortage, Article 27 of the 2002 migration framework law known as the Legge Bossi-Fini (Government of Italy 2002) introduced permanent exemptions from the annual quotas for entry to the Italian labour market for nurses. Overall ceilings on the numbers of foreign nurses were virtually abandoned with effect from 1 May 2004. Moreover, the requirement for non-EU nurses entering the country to work as nurses persists also after the first renewal of their work permit (Chaloff 2008).

The status of many home-care assistants has been regularized following recent EU enlargements, particularly the accession of Romania, Bulgaria and Poland. This has provided more opportunities for families to hire *badante* from abroad legally and many local authorities are working to integrate this spontaneous private care within their systems of elderly care through skill upgrades and support (Chaloff 2008).

The programme that defined immigration policy for 2004–2006 (Presidency of the Council of Ministers 2005) and included a dedicated section on the medical professions (see Mellina et al. 2006 & EMN 2009) appears to be an isolated case. No other documentation was found on Italy's current migration policies relevant to the health professions.

7.3 *Bilateral agreements*

This section focuses on examples of regional and local agreements concerning education and capacity building within the health professions. Indeed, an increasing number of regions have agreed bilateral programmes with foreign nursing institutes in order to guarantee the recruitment of qualified professionals. Distance learning is a particular area of collaboration that has been growing recently. For example, SkyNurse is an experimental project involving 180 candidates in a fourteen-month training programme that includes three months of distance learning between classrooms in Padua and the partners' institutes in Bucharest and Pitesti. The final training is organized in the Veneto Region. This programme is especially designed to guarantee the language and technical skills required for future enrolment in Italy (Chaloff 2008).

The Cluj nursing programme is another good example of cooperation concerning the health workforce. With the support of Parma Province and the Parma Nursing College, this has added training modules covering especially the Italian language and Italian health regulations and professional standards. The Veneto Region and Timis County in Romania have established a similar cooperation agreement that has organized nursing degree courses in Romania since 2002 and developed distance learning modules in conjunction with the

University of Padua – 42 Romanians received nursing degrees at this university in 2006 (Chaloff 2008).

Additionally, an agreement signed on 22 March 2006 authorized an Italian doctor from Treviso Public Health Authority to be sent to Timisoara in order to serve the Italian community comprising many Venetian entrepreneurs who live part- and full-time in Timis (Chaloff 2008).

8. *Conclusion*

Whether at provincial, regional or national level, it remains a challenge for Italian institutions to obtain reliable data on health professional mobility. The data that are available indicate that Italy is mainly a destination country that imports health professionals to alleviate structural shortages in certain areas. To a lesser degree, it is also a source country – exporting supernumerary health professionals. The proportion of the nursing workforce that is of foreign origin has risen from 2% in 2005 to 10% today and the home-care sector relies heavily on mainly undocumented, informal carers who provide services for older people and people with disabilities. The most important inflows of professional nurses migrate from the new EU accession countries, in particular Romania and Poland. With demographic changes, the need for nurses and carers is only likely to continue toincrease.

Outflows of medical doctors are probably negligible, although there is a need for reliable data on general practitioners practising abroad for limited periods as the phenomenon may be expanding. Unemployment and job insecurity among medical doctors make Italy unattractive for both foreign-trained and domestic medical doctors. Medical researchers and prospective and qualified specialists are migrating particularly to the United Kingdom and the United States. These outflows are outnumbering inflows due to an oversupply of medical specialists in Italy and/or a lack of funding for biomedical research at university level.

The growing phenomenon of recruitment of foreign health professionals (predominantly nurses) through bilateral programmes with foreign training institutes can be seen as part of a new response to changing mobility in a changing Europe. So far, private employers have adjusted more quickly to new requirements than the public sector. Recruitment of foreign health professionals is an opportunity for individuals/countries to develop skills, experience and knowledge and to add value to the professions. However, if Italy is to benefit from such opportunities, there is a need to adapt health workforce planning and migration policies to take account of the realities of its system and the population's needs.

References

Binello D (2010). Parola chiave: integrazione possibile [Key word: integration possible]. *L'Infermiere*, 2/2010:17–19. (http://www.ipasvi.it/pubblicazioni/ArchivioRiviste/Indici/files/ 1034/attualità%205.pdf, accessed 2 February 2011).

Camber R (2010). Foreign GPs who commute to Britain: £100-an-hour Poles and Lithuanians fly in for shifts our doctors won't do. *Mail Online*, 26 February 2010 (http://www.dailymail.co.uk/news/article-1208663/Test-foreign-doctors-coming-practice-Britain-say-GP-leaders.html#ixzz0SgMP2MQf, accessed 20 February 2011).

Chaloff J (2008). Mismatches in the formal sector, expansion of the informal sector: immigration of health professionals to Italy. Paris, Organisation for Economic Co-operation and Development (OECD Health Working Paper No. 34).

Di Marzio S (2003). Il NHS Inglese lancia il reclutamento in Italia [The English NHS launches recruitment in Italy]. *Doctor*, 1(16):6–9 (http://www.medweb.it/riviste/Archivio/old /doctor/2003/0703p06.pdf, accessed 20 February 2011).

DoctorNews (2007). Medici Italiani al servizio di sua Maestà…Bianco, riforma universitaria contro fuga medici all'estero…..Psichiatri, stipendi ridicoli ci spingono all'estero [Italian medical doctors to the service of her Majesty… Bianco, university reform against the drain of doctors going abroad… Psychiatrists, ridiculous salaries push them abroad]. *Ordine dei Medici e Chirurghi della Provinci di Latina*, 28 February 2007 (http://www.ordinemedicilatina.it/1244, accessed 3 February 2011).

EMN (2009). *Politiche migratorie, lavoratori qualificati, settore sanitario. Primo Rapporto EMN Italia* [Migration policies, qualified workers, health sector. First EMN Report Italy]. Rome, European Migration Network.

Government of Italy (1997). Legge 15 marzo 1997 n. 59. Delega al governo per il conferimento di funzioni e compiti alle Regioni ed enti locali, per la riforma della Pubblica amministrazione e la semplificazione amministrativa [Law of 15 March 1997 no. 50. Delegation to the government for the transfer of functions and tasks to the regions and local authorities, the public administration reform and administrative simplification]. *Gazzetta Ufficiale* [*Official Gazette*], No. 63, 17 March 1997.

Government of Italy (2002). Legge 30 luglio 2002, n.189. Modifica alla normativa in materia di immigrazione e di asilo [Law 30 July 2002, n.189. Changing the rules on immigration and asylum]. *Gazzetta Ufficiale* [*Official Gazette*], No. 199, 26 August 2002.

INPS (2009a). Diversità culturale, identità di tutela [Cultural diversity, identity protection]. Rome, Istituto Nazionale Previdenza Sociale (III° Rapporto INPS sui lavatori immigrati e previdenza negli archivi Inps [Third report on immigrants and protection in the INPS archives]) (http://www. inps.It/informazioni/template/ migranti/repository/node/N123456789/III_ Rapporto.pdf, accessed 11 March 2011).

INPS (2009b). *Rapporto Annuale 2009* [*Annual report 2009*]. Rome, Istituto Nazionale Previdenza Sociale (http://www.inps.it/Doc/informazione/ rapporto_annuale/INPS_ RappAnnuale09.pdf, accessed 16 February 2011).

IPASVI (2005). Indagine sulla formazione universitaria degli infermieri, Rapporto 2004–2005 [Survey on the university education of nurses, Report 2004–2005]. Rome, Federazione Nazionale Collegio (http://www.ipasvi.it/ content/osservatorio/Indagine%202004-2005.pdf, 3 February 2011).

Macrae F, Pisa N (2007). NHS picks up the bill for an Italian doctor flown 1000 miles. *Mail Online*, 2 January 2007 (http://www.dailymail. co.uk/news/article-426066/NHS-picks-Italian-doctor-flown-1000-miles. html#ixzz0SgLl7v1u, accessed 20 February 2011).

Mellina C et al. (2006). Le migrazioni di infermieri in Italia [The migrations of nurses in Italy]. In: *Atti IX Consensus Conference Sulla Immigrazione – VII Congresso Nazionale SIMM* [Acts from the IX Conference on Immigration – VII National Congress of the Italian Society for Migration Health], *Palermo, 27–29 April* 2006 (http://www.emnitaly.it/down/ev-15-03.pdf, accessed 3 February 2011).

Ministry of Education, Universities and Research (2010). Decreto Ministeriale 21 ottobre 2010. Ampliamento numero posti per immatricolazioni al corso di laurea magistrale in Medicina e Chirurgia, ed ai corsi di laurea in Ostericia e in Tecnica della Riabilitazione Psichiatrica per l'anno accademico 2010/2011 [Ministerial Decree of 21 October 2010 increasing student enrolment numbers for the Bachelor of Science degree in medicine and surgery and degree courses in obstetrics and psychiatric rehabilitation for the 2010/2011 academic year]. Rome, *Gazzetta Ufficiale* [*Official Gazette*], No. 247, 21 October 2010 (http:// attiministeriali.miur.it/anno-2010/ottobre/dm-21102010.aspx, accessed 2 February 2011).

Ministry of Health (2010). Decreto 30 marzo 2010. Determinazione del numero globale dei medici specialisti da formare ed assegnazione dei contratti di formazione specialistica, per l'anno accademico 2009/2010 [Decree of 30 March 2010. Decision on the global number of specialist doctors to be trained and assignment of contracts for specialized training for the academic year 2009/2010]. Rome, *GU Serie Generale*, No. 225, 25 settembre 2010 (http://

www.normativasanitaria.it/jsp/dettaglio.jsp?aggiornamenti=&attoCompleto=s
i&id=35332&page=&anno=null, accessed 2 February 2011).

Ministry of Health (2011). Professioni sanitarie. Modulistica per il
riconoscimento titoli [Health professions. Forms for the recognition of
titles]. Rome (http://www.salute.gov.it/professioniSanitarie/paginaInterna.
jsp?id=92&menu =strumentieservizi, accessed 2 February 2011).

OECD (2008). *The looming crisis in the health workforce: how can OECD
countries respond?* Paris, Organisation for Economic Co-operation and
Development (OECD Health Policy Studies).

OECD (2010). *International migration of health workers.* Paris, Organisation
for Economic Co-operation and Development (Policy Brief) (http://www.
oecd.org/dataoecd/8/1/44783473.pdf, accessed 24 February 2011) including
data on foreign health workforce in OECD countries http://www.oecd.org/
dataoecd/8/0/44783714.xls (accessed 24 February 2011).

Osservatorio Regionale Immigrazione,Regione Veneto (2008). *Donne migranti,
famiglie, anziani: Welfare domestico in Veneto* [Migrant women, families, elderly:
domestic welfare in Veneto]. In: Immigrazione straniera in Veneto. Rapporto
2008 [Foreign immigration in Veneto. 2008 Report].

Presidency of the Council of Ministers (2005). *Documento programmatico
relativo alla politica dell'immigrazione e degli stranieri nel territorio dello Stato per
il 2004–2006* [Programming document regarding the policy on immigration
and on foreigners within the state territory for the years 2004–2006]. Rome.

Regione del Veneto (undated). Rapporto Statistico 2008: Il Veneto si racconta,
il Veneto si confronta [Statistical Report 2008 Veneto: sharing facts, Veneto:
comparing facts]. Veneto (http://statistica.regione.veneto.it/Pubblicazioni/
RapportoStatistico2008/index.jsp, accessed 16 February 2011).

Silvestro A (2010). Crisi, pensioni e carenze [Crisis, pensions and shortages].
L'Infermiere, 3/2010:3 (http://www.ipasvi.it/pubblicazioni/ArchivioRiviste/
Indici/files/1045/editoriale.pdf, accessed 2 February 2011).

Opportunities in an expanding health service: Spain between Latin American and Europe

Beatriz González López-Valcárcel, Patricia Barber Pérez,
Carmen Delia Dávila Quintana

1. Introduction

Health professional inflows and outflows have increased substantially in Spain over the last decade. Market forces have made the country a corridor for health professional mobility between Latin America and Europe – doctors from Latin America have responded to shortages by immigrating to work as general medical doctors and train as specialists. In turn, Spanish doctors and nurses have been leaving for other European Union (EU) countries, presumably attracted by better working conditions. However, outflows have been declining since the mid 2000s and there are indications that Spanish health professionals are now returning.

Recent estimates highlight the importance of foreign[1] inflows for the health workforce and it can be argued that Spain shows some degree of dependency on immigration. Significant and increasing numbers of foreign doctors arrive to take up specialist residencies and some 26 700 foreign degrees in general medicine were recognized between 2003 and 2008, principally from Latin America. In 2007, the authorities recognized 5383 foreign degrees in general medicine; 40% more than the number of medical graduates from Spanish universities (3841). The nursing, dentistry and pharmacy professions also show significant proportions of foreign inflows.

---

1 Foreign refers to nationality unless otherwise specified.

Spain has a population of 46.2 million and is divided into 17 autonomous communities that bear full responsibility for organizing and managing health care. Foreign health professionals in the public sector are employed by the autonomous communities but are licensed to practice by central government.

Limitations of the study

Data on licensing refer to the "authorization to engage in the practice of a profession" (Dussault et al. 2009). The central government is responsible for recognizing diplomas to practise in Spain. Registration data from the professional councils (*Colegios*) is another source of information on the stock of professionals and the National Statistics Institute (*Instituto Nacional de Estadística* – INE) reports data by sex and age (except for dentists, whose council provides data only by sex), distinguishing between retired and active professionals. However, professionals in the public sector are not required to register with professional councils and a doctor's registration reports only the basic medical degree, not specialty degrees. While not all Spanish doctors are registered, practically all recognized foreign doctors register as soon as possible for reasons of social prestige and professional credibility. Therefore, the numbers of foreign doctors may be overrepresented. Registration figures for dentists and nurses are more complete – almost all dentists are in private practice and therefore registered; and a strong sense of professional identity encourages nurses to register in great numbers.

Data on practising doctors come from several sources. Health professionals entering Spain can be quantified from two sources of microdata, both compiled by the INE. The Economically Active Population Survey (EAPS) is a quarterly survey of households with the main objective to obtain data on the labour force. It allows comparison of data on foreign-origin health professionals and all health professionals. The National Immigrant Survey (NIS) 2007 provides information on the social and demographic characteristics of persons born abroad[2] and in relation to the establishment and significance of the composition of the family group in migratory decisions and strategies. The main sources of data and their limitations are shown in the annex (Table 7.13).

There are no official registers on the emigration of any categories of Spanish health professionals.

2. Mobility profile of Spain

Health professional traffic in Spain is two-way (Dumont & Zurn 2007,

---

2 NIS defines foreign as an immigrant – anyone born outside Spain who was 16 years or over at the time of the survey and had been residing in Spain for more than one year or had the intention to do so.

González López-Valcárcel & Barber Pérez 2007 & 2009). Increasing numbers of Latin American doctors and nurses are immigrating and some Spanish doctors (generalists and specialists) and nurses are emigrating to work in other EU countries. However, emigration has been declining since 2003 when shortages began to appear (see section 5). This section will show that Spain acts as a corridor between Latin America and Europe, a situation that has evolved in the absence of a well-defined government immigration policy.

2.1 *Medical doctors*

Using data from 2001 and birthplace as a criterion, Dumont and Zurn (2007) report that 7.5% of doctors working in Spain were foreigners. Conversely, 8530 Spanish doctors were registered in other countries – equivalent to 5.9% of all practising doctors in Spain. Of these, 3960 were practising in the EU and most of the rest were practising in the United States. In the mid 2000s, Spain ranked 13th in Europe in terms of the percentage of foreign-born medical doctors (Garcia- Pérez et al. 2007). Recent estimates of foreign inflows; foreign medical doctor stocks; and numbers with emigration intentions as proportions of total medical stock highlight Spain's importance as a destination for foreign medical doctors and for returning Spanish medical doctors.

Inflows

Each region of Spain has a medical council but most do not report whether their members hold foreign diplomas and/or nationality. Their umbrella organization, the Organization of Medical Colleges (*Organización Médica Colegial* – OMC), estimates that in 2007 about 12.5% of the 203 305 doctors registered were of foreign origin. Table 7.1 shows the stocks of foreign[3] doctors within all doctors registered in each autonomous community. The percentage of foreigners varies from 0.2% in the Basque Country to 14.2% in the Canary Islands and 15.4% in the Balearic Islands.

Between 1998 and 2002, 4318 degrees in general medicine (*licenciaturas*) from countries outside the EU were recognized (Table 7.2), most from Latin America. Between 2003 and 2008 the number jumped almost six-fold to 24 330. In recent years, regional health services have compensated for shortages of doctors in some specialties by hiring non-EU medical doctors whose specialty degrees have not yet been recognized by the Ministry of Education (del Burgo 2009). The OMC (2009) estimates that between 10 000 and 12 000 medical doctors are working in Spain under these irregular conditions. In 2007, 5383 (4811 from outside the EU) degrees in general medicine were recognized; 40% more than the number of medical graduates in Spanish universities (3841).

---

3 Foreign refers to nationality unless otherwise specified.

Table 7.1 *Registered doctors (stock) in autonomous regions in Spain, 2007*

Autonomous regions[k]	Foreign doctors No.	%	Total registered doctors
Andalucia[a]	857	2.7	31 592
Aragon[b]	156	2.0	7 667
Balearic Islands[c]	697	15.4	4 526
Basque Country[d]	24	0.2	10 921
Canary Islands[e]	1 148	14.2	8 060
Catalonia (Barcelona only)[f]	3 454	12.4	27 883
Extremadura[g]	118	1.5	7 568
Galicia (2008)[h]	584	5.8	10 068
Madrid (2008)[i]	1 872	5.6	33 185
Valencian Community (Alicante only)[j]	564	8.8	6 347

Sources: [a] Medical Council of Andalucia 2009; [b] Medical Council of Huesca 2009, Medical Council of Saragossa 2009 & Medical Council of Teruel 2009; [c] Medical Council of Metges, Balearic Islands 2009; [d] Medical Council of Gipuzkoa 2009; [e] Medical Council of Santa Cruz 2009 & Medical Council of Las Palmas; [f] Medical Council of Metges, Barcelona; [g] Medical Council of Cáceres 2009 & Medical Council of Badajoz 2009; [h] elCorreoGallego.es 2009; [i] Medical Council of Madrid 2009; [j] Medical Council of Valencia 2009. *Note*: [k] No data available for Asturias, Cantabria, Castile la Mancha, Castile and Leon, Murcia, Navarre, La Rioja.

Table 7.2 *Foreign degrees in general medicine recognized in Spain, 1998–2008*

Year	Non-EU countries	EU countries (recognition under EU directive)	Total	Proportion of all diplomas delivered in Spain
1998	674	213	887	18%
1999	715	227	942	22%
2000	763	260	1 023	24%
2001	1 342	203	1 545	38%
2002	824	211	1 035	25%
2003	3 352	257	3 609	90%
2004	2 629	240	2 869	65%
2005	2 614	343	2 957	69%
2006	3 218	408	3 626	93%
2007	4 811	564	5 375	140%
2008	7 706	576	8 282	213%

Sources: INE database 2009, Ministry of Education 2002–2008.

The number of degrees recognized through European Directive 2005/36/EC (European Parliament and Council of the European Union 2005) averaged 230 per year between 1998 and 2004 but the trend has been upward since then.

Far fewer medical specialty degrees are recognized – 702 in 2007, the equivalent of 13% of the specialist medical resident (médico interno residente – MIR) slots for that year. The trend has been increasing but is much less striking than that of general medicine – 1154 specialty degrees were recognized in 1998–2002; 2633 in 2003–2007.

The INE (2009) reports that 75% of foreign doctors and dentists in Spain in 2007 came from Latin America. Of these, 45% arrived between 1995 and 2002 and 19% between 2003 and 2007.

Outflows

Within the EU, most migrating Spanish doctors go to Portugal (Dumont & Zurn 2007), France and the United Kingdom. The Association of Spanish Health Professionals in Portugal (*Associação de Profissionais da Saúde Espanhóis em Portugal* – APSEP) estimates that 1870 doctors from Spain were working in Portugal in 2008, most in the public health system. A considerable number of Spanish doctors continue to live in Spain while working in Portugal. APSEP notes a trend towards returning to Spain that began in 2008 (Periodista Digital 2008). Returnees are attracted by a Spanish labour market that moved from a surplus to a shortage of doctors in the mid 2000s.

Spanish doctors who want to work in other countries must obtain a certificate from the OMC. The number of certificates issued is an indication of intention to work outside Spain. There were 650 certificate requests in 2007, only 0.34% of all practising registered doctors. A total of 6194 medical doctors requested certificates in 2000–2007, the equivalent of 0.32% of the active doctors registered in 2007 (OMC 2008).

Furthermore, between 2002 and 2007 the Ministry of Education recognized far fewer general medicine and specialty degrees than the number of certificates issued by the OMC. There is a noticeable decline after 2004. Between 2002 and 2007, the Ministry of Education recognized 507 specialty degrees but more than twice that number of general medicine decrees (1236).

2.2 Nurses

Inflows

The EAPS shows that only around 1% of nurses working in Spain are foreign nationals, half of whom come from Latin America (Table 7.3) (INE database

2004–2008). Combined EAPS data for 2004–2008 by zone of origin shows that 39% of nurses came from the EU, 18% from Andean countries, 30% from other countries in Latin America, 10% from Africa and 3% from the rest of the world. Spanish and foreign-national nurses have similar age profiles with the average around 40 years old (INE database 2004–2008). The inflows of Latin American nurses have increased since 2000 but outflows of Spanish nurses to EU countries peaked in 2002–2003 and have been declining since. The large drop in 2007 could be due to sampling errors, as the EAPS is a small sample of the full population of nurses.

Table 7.3 *Registered nurses (stock) working in Spain, 2004–2008*

	2004	2005	2006	2007	2008
Nurses working in Spain, registered with Council of Nurses[a]	192 562	200 203	210 045	216 238	223 655
Foreign nurses (%)[bc]	3 184 (1.7)	3 279 (1.6)	2 477 (1.2)	1 251 (0.6)	2 295 (1.0)

Sources: [a] Council of Nurses 2009, [b] EAPS unpublished data 2009. *Note*: [c] Foreign nationals and holders of dual citizenship (Spanish/foreign).

There has been an upward trend in nurse inflows (Fig. 7.1). Recognized or homologated foreign nursing degrees represented the equivalent of 20% of new nursing graduates in 2007, up from 3% in 2002. Ministry of Education data (Periodista Digital 2008) show that the diplomas of a total of 1195 nurses and midwives from the EU were recognized for practise in Spain in 2002–2007. Of these, 23% came from the United Kingdom (280 nurses and midwives, including the largest number of foreign European midwives); 20% (237) from Germany; and 18% from Portugal (221 – including 195 in 2007 alone).

Outflows

The number of Spanish nurses who validated their degrees to work in the EU increased sharply in 2002 (1621 for the year, equivalent to 19% of that year's nursing school graduates).[4] However, the increase in internal demand has led numbers to decline sharply since 2003 (Fig. 7.1), falling to 275 or only 3% of nursing graduate numbers in 2007. The same trend was observed for medical doctors (see section 2.1). According to APSEP, about 1500 Spanish nurses were working in Portugal in 2007, many living in Spain and commuting daily (Policlínica Miramar 2007).

Fig. 7.1 *Nursing degrees homologated or recognized in Spain, 2002–2007*

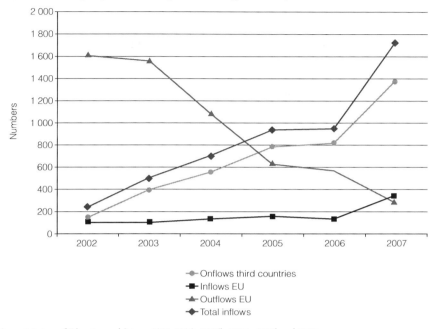

Onflows third countries
Inflows EU
Outflows EU
Total inflows

Source: Ministry of Education and Science 2005, 2006a, 2006b, 2007a, 2007b and 2009.

2.3 *Dentists*

The number of registered dentists has increased threefold in Spain, from 7471 in 1988 to 24 515 in 2007 – 1 for every 1917 inhabitants (INE 2007). There are significant proportions of foreign dentists in tourist areas. Before 1995, all dentists were medical doctors and the number of medical graduates far exceeded demand. This precipitated a market solution to a serious planning failure – an exodus of Spanish doctors in the 1980s, migrating to study dentistry in Latin America and then returning to practise. This explains why 18% of dentists registered in Valencia in 2007 held foreign degrees (ICOEV 2007a).

Professional associations anticipated that overwhelming numbers of dentists would immigrate from the 2004 and 2007 accession countries (ICOEV 2007b). Yet only a small number of degrees from these countries were recognized in Spain in 2005–2007. Between 2002 and 2007 a total of 2145 dentists with foreign diplomas obtained recognitions to practise in Spain (Periodista Digital 2008) (Table 7.4).

Information provided by the dental councils of Madrid, Catalonia and Valencia indicates that about 20% of dentists are foreign nationals with foreign degrees. Percentages are higher in tourist areas such as Las Palmas where 34% of registered dentists are foreign nationals – 55% from Latin America and the rest from Europe (INE 2007). In 2004, 34.5% of registered dentists in Catalonia had obtained their degrees outside Spain but were not necessarily foreign nationals (Table 7.4).

Table 7.4 *Nationality of dentists and origin of dental degree, 1998 and 2007*

Year and place of practice	1998 (Catalonia)[a]	2007 (Madrid and Valencia)[b]
Spanish with Spanish degree	69 %	80.4%
Spanish with foreign degree	18 %	
Foreign with foreign degree	13 %	19.6 %

Sources: [a] COEC 1997, [b] COEM 2007, ICOEV 2007a.

There is a positive balance between dentists with foreign degrees who are licensed to practise in Spain and Spanish dentists who have obtained recognition to practice in another EU Member State (Table 7.5). In 2007, 303 dental diplomas from outside the EU and 118 European dental degrees were recognized. These 421 dentists were the equivalent of 37% of Spanish dental school graduates that year. The main sources were countries in Latin America and the EU.

The United Kingdom was the main destination for Spanish dentists, following the signing of a bilateral agreement in 2001 (see section 7). The ratio between inflows and outflows (intentions) is in the order of 3:1 (Table 7.5).

Table 7.5 *Inflows and outflows of dentists in Spain, 2002–2007*

	2002	2003	2004	2005	2006	2007
Dentists newly registered	785	713	1 050	1 095	1 150	1 215
Non-EU degrees recognized (a)	162	150	269	318	259	303
European Economic Area (EEA) degrees recognized (b)	114	107	124	116	105	118
Total foreign inflows (c=a+b)	276	257	393	434	364	421
Spanish degrees recognized for practise in EU (outflow intentions) (d)	25	115	112	177	160	125
Inflow/outflow (intentions) (c/d)	11.0	2.2	3.5	2.5	2.3	3.4
Spanish dental school graduates (e)	1 059	954	1 138	1 111	1 072	1 138
Total foreign inflows as proportion of Spanish graduates (c/e X 100)	26.1%	26.9%	34.5%	39.1%	34.0%	37.0%

Sources: INE 2007, Ministry of Education and Science 2005, 2006a, 2006b, 2007a, 2007b & 2009.

2.4 Pharmacists

Pharmacist inflows are smaller than those of doctors, nurses and dentists. Of the 247 foreign pharmacists whose degrees were recognized in 2007, 89% (220) came from countries outside the EEA (Periodista Digital 2008, Policlínica Miramar 2007). In the same year, 242 Spaniards obtained degree validations for use in Europe (the equivalent of 10.7% of Spanish pharmacy school graduates for the year) (Table 7.6). There is no risk of a shortage, rather the risk of unemployment is pushing some professionals (both foreign and nationals) to look for work elsewhere (Meneu 2006).

Table 7.6 *Inflows and outflows of pharmacists in Spain, 2002–2007*

	2002	2003	2004	2005	2006	2007
New registrations	2 069	1 791	1 444	1 306	1 330	719
Non-EU degrees recognized (a)	85	212	216	157	214	220
EEA degrees recognized (b)	15	21	12	29	23	27
Total foreign inflows (c=a+b)	100	233	228	186	237	247
Spanish degrees recognized for work in EU (outflow intentions) (d)	479	488	354	320	299	242
Inflow/outflow (intentions) (c/d)	0.2	0.5	0.6	0.6	0.8	1.0
Spanish pharmacy school graduates (e)	3 092	2 832	2 691	2 641	2 244	2 254
Total foreign inflows as proportion of Spanish graduates (c/e X 100)	3.2%	8.2%	8.5%	7.0%	10.6%	11.0%

Sources: INE 2007, Ministry of Education and Science 2005, 2006a, 2006b,2007a, 2007b & 2009.

3. Vignettes on health professional mobility

Spanish doctor commuting between Spain and Portugal

Dr G lives in Galicia near the Portuguese border, his children attend school in Spain and his wife has a job there. Since 2001 Dr G has commuted daily to work as a general practitioner at the health clinic in Viana do Castelo in Portugal. In the early 2000s it was hard to be a family doctor in Spain as the only jobs were short-term locum posts on weekly contracts. In Portugal he has professional status, a higher salary, more autonomy and his patients' respect. The language has caused little problem as it resembles his native Galician. He does not rule out returning to work in Spain when he can get a secure and satisfying job with decent pay. Now that there is a shortage of doctors and nurses in Spain fellow members of the APSEP (which includes about 1900 doctors and 1500 nurses) are beginning to negotiate returning to their home country.[5]

---

5 Interview 12 January 2009.

Immigrant to permanent resident

Dr Y was born and studied medicine in Venezuela, the granddaughter of a Spaniard who emigrated in the 1940s. She applied for and was granted Spanish citizenship in 2006. Her basic medical degree (*licenciatura*) was recognized in Spain following a long and complicated process – a year of paperwork followed by an exam in legal and forensic medicine (a subject not covered in her Venezuelan degree) in a Spanish university of her choice. This year, she will take the MIR exam in order to train for a specialty but will not have to compete for the limited quota of slots for foreigners. There were more than 6000 residency places but fewer than 4000 medical graduates in 2007. This surplus means that she is certain to obtain a specialist training place but it is not certain that she will achieve the grade required for her chosen specialty – paediatrics. Her second choice is family and community medicine.[6]

---

4. Dynamics of enlargement

There have been no significant inflows from the 2004 and 2007 accession countries (although flows appear to be increasing). The exception was Polish medical doctors whose numbers increased significantly in 2007. In 2008, doctors from the new EU Member States acquired recognition of 268 general medical degrees and 202 specialty degrees. These constitute 3.2% and 36.5% respectively of all the degrees recognized in 2008 and, in 2007, represented 4.3% and 35.5% of all inflows (Table 7.7). As yet, there have been no similar influxes of dentists, nurses and pharmacists.

Table 7.7 *Inflows of health professionals from new Member States, 2005–2008*

Year	2004 accession countries				2007 accession countries		Proportion of total inflows[a]	
	2005	**2006**	**2007**	**2008**	**2007**	**2008**	**2007 (%)**	**2008 (%)**
General medical doctors	43	154	227	185	6	83	4.3	3.2
Medical specialists	34	135	199	150	4	52	35.5	36.5
Nurses	4	6	8	23	0	3	0	0
Dentists	5	6	10	9	0	10	0	0
Pharmacists	1	0	2	3	0	0	0	0

Sources: Ministry of Education and Science 2007a, 2007b, 2009 & 2010.
Note: [a] Total inflows were 5947 (5375 basic medical degrees + 572 specialty degrees) in 2007 and 8835 (8281 basic medical degrees + 554 specialty degrees) in 2008.

Shortages of health professionals in Spain have led to the emergence of companies that recruit health professionals in the new EU countries, especially Poland

---

6 Interview 19 March 2009.

and Romania (González López-Valcárcel & Barber Pérez 2008). Autonomous communities have also embarked on recruiting expeditions, some of which have been led by the head of the regional health service.

5. Impacts on the Spanish health system

International health professional mobility has had an impact on the Spanish health system. The inflow of foreign professionals, particularly medical doctors, relieved the acute shortages in 2000–2005 and added flexibility to the market (González López-Valcárcel & Barber Pérez 2007 & 2009). But it also led to public debate (Bruguera 2009, Mayol 2009) about the quality of some foreign professionals (Ortún et al. 2008). There is no defined national strategy for health in Spain (González López-Valcárcel 2009) and therefore the recruitment and training of foreign professionals is improvised rather than planned. However, foreign professionals bring cultural diversity to an increasingly international population and improve doctor-patient communications by lowering cultural barriers (Montero 2007).

5.1 *Stewardship*

The high rates of unemployment caused by a surplus of doctors in the 1990s changed to shortages in some specialties and regions in 2001–2002 (González López-Valcárcel & Barber Pérez 2008]. This deficit entered an acute phase between 2003 and 2006 due to the combination of three demand shocks. The first was internal, the result of responsibility for health moving from central government to Spain's autonomous communities that invested in new hospitals and clinics. The second was also internal as the buoyant economy supported a flourishing of the private sector, particularly for medical services for the well-off whose demand is largely income sensitive. The third demand shock was external as doctors were attracted by European countries with similar doctor shortages (particularly the United Kingdom, Portugal and France). The symptomatic evidence of shortages stimulated reconsideration of the planning process by adjusting the number of MIR places (González López-Valcárcel & Barber 2005).

5.2 *Service delivery*

The inflows of foreign professionals enrich cultural variety in the health network and provide a solution for shortages, especially among doctors and nurses (ParaInmigrantes.info 2008). Thus, they contribute to social fairness by helping to ensure that all the population has access to health assistance.

There is concern over the risk of producing a clustered supply in which doctors with deficient training work in less attractive positions (Ortún et al. 2008). This quality problem arises because as yet there is no mechanism to guarantee the recognition of degrees from non-EU countries or to identify the skills and qualities that are needed.

5.3 *Financing*

The salary levels of health professionals in Spain have not risen to the levels that would be expected in a closed market. This is due to foreign professionals, mainly from Latin America, who are willing to accept lower salaries and poorer working conditions (González López-Valcárcel & Barber Pérez 2007 & 2008). Since 70% of health financing is funded by taxes, foreign professionals have produced savings for Spanish taxpayers. Nevertheless, medical salaries have risen considerably over the last five years as a consequence of the triple demand shock caused by competition from private health-care providers, infrastructure changes and pull pressure from other countries (see section 5.1). In the mid 2000s, the professional organizations were pressing hard in the collective negotiations on reimbursements in all the regions (CESM 2006). Reimbursement models changed regions such as Catalonia (ABC.es 2008) and salaries rose everywhere. However, the cost increase would be considerably larger if no foreign professionals were willing to immigrate.

6. Relevance of cross-border health professional mobility

In the short term, Spain has middle to high dependence on foreign doctors and, to a lesser extent, on foreign nurses (see section 2). It does not appear that the country needs to import dentists but market forces attract dentists from Latin America. In turn, this helps to moderate the pace of increases in incomes. Increasingly, dentists are changing from self-employed professionals to salaried employees and dental franchises are spreading. It is possible that the expansion of dental coverage in the public health system also increases demand (Pinilla & González 2009).

6.1 *Distribution issues affecting composition of the health workforce*

Generally, international health professional migration has helped to relieve imbalances in supply, both geographical and for certain categories of health professionals. The situation has changed from a surplus of doctors that began in the 1980s to a shortage that started around 2003 (Barber Pérez & González López-Valcárcel 2008).

Variation in the availability of professionals among autonomous communities is less marked than in other western European countries (González López-Valcárcel & Barber Pérez 2009). Nevertheless, isolated and rural areas and the smaller islands find it difficult to recruit sufficient doctors and nurses.

There are shortages of specialists in anaesthetics, orthopaedic and traumatic surgery, paediatric surgery, reconstructive surgery, family and community medicine, paediatrics, radiology and urology (González López-Valcárcel & Barber Pérez 2009). Family medicine has the greatest shortages although the problem is relieved to some extent by immigrating family doctors or by foreign doctors who train as specialists in Spain.

Spain has one of the lowest nurse/medical doctor ratios (about 1:1 in primary care centres and 1.8:1 in public hospitals) in Europe. As elsewhere in Europe, the market for nurses is complex and fluctuating (Dussault 2009). The public and private sectors compete for health professionals, offering different incentives – job security in the public sector; higher pay and more clinical freedom in the private sector. The resulting sharp jump in demand has seen a considerable increase in public-sector doctors' pay in recent years (see section 4). Many professionals work in both sectors.

6.2 *Factors influencing size and composition of the health workforce*

Education system and specialist training

Few nurses, pharmacists or dentists move to Spain to undertake specialist training but Spain has become a net trainer of medical specialists, with residency programmes that are recognized internationally for their high quality.

The presence of foreign doctors in specialist training is possibly one of the clearest examples of Spain's attraction for the medical profession and its growing relevance as a training ground for foreign doctors, particularly from Latin America. This is reflected in the marked increases in the number of foreign candidates sitting the medical residency exam in recent years. In 2008, the total number of exam candidates increased by 5% but the number of foreign candidates jumped by 29% (Table 7.8). In 2007, foreign candidates gained 16% of the MIR places. The main source countries are in Spanish America, especially Peru (36.3%), Argentina (19.8%), Colombia (14%) and Venezuela (9.8%).

Spanish universities are mainly public, with subsidized fees and increasing numbers of scholarships. Dentistry is an exception and only 47% of new students attend public universities (Table 7.9). Central government sets enrolment

Table 7.8 *MIR entrance exam candidates, 2007 and 2008*

	2007	2008
Spanish	7 568	7 209
Foreign	3 204	4 122
Total	10 772	11 331
Proportion of foreign candidates	30%	36%
Annual increase in foreign candidates	–	29%

Source: Ministry of Health unpublished data 2009.

Table 7.9 *University degrees in the health professions: students, universities and graduates, 2007–2008*

	First-year students	First-year students in public universities	Public/ private universities	Total students	Total graduates	Women graduates
Medicine	5 223	95%	27/2	29 967	3 922	72.4%
Nursing	10 695	80%	87/14	28 887	8 987	85.3%
Pharmacy	3 000	88%	11/4	19 175	2 059	76.4%
Dentistry	1 703	47%	12/5	8 276	1 475	69.0%

Source: Ministry of Education 2008.

limits for certain professions including medicine, nursing, pharmacy and dentistry. Nursing is an academic university degree; assistant nurses or nursing care auxiliaries complete a 1400 hour vocational training course (Government of Spain 1995).

Enrolment limits have caused imbalances between the production of medical graduates and the demand for specialists. The number of students seeking to study medicine has been growing exponentially – there were seven applicants for each public medical school place in 2007, far above the demand for other university disciplines (González López-Valcárcel & Barber Pérez 2008, Ministry of Education 2008, Ministry of Science and Innovation 2006).

There are no official data on the number of foreign students in universities and technical colleges but internal data from several universities indicate that their numbers are generally negligible. Newspapers report that a significant number of foreign students have been admitted to Spanish universities since 2007–2008, particularly in the border regions (Álvarez 2008).

The fixed enrolments introduced to reduce the overloading of medical schools at the end of the 1970s resulted in drastic reductions in the numbers of new students, stabilizing at about 4500 each year. A graduated increase in enrolments began in the 2006–2007 academic year, with the goal of 7000 new medical students in 2012.

Fig. 7.2 *Evolution of the number of new students in medical schools 1964–2009*

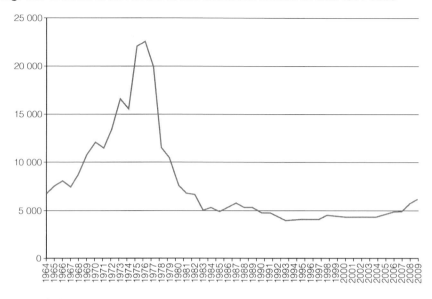

Source: INE database 2009.

The historical dynamic of medical school entry driven by enrolment limits gives a peculiar shape to the population pyramid of student doctors in Spain (Fig. 7.2). In 1976, 22 554 first-year students started studying medicine, almost five times more than the current number.

After six years of medical studies, a specialty is required in order to practise in the public health network. Those seeking to work as general practitioners must undertake a four-year specialization in family and community medicine. This is not required for private practice. Demand for specialists has led to increases in the numbers of MIR places but there will still be too few Spanish candidates unless there is a parallel increase in the number of new medical graduates. MIR training has attracted foreign doctors but the number of unfilled places has been increasing every year since 2005–2006 (87 in 2005–2006; 244 in 2006–2007; 301 in 2007–2008).

Demographics and retirement

Pharmacy and nursing are feminized professions (Fig. 7.3). In 2008, 83% of the 243 000 registered nurses were women. Three in four medical students and MIRs are women. There are no data on registered dentists by age and sex but the profession has a young profile, given the number of new dental schools from which the first dentists (no longer doctor-dentists) graduated in 1990. Nurses working in Spain have a young demographic profile than other countries. Registered medical doctors are older; the most frequent age interval is 45–54 years of age (35%).

Ageing of the workforce is particularly problematic for the medical profession. The retirement age for doctors in the public health system is 65 but this can be extended to 70 on a case-by-case basis; the private sector has no mandatory retirement age. Four of every ten specialists will retire in the next 15 years. In some of the most traditional specialties more than half of the doctors are over 50 years old. It is estimated that those retiring will exceed new medical graduates from 2016 onwards (González López-Valcárcel & Barber Pérez 2007 & 2009).

7. Factors influencing health professional mobility

Table 7.10 summarizes the main factors influencing health professional mobility. The summaries give a useful overview of what is a complex phenomenon.

Table 7.10 *Factors influencing health professional mobility in Spain*

Factors	Description and comments
Instigating factors	1990s and early 2000s: unemployment (Amaya & Garcia 2005, González López-Valcárcel et al. 2006); low salaries in comparison to other EU countries (Barham & Bramley-Harker 2004); temporary contracts and job instability; low prestige and social recognition These factors have been mitigated in recent years: pay has risen and temporary and locum professionals have better working conditions (see section 5)
Activating factors	Attraction of the United Kingdom (until 2006), Portugal and France – outreach to Spanish professionals; facilitation of adaptation (language classes, etc); social and professional safety net of Spaniards settled in the country; job security (Portugal); social and professional recognition (Periodista Digital 2008, Policlínica Miramar 2007)
Facilitating factors	Bilateral agreements (with United Kingdom in 2001)
Inhibiting factors	Foreign language; settling family in host country

8. Policy, regulation and interventions

8.1 *Workforce planning and development*

Generally, policies dealing with professional mobility have been reactive rather than proactive, relying on short-term instruments to alleviate obvious imbalances (González López-Valcárcel & Barber Párez 2006). Without any monitoring of professional employment, problems could not be anticipated and imbalances were recognized only when they had become serious. A formal planning process for doctors (based on analysis of needs and supply with a temporal horizon to 2025) was only set up in 2005. It is not easy to supervise and coordinate such a decentralized system – the professional planning process is complex and includes many actors with conflicting interests.

Table 7.11 *National-level instruments for guiding and managing health professional mobility*

Instrument	Description
Bilateral agreements	Signed 2001 between Spanish Ministry of Health and United Kingdom to send Spanish medical doctors, nurses and other health professionals to work in the National Health Service
Royal decree on the homologation of the medical specialty degree from non EU-countries (Government of Spain 2010)	Homologation of specialty degrees
Studies of the need for health professionals	Ministry of Health (González López-Valcárcel & Barber Pérez 2009); Senate holds special hearings on the needs for, and shortages of, health professionals*
Streamlined work visas for non-EU citizens in shortage professions	Labour ministry publishes quarterly list of shortage occupations by autonomous community
Historical Memory Law (Government of Spain 2007)	Acquisition of Spanish nationality for children and grandchildren.

* From December 2008 to November 2009 the Senate hearing called on witnesses representing various associations and organizations, including one of the authors of this chapter (González López-Valcárcel 2009).

Current challenges facing the Spanish health-care system include coordination; funding; the management search for improved efficiency; and workforce planning (Lisac et al. 2008). A simulation model has been used to estimate the shortages and surpluses of medical specialists for each specialty in order to set adequate enrolment limits in medical schools and to establish the individual specialty numbers in the annual residency competition on the basis of need (González López-Valcárcel & Barber 2005). The need for a register of health professionals is universally recognized. This is being set up and funded by the Ministry of Health with the participation of the autonomous communities.

8.2 *Recognition of diplomas*

The application of European Community directives for the recognition of diplomas is a competency of the Ministry of Education. Directive 2005/36/ ED for the mutual recognition of professional qualifications (Parliament and Council of the European Union 2005) was applied by Royal Decree 183/2008 (Ministry of Education and Science 2008a, 2008b, 2008c and 2008d).

"Spain, which is supposed to have a surplus of nurses, has signed bilateral agreements, notably with France and the United Kingdom" (Dumont &

Zurn 2007). Spain has signed mutual recognition agreements with numerous other countries too. From 1996, the law as interpreted by the Supreme Court established that these agreements do not exempt the administration from checking a foreign degree's equivalence to the corresponding Spanish degree. That is, non-EU country degrees must be recognized on an individual basis, comparing the content and the length of training. Non-EU citizens require a residence permit in order to practise a profession in Spain. An important number of Spanish nationals were born and lived in Latin America, the offspring of Spaniards – they have full citizenship rights. Dual citizenship is permitted under Spanish law and has been acquired by an undetermined but substantial number of people, particularly from Argentina, Cuba, Uruguay and Venezuela.

The Ministry of Education recognizes basic medical degrees but specialty degrees fall under the Ministry of Science and are put before the national commission for each specialty on a case-by-case basis. Having evaluated the curriculum and experience of a candidate, these commissions can issue a report that is favourable, unfavourable, or conditional upon passing the theoretical and practical examination that is held annually (Ministry of Education 2011). A royal decree for the professional recognition of health specialists from outside the EU was published in May 2010 (Ministry of Health and Social Policy 2010).

There is tension between the Spanish medical organizations and the autonomous communities as the latter need specialists and hire them before their degrees have been recognized.

9. Conclusion

The health professional market is sensitive to shocks external to the health sector and to the country. Over a very few years Spain has moved from a surplus of medical doctors to a deficit; from doctor unemployment and an exodus of health professionals to Europe to the need to recruit professionals from other countries. Now Spain is training foreign specialists and in the process resolving the numerical imbalance between the numbers of graduating students and specialist residency places (Tribunalatina.com 2008).

Foreign specialists alleviate shortages in the short run, bring cultural variety to the system, keep salaries in the public sector at a fiscally sustainable level and improve the equitable distribution of health services over the national territory. But the lack of effective quality control mechanisms could lead to a two-tier system comprising doctors who are excellent and doctors with deficient training. There is a legal problem with doctors from non-EU countries working as specialists without specialty degrees validated in Spain. A recently approved royal decree addresses this problem (Ministry of Health and Social Policy 2010). In addition, anecdotal evidence suggests that Spanish professionals who moved to other European countries during the years of internal unemployment may be beginning to return but data are lacking on this as on many other matters.

A trend of increasing inflows has been observed for nurses. The numbers of foreign nurses who obtained licences to work in Spain in 2007 numbers had reached in 2007 numbers had reached amounted to 3% of new graduates from nursing schools in Spain in 2002 but were 20% in 2007. Private and public health facilities compete to attract these nurses as well as medical doctors; this pushes up salary levels.

The net inflow of doctors from non-EU countries is increasing sharply. This increases the flexibility of the market but raises quality problems as Spain does not have a consolidated reliable system of diploma recognition for health professionals. Spain is in need of a national strategy to guarantee a minimal level of professional skills in degree holders. Spare capacity in the MIR system offers the opportunity to pursue a proactive policy of specialist training. However, there has been no consistent policy for regulation or any strategy in planning as the latter requires technical difficulties to be overcome and good information. In addition, the goals of Spain's administrations and the protagonists do not coincide. More systematic planning is required, based on more comprehensive and reliable data. This should begin by meeting the urgent need for a national registry of active health professionals.

References

ABC.es (2008). Los médicos catalanes tendrán un nuevo modelo retributivo pionero [A new reimbursement model for Catalonian doctors]. *ABC.es*, 18 March 2008 (http://www.abc.es/hemeroteca/historico-18-03-2008/abc/Catalunya/los-medicos-catalanes-tendran-un-nuevo-modelo-retributivo-pionero_1641729703468.html, accessed 8 February 2011).

Álvarez E (2008). Alumnos extranjeros copan cien de las 350 plazas de primero de Medicina [Foreign students get 100 out of 350 seats in the medical school]. *La Voz de Galicia.es*, 12 September 2008 (http://www.lavozdegalicia.es/galicia/2008/09/13/0003_7135768.htm, accessed 13 January 2011).

Amaya C, Garcia MA (2005). *Demografía médica en España. Mirando al futuro* [*Medical demography in Spain. Looking at the future*]. Madrid, Confederación Estatal de Sindicatos Médicos.

Barber Pérez P, González López-Valcárcel B (2008). ¿Hay suficientes profesionales sanitarios en España? Desequilibrios, déficits, movilidad internacional y acreditación de los médicos [Are there enough health professionals in Spain? Imbalances, shortages, international mobility and medical certification]. *Humanitas Humanidades Médicas*, No. 23 (http://www.fundacionmhm.org/revista.html, accessed 13 January 2011).

Barham L, Bramley-Harker E (2004). *Comparing physicians' earnings: current knowledge and challenges. A report for the Department of Health.* London, NERA.

Bruguera M (2009). Hace falta un proceso de homologación de titulaciones ágil, justo y riguroso [An agile, fair and rigorous degree approval process is necessary]. *Tribuna*, 21 January 2009 (http://www.comb.cat/ cat/ actualitat/ noticies/homologacion.pdf, accessed 13 January 2011).

del Burgo P (2009). La OMC exige a Sanidad un censo de los médicos extranjeros contratados que carecen de la especialidad [The Medical Association requests the Ministry of Health for a census of foreign doctors working without diplomas]. *Levante-EMV.com*, 27 January 2009 (http://www.levante-emv.com/ secciones/noticia.jsp? pRef=2009012700 19_547889__ComunitatValenciana-exige-Sanidad-censo-medicos-extranjeros-contratados-carecen-especialidad, accessed 12 January 2011).

CESM (2006). *Los salarios de los médicos varían más de un 30% según la Comunidad en la que trabajan [Physicians' salaries vary more than 30% among autonomous communities].* Madrid, Confederacion Estatal de Sindicatos Medicos (http://www.cesm.org/nueva/ index.asp?pag=detallenoticia.asp&formid =502187&categoria=2, accessed 13 January 2011).

COEC (1997). *Presente y futuro socioeconómico del sector odontoestomatológico en Cataluña. Años 1996–2005 [The socioeconomic present and future of odontology in Catalonia 1996–2005].* Barcelona, Collegi Oficial d'Odontòlegs i Estomatòlegs de Catalunya.

COEM (2007). *Libro Blanco de la Profesión: Odontólogos y Estomatólogos de la Comunidad de Madrid [White Paper of the profession: odontologists and physicians specialized in dentistry in Madrid].* Madrid, Odontólogos y Estomatólogos de la Comunidad de Madrid.

elCorreoGallego.es (2009).Cerca de 600 médicos extranjeros trabajan en la sanidad gallega [Nearly 600 foreign doctors working in health services in Galicia]. *elCorreoGallego.es*, 6 April 2009 (http://www.elcorreogallego.es/ galicia/ecg/ cerca-600-medicos-extranjeros-trabajan-sanidad-gallega/idNoticia-413716/, accessed 23 February 2011).

CGE (2009) [web site]. Madrid, Consejo General de Enfermería [General Council of Nurses]. (http:\\www.cge.enfermundi.com, accessed 23 February 2011).

Dumont J, Zurn P (2007). Immigrant health workers in OECD countries in the broader context of highly skilled migration. In: *International migration outlook*. Paris, Organisation for Economic Co-operation and Development.

Dussault G et al. (2009). *The nursing labour market in the European Union in transition. Scoping paper: series of policy dialogues on the nursing and social care workforces in Europe*. Brussels, European Observatory on Health Systems and Policies.

European Parliament and Council of the European Union (2005). Directive 2005/36/EC of the European Parliament and of the Council of 7 September 2005 on the recognition of professional qualifications. *Official Journal of the European Union*, 255(48):22–142.

García-Pérez MA et al. (2007). Physicians' migration in Europe: an overview of the current situation. *BMC Health Services Research*, 7:201.

González López-Valcárcel B (2009). Senate testimony 8 September 2009. *Boletín Oficial de las Cortes Generales Senado*, No. 483, 18 June 2010 (http://www.senado.es/legis9/publicaciones/html/textos/I0483.html, accessed 8 February 2011).

González López-Valcárcel B, Barber P (2005). El programa MIR como innovación y como mecanismo de asignación de recursos humanos [The medical residency programme as innovation and as a mechanism for allocating resources]. In: Meneu R et al. (eds.). *Innovaciones en gestión clínica y sanitaria [Innovations in clinical and health management]*. Barcelona, Masson.

González López-Valcárcel B, Barber Párez P (2006). Los recursos humanos y sus desequilibrios mitigables [Human resources and their mitigating unbalances]. *Gaceta Sanitaria*, 20(Suppl.1.):103–109.

González López-Valcárcel B, Barber Pérez P (2007). *Oferta y necesidad de médicos especialistas en España 2006–2030 [Supply and demand of medical specialists in Spain 2006–2030]*. Madrid, Ministerio de Sanidad y Consumo [Ministry of Health, Social Affairs and Equality].

González López-Valcárcel B, Barber Pérez P (2008). Dificultades, trampas y tópicos en la planificación del personal médico [Difficulties, pitfalls and stereotypes in physician workforce planning]. *Gaceta Sanitaria*, 22(5):393–395.

González López-Valcárcel B, Barber Pérez P (2009). *Oferta y necesidad de médicos especialistas en España 2008–2025 [Supply and demand of medical specialists in Spain 2008–2025]*. Madrid, Ministerio de Sanidad y Consumo [Ministry of Health, Social Affairs and Equality].

González López-Valcárcel B et al. (2006). Spain. In: Rechel B et al. (eds.). *The health care workforce in Europe. Learning from experience*. Copenhagen, WHO Regional Office for Europe on behalf of the European Observatory on Health Systems and Policies.

Government of Spain (1995). Real Decreto 558/1995, de 7 de abril, por el que se establece el curriculo del ciclo formativo de grado medio correspondiente al título de Técnico en Cuidados Auxiliares de Enfermería [Royal Decree 558/1995 of 7 April setting the training curriculum for the Technician in Auxiliary Nursing Care diploma]. *Boletin Oficial del Estado* [*Official State Bulletin*], No. 134, 6 June 1995.

Government of Spain (2005). Orden SCO/2920/2005, de 16 de septiembre. Convocatoria de pruebas selectivas 2005, para el acceso en el año 2006, a plazas de formación sanitaria especializada para Médicos, Farmacéuticos, Químicos, Biólogos, Bioquímicos, Psicólogos y Radiofísicos en hospitales [Official announcement in 2005 to access in year 2006 to fill positions in health specialist training for physicians, pharmacists, chemists, biologists, biochemists, psychologists and radiophysicists in hospitals]. *Boletín Oficial del Estado* [*Official State Bulletin*], No.227, 22 September 2005. (www.boe.es/ boe/ dias/2005/09/22/pdfs/A31478-31554.pdf, accessed 8 February 2011).

Government of Spain (2007). Ley de la Memoria Histórica Ley 52/2007, December 26. [Historical Memory Law] DISPOSICIÓN ADICIONAL SÉPTIMA. *Boletin Oficial del Estado* [*Official State Bulletin*], No. 310, 27 December 2007.

Government of Spain (2010). Real Decreto 459/2010, de 16 de abril, por el que se regulan las condiciones para el reconocimiento de efectos profesionales a títulos extranjeros de especialista en Ciencias de la Salud, obtenidos en Estados no miembros de la Unión Europea [Royal Decree 459/2010 of 16 April regulating the conditions for professional recognition of foreign diplomas in health science specialties obtained in non-EU Member States]. *Boletin Oficial del Estado* [*Official State Bulletin*]. No. 107, 3 May 2010.

ICOEV (2007a). La memoria anual 2007 [Annual report 2007]. Valencia, Illustre Colegio Oficial de Odontólogos y Estomatólogos de Valencia.

ICOEV (2007b). *Título de grado en odontología en la Universitat de Valencia.* [*Degree diploma in odontology, University of Valencia*]. Valencia, Informe del Ilustre Colegio Oficial de Odontólogos y Estomatólogos de Valencia (http:// centros.uv.es/web/departamentos/D285/data/tablones/tablon_general/PDF9. pdf, accessed 13 January 2011).

INE (2007). *Profesionales sanitarios colegiados por tipo de profesional, años y sexo 2007* [*Collegiate health professionals by type of professional, years and sex 2007*]. Madrid, Instituto Nacional de Estadística [National Statistics Institute] (http://www.ine.es/jaxi/tabla.do?path=/t15/p416/a2007/l0/&file=s1001. px&type=pcaxis&L=0, accessed 8 February 2010).

INE (2009). *National immigrant survey 2007*. Madrid, Instituto Nacional de Estadística [National Statistics Institute] (http://www.ine.es/en/prodyser/ pubweb/eni07/eni07_en.htm, accessed 18 February 2011).

INE database (2004–2008) [online database]. Economically active population survey. Madrid, Instituto Nacional de Estadística [National Statistics Institute] (http://www.ine.es/jaxi/ menu.do?type=pcaxis&path=%2Ft22 %2Fe308mnu &file=inebase&L=1, accessed 18 February 2011).

INE database (2009) [online database]. Estadística de la Enseñanza Universitaria en España. Curso 2006–2007 [Higher education statistics in Spain. Academic year 2006–2007]. Madrid, Instituto Nacional de Estadística [National Statistics Institute] (http://www.ine.es/jaxi/menu.do?type=pcaxis&path =%2Ft13%2Fp 405&file=inebase&L=0, accessed 18 February 2011).

Lisac MB et al. (2008). Health systems and health reform in Europe. *Intereconomics*, 43(4):184–218.

Mayol J (2009). El MIR los médicos extranjeros [The MIR for foreign physicians]. *Medicblogs*, 26 January 2009 (http://medicablogs.diariomedico. com/desdeelpuente/2009/01/26/el-mir-y-los-medicos-extranjeros/, accessed 13 January 2011).

Medical Council of Andalucia (2009) [web site]. (http://www. consejomedicoandaluz.org/, accessed 23 February 2011).

Medical Council of Badajoz (2009) [web site]. (http://www.combadajoz.com/, accessed 23 February 2011).

Medical Council of Cáceres (2009) [web site]. (http://www.comeca.org/, accessed 23 February 2011).

Medical Council of Gipuzkoa (2009) [web site]. (http://www.gisep.org/, accessed 23 February 2011).

Medical Council of Huesca (2009) [web site]. (http://www.colmedhuesca. com/, accessed 23 February 2011).

Medical Council of Las Palmas (2009) [web site]. (http://www.medicoslaspalmas. es/, accessed 23 February 2011).

Medical Council of Madrid (2009) [web site]. (http://www.icomem.es/, accessed 23 February 2011).

Medical Council of Metges, Balearic Islands (2009) [web site]. (http://www.comib.com/, accessed 23 February 2011).

Medical Council of Metges, Barcelona (2009) [web site]. (http://www.comb.cat/, accessed 23 February 2011).

Medical Council of Santa Cruz (2009) [web site]. (http://www.comtf.es/, accessed 23 February 2011).

Medical Council of Saragossa (2009) [web site]. (http://www.comz.org/, accessed 23 February 2011).

Medical Council of Teruel (2009) [web site]. (http://www.comteruel.org/, accessed 23 February 2011).

Medical Council of Valencia (2009) [web site]. (http://www.comv.es/, accessed 23 February 2011).

Meneu R (2006). Pharmaceutical distribution and retail pharmacy. *Gaceta Sanitaria*, 20 (Suppl.1.):154–159.

Ministry of Education (2002–2008). *Homologación de títulos* [*Homologation of titles*]. Madrid, Office of Degrees, Validations, and Homologations [http://www.educacion.es/educacion/universidades/educacion-superior-universitaria/titulos/homologacion-titulos.html, accessed 18 February 2011).

Ministry of Education (2002–2009). *Notas de corte universidad* [*Grades required for university entrance*]. Madrid (https://www.educacion.es/ notasdecorte/jsp/menuDo.do?rama=431001&tipoEns=CICLO&pintaCcaa=&codAut=00&codProv=00, accessed 17 February 2011).

Ministry of Education (2008). *Cifras del sistema universitario. Curso 2007–08* [*Figures for the university system, year 2007–08*). http://www.educacion.es/educacion/universidades/estadisticas-informes/datos-cifras.html, accessed 18 February 2011).

Ministry of Education (2011). *Homologación de títulos extranjeros de educación superior a títulos universitarios y grados académicos Españoles* [*Standardization of foreign studies with university degrees and academic grades in Spain*]. Madrid (http://www.educacion.es/educacion /universidades/educacion-superior-universitaria/titulos/homologacion-titulos/homologacion-titulos-universitarios.html, accessed 23 February 2011).

Ministry of Education and Science (2005). *La homologación, convalidación y reconocimiento de estudios extranjeros, año 2002* [*The standardization, validation and recognition of foreign studies, 2002*]. Madrid [http://www.educacion.es/mecd/estadisticas/educativas/cee/2005/G3-Titulos.pdf, accessed 17 February 2011).

Ministry of Education and Science (2006a). *La homologación, convalidación y reconocimiento de estudios extranjeros, año 2003* [*The standardization, validation and recognition of foreign studies, 2003*]. Madrid (http://www. educacion.es/mecd/estadisticas/educativas/cee/2006/G3-Titulos.pdf, accessed 17 February 2011).

Ministry of Education and Science (2006b). *La homologación, convalidación y reconocimiento de estudios extranjeros, año 2004* [*The standardization, validation and recognition of foreign studies, 2004*]. Madrid (http://www.educacion.es/mecd/estadisticas/educativas/cee/2006A/G3-Titulos.pdf accessed 17 February 2011).

Ministry of Education and Science (2007a). *La homologación, convalidación y reconocimiento de estudios extranjeros, año 2005* [*The standardization, validation and recognition of foreign studies, 2005*]. Madrid (http://www.educacion.es/mecd/estadisticas/educativas/cee/2007/G3-Titulos.pdf, accessed 17 February 2011).

Ministry of Education and Science (2007b). *La homologación, convalidación y reconocimiento de estudios extranjeros, año 2006* [*The standardization, validation and recognition of foreign studies, 2006*]. Madrid http://www.educacion.es/mecd/estadisticas/educativas/cee/20061/G3-Titulos.pdf, accessed 17 February 2011).

Ministry of Education and Science (2008a). Orden EC1/332/2008, de 13 de febrero, por la que se establecen los requisitos para la verificación de los títulos universitarios oficiales que habiliten para el ejercicio de la profesión de Médico [EC1/332/2008 Order of 13 February, laying down the requirements for verification of university degrees that qualify for the practice of the medical profession]. *Boletin Oficial del Estado* [*Official State Bulletin*], No. 40, 15 February 2008.

Ministry of Education and Science (2008b). Resolución de 14 de febrero de 2008, de la Secretaría de Estado de Universidades e Investigación, por la que se da publicidad al Acuerdo de Consejo de Ministros de 8 de febrero de 2008, por el que se establecen las condiciones a las que deberán adecuarse los planos de estudios conducentes a la obtención de títulos que habiliten para el ejercicio de la profesión regulada de Dentista [Resolution of 14 February 2008, Secretary of State for Universities and Research, which publicises the Council of Ministers Agreement of 8 February 2008, laying down the conditions which should suit the curricula leading to the award of a qualification of the regulated profession of dentist]. *Boletin Oficial del Estado* [*Official State Bulletin*], No. 50, 27 February 2008.

Ministry of Education and Science (2008c). Resolución de 14 de febrero de 2008, de la Secretaría de Estado de Universidades e Investigación, por la que se da publicidad al Acuerdo de Consejo de Ministros de 8 de febrero de 2008, por el que se establecen las condiciones a las que deberán adecuarse los planos de estudios conducentes a la obtención de títulos que habiliten para el ejercicio de la profesión regulada de Enfermería [Resolution of 14 February 2008, of the Secretary of State for Universities and Research, which publicises the Council of Ministers Agreement of 8 February 2008, laying down the conditions which should suit the curricula leading to the award of a qualification of the regulated profession of nursing]. *Boletin Oficial del Estado* [*Official State Bulletin*], No. 50, 27 February 2008.

Ministry of Education and Science (2008d). Resolución de 14 de febrero de 2008, de la Secretaría de Estado de Universidades e Investigación, por la que se da publicidad al Acuerdo de Consejo de Ministros de 8 de febrero de 2008, por el que se establecen las condiciones a las que deberán adecuarse los planos de estudios conducentes a la obtención de títulos que habiliten para el ejercicio de la profesión regulada de Farmacéutico [Resolution of 14 February 2008, Secretary of State for Universities and Research, which publicises the Council of Ministers Agreement of 8 February 2008, laying down the conditions which should suit the plans of study leading to the attainment of titles that qualify for the exercise of the regulated profession of pharmacist]. *Boletin Oficial del Estado* [*Official Bulletin of Spain*], No. 50, 27 February 2008.

Ministry of Education and Science (2009). *La homologación, convalidación y reconocimiento de estudios extranjeros, año 2007* [*The standardization, validation and recognition of foreign studies, 2007*]. Madrid (http://www.educacion.es/mecd/estadisticas/educativas/cee/2009/G3.pdf, accessed 17 February 2011).

Ministry of Health and Social Policy (2010). Real Decreto 459/2010, de 16 de abril, por el que se regulan las condiciones para el reconocimiento de efectos profesionales a títulos extranjeros de especialista en Ciencias de la Salud, obtenidos en Estados no miembros de la Unión Europea [Royal Decree 459/2010 of 16 April, regulating the conditions for professional recognition of foreign diploma in health science specialties, obtained in non-EU Member States. *Oficial del Estado* [*Official State Bulletin*], No. 107, 3 May 2010 (www.boe.es/ boe/dias/2010/05/03/pdfs/BOE-A-2010-6960.pdf, accessed 8 February 2010).

Ministry of Science and Innovation (2006). *Estudio de la oferta, la demanda y la matrícula de nuevo ingreso en las universidades públicas y privadas* [*Study of the supply, demand and enrolment of new entrants to the public and private universities*]. Madrid (http://www.educacion.es/dctm/mepsyd/educacion/universidades/estadisticas-informes/informes/convocatoria-2006-2007/ofertademanda200607.pdf?documentId=0901e72b8004a994, accessed 18 February 2011).

Montero Y (2007). Contar con médicos extranjeros bien formados enriquece un país [Having well-trained foreign doctors enriches a country]. *ELPAIS.com*, 2 January 2007 (http://www.elpais.com/ articulo/pais/vasco/Contar/medicos/extranjeros/bien/formados/enriquece/pais/elpepuesppvs/20070102 elpvas2/Tes, accessed 13 January 2011).

OMC (2008). *La OMC acoge al grupo europeo de trabajo sobre reconocimiento seguro de profesionales sanitarios* [*The OMC welcomes the European working group on secure recognition of health professionals*]. Madrid, Organización Médical Colegial [Organization of Medical Colleges] Press Release, 10 April 2008 (http://www.acceso.com/display _release.html?id=44983, accessed 12 January 2011).

OMC (2009). Informe sobre homologación de títulos de Medicina obtenidos en países extracomunitarios [Report on approval of medical titles obtained in countries outside the EU]. Madrid, Organización Médical Colegial [Organization of Medical Colleges].

Ortún V et al. (2008). Determinantes de las retribuciones médicas [Determinants of physicians' compensation]. *Medicina Clinica (Barcelona)*, 131(5):180–183.

ParaInmigrantes.info (2008). Cataluña necesita médicos extranjeros [Catalonia needs foreign doctors]. *ParaInmigrantes.info*, 2 June 2008 (http://www.parainmigrantes.info/cataluna-necesita-medicos-extranjeros/, accessed 13 January 2011).

Periodista Digital (2008). Los médicos españoles abandonan Portugal con mejoras laborales [Spanish doctors leave Portugal with improvements in working conditions]. Periodista Digital, 19 June 2008 (http://blogs. periodistadigital. com/vidasaludable.php/2008/06/19/los-medicos-espanoles-abandonan-portugal, accessed 12 January 2011).

Pinilla J, González B (2009). Exploring changes in dental workforce, dental care utilisation and dental caries levels in Europe, 1990–2004. *International Dental Journal*, 59(2):87–95.

Policlínica Miramar (2007). *Sanidad afirma que en 2007 un total de 920 médicos extranjeros obtuvieron plaza MIR, casi el doble que hace dos años.* [*Department of Health reports a total of 920 foreign doctors with MIR places, nearly twice the number of two years before*]. Palma de Mallorca (http://www.policlinicamiramar.

com/noticias.asp?tipo=INT&idioma=ES&noticia =19, accessed 22 February 2011).

Tribunalatina.com (2008). La Generalitat podrá contratar médicos extranjeros con el título pendiente de homologar [The Generalitat may hire foreign doctors with the title approved pending]. *Tribunalatina.com*, 3 June 2008 (http://www.tribunalatina.com/es/notices/lageneralitat_podra_contratar_ medicosextranjeros_con_el_titulo_pendiente_de_homologar_11801.php, accessed 13 January 2011).

Annex

Definitions

Foreign health professionals

Within this study, foreign is used differently in different contexts but refers to nationality unless otherwise stated.

In the tables compiled from the EAPS, foreign includes both foreign nationals and those with dual Spanish and foreign citizenship.

The National Immigrant Survey (NIS) (2007) uses foreign to mean immigrant –anyone born outside Spain who, at the time of the survey, was 16 years or over and had been residing in Spain for more than one year or had the intention to do so.

Source country/destination country

The NIS 2007 groups countries of origin in five zones (Table 7.12). For the EAPS data, this study has classified nationality by the country of origin (although this does not necessarily coincide with the country of birth) and countries have been grouped in the same five zones used in Table 7.12.

Table 7.12 *Country zones used with EAPS microdata*

EU-27 and developed countries	EU-15 + EEA + Switzerland + Japan + Republic of Korea + United States of America + Canada + Australia + New Zealand.
Andean countries	Colombia, Ecuador, Peru, Bolivia
Rest of Latin America	Rest of Latin America
Africa	Africa
Rest of Europe and the world	Rest of Europe and the world

Classification of health professionals

A classification problem arises because the EAPS and the NIS use the National Classification of Occupations (CNO-94) which includes doctors and dentists in the same category (no. 214). Other sources (professional councils, Ministry of Health) provide data that allows licensing and registration figures to be shown separately for doctors and for dentists. Figures that are not statistically

Table 7.13 *Main data sources for stock and flows of health professionals in Spain*

	Primary source	Observations and links
Licensing	Ministry of Education and Ministry of Health registers of degrees. Homologation and recognition of foreign degrees	Ministry of Education. Subsecretariat of the Ministry of Education, Social Policy and Sports (Office of Degrees, Validations and Homologations) (http://www.educacion.es/educacion/universidades/educacion-superior-universitaria/titulos/homologacion-titulos.html)
	Ministry of Health. Specialist residency competitions	Microdata database provided by the Ministry of Health (unpublished)
Registration	Official councils of medical doctors, dentists, nurses and pharmacists	Annual census (31 December) (http://www.ine.es/inebmenu/mnu_salud.htm)
		Data on intention to migrate. Requests to the Councils for certification (unpublished)
		Limitations: In some autonomous communities, registration is not obligatory for those working in the public health system but is compulsory for all in private practice)
		Almost all foreign national professionals register and this causes a positive bias in their percentages
		Most councils do not report their members' nationalities
Practising	EAPS (2004–2008)	Quarterly
		Microdata broken down specifically for this case study (http://www.ine.es/jaxi/menu.do?type=pcaxis&path=%2Ft22%2Fe308_mnu&file=inebase&L=1)
	NIS 2007	Microdata broken down specifically for this case study (INE 2009)
	Employment data from the autonomous communities' regional health services	No public registers record nationality or place where title was obtained. Some autonomous communities report information on foreign health professionals
	Health professional recruitment agencies	Private sources. Available on the Internet and through personal contacts
	Professional associations	APSEP; Association of Doctors from Outside the EU (ASOMEX)

significant are omitted from the tables based on the EAPS and the NIS. Neither survey has information on medical specialties. The data in the tables were calculated with survey weights and so are estimates for the total population. The EAPS and the NIS both have a very small sample size when broken down by profession. This is a serious limitation that causes the numbers to vary considerably from year to year.

Table 7.14 *Application requirements for MIR candidates*

- Applicants must be Spanish or a national of an EU country, Switzerland or Andorra.
- Applicants who are nationals of non-EU countries may also participate in the selection exams following the rules below, documenting their membership in one or another group.

	1) Spouse or offspring of nationals of an EU country, Switzerland or Andorra[a]	2) Holds valid residence permit/work and residence permit at date of application	3) Holds study permit at date of application	4) Other
Doctors	Yes	Yes	Yes	Yes[b]
Pharmacists	Yes	Yes	Yes	Yes[b]
Chemists	Yes	Yes	Yes	No
Biologists	Yes	Yes	Yes	No
Psychologists	Yes	Yes	Yes	No
Radiologists	Yes	Yes	Yes	No
Nursing specialties	Yes	Yes	Yes	Yes[b]
Submits sworn declaration for foreigners	No	No	No	Yes
Subject to quotas	No	No	No	Yes[c]

[a] Must be confirmed with an authenticated photocopy of the ID card of the EU-resident relative.
[b] Applicant's native country must have an ongoing agreement for cultural cooperation with Spain.
[c] Maximum quotas for these applicants: 657 doctors, 12 pharmacists and 11 for nursing specialties.

Source: Government of Spain 2005.

Fig. 7.3 *Age-sex pyramids of professionals registered in Spain, 31 December 2009*

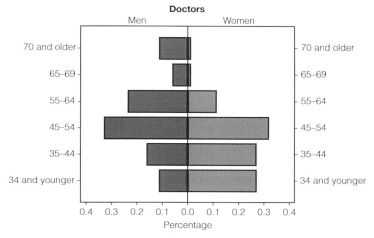

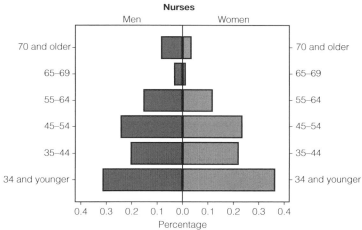

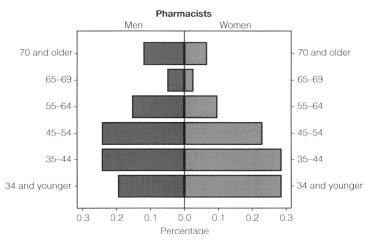

Source: INE 2009.

Chapter 8

A major destination country: the United Kingdom and its changing recruitment policies

Ruth Young

1. Introduction

The United Kingdom's history as a destination country for health professionals began in the 1950s. In areas such as hospital medicine, the National Health Service (NHS) has consistently depended on immigrants (Kelly et al. 2005, Raghuram & Kofman 2002, Smith 1980). In specialties such as nursing and general practice, the reliance has fluctuated with domestic shortages (Aiken & Buchan 2004, Buchan & O'May 1999, Taylor & Esmail 1999). Today, more than a third of medical doctors and every tenth nurse registered in the United Kingdom are internationally trained; the main source countries are India, Pakistan, Nigeria and South Africa as well as Australia and New Zealand. Such trends indicate how old colonial ties influence migration patterns and the importance of English as common language. The numbers of health professionals leaving the United Kingdom appear to be significantly lower than inflows but data on outflows are scarce.

The British government began a policy of massive NHS workforce expansion across all health professions in the late 1990s (Department of Health 2000a). This instigated a period of active international recruitment on an unprecedented scale (Bellingham 2001, Buchan 2004). At the same time many immigrant health professionals were recruited into private sector hospitals, nursing homes and social care (Smith et al. 2006). The policy of active international recruitment was reversed in 2006 and more restrictive immigration rules were introduced as earlier expansion in United Kingdom training numbers came on stream. These changing policy attitudes are a key element of this case study.

The other aspect of the United Kingdom's story is the increasingly complex picture of migration patterns. The majority of internationally qualified health professionals still come from outside the European region but European Union (EU) enlargement in 2004 and 2007 provided a new migration source, particularly from Poland, Romania and Bulgaria. Migration patterns have therefore shifted towards relatively more significant flows from the EU.

This case study will first assess the scale of health professional mobility in the United Kingdom and how the 2004 and 2007 EU enlargements affected the composition of the foreign workforce. This will be followed by a discussion of how migration impacts on the British health system and the relevance of health professional mobility vis-à-vis other domestic workforce issues. The personal factors that activate, instigate or mitigate health professional flows will then be outlined in order to provide an individual's perspective. Finally, recent United Kingdom policies on the health workforce and current workforce planning practice will be set in context, with particular emphasis on policy developments over time and how such changes impact on migration patterns.

Limitations of the study

A wide range of United Kingdom data sources contain information on health professional migration. These provide a good overview of the country's mobility profile but there are key shortcomings (Table 8.1). It is difficult to assess the number of health professionals leaving or returning to the United Kingdom; numbers working in sectors outside the NHS; and workforce activity as opposed to professional registration. It is hard to obtain longitudinal data and comparable data across professions (EMN 2006, Pollard et al. 2008). Most data cover the entire United Kingdom but certain sources deal separately with England, Scotland, Wales and Northern Ireland. As a general rule the most data are available for medical doctors, then for nurses/midwives and for dentists. Published data on allied health professionals and pharmacists are more limited. Until now, there has been less interest on intra-EU mobility to and from the United Kingdom and this may explain why health professional migration from outside Europe has been researched more extensively. The remainder of the chapter draws on the most comprehensive nationwide data sources in the United Kingdom – registration and work permit data.

Table 8.1 *Data sources on mobility: coverage, availability and limitations*

Professional registration	Comprehensive information but has limitations.
	Lack of comparability across professions – the General Medical Council (GMC) and General Dental Council (GDC) provide all data by *country of qualification*; the Nursing and Midwifery Council (NMC) and Royal Pharmaceutical Society of Great Britain (RPSGB) use both *country of qualification* (inflows) and domicile (stocks). NMC data prior to 2004 record only European Economic Area (EEA), not individual, countries. RPSGB data cover England, Scotland and Wales only. Northern Ireland (part of the United Kingdom but not of Great Britain) registers pharmacists separately.
	Lack of longitudinal data – the GMC has held the specialist and general practice medical registers since only 1997 and 2006 respectively. The NMC and the Health Professions Council (HPC) (latter registers allied health professionals) were not set up until 2002 and 2004 respectively. There are some data from previous data holders but they are not computerized and, for allied health professionals, do not cover all groups or give country sources.
	Limited data on outflows – information relates to checks made by EEA/overseas regulators on an individual's intention to leave the United Kingdom rather than actual migration.
NHS workforce censuses	Public sector staffing numbers across all professional groups, grades and service areas – but country of qualification for medical doctors only. Separate organizations hold data for different parts of United Kingdom.
Immigration statistics	Work permit data include occupation of non-EEA applicants but only from 1998 until 2008 when a new system was introduced. After 2004 and 2007 a different worker registration scheme covered central and eastern Europe (CEE) countries joining the EU, but data on particular occupational groups are not published.
Labour Force Survey	Detailed occupation data at the level of individual health professions by country of birth and nationality – but only from 1992 (quarterly) and 1998 (annually) and with variable inconsistencies over the periods.
Population census	Information on occupation but little on migration. The 2001 census contains no information on respondents' domicile prior to one year before or the length of time resident in the United Kingdom. However, it is proposed that the 2011 census will contain more detailed migration questions.
Household Panel Survey	Information on occupation and country of origin when people arrived in United Kingdom but numbers in health professional employment are small given overall sample size. A new, larger survey (40 000 households) is being undertaken but results are not yet available.
International Passenger Survey	As there is no comprehensive registration of migration, estimates are drawn from this survey of principal air and sea routes and the Channel Tunnel. However, the survey does not cover all migration types, is completed voluntarily and highlights only generic occupation types.

2. Mobility profile of the United Kingdom

The United Kingdom health system has always been, and continues to be, largely reliant on immigrants. Foreign-trained medical doctors accounted for 36.8% among all registered medical doctors in 2008, around one quarter of whom came from the EEA and three quarters from the rest of the world. The share of foreign-trained nurses/midwives was smaller but still represented more than 12% of those registered (Tables 8.2 and 8.3). The main countries of origin lie outside Europe but the relatively small share of health professionals from the European region has increased in recent years.

2.1 *Overall stocks and inflows*

The United Kingdom's health system has always relied on immigrants. For instance, 57 575 of all registered medical doctors in 1988 had gained their primary qualification abroad (Table 8.2). However, the proportions of internationally qualified health professionals have risen even further in recent years – between 1988 and 2008 the numbers of medical doctors rose by more than 34 000, from 34.5% to 36.8% of those registered (Table 8.2). Similarly, new nursing registrants who had qualified abroad rose from just over 2808 (9.2%) in 1988 to 4099 (15.8%) in 2008 (Table 8.3).

All world regions are represented in the United Kingdom's mobility profile. Historical immigration sources such as Asia, Africa and Oceania remain numerically more significant but EEA numbers are growing (Tables 8.2 and 8.3). Equal numbers of new registrations from EEA and non-EEA sources have been recorded for the first time, following the 2006 policy/immigration changes. Overall, EEA-qualified medical doctors accounted for 6% of those registered in 1998, 7.6% in 2003 and 9% in 2008 – an increase of 5434 registered EEA doctors (Table 8.2). Numbers of EEA-qualified nurses/midwives rose by 1654 between 2003 and 2008 alone (Table 8.3).

Source countries

Historically, migration of internationally qualified health professionals was based on old colonial ties and on English as a common language. Such links are still reflected in the continuing predominance of India, Pakistan, Nigeria and South Africa in the United Kingdom's top ten source countries for medical doctors (Table 8.4). The same applies to nurses/midwives from Australia, New Zealand, South Africa, Nigeria, Zimbabwe and the West Indies (Table 8.5). However, there are some changes in overall health professional migration to the United Kingdom from such non-EU/EEA sources. For example, numbers of medical doctors from Australia and New Zealand and countries with former colonial links (such as Hong Kong) have fallen since the 1980s whereas the

Table 8.2 Total and newly registered medical doctors from United Kingdom, EEA and other world regions, 1988 and 2003–2008

Source – primary qualification	1988	2003	2004	2005	2006	2007	2008
Stock – total registered							
All sources	167 096[a]	222 923	231 140	239 287	240 363	244 590	247 638
United Kingdom (%)	108 593 (65.0)	142 847 (64.0)	144 407 (62.5)	146 964 (61.4)	149 048 (62.0)	153 293 (62.7)	156 574 (63.2)
EEA (%)	10 003 (6.0)	16 876 (7.6)	19 216 (8.3)	21 908 (9.2)	22 424 (9.3)	22 759 (9.3)	22 310 (9.0)
Rest of world (%)	47 572 (28.5)	63 199 (28.4)	67 516 (29.2)	70 415 (29.4)	68 891 (28.7)	68 538 (28.0)	68 754 (27.8)
Of which:							
EU-15	9 258	15 272	16 467	17 390	17 025	16 800	16 051
EU-12	707	1 446	2 554	4 288	5 175	5 727	6 029
Remaining EEA	23	123	149	188	188	196	195
Other Europe	202	810	1004	1 233	1 372	1 489	1 611
Asia	28 262	36 712	41 342	44 864	44 818	45 063	45 370
Africa	7 389	17 099	17 294	17 243	16 546	16 306	16 345
Oceania	10 307	6 489	5 780	4 950	4 100	3 670	3 402
Americas	1 410	2 094	2 106	2 125	2 055	2 015	2 021

Table 8.2 *contd*

Source – primary qualification	1988	2003	2004	2005	2006	2007	2008
Inflow – new registrants							
All sources	7 107	18 684	14 736	15 092	11 777	11 189	11 794
United Kingdom (%)	3 722 (52.4)	4 731 (25.3)	4 732 (32.1)	5 164 (34.2)	5 620 (47.7)	6 134 (54.8)	6 770 (57.4)
EEA (%)	800 (11.3)	1 956 (10.5)	3 674 (24.9)	4 103 (27.2)	2 994 (25.4)	2 446 (21.9)	2 181 (18.5)
Rest of world (%)	2 186 (30.8)	11 996 (64.2)	6 330 (43.0)	5 825 (38.6)	3 163 (26.9)	2 609 (23.3)	2 841 (24.1)
Of which:							
EU-15	759	1 732	2 437	2 249	1 703	1 364	1 166
EU-12	32	175	1 172	1 792	1 251	1 039	970
Remaining EEA	9	49	65	62	40	43	45
Other Europe	25	109	211	239	195	162	161
Asia	1 041	4 974	5 366	4 670	2 232	1 706	1 705
Africa	599	3 707	590	665	457	530	706
Oceania	390	2 685	16	80	132	80	96
Americas	131	521	147	169	147	131	131

Source: GMC unpublished data 2009 *Note:* [a] There were 928 doctors with unspecified country of primary medical qualification in 1988

Table 8.3 Total and newly registered nurses/midwives from United Kingdom, EEA and other world regions, 1988 and 2003–2008

Source – nursing qualification	1988/1989	2003	2004	2005	2006	2007	2008
Stock– total registered							
All sources	nd	645 528	660 444	672 916	682 197	686 370	676 542
United Kingdom (%)	nd	583 809 (90.4)	586 771 (88.8)	590248 (87.7)	592 837 (86.9)	595 757 (86.8)	589 595 (87.1)
EEA (%)	nd	7 069 (1.1)	7 153 (1.1)	7 371 (1.1)	8 323 (1.2)	8 810 (1.3)	8 723 (1.3)
Rest of world (%)	nd	54 650 (8.5)	66 520 (10.1)	75 297 (11.2)	81 037 (11.8)	81 803 (11.9)	78 224 (11.6)
Inflow – new registrants							
All sources	30 675	31 696	34 522	33 203	31 342	27 641	25 336
United Kingdom (%)	27 867 (90.8)	18 212 (57.5)	19 457 (56.4)	20 584 (62.0)	20 946 (66.8)	21 380 (77.3)	21 612 (85.3)
EEA (%)	824 (2.7)	889 (2.8)	1 125 (3.3)	1 273 (3.8)	1 833 (5.8)	1 549 (5.6)	1 390 (5.5)
Rest of world (%)	1 984 (6.5)	12 595 (39.7)	13 940 (40.4)	11 346 (34.2)	8 563 (27.3)	4 712 (17.0)	2 334 (9.2)
Of which:							
EU-15	nd	782	1 007	923	940	558	437
EU-12	nd	84	87	305	848	958	932
Remaining EEA	nd	23	31	45	45	33	21
Other Europe	nd	48	44	15	15	14	8
Asia	nd	7 872	7 860	6 793	5 654	3 640	1 541
Africa	nd	3 156	3 761	2 709	1 503	632	399
Oceania	nd	1 222	1 676	1 273	967	376	329
Americas	nd	345	643	571	439	64	65
Others – unspecified	nd	13	31	45	49	39	63

Source: NMC unpublished data 2009; UKCC 1989. *Notes:* Data are as at 31 March each year (nd indicates no data). It is not possible to break down numbers registered (stocks) for the EU-15, EU-12 and other world regions. New registrations (inflow) specifically for 1988 are also not available by world region. However, a detailed breakdown of applications to be entered in the register for 1988/1989 is available: of the 3531 applications from abroad, 865 (24.5%) were from Africa, 1390 (39.4%) from Oceania (Australia and New Zealand), 125 (3.5%) from the United States and 839 (23.8%) from other countries (in the EEA or elsewhere). Ireland accounted for 312 (8.9%) of all applications from abroad and by far the largest proportion of applications from the EEA.

numbers from India have substantially increased (Table 8.4). Major source countries for nurses are India and the Philippines (Table 8.5). All these trends are reinforced by evidence from work permit data, the other main source of information on individual source countries (Table 8.6).

With the exception of Ireland, EU-15 countries were not particularly significant migration sources for the United Kingdom (Brazier et al. 1992, Buchan & Maynard 2006, Buchan & Rafferty 2004). However, recent international recruitment has made the EU-15 relatively more important. In addition to negotiating access outside Europe, the British government also signed recruitment agreements targeting (for instance) general practitioners, nurses and pharmacists in Spain; nurses in Greece; nurses and general practitioners in Germany; hospital doctors and general practitioners in Italy and Austria; and general practitioners in France. Scandinavian countries were the other main sources targeted. Such policies are clearly reflected in the country-level rankings of total new registrations between 2003 and 2008 (Tables 8.4 and 8.5).[1] Overall, Germany is now the most significant EU-15 source country with 3201 more medical doctors registered in 2008 than in 1988 (Table 8.4) and new nurse/midwife registrants between 2003 and 2008 (Table 8.5). Ireland remains a major migration source but numbers are declining (see Table 8.4 for medical doctors; Young et al. 2010 for other professional groups).

2.2 Outflows

There is little quantitative information about outflows of health professionals from the United Kingdom. Data on verifications of qualifications are available but can only approximate the number of health professionals leaving the United Kingdom as they show intention to leave rather than actual outflows. United Kingdom regulators for nurses/midwives and for medical doctors issue ten times more verifications for Ireland than for any other EU country, indicating that this is the main destination within Europe The next most significant European destinations are Spain and France (Tables 8.7 and 8.8).

Outside Europe, Australia is the main destination country for both nurses and medical doctors; other major destinations are New Zealand, the United States, Canada and the Middle East. Several African countries are also destinations for medical doctors. It is not known how much of this overall movement is due to emigrating United Kingdom nationals or to foreign-qualified professionals returning home or moving onto a third country for which the United Kingdom

---

1 In addition, Spain had the largest total of new registrant pharmacists (974) and Sweden had the largest total of new registrant dentists (830) from individual EU countries between 2003 and 2008 (RPSGB and GDC unpublished data 2009).

Table 8.4 *Medical doctors from EEA and other international source countries on the GMC Medical Register: total new registrants 2003–2008 and change in numbers registered 1988–2003*

Country of primary medical qualification[a]	Countries ranked by total new registrants 2003–2008	Numerical change on register +/ - 1988–2008
EU-15		
Germany	3 064	+3 201
Italy	1 692	+1 354
Greece	1 960	+1 273
Ireland	857	-1 963[b]
Spain	620	+906
Netherlands	374	+439
France	583	+418
Sweden	402	+382
Belgium	411	+265
Austria	360	+262
Denmark	152	+121
Portugal	112	+80
Finland	64	+55
EU-12		
Poland	2 336	+1 750
Hungary	1 141	+965
Romania	671	+742
Czech Republic	782	+669
Bulgaria	338	+376
Slovakia	381	+314
Lithuania	293	+206
Malta	244	+134
Latvia	126	+106
Estonia	61	+44
Slovenia	26	+16
Other EEA		
Switzerland	217	+120
Norway	54	+52
Iceland	33	+20
Other Europe		
Russian Federation	436	+578
Ukraine	282	+320
Serbia	104	+158
Turkey	114	+132
Others (6 countries)	141	+221
Rest of world[c]		
Six most increasing sources:		
India	12 007	+11 165
Pakistan	4 041	+5 169
South Africa	3350	+2 226
Nigeria	1409	+2 948
Iraq	724	+1 575
Egypt	709	+1 638
Three most declining sources:		
Australia	2 431	-5 523
New Zealand	657	-1 386
Hong Kong	529	-1 224
Other (106) countries in Middle East, south and east Asia, Americas, West Indies, Pacific Islands etc.	5 971	+3 406

Source: GMC unpublished data 2009. *Notes*: [a] 928 doctors with unspecified country of primary medical qualification in 1988, [b] Total numbers registered grew between 1988 and 2008 for all EEA countries; Ireland was the exception – numbers declined by 1963. [c] Countries for which total numbers registered increased or declined by >1000 between 1988 and 2008.

Table 8.5 *Nurses/midwives from EEA and other international source countries: total new registrants on NMC register, 2003–2008*

Country of qualification	Countries ranked by total new registrants 2003–2008 [a]
EU-15	
Spain	1 091
Germany	1 000
Ireland	750
Italy	346
Finland	303
Sweden	255
Netherlands	158
France	156
Denmark	152
Austria	135
Portugal	116
Greece	106
Belgium	76
Luxembourg	3
EU-12	
Poland	1 561
Romania	493
Bulgaria	227
Slovakia [b]	208
Czech Republic [b]	194
Lithuania	173
Hungary	159
Malta	68
Latvia	40
Estonia	29
Cyprus	25
Slovenia	3
Other EEA	
Norway	99
Switzerland	77
Iceland	22
Rest of world	
Top ten countries	
India	15 595
Philippines	14 923
Australia	4 544
South Africa	4 431
Nigeria	2 278
Zimbabwe	1 488
New Zealand	1 270
Ghana	1 135
Pakistan	909
Zambia	678
Other (96) countries in Middle East, south and east Asia, Americas, West Indies, Pacific Islands etc.	6 239

Source: NMC unpublished data 2009. *Notes*: [a] Overall, lack of data makes it impossible to illustrate long-term numerical changes in totals registered from different countries. [b] An additional 40 nurses recorded as registered from Czechoslovakia (i.e. the data do not differentiate between the Czech Republic or Slovakia in these cases) between 2003 and 2006.

Table 8.6 *Cleared, individual work permit applications for health professional groups – by world region and main countries, 2003–2008*

Application source	Total work permits issued 2003–2008				
	Medical doctors	Dentists	Nurses	Midwives	Pharmacists
EU/EEA (joined 2004–2007)	262	30	795	9	69
Of which:					
Romania	125	6	315	0	47
Bulgaria	66	4	250	7	12
Poland	21	16	80	0	0
Others (9 countries)	50	4	150	2	10
Other Europe	195	20	189	10	72
Of which:					
Russian Federation	48	4	14	0	4
Serbia	44	4	21	0	28
Turkey	34	4	32	0	0
Ukraine	31	0	42	6	6
Others (8 countries)	38	8	80	4	34
Asia	16 454	649	71 985	83	1 995
Of which:					
India	9 662	412	33 845	10	785
Philippines	63	11	32 010	9	16
Other south Asia (3 countries)	3 100	32	2 885	2	226
Other east Asia (14 countries)	2 445	115	2 783	29	833
Others (26 countries)	1 184	79	462	33	135
Africa	5 013	800	40 757	388	1 882
Of which:					
South Africa	2 595	592	10 910	18	230
Zimbabwe	143	11	12 605	195	185
Nigeria	612	60	5 800	62	565
Others (37 countries)	1 663	137	11 442	113	902
Americas	752	80	4 296	86	130
Of which:					
United States	132	19	340	4	30
Canada	98	22	260	7	39
West Indies (14 countries)	361	25	2 509	71	30
Central Americas (7 countries)	51	0	57	2	2
South Americas (10 countries)	82	14	1 130	2	29
Oceania	626	135	2 750	50	431
Of which:					
Australia	498	94	1 985	32	245
New Zealand	128	41	725	16	180
Others (3 countries)	0	0	40	2	6

Source: UK Border Agency unpublished data 2009. *Notes*: (i) Figures provided were either rounded to the nearest 5 or made no distinction between 1 and 2 work permits issued by country. In the latter instance the figure 2 was assumed for purposes of this analysis. In addition, the figures do not equate to the number of individuals granted work permits as they include applications approved to extend or amend an existing work permit or for individuals moving to a different employer. Not all those who were granted work permits took up jobs and some may have been refused entry clearance or further leave to remain; (ii) "doctor" is an amalgamation of the following occupational categories: doctor, hospital consultant, medical practitioner, psychiatrist and, from 2006 onwards, foundation programme doctor, GP registrar, senior house officer and specialist registrar; (iii) "dentist" includes dental surgeons and assistant dentists; (iv) the work permit system no longer applied to EU-12 countries that joined the EU in 2004 and 2007, therefore EU-12 figures do not account for all mobility from those countries; (v) some permits were issued to overseas British nationals/citizens, stateless people etc (including 43 doctors, 13 dentists, 43 nurses and 109 pharmacists).

Table 8.7 *Verification applications from nurses/midwives considering work abroad – main European and other international destinations*

Destination country	2002/ 2003	2003/ 2004	2004/ 2005	2005/ 2006	2006/ 2007	2007/ 2008
Australia	2 602	2 708	3 296	3 047	4 764	5 581
United States	2 224	2 082	1 729	1 338	1 613	1 701
New Zealand	958	980	1 097	1 423	1 336	1 237
Canada	452	376	461	404	739	898
Saudi Arabia (United Arab Emirates in 2006/2007–2007/2008)	74	38	28	18	42	66
EEA total	1 622	1 294	1 284	nd[a]	nd	nd
Of which:						
Ireland	1 177	916	847	1 009	999	1 011
Spain	73	103	124	132	142	164
France	50	74	87	60	56	62
Other – worldwide	469	333	375	341	384	458
OVERALL TOTAL	**8 079**	**7 610**	**8 044**	**7 772**	**10 033**	**11 178**

Sources: NMC 2003, 2004, 2005a, 2006, 2007 & 2008. *Notes*: Table provides details of the number of verification checks made by regulators outside the United Kingdom for individuals on the NMC register. These statistics provide an indication of the numbers intending to practice abroad as it does not follow that all those who applied for verification went on to work in the countries concerned. In addition, a separate verification check is required for each application outside the United Kingdom – one nurse or midwife may make several applications. N.B. The NMC publishes this information only for the countries shown. No detailed data are available for 1988. However, the UKCC (1989) annual report noted that verification requests had "doubled since 1985, with the largest increase in applications to register and practice in Australia. [a] nd indicates no data.

is simply a stepping stone. It is suggested that this depends upon the destination (Ball & Pike 2004, Blitz 2005, Buchan 2003, Buchan & Seccombe 2006a, Hassell et al. 2008, NMC 2004, Petchey & Needle 2008, Young et al. 2003 & 2008).

Overall the United Kingdom can be characterized primarily as a destination country, with anecdotal evidence suggesting that it may also be a stepping-stone – particularly to the United States. Reliance on mobile health professionals from different sources differs across the professional groups (Table 8.6). For example, it appears that certain health professions (e.g. dentistry, midwifery, general practice) are proportionally more reliant on European migrants, especially following the 2006 introduction of restrictions on other sources (Young et al. 2010). Another key feature of the United Kingdom's mobility profile is the sheer range of countries and world regions from which health professionals migrate (Tables 8.4, 8.5 and 8.6). The *relative* increase in EU/EEA-qualified health professionals registered in the last ten years is also noteworthy although the numbers remain lower than for non-EEA sources.

Table 8.8 *Certificates of good standing (CGSs) issued for medical doctors to work abroad – main European and other international destinations, 2007–2009*

Destination country	Total November 2007–May 2009[a]
Australia	4 936
New Zealand	1 135
Canada	919
South Africa	234
United States	222
Singapore	207
Malaysia	135
United Arab Emirates	106
Other (50) countries in Africa, Middle East, east Asia, Americas, West Indies etc	576
EEA total	**1 350**
Of which:	
EU-15	
Ireland	786
Spain	86
France	53
Germany	43
Sweden	43
Netherlands	33
Greece	32
Belgium	22
Italy	21
Denmark	16
Portugal	12
Austria	5
EU-12	
Cyprus	38
Poland	27
Malta	20
Lithuania	4
Bulgaria	3
Czech Republic	3
Hungary	2
Other EEA	
Norway	21
Switzerland	10
OVERALL TOTAL	**9 820**

Source: GMC unpublished data 2009. *Note*: [a] 161 certificates were sent to unspecified countries between November 2007 and May 2009, the period in which the CGS system was in place. The GMC was unable to locate equivalent statistics for previous years.

3. Vignettes on health professional mobility

> ### *Contrasting experiences of Indian doctors in NHS hospitals*
>
> Postgraduate training has always been a key motivation for Indian doctors migrating to the United Kingdom. However, many like Dr M have experienced difficulties accessing their chosen specialty and/or a recognized training post. Without such a post (having a training number that affords specialist accreditation), doctors cannot climb the NHS career ladder to reach the higher grades such as hospital consultant (Grant et al. 2004). Commentators argue that this situation stems from discrimination within the system that has favoured United Kingdom-educated graduates (Esmail & Carnall 1993, Esmail & Everington 1997).*
>
> By contrast, Dr K was appointed via active international recruitment of Indian doctors and felt much more "valued" (Young et al. 2008). Consultants/senior specialists in shortage specialties were recruited via a dedicated International Fellowship Programme (IFP) launched in 2002 offering generous financial and practical (such as finding accommodation and children's schools) relocation support; continuing professional development (CPD) and other career opportunities (including professional network building, clinical research, teaching); and the prospect of remaining in the United Kingdom under normal NHS terms, if offered a substantive post by the recruiting, or another, Trust.
>
> * For nurses, see also Allan et al. 2004, Larsen 2007 and Smith et al. 2006.

> ### *Contrasting routes into nursing in the United Kingdom*
>
> A significant proportion of overseas nurses have struggled to find suitable jobs in the NHS. Ms W is typical of many, having moved from Poland and entered the independent nursing home sector – looking after older people and others in long-term care (Allan & Larsen 2003). There is consensus that nursing homes do not provide adaptation (required for NMC registration) and work experience of the quality offered in the NHS and the work is relatively lower paid. Another concern is (so-called) back door recruitment by which some nursing homes provide the required adaptation but no longer-term job prospects because it is assumed that nurses will move into the NHS when they achieve full registration (Buchan et al. 2008). Such nurses are generally left to deal with the practicalities of moving to the United Kingdom, finding jobs, establishing social networks and so on.
>
> By contrast, Mr P from the Philippines and his colleague Ms G from Spain are typical of nurses who responded to the NHS's dedicated international recruitment initiatives of 1998–2006. They had good employment prospects and received much more support. Trusts typically provided in-service support (including dedicated induction and ongoing training); some initial financial support for relocation; and pastoral support (such as meeting individuals at airports; arranging initial accommodation and bank accounts) in order to "get them started" in the United Kingdom (Young et al. 2008).

> ### General practitioners and dentists from Poland and other CEE countries
>
> Both general practice and dentistry have received recruits from CEE countries in recent years, particularly from Poland. Mr R is typical of many who entered full-time, permanent posts as part of an agreement between the British and Polish governments. Primarily recruited into previously underserved local areas they have provided much needed improvements in patient access to NHS services. However, working independently in communities (usually in a one-on-one relationship with patients) is a very different experience to that of internationally-recruited health professionals in other NHS organizations (Young et al. 2008).
>
> Another high-profile (though not fully quantified) phenomenon is the (so-called) Easyjet dentists and general practitioners from eastern Europe. They take advantage of EU regulations on free labour movement by maintaining their primary jobs in their home countries and using cheap airlines to fly into the United Kingdom to undertake locum work. This can be for short periods of a few weeks/months or even just weekends (Harding et al. 2005, Johnson 2005, Sears 2008). Such arrangements are possible because the British system requires general practitioners and dental practices to provide 24-hour emergency cover (evenings and weekends) but many subcontract this work to out-of-hours services employing doctors in a temporary/short-term capacity. There are therefore opportunities for individuals such as Mr S to supplement main (country-of-origin) incomes with additional earnings in the United Kingdom.

4. Dynamics of enlargement

The numbers of EU health professionals registered in the United Kingdom increased following the accession of the EU-12 – ten new Member States in 2004 and Bulgaria and Romania in 2007 (Home Office et al. 2006) (Tables 8.2 and 8.3). The EU-15 countries still account for most of the registered EEA health professionals but numbers from EU-12 countries are rapidly catching up. In 2008 alone the EU-15 and the EU-12 accounted for 1166 and 970 new registrant medical doctors respectively. Among newly registered nurses/midwives in 2008, 932 were from the EU-12 and just 437 from the EU-15.

It is expected that this trend will continue as numbers from non-EU countries fall following the 2006 abandonment of active international recruitment but EU residents continue to exercise their right to free movement (Young et al. 2010). By far the largest increases in numbers of EU-12 medical doctors and nurses/midwives have come from Poland,[2] the country most heavily targeted

2 Poland was also the most significant EU-12 source country for pharmacist and dentist migrants, accounting for 928 and 664 new registrants respectively in each of those professions between 2003/2007 and 2003/2008 (Source: RPSGB and GDC unpublished data 2009).

for international recruitment, but several other countries have been heavily represented. These include Hungary, the Czech Republic, Romania, Slovakia, Bulgaria and Lithuania (Tables 8.4 and 8.5).

Overall, it is impossible to separate out the precise effects of accession *per se* from the United Kingdom's targeted recruitment in certain countries. However, it is clear that the 2004 EU enlargement did provide a new migration source that the United Kingdom was quick to tap into. Even without active recruitment, the post-2007 increase in health professionals from Bulgaria and Romania is significant in relative terms (see also work permit data in Table 8.6) (Bach 2008, EMN 2006, Pollard et al. 2008). For doctors and, to some extent, nurses there are also other European sources outside the EU. These include the Russian Federation, Ukraine, Serbia and Turkey (Tables 8.4 and 8.6).

5. Impacts on the United Kingdom's health system

The benefits and challenges of health professional mobility are acknowledged but none has been systematically quantified and evidence on causal relationships cannot be given. Nevertheless, certain observations can be made. First, the United Kingdom's recent openness to mobility fulfilled its purpose of improving staff coverage rates. In turn this was perceived to have contributed to reductions in waiting times for NHS treatment (Young et al. 2008). Second, NHS organizations were able to make financial savings on agency fees for temporary staff and greater workforce stability also enabled increases in the United Kingdom's training capacity. For example, recruitment from Germany, Greece and Scandinavia helped free up supervisors' time to expand midwifery training in London and the south east (Young et al. 2008). More generally, mobility clearly has resource benefits for the British system because it reduces domestic spending on health professional education and postgraduate training (Young et al. 2008) – the United Kingdom has always educated fewer medical doctors than would be necessary without immigration (Bloor et al. 2005).

These service and resource benefits must be weighed against the potential challenges associated with mobility (Young et al. 2010). One challenge is the potential impact on practice caused by different cultural perceptions of professional roles. Across all professional groups from Europe and elsewhere there are (for instance) differing levels of autonomy, holistic versus task-oriented care delivery or multiprofessional team-working. Language skills and different styles of communication also impact on patient/carer experiences (Young et al. 2008). One major lesson of recent years is the high input required to support internationally qualified individuals to integrate effectively into the NHS, regardless of previous experience (Atherton & Mathie 2002, Ballard &

Laurence 2004, Dye & Gajewska 2001, Winkelmann-Gleed & Seeley 2005). Questions have also been raised about the "real equivalence" of training and experience and the related difficulties of ensuring service standards (Meikle 2009, Meikle & Connolly 2009).

Professional mobility influences system stewardship and financing by providing opportunities to improve United Kingdom service provision and, conversely, by the need to restrict the *potential* negative impacts of importing staff. While it is not relevant for overall system financing, the opportunity to capitalize on mobility has brought about more imaginative thinking – around service purchasing, for example. Specifically, whole clinical teams were imported from 2001 to 2005 to provide services that directly tackled long waiting lists (Department of Health 2002a, Moore 2002). In the context of stewardship, the United Kingdom has always called on international staff when workforce shortfalls and associated capacity problems in service provision are identified (Taylor & Esmail 1999). However, the potential negative impacts on migration source countries are also acknowledged (Mellor 2003).

Finally, there can be little doubt that deploying internationally qualified staff to expand capacity must have wider system impacts from follow-through benefits concerning population health, service responsiveness and improved patient access (Davis 2007, Leatherman & Sutherland 2008). One example is the reduction in inequalities in access achieved by facilitating NHS primary care (general practitioner and dental) in areas previously lacking such provision but again there is a lack of empirical research documenting such outcomes.

6. Relevance of cross-border health professional mobility

International mobility has undoubtedly had a major influence on health workforce supplies in the United Kingdom – both historically and in the particular policy circumstances of recent years. Alongside fluctuations in United Kingdom domestic training, the supply-side factor can affect NHS workforce supplies by many thousands – and on a much shorter timescale than it takes for domestic training numbers to feed through. For example, the most recent international recruitment saw 17 000 internationally qualified doctors enter the NHS workforce between 2001 and 2003 and the registration of 68 000 nurses between 2001 and 2006 (Hann et al. 2008). Another illustration of the potential pace of international recruitment's contribution is shown by the fact that only 53 Filipino nurses were registered in the United Kingdom in 1998, compared with 7235 at the height of the active recruitment drive in 2005. Thus, mobility and/or international recruitment has been an important workforce solution in absolute terms. Significantly, however, the various demographic and distributional challenges underpinning the United Kingdom's health workforce supply problems still remain. They have not been resolved by either international recruitment or by any of the other solutions to improve recruitment, retention and workforce deployment.[3]

Those other challenges influence the overall United Kingdom workforce supplies and have implications for different parts of the health workforce – i.e. certain professions, specialties and local/regional labour markets (Wanless 2002). One key issue is the ongoing trend of workforce ageing and increasing retirement rates set against inadequate recruitment to replenish workforce losses. These problems are known particularly to affect certain workforce groups such as general practitioners in underserved areas and district nurses (MAC 2009a, Taylor & Esmail 1999). A second challenge is the trend for part-time working, which stems from the changing workforce gender balance and the general need for both women and men to balance work with other aspects of their lives. This effectively means that more health professionals are required just to provide the same level of service (Young & Leese 1999; Young et al. 2001). Such demographic factors compound existing problems in the geographical areas and specialties that are already less attractive for new recruits because of the nature of the work, irregular hours, high living costs etc. (NHS Information Centre 2008).

In addition, the United Kingdom has experienced workforce challenges resulting from EU policies such as the Working Time Directive (WTD) (Department of Health 2010). The NHS has always relied heavily on junior doctors working extremely long hours in order to underpin service delivery. The WTD restriction to a 48-hour week has reduced their contribution to the workforce and required adjustments and redesign of roles and services in order for the NHS to comply with the changes (Mahon & Harris 2003). Yet problems remain (BMA 2009a, MAC 2009a, Reid 2009, Santry 2009, WRT 2009c & 2009d).

Mobility inflows are clearly seen to have most effect on the United Kingdom's health workforce; there have been few expressions of concern about outflows of qualified staff, whether domestic or international. However, there is growing interest in the potential implications of EU students' entitlement to apply for

---

3 Other measures to address supply-side numerical challenges for the United Kingdom's health workforce have included the expansion of professional education and training to increase domestic recruitment and various initiatives to encourage the retention and return of mid-career health professionals and potential retirees. The latter include measures such as pay improvements, flexible working and childcare provision. In addition, role redesign and skill-mix changes have been designed to ensure better deployment of the existing workforce by sharing overall task bundles more effectively within and between different professionals and other staff (Bach 2008, Department of Health 2000b, Mahon & Harris 2003, NHS Modernisation Agency 2003).

undergraduate and postgraduate places. This may affect workforce planning and the future capacity of the permanent NHS workforce since many do not remain in the United Kingdom beyond their initial training (Goldbart et al. 2005, Pitts et al 1998, Winyard 2007).

Mobility within the United Kingdom has also gained significance following political devolution. On the one hand it appears that England (particularly the south east) benefits most from internal migration/circulation and that Scotland, for instance, is a net exporter (BBC 2008, Waite et al. 1990). On the other hand, a study of the employment location of nurses three years post-qualification indicated that London and south-east England tend to lose nurses to the north and north west (NNRU 2007). Again, there is a lack of clear, quantified data on which to base health workforce-related policy decisions within the devolved administrations (Buchan 2004).

Policy-makers in the United Kingdom have largely used mobility as an approach to influence numbers in the health workforce in absolute terms. Unlike countries such as Australia and the United States, it has not channelled migrants specifically to address geographical maldistribution (Young et al. 2003). While important, to date mobility has been more significant as a solution to workforce supply problems generated as a result of demographic and distributional challenges within the United Kingdom. The supply-side challenges caused by mobility – outflows rather than inflows – have been less relevant in the United Kingdom context. However, this situation may well change due to the increasing contribution of EU/EEA health professionals and the fact that there is less control over this migration than over migration from non-EEA sources.

7. Factors influencing health professional mobility

It is not possible to identify a single factor influencing foreign health professionals seeking employment in the United Kingdom, nor can particular professional groups or source countries be categorized easily. Nevertheless, certain points about the drivers and constraints to health professional migration can be determined from the literature. The macro-, meso- and micro-level factors summarized in Table 8.9 are seen to have overall relevance.

Table 8.9 *Factors attracting health professionals to the United Kingdom*

Macro-level drivers – national economic and sociopolitical factors that exert influence across all international labour markets and also affect the health system dynamics relevant to health professionals

Economic	• prospect of generally improved standard of living for self/family
	• means to send remittance income to country of origin
Health system	• un/underemployment amongst health professionals in home country
	• poor salaries and working conditions generally in health sector in home country
Political	• political instability in home country versus stability in United Kingdom

Meso-level drivers – profession-specific factors (education/training, job conditions etc) that frame perceived opportunities in a given occupational sector

Progression opportunities	• shortage of postgraduate training opportunities and/or posts in particular specialty/profession in home country
Additional skills/ experience	• chance to experience work in different system rather than learning from theory
	• learn to use state-of-the-art equipment and generally broaden knowledge
Career development	• professional challenge associated, for instance, with different ways of working
	• reputation and status of the British system, specific organization or particular clinical field
	• opportunity for involvement in cross-cultural research and/or general networking

Micro-level drivers – individual circumstances and attitudes through which macro- and meso-level drivers are viewed but which also influence migration decision-making in their own right

Family/social network	• perceived better quality of life for family
	• desire to give children quality education and cultural experience
	• partner's decision to work in the United Kingdom
	• choices possible within context of social/migrant networks in United Kingdom
Personal fulfilment	• desire for a life change; excitement; a break from predictable pathway
	• career stage – taking opportunities at particular point
	• experience different culture; looking for opportunities to travel; restlessness
	• United Kingdom provides gateway to Europe and/or adds to other overseas experience
Language skills	• desire to improve own/ family's/children's English language proficiency
	• English first language so easier to work in United Kingdom /Anglophone country

Opportunity window – one-off opportunity provided by the United Kingdom's policy of active international recruitment (a step-jump in mobility but for a limited period)

United Kingdom policy	• response to positive recruitment strategy from British government and Department of Health
Recruitment incentives	• perception of United Kingdom in international marketplace – barriers to/ ease of entry, nature of support at recruitment and settling-in stages
Migration stepping stone	• work in United Kingdom attractive as potential stage in migration, primarily to the United States

Sources: Young et al. 2008 & 2010 (see Bach 2007, Buchan & Rafferty 2004 for similar categorizations).

Overall, the most important instigating factors for migration to the United Kingdom are the potential economic and professional/career development opportunities in comparison to source countries. This applies to differing degrees to individuals from developing and CEE countries and to richer countries such as the EU-15 (Hassell 2003, Larsen et al. 2005, Pollard et al. 2008, Young et al. 2003 & 2008). The interaction of economic and family circumstances also appears to be important – whether the need to generate remittances to pay for children's schooling in the country of origin or the perception that the family will have a better life in the United Kingdom (Daniel et al. 2001, Winkelmann-Gleed 2006, Young et al. 2008). The general political situation is another macro-level factor considered to be driving migration, from countries neighbouring the EU such as Ukraine, Georgia and various states of the former Yugoslavia, for example (Young et al. 2010).

The main activating and facilitating factor of recent years has been the international recruitment policy and its associated incentives to move to the United Kingdom (see section 8). These included financial relocation packages, language training and outside-work/pastoral support. This policy led to massive increases in the numbers of health professionals moving to the United Kingdom and opened up new migration sources. It seems unlikely, for instance, that NHS organizations would have targeted the Philippines and European countries (such as Spain, Germany, Poland) on such a large scale without government-to-government agreements and the national department of health recruitment schemes (Young et al. 2008).

Whether from within Europe, or from outside, mobility has always been facilitated by linguistic and cultural ties and by shared traditions in educational curricula and professional practice (Buchan 2006, Pitts et al. 1998, Young et al. 2003). The use of English as a universal language is a related facilitating factor that attracts migrants to the United Kingdom as they consider that their relevant language skills will enable them to slot into the British system more quickly and more easily. Conversely, from the United Kingdom perspective, an individual's language skills are seen as a key mitigating factor working against successful migration and integration. Similarly, potential migrants are seen to be discouraged by intercountry differences in professional cultures, working methods and the task content of specific roles. These include differences in the scope of practice, levels of professional autonomy, experience of multidisciplinary team-working and interaction with patients (Bola et al. 2003, Buchan & Seccombe 2004, Close 2002, Grant et al. 2004, Magnusdotir 2005, Sales 2002). These are entirely separate considerations from mutual recognition of qualifications (Young et al. 2010).[4]

---

4 See also Ballard et al. 2004, Buth et al. 2000, Cashman & Slovak 2005, Cowan 2005 & 2006, Gerrish & Griffith 2004, Grisold et al. 2007, Mathie 2002, McKendrick 2005, O'Dowd 2003, Palese et al. 2006, Petchey & Needle 2007, Porter &

Many of the factors discussed (Table 8.9) are also relevant to outmigration from the United Kingdom. For example, personal incentives related to professional development and perceived improvements in the quality of life are seen as key activating factors for British-qualified staff (Young et al. 2010). In addition, active recruitment by countries such as Australia and the United States attracts both home- and internationally qualified staff away from the United Kingdom (Buchan 2003, Finch et al. 2009, NMC 2004, Travis 2009). Finally, language and practice differences are seen as key constraints (mitigating factors) on outmigration.

8. Policy, regulation and interventions

Several distinct policies on migration and the recruitment of internationally qualified health professionals have been in place in the United Kingdom, most recently moving from active recruitment policies to a more restrictive approach.

8.1 *Policies and policy development on health professional mobility*

Policy relating to mobility first became an issue in the 1950s and 1960s. Since that time it has always been set in response to the changing domestic workforce situation and/or related lobbying by professional groups with perceived shortages (Aiken & Buchan 2004, Buchan & Rafferty 2004, Department of Health 2002a, Goodman 2005, Kelly et al. 2005, Raguhuranm & Kofman 2002). Three distinct policy periods can be identified in the last decade (Table 8.10):

- 1998–2006: openness to mobility

- 2006–2008: restrictions introduced

- November 2008 onwards: further tightening of immigration.

In the 1998–2006 period, policy centred on the government's ambitious plan of NHS investment and related workforce expansion targets. Increased domestic training capacity alone was not sufficient for the timescale required (Department of Health 2000a). This led to the United Kingdom's high-profile recruitment policy and its openness to immigration across the major health professions (Table 8.10). At a time of economic growth, this also led the United Kingdom to open up to immigrating health and other workers from the ten countries which joined the EU in 2004. Specifically, the United Kingdom imposed no restrictions on immigrants from Malta and Cyprus and only required citizens of the CEE countries in the EU-10 to register under a worker registration scheme. Individuals who worked legally for 12 months with no more than 30 days break could obtain a residence permit confirming their right (alongside other EEA citizens) to live and work in the United Kingdom. This policy contrasted markedly with the more restrictive transition arrangements in the majority of EU-15 countries (MAC 2009b).

In 2006, policy-makers recognized that the United Kingdom's training expansion was coming on stream. International recruitment became an option to fill a far more restrictive set of vacancies, NHS organizations were no longer able to access national-level recruitment programmes and immigration rules for non-EEA health professionals were tightened. Employer organizations were required to recruit from resident workers (and EEA nationals) before looking to other candidates and several health professional categories were removed from the shortage occupation list (official list of occupations with acute shortages of suitably qualified and skilled workers within the resident labour market) (Table 8.10). Also, the 2007 accession countries faced slightly more restrictive arrangements than those for the EU-10. For example, Bulgarian and Romanian nationals were required to be able to support themselves and their families without the help of public funds (i.e. social security benefits) and had to apply to the UK Border Agency for prior permission to work. However, individuals who work legally as an employee for 12 months without a break are granted full rights of free movement (MAC 2008).

The latest changes were introduced in 2008/2009 within the context of the "biggest shake up of the [United Kingdom] immigration scheme for 45 years" (NHS Employers 2008). These changes streamlined the employment categories that afford eligibility for immigration (from 80 routes into 5 tiers) within a new points-based system. The shortage occupation list was tightened further (Table 8.10) and is now reviewed every six months. In addition, employing organizations require a sponsorship licence to recruit skilled/temporary migrants such as health professionals wishing to take up short-term clinical attachments (MAC 2009a). The current view is: "… an NHS Trust is unlikely to go through the time consuming and expensive process of international recruitment if they cannot fill posts in the United Kingdom. International recruitment is normally only considered as an option when all domestic recruitment opportunities have been exhausted, including using return to practice or recruiting UK-based qualified refugees" (NHS Employers 2009).

Table 8.10 *Timeline of immigration and mobility policy for health professionals**

1. 1998–2006: openness to mobility	2. 2006–2008: restrictions introduced	3. From November 2008: further tightening of immigration
During this period **qualified** health professionals from the EU and elsewhere were actively recruited under the auspices of bilateral agreements. Those targeted included medical doctors (general practitioners and senior hospital doctors in shortage specialties); nurses (entry bands 5/6 to more senior bands 7/8 across all specialties); dentists; pharmacists; and allied health professionals Countries targeted included India, the Philippines, Spain, Germany, Austria, Italy and Poland. Midwives were not targeted nationally but local Trusts recruited in Germany, Scandinavia and Greece. Trusts targeted other countries including Australia and New Zealand. United Kingdom also opened up to health professionals from the EU-10 and non-EEA migrants (e.g. junior doctors) were free to work or train in the United Kingdom.	**Medical doctors and dentists** from outside the EEA now required to meet the requirements of an employment category of the Immigration Rules (e.g. work permit provisions). Access to postgraduate training restricted for non-EEA nationals unless they had trained at United Kingdom medical schools. Senior **nursing** positions and shortage specialties remained on the shortage occupation list but entry grades were removed to ensure that United Kingdom resident nurses could fill NHS posts. NHS organizations required to advertise vacancies first and only turn to international recruitment if this failed. Non-EEA **midwives** continued to need a job offer in order to qualify under the overseas nurses and midwives immigration category.	**Shortage occupation list** – only restricted specialties and grades of **medical doctors, dentists, nurses and pharmacists** remain on the list. **Midwives** are not included because "overseas recruitment is not [seen as] a sensible mechanism for alleviating shortages" – due to the particular (autonomous) nature of United Kingdom practice (MAC 2009a). **Other categories:** • Non-EEA medical doctors applying for **specialty training** are now subject to the resident labour market test (i.e. employers must show that they cannot fill posts from United Kingdom/EEA candidates) (Department of Health 2008a). • Non-EEA nurses can enter United Kingdom as a **sponsored skilled worker** only if they have a job offer from a licensed NHS sponsor. • Doctors undertaking United Kingdom's medical equivalence exam or clinical attachment and dental observer posts are **business and special visitors** – granted United Kingdom entry for only six weeks at a time, up to six months maximum.

* Compiled from:
http://www.nhscareers.nhs.uk, accessed 3 April 2007.
http://www.nursinguk.nhs.uk/index.asp, accessed 22 November 2005.
http://www/nhsemployers.org/RecruitmentAndRetention/InternationalRecruitment/Specific-guidance, accessed 22 May 2009.
http://www.ukba/homeoffice.gov.uk/workingintheuk/, accessed 22 May 2009.

8.2 *Workforce planning and development*

Historically, most workforce planning has concerned medical doctors and other professions were underserved by comparison (Buchan 2004). Even so, the contribution of internationally qualified medical doctors was not factored in adequately (Bloor & Maynard 2003, Bloor et al. 2005). Planning models focussed on quotas for undergraduate education and postgraduate specialist and general practitioner training with the aim of achieving appropriate throughput to allow the required numbers onto the career ladder in different service/specialty areas. Thus, the thousands of overseas doctors in NHS posts who lacked the postgraduate training accreditation necessary to achieve promotion were overlooked. Some would argue that they were regarded as a dispensable resource supplementary to the main medical workforce (Esmail & Everington 1997, Grant et al. 2004).[5]

In addition, workforce planning has not eliminated cyclical shortages/surpluses and the recruitment/retention problems of less popular specialties and geographical areas. As a national service with national pay scales, the NHS has no other market mechanisms to encourage redistribution (Bloor et al. 2005, Buchan & Seccombe 2004 & 2006b, Hall 2005). Planning also took little account of the need to pace international recruitment and reduce it in line with the increases in United Kingdom training numbers that began to feed into the system in 2006 (Health Committee 2007, Young et al. 2008). Coinciding with NHS budget cuts, this resulted in high unemployment among nurses, medical doctors and allied health professionals who had qualified in the United Kingdom. In turn, this triggered the rapid policy reversal on mobility (Table 8.10) that caused significant uncertainty amongst affected groups (Casciani 2006a & 2006b).

Such shortcomings have been recognized (Curson et al. 2008, Darzi 2008) and planning is moving from a national system based on supply-side inputs to one in which the commissioning of education/training is employer-driven, based on demand-side needs identified locally (Department of Health 2008b & 2008c, Health Committee 2007). At the time of writing, it is planned that such local signals will integrate into regional plans that in turn will feed into national workforce needs assessment. A centre of excellence for workforce planning has also been established to provide intelligence and develop planning capacity at all levels.

Nationally, all the health professions have come under the auspices of the Workforce Review Team (WRT). This is responsible for identifying development priorities for the different professions; their constituent specialties; and wider,

---

5 For nurses see also Allan et al. 2004, Smith et al. 2006.

cross-professional service areas such as cancer, diabetes, accident and emergency and mental health. The latter approach is increasingly necessary as professional boundaries are blurring within multidisciplinary teams (for example see WRT 2008a & 2008b). Together with both NHS Employers and Skills for Health, the WRT provides annual evidence to the Home Office's Migration Advisory Committee (MAC) that reviews the shortage occupation list. This arrangement enables far clearer links between health professional mobility and NHS workforce analysis and planning (see for example WRT 2009c, 2009e, 2009f, 2009g, 2009h & 2009i). It also allows for the needs of the individual countries within the United Kingdom (such as Scotland) to be assessed separately from those of the United Kingdom as a whole (Department of Health 2009, MAC 2009a).

It should be noted that EU-linked flows cannot be controlled by United Kingdom policy-makers although non-EU flows can be influenced by immigration regulations. Therefore, increasing migration from EU countries is arguably a bigger challenge for health workforce planning than the mobility patterns previously typical in the United Kingdom.

8.3 *Cross-border regulatory frameworks and interventions*

To a certain extent, mechanisms to manage cross-border flows can also be viewed in the context of government mobility policy. For example, a tightening of professional registration requirements for non-EEA health professionals coincided with moves away from active international recruitment. The changes included more stringent language requirements for non-EEA nurses; the removal of top-up courses for midwives lacking equivalent qualifications; and the removal of reciprocal recognition for Australian and New Zealand pharmacists.[6] However, professional regulatory bodies would consider that such moves as more concerned with their role of ensuring quality and patient safety in the face of large-scale health professional migration. The United Kingdom fully transposes the directive on the recognition of professional qualifications (European Parliament and Council of the European Union 2005) but imposes certain profession-specific restrictions (such as additional adaptation requirements or minimum lengths of practice) on individuals from CEE countries, for instance. United Kingdom professional organizations have several quality/safety issues with EU mobility. These centre around: (i) the real equivalence of education and training; (ii) regulatory bodies' lack of ability to test for language competency as part of the registration process; (iii) the need for EU mobility legislation to require CPD in order to ensure continuing fitness and suitability to practice in potentially mobile health professionals;

---

6 For more details see NHS Careers 2009.

and (iv) the need for more effective information sharing between regulators in order to restrict the movement of unsafe individuals within Europe (BMA 2009b, Griffiths 2002, Hazell 2009, Mead 2003, NMC 2005b, Young et al. 2010). These concerns are reflected in the United Kingdom's instigation of the cross-EU initiative on Healthcare Professionals Crossing Borders (AURE 2005, HPCB 2007).[7]

National-level mechanisms to manage cross-border mobility include bilateral agreements between the United Kingdom and several overseas governments. A high-profile code of practice for international recruitment was introduced in England in 2001 (Department of Health 2001) and later revised to encourage the involvement of the independent sector as well as the NHS (Department of Health 2004).[8] This code of practice aims to prevent recruitment from over 150 countries experiencing health professional shortages. These include developing economies in Africa, east and south Asia, the Middle East, the Caribbean, South America and the Pacific Islands. It also includes EU candidate countries (such as Croatia) and other countries in what might be termed wider Europe (such as Albania). Elsewhere under the code (China, India, the Philippines) recruitment was restricted to particular professional groups and/or geographical areas. Another main set of bilateral agreements was signed in the context of the United Kingdom's active recruitment policy in Europe, for example with Spain, Germany, Austria, Italy and Poland between 2001 and 2005.

Increasingly, such arrangements are set within the context of the wider policy on international development (Buchan & Dovlo 2004, Crisp 2007, Department of Health 2007, Department of Health & DfID 2008, Robinson & Clark 2008). This approach was clearly reflected in the bilateral agreement signed with South Africa in 2003 that focused on sharing expertise through time-limited placements of health-care staff. Similarly, at sub-national level there are Royal College sponsorship schemes for medical doctors as well as exchange agreements and twinning or staff volunteering partnerships between local NHS organizations and overseas providers and regional governments (Sloan 2005).[9] It is difficult to measure how these impact on both mobility and international development as the evidence on all these mechanisms is equivocal and difficult to monitor (Buchan et al. 2008; Department of Health & DfID 2008). For example, qualitative evidence suggests that NHS organizations and private agencies were influenced against targeting countries covered by the code of practice on international recruitment (e.g. African and non-EU European countries) but applications for United Kingdom professional registration still

---

7 See HPCB web site (http://www.hpcb.eu/, accessed 23 November 2010).

8 A separate code for Scottish health care was launched in 2006 (Scottish Executive 2006).

9 Such arrangements will be facilitated by the temporary worker strand of the new Immigration Rules. This allows NHS organizations to employ individuals from outside the UK and EEA for up to 24 months as part of a government-authorized exchange programme (NHS Employers 2008).

continued from individuals in those countries (Young et al. 2008 & 2010). In addition, some private-sector nursing homes encouraged back-door recruitment that circumvented the code. This was a problem because these nursing homes provided adaptation to the United Kingdom system but no longer-term job prospects, under the assumption that nurses who achieved full registration would move into the NHS (Buchan et al. 2008).

8.4 *Political force field of regulating and managing health professional mobility*

Besides the national government and the relevant devolved administrations, the main political stakeholders in the United Kingdom are the professional regulatory and representative bodies; the NHS itself; the trade unions; and mutual support associations for different immigrant health professional groups. The professional stakeholders work to defend migrants' interests in, for example, workplace equality and immigration rule changes (BMA 2009b, BBC 2009, Carlisle 2005, Casciani 2006a & 2006b). The professional bodies also work to ensure the protection of services and patients by lobbying for only competent health professionals to be allowed to enter practice in the United Kingdom. Such issues have been highlighted by certain high-profile cases that have been associated with free movement in the EU (Meikle 2009, Meikle & Connolly 2009). There is a view that EU arrangements allow health professionals to practice in the United Kingdom although lacking relevant experience and quality safeguards concerning, for example, language skills (AURE 2005, Harding et al. 2005, HPCB 2007, NMC 2009).

More broadly, the NHS holds immense significance for the United Kingdom population and receives widespread media coverage. Different political parties have different priorities and approaches but all consider the perceived successes/failures of the NHS to be key to their ongoing electoral prospects. In turn, the shape of the NHS changes with the policies of different governments. For example, the post-1997 Labour government's *political* commitment to expand the NHS workforce necessitated the policy of active international recruitment and openness to health professional mobility (Department of Health 2000c, Jenkins 2004). In addition, health professional mobility becomes an important issue in debates about the British economy. The United Kingdom opened up immediately to migrants from the EU-10 as there was then some consensus that the country needed additional workers (Blanchflower et al. 2007, Pollard et al. 2008). However, the economic situation and public/media opinion had changed by the time Bulgaria and Romania joined the EU in 2007 and led to the more restrictive transitional arrangements for migrants, including health professionals, from those countries.

The debate around professional mobility includes the view that the United Kingdom should become self-sufficient in the production of health professional labour (Mellor 2007 [personal communication]). This is not least because of the need to reduce risk as, for example, migrants are by definition a less constant workforce (given their potential to re-migrate). Also, policy-makers are more aware of the need to consider the potentially vulnerable health systems that are the main United Kingdom migration sources (Jenkins 2004, Mellor 2003). This realization – triggered by complaints from countries such as South Africa and Ghana – led to the various codes of practice on international recruitment (Department of Health 2001 & 2004, Scottish Executive 2006) and the subsequent linking of health-care mobility and international development policy (Crisp 2007). Of course, there is continuing debate about the extent to which the United Kingdom will remain self-sufficient and whether ethical recruitment can ever really work (Bundred & Levitt 2000, Deeming 2004, Khan 2005, Sartorius 2005).

9. Conclusion

As the mobility profile has shown, the United Kingdom has always relied on internationally qualified health professionals to address workforce supply needs. Historically, most professional mobility came from outside Europe but European sources have recently started to become more important – at least in relative terms. Active international recruitment targeting the EU-15 and EU-12 have increased professional registration applications from these countries (such as Spain, Germany, Greece, Italy and Poland) but numbers generally have risen in the last five years, particularly from CEE countries that have newly joined the EU.

Such trends make it vital that debates about the employment of foreign-trained health professionals and their impact on the NHS and its workforce give greater prominence to the EU dimension. For example, the continuing moral question regarding the ethical recruitment policy's ability to restrict negative impacts on source countries, including those in Europe. More practically, the sheer variety of countries and professional cultures represented in EU-United Kingdom migration makes effective induction and workforce integration measures a major challenge for NHS employers.

In addition, EU/EEA and other international mobility has implications for United Kingdom workforce planning. The potential impact of return migration to source countries has not been factored in to date due to the lack of accurate information on outflows. Similarly, lack of information about mobility within the United Kingdom and the differences in levels of dependency on internationally qualified staff (e.g. between England and other parts of the United Kingdom) pose major challenges for United Kingdom policy-makers addressing health professional workforce issues.

References

Aiken L, Buchan J (2004). Trends in international nurse migration. *Health Affairs*, 23(3):69.

Allan H, Larsen JA (2003). We need respect: experiences of internationallly recruited nurses in the UK. London, Royal College of Nursing.

Allan HT et al. (2004). The social reproduction of institutional racism: internationally recruited nurses' experiences of the British health services. *Diversity in Health and Social Care*, 1(2):117–126.

Atherton S, Mathie T (2002). GP and consultant planning and quality assurance. *Conference on International Recruitment and Co-operation: A Global Perspective, London, 1 May 2002.*

AURE (2005). *Healthcare Professionals Crossing Borders. UK Presidency Patient Safety Initiative*. London, Alliance of UK Health Regulators on Europe (AURE) and Department of Health.

Bach S (2007). Going global? The regulation of nurse migration in the UK. *British Journal of Industrial Relations*, 45(2):383–403.

Bach S (2008). *Staff shortages and immigration in the health sector. A paper prepared for the Migration Advisory Committee*. London, Home Office (http://www.ukba.homeoffice.gov.uk/sitecontent/documents/aboutus/workingwithus/mac/239769/bach2008, accessed 23 November 2010).

Ball J, Pike G (2004). Stepping stones: results from the RCN membership survey 2003. London, Royal College of Nursing (http://www.rcn.org.uk/__data/ assets/pdf_file/0003/78600/002235.pdf, accessed 23 November 2020).

Ballard K, Laurence P (2004). An induction programme for European general practitioners coming to work in England: development and evaluation. *Education for Primary Care*, 15(4):584–595.

Ballard K et al. (2004). Why do general practitioners from France choose to work in London? A qualitative study. *British Journal of General Practice*, 54(507):747–752.

BBC (2008). NHS trust looks north for nurses. *BBC News,* 6 February 2008 (http://news.bbc.co.uk/1/hi/england/southern_counties/7230984.stm, accessed 19 March 2009).

BBC (2009). Immigration change will hurt NHS. *BBC News*, 14 May 2009 (http://news.bbc.co.uk/2/hi/health/8048744.stm, accessed 22 May 2009).

Bellingham C (2001). Facing the recruitment and retention crisis in pharmacy: looking abroad. *Pharmaceutical Journal*, 267(7156):45–46.

Blanchflower D et al. (2007). *The impact of the recent migration from eastern Europe on the UK economy*. London, Bank of England (http://www.bankofengland.co.uk/ publications/speeches/2007/speech297.pdf, 23 November 2010).

Blitz B (2005). "Brain circulation": the Spanish medical profession and international medical recruitment in the UK. *Journal of European Social Policy*, 15(4):363–369.

Bloor K, Maynard A (2003). *Planning human resources in health care: towards an economic approach. An international comparative review*. Ottawa, Canadian Health Services Research Foundation (http://www.chsrf.ca/final_research/commissioned _research/programs/pdf/bloor_e.pdf, accessed 23 November 2010).

Bloor K et al. (2005). *Medical school intakes and the implications of expansion: a literature review and policy overview*. Department of Health Sciences, University of York.

BMA (2009a). *BMA concerned about NHS preparedness for new working time regulations*. London, British Medical Association (http://web.bma.org.uk / pressrel.nsf/wlu/SGOY-7UFHA2?OpenDocument&vw=wfmms, accessed 23 November 2010).

BMA (2009b). *BMA response to the European Commission Green Paper on the European workforce for health*. London, British Medical Association (http://www.bma.org.uk/images/bmaresponsegreenpapereuropeanhealthworkforce_tcm41-183022.pdf, accessed 23 November 2010).

Bola T et al. (2003). Foreign-educated nurses: strangers in a strange land? *Nursing Management*, 34(7):39–42.

Brazier M et al. (1992). Professional mobility and the single European market: the case of doctors. *Journal of Area Studies*, 19(1):115–24.

Buchan J (2003). *Here to stay? International nurses in the UK*. London, Royal College of Nursing.

Buchan J (2004). Commentary: nurse workforce planning in the UK. Policies and impact. *Journal of Nursing Management*, 12(6):388–392.

Buchan J (2006). Migration of health workers in Europe: policy problem or policy solution? In: Dubois C-A et al. (eds.). *Human resources for health in Europe*. London, Open University Press (European Observatory on Health Systems and Policies Series).

Buchan J, Dovlo D (2004). *International recruitment of health workers to the UK: a report for DFID*. London, DFID Health Systems Resource Centre.

Buchan J, Maynard A (2006). United Kingdom. In: Rechel B et al. (eds.). *The health care workforce in Europe: learning from experience*. London, European Observatory on Health Systems and Policies.

Buchan J, O'May F (1999). Globalisation and healthcare labour markets: a case study from the United Kingdom. *Human Resources for Health Development Journal*, 3:3.

Buchan J, Rafferty AM (2004). Not from our own backyard? The United Kingdom, Europe and international recruitment of nurses. In: McKee M et al. (eds.). *Health policy and European enlargement*. London, Open University Press (European Observatory on Health Systems and Policies Series).

Buchan J, Seccombe I (2004). *Fragile future? A review of the UK nursing labour market in 2003*. London, Royal College of Nursing (RCN Labour Market Review).

Buchan J, Seccombe I (2006a). *Worlds apart? The UK and international nurses*. London, Royal College of Nursing (RCN publication 003 049).

Buchan J, Seccombe I (2006b). *From boom to bust? The UK nursing labour market review 2005/6*. London, Royal College of Nursing.

Buchan J et al. (2008). Does a code make a difference – assessing the English code of practice on international recruitment. *Human Resources for Health*, 7:33.

Bundred PE, Levitt C (2000). Medical migration: who are the real losers? *Lancet*, 356(9225):245–246.

Buth J et al. (2000). Harmonization of vascular surgical training in Europe. A task for the European Board of Vascular Surgery (EBVS). *Cardiovascular Surgery*, 8(2):98–103.

Carlisle D (2005). Immigrant workforce. Needed by the NHS but denigrated by the politicians. *Health Service Journal*, 115(5954):12–13.

Casciani D (2006a). Overseas NHS doctors "betrayed". *BBC News*, 21 April 2006 (http://news.bbc.co.uk/1/hi/health/4928954.stm, accessed 22 May 2009).

Casciani D (2006b). "Let down by UK" – foreign doctors. *BBC News*, 21 April 2006 (http://news.bbc.co.uk/1/hi/health/4929902.stm, accessed 22 May 2009).

Cashman C, Slovak A (2005). The occupational medicine agenda: routes and standards of specialization in occupational medicine in Europe. *Occupational Medicine*, 55(4):308–311.

Close A (2002). Recruits from overseas need better assessment and support. *British Journal of Nursing*, 11(15):994.

Cowan D (2005). A project to establish a skills competency matrix for EU nurses. *British Journal of Nursing*, 14(11):613–617.

Cowan D (2006). Cultural competence in nursing: new meanings. *Journal of Transcultural Nursing*, 17(1):2–88.

Crisp N (2007). Global health partnerships: the UK contribution to health in developing countries – summary and recommendations. London, Department for International Development (http://dfid.gov.uk/pubs/files/ghp.pdf, accessed 2 February 2008).

Curson J A et al. (2008). Who does workforce planning well? Workforce review team rapid review summary. *International Journal of Health Care Quality Assurance,* 23(1):110–119.

Daniel P et al. (2001). Expectations and experiences of newly recruited Filipino nurses. *British Journal of Nursing*, 10(4):254–265.

Darzi A (2008). *High quality care for all: next stage review final report – summary.* London, Department of Health.

Davis K (2007). *Mirror, mirror on the wall: an international update on the comparative performance of American healthcare.* New York & Washington, The Commonwealth Fund (Volume 59).

Deeming C (2004). Policy targets and ethical tensions: UK nurse recruitment. *Social Policy and Administration*, 38(7):775–792.

Department of Health (2000a). *The NHS Plan: a plan for investment, a plan for reform.* London, The Stationery Office.

Department of Health (2000b). *A health service for all our talents: developing the NHS workforce.* London.

Department of Health (2000c). *NHS aims to recruit up to 5000 Spanish nurses.* Press release, London, 7th November 2000.

Department of Health (2001). *Code of practice for NHS employers involved in the international recruitment of healthcare professionals.* London (http://webarchive. nationalarchives.gov.uk/+/www.dh.gov.uk/en/Publicationsandstatistics/ Publications/PublicationsPolicyAndGuidance/DH_4006781, accessed 23 November 2010).

Department of Health (2002a). *A new role for overseas and independent healthcare providers in England.* Press release, London, 25 June 2002 (http:// tap.ukwebhost. eds.com/doh/intpress.nsf/page/202-0283?OpenDocument, accessed 14 December 2003).

Department of Health (2004). *Code of practice for the international recruitment of healthcare professionals.* London (http://www.dh.gov.uk/assetRoot/04/09/77 /34/04097734.pdf, accessed 23 November 2010).

Department of Health (2007). *Stopping the brain-drain: £1 million boost for global health workers.* Press release, London, 13 February 2007 (http://www. egovmonitor.com/node/9401, accessed 23 November 2010).

Department of Health (2008a). *New immigration rules to restrict international medical graduates' access to UK postgraduate medical training.* London (www. gnn/gov.uk /environment/fullDetail.asp?ReleaseID=350762&NewsAreaID=2, accessed 21 February 2008).

Department of Health (2008b). *NHS next stage review: quality workforce – strategy impact assessment.* London.

Department of Health (2008c). *A high quality workforce: NHS next stage review.* London.

Department of Health (2009). *Review body on doctors' and dentists' remuneration – review for 2010. Written evidence from the health departments for the United Kingdom.* London (http://www.dh.gov.uk/en/Publicationsandstatistics/ Publications/PublicationsPolicyAndGuidance/DH_106057, accessed 23 February 2011).

Department of Health (2010). *European working time directive* (http://webarchive. nationalarchives.gov.uk/+/www.dh.gov.uk/en/ Managingyourorganisation/Workforce/Workforceplanninganddevelopment/ Europeanworkingtimedirective/index.htm, accessed 23 February 2011).

Department of Health and DfID (2008). *Global health partnerships: the UK contribution to health in developing countries – the government response.* London, Department of Health and Department for International Development.

Dye J, Gajewska V (2001). Meeting the needs of non-UK trained European physiotherapists seeking employment within the United Kingdom. *Physiotherapy*, 87(8):424–432.

EMN (2006*). Managed migration and the labour market: the health sector.* Luxembourg, Office for Official Publications of the European Union (European Migration Network Small Scale Study II).

Esmail A, Carnall D (1993). Tackling racism in the NHS. *BMJ*, 314(7081):618.

Esmail A, Everington S (1997). Asian doctors are still being discriminated against. *BMJ*, 314(7094):1619.

European Parliament and Council of the European Union (2005). Directive 2005/36/EC of the European Parliament and of the Council of 7 September 2005 on the recognition of professional qualifications. *Official Journal of the European Union*, 255(48): 22–142.

Finch T et al. (2009). *Shall we stay or shall we go? Re-migration trends among Britain's immigrants – executive summary.* London, Institute for Public Policy Research (http://www.ippr.org.uk/publicationsandreports/publication. asp?id =685&print=yes, accessed 7 August 2009).

Gerrish K, Griffith V (2004). Integration of overseas registered nurses: evaluation of an adaptation programme. *Journal of Advanced Nursing.* 45(6):579–587.

Goldbart J et al. (2005). International students of speech and language therapy in the UK: choices about where to study and whether to return. *Higher Education,* 50(1):89–109.

Goodman B (2005). Overseas recruitment and migration. *Nursing Management*, 12(8):32–37.

Grant J et al. (2004). Overseas doctors' expectations and experiences of training and practice in the UK. Milton Keynes, The Open University.

Griffiths H (2002). EU's proposed policies are unfair and unsafe. *British Journal of Nursing*, 11(19):1234.

Grisold W et al. (2007). One Europe, one neurologist? *European Journal of Neurology,* 14(3):241–247.

Hall J (2005). Health care workforce planning: can it ever work? *Journal of Health Services Research and Policy*, 10(2):55–56.

Hann M et al. (2008). Workforce participation among international medical graduates in the National Health Service of England: a retrospective longitudinal study. *Human Resources for Health*, 6:9.

Harding L et al. (2005). GPs fear "flying doctors" crisis. *The Guardian*, 17 June 2005. (http://www.guardian.co.uk/uk/2005/jun/17/germany.society, accessed 23 November 2010).

Hassell K (2003). The national workforce census: (4) Overseas pharmacists – does the "globalisation" of pharmacy affect workforce supply? *Pharmaceutical Journal*, 271:183–185.

Hassell K et al. (2008). Part of a global workforce: migration of British-trained pharmacists. *Journal of Health Service Research and Policy*, 13(2):32.

Hazell T (2009). *NMC Response – Green paper on workforce for health COM (2008) 725 final*. London, Nursing and Midwifery Council (http://www.nmc-uk.org/ Documents/ EU-nternational%20documents/NMC%20position%20 paper %20Green%20paper%20healthcare%20workforce.pdf, accessed 23 November 2010).

Health Committee (2007). *Workforce planning, fourth report of session 2006-07. Volume I*. London, House of Commons Health Committee (HC 171-I).

Home Office et al. (2006). *Accession monitoring report. May 2004–June 2006*. London (http://www.ind.homeoffice.gov.uk/6353/aboutus/accession monitoringreport9.pdf, accessed 9 July 2009).

HPCB (2007). Healthcare Professionals Crossing Borders Portugal Agreement. London (http://www.hpcb.eu/activities/documents/Portugal_Agreement_ Final-September_2010.pdf, accessed 23 November 2010).

Jenkins C (2004). Ethical international recruitment. *International Psychiatry*, 6:18–19.

Johnson E (2005). Czech doctors getting to London for working weekends. *Monsters and Critics* 27 June 2005 (http://www.monsterandcritics.com/news/ health /news/article_1023171.php/Czech_doctors_jetting_to_london_for-working_weekends, accessed 7 August 2009).

Kelly R et al. (2005). *Migration and health in the UK. An ippr FactFile*. London, Institute for Public Policy Research.

Khan MM (2005). Beyond numbers: the NHS International Fellowship Programme in psychiatry. *International Psychiatry*, 3(1):20–21.

Larsen JA (2007). Embodiment of discrimination and overseas nurses' career progression. *Journal of Clinical Nursing* 16(12):2187–2195.

Larsen J et al. (2005). Overseas nurses' motivations for working in the UK: globalisation and life politics. *Work, Employment and Society*, 19(2):349–368.

Leatherman S, Sutherland K (2008). *The quest for quality in the NHS: refining the NHS reforms*. London, Nuffield Trust.

MAC (2008). *The labour market impact of relaxing restrictions on employment in the UK of nationals of Bulgarian and Romanian EU member states*. London, Migration Advisory Committee (http://www.ukba.homeoffice.gov.uk/sitecontent/documents/   aboutus/workingwithus/mac/a2-report/1208/relaxing-restrictions?view=Binary, accessed 23 November 2010).

MAC (2009a). *Skilled, shortage, sensible. First review of the recommended shortage occupation lists for the UK and Scotland. Spring 2009*. London, Migration Advisory Committee (http://www.ukba.homeoffice.gov.uk/sitecontent/documents/   aboutus/workingwithus/mac/first-review-lists/0409/mac-skilled-shortage-list-2009?view=Binary, accessed 23 November 2010).

MAC (2009b). *Review of the UK's transitional measures for nationals of member states that acceded to the European Union in 2004*. London, Migration Advisory Committee (http://www.ukba.homeoffice.gov.uk/sitecontent/documents/aboutus/workingwithus/mac/a8-report/, accessed 23 November 2010).

Magnusdottir H (2005). Overcoming strangeness and communication barriers: a phenomenological study of becoming a foreign nurse. *International Nursing Review*, 52(4):263–269.

Mahon A, Harris C (2003). *The European working time directive and doctors in training. An early evaluation of 19 pilot projects*. London, Department of Health.

Masters P (2005). *Working out: developing the London physiotherapy workforce*. Report commissioned by the London Physiotherapy Managers' Education Steering Group for South East London Health Authority (SELHA). London, SELHA.

Mathie T (2002). The Spanish acquisitions. *Health Service Journal*, 112:28–30.

McKendrick M (2005). The European Union of Medical Specialties core training curriculum in infectious diseases: overview of national systems and distribution of specialists. *Clinical Microbiology and Infection*, 11(Suppl. 1):28–32.

Mead M (2003). Midwifery and the enlarged European Union. *Midwifery*, 19(2):82–86.

Meikle J (2009). "Rules on EU doctors leave patients at risk", says GMC chief. *The Guardian*, 24 August 2009 (http://www.guardian.co.uk/society/2009/aug/23/rules-eu-doctors-medical-risk, accessed 23 November 2010).

Meikle J, Connolly K (2009). German GP who accidentally killed patient was advised to "go home". *The Guardian*, 23 August 2009 (http://www.guardian.co.uk/uk/ 2009/aug/23/german-gp-ubani-watchdog-findings, accessed 23 November 2010).

Mellor D (2003). Recruitment is ethical. *BMJ*, 327(7420):928.

Moore W (2002). First team of overseas surgeons arrives in England. *BMJ*, 325(7359):297.

NHS Careers (2009) [web site]. *Information for overseas doctors.* (http://www.nhscareers.nhs.uk/img_qa.shtml, accessed 3 April 2007).

NHS Employers (2008). *The points-based system: how the immigration overhaul affects NHS recruitment. Briefing 55.* London & Leeds (http://www.nhsemployers. org/Aboutus/Publications/Documents/The%20points-based%20system.pdf, accessed 23 November 2010).

NHS Employers (2009). *Why use international recruitment?* London & Leeds (http://www.nhsemployers.org/RecruitmentAndRetention/International Recruitment/Pages/Whyuseinternationalrecruitment.aspx, accessed 14 April 2009).

NHS Information Centre (2008). *GP practice vacancies survey 2008.* Leeds (http://www.ic.nhs.uk/webfiles/publications/Vacancy%20Survey%20 %28NHS%20and%20%20GP%29%202008/GP%202008%20FINAL%20 pdf.doc.pdf, accessed 23 November 2010).

NHS Modernisation Agency (2003). *Changing workforce programme. Pilot sites progress reports.* London.

NMC (2003) *The Nursing and Midwifery Council statistical analysis of the register 1 April 2002 to 31 March 2003.* London (http://www.nmc-uk.org/ Documents/ Statistical%20 analysis%20of%20the%20register/NMC%20 Statistical%20analysis%20of%20the %20register%202002%202003.pdf, accessed 23 November 2010).

NMC (2004) *The Nursing and Midwifery Council statistical analysis of the register 1 April 2003 to 31 March 2004.* London (http://www.nmc-uk.org/ Documents/ Statistical%20 analysis %20of%20the%20register/NMC%20 Statistical%20analysis %20of%20the %20register%202003%202004.pdf, accessed 23 November 2010).

NMC (2005a) *The Nursing and Midwifery Council statistical analysis of the register 1 April 2004 to 31 March 2005.* London (http://www.nmc-uk.org/ Documents/ Statistical%20 analysis%20of%20the%20register/NMC%20

Statistical%20analysis %20of%20the %20register%202004%202005.pdf, accessed 23 November 2010).

NMC (2005b). *EU language position a "dangerous farce" says NMC President.* London, Nursing and Midwifery Council (Press release 44/2005).

NMC (2006) The Nursing and Midwifery Council statistical analysis of the register

1 April 2005 to 31 March 2006. London (http://www.nmc-uk.org/Documents/ Statistical %20analysis%20of%20the%20register/NMC%20Statistical%20 analysis%20of%20the%20register%202005%202006.pdf, accessed 23 November 2010).

NMC (2007) The Nursing and Midwifery Council statistical analysis of the register

1 April 2006 to 31 March 2007. London (http://www.nmc-uk.org/Documents/ Statistical %20analysis%20of%20the%20register/NMC-Statistical-analysis-of-the-register-202006-202007.pdf, accessed 23 November 2010).

NMC (2008). *Statistical analysis of the register 1 April 2007 to 31 March 2008.* London (http://www.nmc-uk.org/Documents/Statistical%20analysis%20 of%20the% 20register/NMC-Statistical-analysis-of-the-register-2007-2008. pdf, accessed July 2010).

NMC (2009). *Survey of European midwifery regulators.* London, Nursing and Midwifery Council. (http://www.nmc-uk.org/Documents/EU-International%20documents/Survey%20of%20European%20Midwifery%20 Regulators%20July%202009.pdf, accessed 23 November 2010).

NNRU (2007). Nurses on the move: implications of internal migration in the UK. *Policy*, 3 (http://www.kcl.ac.uk/content/1/c6/03/01/08/PolicyIssue3.pdf, accessed 23 November 2010).

O'Dowd A (2003). How will the UK cope with an influx of EU nurses? *Nursing Times*, 99(21):10–11.

Palese A et al. (2006). Competence of Romanian nurses after their first six months in Italy: a descriptive study. *Journal of Clinical Nursing*, 16(12):2260–2271.

Petchey R, Needle J (2008). Helping hands? The allied health professions in Europe. *Workforce Special Interest Group of the European Health Management Association, EHMA Annual Conference, Athens, June 2008.*

Pitts J et al. (1998). Experiences and career intentions of general practice registrars from the Netherlands. *Medical Education*, 32(6):613–621.

Pollard N et al. (2008). *Floodgates or turnstiles? Post-EU enlargement migration flows to (and from) the UK*. London, Institute for Public Policy Research.

Porter E, Powell G (2005). Recruitment of European Union general practitioners: developing a process for the analysis of English language training needs. Education for Primary Care, 16(1):31–35.

Raghuram P, Kofman E (2002). The state, skilled labour markets, and immigration: the case of doctors in England. *Environment and Planning A*, 34(11):2071-2089.

Reid C (2009). No time for complacency on European working time directive. *Health Service Journal*, 14 May 2009 (http://www.hsj.co.uk/comment/opiniion/wendy-reid-this-is-no-time-for-complacency/5001118.article, accessed 7 August 2009).

Robinson M, Clark P (2008). Forging solutions to health worker migration. *The Lancet*, 371(9613):691–693.

Sales H (2002). Bad accent, good nurse. *Nursing Times*, 98(44):24–25.

Santry C (2009). Trainee NHS doctors being told to lie about long working hours. *Health Service Journal*, 28 May 2009 (http://www.hsj.co.uk/news/workforce/trainee-nhs-doctors-being-told-to-lie-about-long-working-hours/5002032.article, accessed 7 August 2009).

Sartorius N (2005). Ethical international recruitment – a response. *International Psychiatry*, 7:3–5.

Scottish Executive (2006). *Code of practice for the international recruitment of healthcare professionals in Scotland*. Edinburgh.

Sears N (2008). The Polish doctor who makes 12-hour commute to treat patients in Britain. *Mail Online*, 16 January 2008 (http://www.dailymail.co.uk/news/article-508330/The-Polish-doctor-makes-12-hour-commute-to-treat-patients, accessed 7 August 2009.

Simon M et al. (2005). *NEXT – scientific results*. Wuppertal (www.next-study.net, accessed 23 November 2010).

Sloan J (2005). NHS links: a new approach to international health links. *BMJ Careers*, 19 February 2005 (http://careers.bmj.com/careers/advice/view-article.html?id=680, accessed 22 February 2008).

Smith DJ (1980). *Overseas doctors in the NHS*. London, Policy Studies Institute.

Smith PA et al. (2006). *Valuing and recognising the talents of a diverse healthcare workforce*. London, Royal College of Nursing (http://www.rcn.org.uk/__data/assets/ pdf_file/0008/78713/003078.pdf, accessed 23 November 2010).

Taylor DH, Esmail A (1999). Retrospective analysis of census data on general practitioners who qualified in south Asia: who will replace them as they retire? *BMJ*, 318(7179):306–310.

Travis A (2009). Here today, gone tomorrow: new breed of migrants finds grass greener overseas. *The Guardian*, 6 August 2009 (http://www.guardian.co.uk/uk/2009/aug/06/britain-losing-highly-skilled-migrants, accessed 23 November 2010).

UKCC (1989). *Annual report 1988–1989*. London, United Kingdom Central Council for Nursing, Midwifery and Health Visiting.

Waite R et al. (1990). *Career patterns of Scotland's qualified nurses*. Edinburgh, Scottish Office Central Research Unit.

Wang L (2007). Eastern European pharmacists in the UK. *The Pharmaceutical Journal*, 278:7–8.

Wanless D (2002). *Securing our future health: taking a long-term view. Final Report*. London, HM Treasury.

Winkelmann-Gleed A (2006). *Migrant nurses: motivation, integration and contribution*. Oxford, Radcliffe Press.

Winkelmann-Gleed A, Seeley J (2005). Strangers in a British world? Integration of international nurses. *British Journal of Nursing*, 14(18):954–961.

Winyard G (2007). Medical immigration: the elephant in the room. *BMJ*, 335(7620): 593.

Woolf A (2002). Specialist training in rheumatology in Europe. *Rheumatology*, 41(9): 1062–1066.

WRT (2008a). *Workforce summary – nursing. October 2008 – England only*. London, Workforce Review Team (http://www.cfwi.org.uk/intelligence/previous-projects/workforce-summaries/nursing, accessed 23 November 2010).

WRT (2008b). *Workforce summary – pharmacy workforce. Pharmacy and pharmacy technicians. September 2008 – England only*. London, Workforce Review Team (http://www.cfwi.org.uk/intelligence/previous-projects/workforce-summaries/ pharmacy, accessed 23 November 2010).

WRT (2009c). *Migration Advisory Committee Shortage Report. Non-consultant (non-training) posts in all specialties that are not currently WTD compliant*. London, Workforce Review Team (http://www.wrt.nhs.uk/index.php/mac, accessed 9 July 2009)

WRT (2009d). *Migration Advisory Committee Shortage Report. Medical posts in histopathology that are not training posts*. London, Workforce Review Team (http://www.cfwi.org.uk/resources/mac-reports/histopathology-mac-report/at_download/attachment1, accessed 23 November 2010).

WRT (2009e). *Migration Advisory Committee Shortage Report. Nurses SOC 3211 – March 2009.* London, Workforce Review Team (http://www.cfwi.org.uk/resources/ mac-reports/nursing-mac-report, accessed 23 February 2011).

WRT (2009f). *Migration Advisory Committee Shortage Report. Midwives. SOC 3212.* London, Workforce Review Team, (http://cfwi.fry-it.com/resources/mac-reports/midwifery-mac-report, accessed 23 November 2010).

WRT (2009g). *Migration Advisory Committee Shortage Report. Pharmacy workforce. SOC 2213.* London, Workforce Review Team (http://cfwi.fry-it.com/resources/mac-reports/pharmacy-mac-report, accessed 23 November 2010).

WRT (2009h). *Migration Advisory Committee Shortage Report. Health Professions Council (HPC) registered diagnostic radiographers. March 2009.* London, Workforce Review Team (http://cfwi.fry-it.com/resources/mac-reports/diagnostic-radiographers-mac-report, accessed 23 November 2010).

WRT (2009i). *Migration Advisory Committee Shortage Report. Senior speech and language therapists only. SOC 3223. March 2009.* London, Workforce Review Team (http://cfwi.fry-it.com/resources/mac-reports/senior-speech-and-language-therapists-mac-report, accessed 23 November 2010).

Young R, Leese B (1999). Recruitment and retention of general practitioners in the UK: what are the problems and solutions? *British Journal of General Practice,* 49(447):829–833.

Young R et al. (2001). Imbalances in the GP labour market in the UK: evidence from a postal survey and interviews with GP leavers. *Work, Employment & Society,* 15(4):699–719.

Young R et al. (2003). *The international market for medical doctors: perspectives on the positioning of the UK.* MCHM and NPCRDC, University of Manchester.

Young R et al. (2008). *International recruitment into the NHS: evaluation of initiatives for hospital doctors, general practitioners, nurses, midwives and allied health professionals.* FNSNM, King's College, London; Open University Centre for Education in Medicine; Manchester Business School and NPCRDC, University of Manchester.

Young R et al. (2010). *Health professional mobility in Europe and the UK: a scoping study of issues and evidence. Research report for the National Institute for Health Research Service Delivery and Organisation programme.* http://www.sdo.nihr.ac.uk/files/project/134-final-report.pdf, accessed 23 February 2011)

Part III

Case studies from countries that joined the EU in 2004 or 2007

Chapter 9

Migration and attrition: Estonia, its health sector and cross-border mobility

Pille Saar, Jarno Habicht

1. Introduction

Both medical education and health professional mobility have a long history in Estonia. The University of Tartu was founded in 1632 and, over the centuries, Estonian health professionals have gained education and work experience in Scandinavia and other countries in the east and west. Thus, the phenomenon of health-care professionals working abroad is not new.

Estonia is predominantly a source country. Since European Union (EU) accession the outflow of health professionals to foreign countries appears to have been moderate, especially in comparison to other human resource issues such as ageing of the workforce or attrition. Inflows from other countries have remained insignificant – only a small number of medical doctors and dentists have migrated to Estonia in recent years, mostly from the Russian Federation.

Since accession to the EU, medical doctors, nurses and dentists in Estonia have shown similar and relatively stable levels of interest in seeking work opportunities in other countries. The five most popular destination countries are Finland, the United Kingdom, Sweden, Germany and Norway. Health system reforms have improved the service delivery and financing structures of primary care and hospitals and provided a good working environment for health professionals (Atun et al. 2006, Habicht & Habicht 2008, Koppel et al. 2008). However, higher salaries and better working conditions in other countries are the main reasons for emigration (Rechel et al. 2006).

It is likely that the constant rises in salaries since 2005 have made working abroad less attractive for the Estonian health workforce. However, the active recruitment practices of Scandinavian, especially Finnish, health-care institutions may pose a threat in the near future by significantly increasing the numbers of health professionals leaving Estonia.

This case study aims to provide the best available and comparable information on health professional mobility with a focus on the period since accession to the EU in 2004. It will assess the relative importance of mobility compared to other workforce factors such as ageing and professionals working outside the health system. Moreover, it will describe the impact of international mobility on the health system as well as the motivational factors for migration. Finally, the study will describe recent human resource policies, workforce planning and other policy-related issues.

Limitations of the study

Data on the mobility of health professionals are based on the Ministry of Social Affairs annual reports on health-care statistics and the Health Care Board (HCB) registry of health-care professionals. Registration does not have to be renewed and therefore it cannot be presumed that all registered health-care professionals are working in the health-care sector. However, the number of active health professionals was obtained from the National Institute for Health Development (NIHD) annual reports on health-care statistics.

Data on the outflows of health professionals are not available in Estonia. However, data on the intention to migrate to another country do exist in the form of certificates on the mutual recognition of diplomas issued by the HCB. These certificates facilitate the recognition process for degrees and diplomas and thus health professionals' mobility between Member States of the EU (HCB 2008).

To date, only a few studies have analysed professional mobility but research interest has been growing since EU accession (Buchan et al. 2006). In this study the authors complement the published research with statistical data on the health system (from the HCB and NIHD, for example) and individual contacts with managers and policy-makers. One major weakness of this study is a lack of information on the number of health professionals who emigrated but returned, therefore the number of returnees cannot be estimated correctly.

For better interpretation of the data it is necessary to know that the new Health Services Organization Act came into force in 2001. Also, the overall system of registration changed with the establishment of the HCB registry in 2002 which introduced legal changes requiring all health professionals to reregister within a transitional period of three years (2002–2005).

2. Mobility profile of Estonia

Estonia is mainly a source country for health professionals. The EU accession in 2004 led to a significant rise in the number of medical doctors and nurses moving to neighbouring EU countries, principally Finland, but numbers stabilized over the following years. Inflows to Estonia are relatively insignificant (HCB 2008).

2.1 *Medical doctors*

Inflows

There has been little inflow of medical doctors to Estonia over the last few years. Since 2002, the year in which statistics on inflows first became available, the HCB has registered a total of 25 medical doctors from EU countries and 45 medical doctors from elsewhere (Table 9.1). Medical doctors from EU countries are mostly of Finnish and Latvian origin; those from outside the EU come mainly from the Russian Federation and Ukraine. There are no significant differences in age and sex between the migrants from EU and third countries, most are middle-aged (48–50 years) or older male medical doctors (HCB unpublished data 2008).

Among registered doctors, Estonia has higher numbers of foreign-trained anaesthetists, radiologists, general surgeons, psychiatrists and medical graduates without specialization (basic training only). Some of the small number of foreign-trained health professionals use the country as a transition point – around half of the registered foreign-trained doctors leave Estonia after some years. There are no exact data on the destination countries (HCB 2008) but work experience in an EU Member State is considered beneficial for achieving recognition in another, more attractive target country such as Finland or the United Kingdom. Doctors who have remained in Estonia are mainly from the Russian Federation (HCB 2008).

The percentage of foreign-trained doctors is insignificant in comparison to that of domestic medical doctors registered and working in Estonia. Between 2004 and 2008 foreign-trained doctors comprised 0.1%–0.2% (2–8 individuals) of the total number of active doctors. Foreign-trained medical doctors usually provide services in small hospitals or private practices. For geographical and cultural reasons (mainly Russian-speaking population) the majority of the

Table 9.1 *Registry data on domestic and foreign-trained medical doctors in Estonia according to activity, 2003–2009*

	2003	2004	2005	2006	2007	2008	2009
Registered medical doctors	4 052	5 012	5 201	5 334	5 418	5 524	5 636
Foreign-trained	1	6	12	10	10	15	16
EU countries	0	4	8	4	4	4	1
other countries	1	2	4	6	6	11	15
Practising registered medical doctors		4 335	4 306	4 319	4 400	4 503	4 414
Foreign-trained	1	3	8	3	2	6	na
EU countries	0	1	4	0	0	1	
other countries	1	2	4	3	2	5	
Active foreign medical doctors among active Estonian medical doctors (%)		0.07	0.19	0.07	0.05	0.13	

Sources: HCB unpublished data 2008 & 2009, NIHD 2008 & 2009a. *Note*: na – not available

medical doctors from Russia or the Ukraine work in north-eastern Estonia (HCB 2008).

Outflows

Between 2004 and 2009 the HCB issued 709 mutual recognition of diploma certificates to medical doctors (Table 9.2). In 2004, 283 certificates were issued but numbers dropped significantly (between three- and fourfold) and stabilized in the following years before rising again in 2009. The major destination countries were Finland (74%), the United Kingdom (10%), Sweden (6%) and Germany (6%).

Table 9.2 *Mutual recognition of diploma certificates issued to practising registered medical doctors in Estonia, by intended destination country, 2004–2009*

Destination country	2004	2005	2006	2007	2008	2009	Total
Finland	203	59	60	61	61	81	**525**
United Kingdom	30	10	8	7	8	10	**73**
Sweden	23	4	6	1	1	4	**39**
Germany	7	3	3	1	0	4	**18**
Norway	7	1	2	1	2	0	**13**
Others	13	2	8	4	7	7	**41**
Total	**283**	**79**	**87**	**75**	**79**	**106**	**709**

Source: HCB unpublished data 2008 & 2009.

The largest numbers of emigrants (190) are doctors with no specialization (including resident doctors). These are followed by family physicians (118), anaesthetists (72), radiologists (58) and general surgeons (44) (HCB unpublished data 2009). The doctors with no specialization are usually residents studying for specialization and practising medicine after basic studies. The HCB assumes that certificates are requested mostly by residents interested in practising abroad before acquiring their diplomas (HCB 2008). The annual percentage of Estonian doctors wishing to emigrate fell from 6.5% to 1.8% between 2004 and 2008 but rose to 2.4% in 2009 (Table 9.3). HCB analysis shows that not all doctors with certificates leave the country – between 2004 and 2008 around 52% of these doctors continued to provide health-care services in Estonia.

There are various cross-border practices in Estonia. For example, some radiologists residing in Estonia provide their services abroad over the Internet (HCB 2008). The numbers of medical doctors who leave include commuters who work in Finland over weekends and in Estonia during the week (HCB 2008, NIHD 2009). In several cases, Scandinavian health-care providers have targeted Estonian health professionals through active recruitment practices such as free language courses and information days for doctors.

Comparison of the workforce outflow to foreign states and the workforce outflow from the health-care sector shows that migration to other countries is less significant than the number of non-practising doctors in Estonia who do not provide health-care services (Table 9.3).

Table 9.3 *Mutual recognition of diploma certificates issued to practising registered medical doctors in Estonia, 2004–2009*

Medical doctors	2004	2005	2006	2007	2008	2009
Total registered	5 012	5 202	5 334	5 418	5 524	5 636
Practising and registered	4 335	4 306	4 319	4 400	4 503	4 414
Not practicing (%)	677 (14)	896 (17)	919 (17)	914 (17)	1 080 (20)	1 165 (21)
Certificates issued (% among practising MDs)	**283 (6.5)**	**79 (1.8)**	**87 (2.0)**	**75 (1.7)**	**79 (1.8)**	**106 (2.4)**

Sources: HCB unpublished data 2008 & 2009, NIHD 2008 & 2009a.

2.2 Nurses

Inflows and outflows

There is barely any inflow of nurses. Since 2002, it is reported that only one nurse (from Latvia) has moved to Estonia. Conversely, a number of Estonian nurses have shown interest in migrating in recent years. This may have been influenced by the specific activity of Finnish and Norwegian recruitment companies since 2007 (Ilves 2007). Since EU accession, the HCB has issued 605 certificates to nurses wishing to work abroad. Between 2004 and 2009, the three most popular destination countries were Finland (61%), Norway (12%) and the United Kingdom (9%) (Table 9.4).

Table 9.4 *Mutual recognition of diploma certificates issued to practising registered nurses[a] in Estonia, by intended destination country, 2004–2009*

Destination country	2004	2005	2006	2007	2008	2009	Total
Finland	61	50	49	52	71	84	**367**
Norway	10	4	5	29	15	8	**71**
United Kingdom	11	11	8	8	8	6	**52**
Sweden	26	6	3	1	0	2	**38**
Ireland	3	11	1	5	3	1	**24**
Netherlands	4	0	0	0	0	1	**5**
Others	3	7	1	5	0	32	**48**
Total	**118**	**89**	**67**	**100**	**97**	**134**	**605**

Source: HCB unpublished data 2008 & 2009. *Note*: [a] One per professional, duplicates for one individual have been removed.

The share of Estonian nurses wishing to emigrate declined from 1.4% in 2004 to 0.8% in 2006 but rose to 1.6% in 2009 (Table 9.5). As with doctors, only around 56% of the nurses issued with recognition certificates actually left the country (HCB unpublished data 2008). Similarly, attrition is a continuous problem since a large number of registered nurses work outside the health-care sector (25% in 2009). Despite increases in health professional salaries between 2004 and 2008 many nurses choose to work in spas, beauty salons or elsewhere in the service sector.

Table 9.5 *Mutual recognition of diploma certificates issued to practising registered nurses in Estonia, 2004–2009*

Nurses	2004	2005	2006	2007	2008	2009
Total registered	9 365	9 772	10 264	10 541	10 776	11 027
Practising registered	8 420	8 530	8 556	8 603	8 297	8281
Not practising (%)	945 (10.)	1 242 (13)	1 708 (17)	1 938 (18)	2 479 (23)	2746 (25)
Number of issued certificates (% practising nurses)	**118 (1.4)**	**89 (1.0)**	**67 (0.8)**	**100 (1.2)**	**97 (1.2)**	**134 (1.6)**

Sources: HCB unpublished data 2008 & 2009, NIHD 2008 & 2009a.

2.3 Dentists

Inflows

Between 2002 and 2009, the HCB recognized and registered 5 dentists from EU countries and 17 from elsewhere. Like doctors, dentists who migrate to Estonia are mostly middle-aged (45–46 years) males; the majority from Finland and the Russian Federation. Unlike medical doctors, dentists from the Russian Federation who register in Estonia are more likely to stay in the country (more than half have done so).

Table 9.6 *Registry data on domestic and foreign dentists in Estonia, 2003–2009*

Dentists	2003	2004	2005	2006	2007	2008	2009
Registered	1 247	1 300	1 349	1 390	1 424	1 465	1495
Foreign-trained and registered	3	3	5	8	2	1	2
EU countries	0	0	1	3	1	0	0
other countries	1	3	4	5	1	1	2
Practising and registered		1 166	1 202	1 194	1 164	1 237	1 196
Practising foreign-trained and registered	2	3	1	6	1	0	na
EU countries	0	0	0	1	0	0	
other countries	2	3	1	5	1	0	
% of active foreign dentists (working in Estonia) among active Estonian dentists		0.26	0.08	0.50	0.09	0.00	

Sources: HCB unpublished data 2008 & 2009, NIHD 2008 & 2009a. Note: na – not available.

Outflows

Between 2004 and 2009 a total of 174 Estonian dentists obtained certificates allowing them to work in the EU. Analysis of the intended destination countries shows that most dentists planned to migrate to Finland (67%) and the United Kingdom (14%) (Table 9.7). This is in line with the major destination countries of medical doctors and nurses.

From 2004 to 2009, 174 dentists (between 1.4% and 3.4% per year) applied for certificates enabling them to begin the recognition procedure in a foreign state (Table 9.8).

Like doctors and nurses, increasing numbers of dentists are not actively providing health-care services – from 9% in 2004 to 21% in 2009 (Table 9.8). Estonia has had high numbers of dentists for many years and these have increased further since 1990 (89 dentists per 100 inhabitants in 2007). For this

Table 9.7 *Mutual recognition of diploma certificates issued to practising registered dentists in Estonia, by intended destination country, 2004–2009*

Destination country	2004	2005	2006	2007	2008	2009	Total
Finland	15	12	23	15	16	36	**117**
United Kingdom	7	4	6	3	2	2	**24**
Sweden	0	0	5	6	0	1	**12**
Others	7	1	3	4	5	1	**21**
Total	**29**	**17**	**37**	**28**	**23**	**40**	**174**

Source: HCB unpublished data 2008 & 2009.

Table 9.8 *Mutual recognition of diploma certificates issued to practising registered dentists in Estonia, 2004–2009*

Dentists	2004	2005	2006	2007	2008	2009
Total registered	1 286	1 335	1 381	1 424	1 465	1 495
Practising registered	1 166	1 202	1 194	1 164	1 237	1 196
Not practising (%)	120 (9)	133 (10)	185 (13)	257 (18)	281 (19)	314 (21)
Certificates issued (% of practising dentists)	29 (2.5)	17 (1.4)	37 (3.1)	28 (2.4)	23 (1.9)	40 (3.4)

Sources: HCB unpublished data 2008 & 2009, NIHD 2008 & 2009a.

reason, migration and attrition to other sectors have no remarkable influence on the availability of dental health-care services within the country.

Medical doctors, nurses and dentists leaving or working temporarily

One feature that characterizes the outflow of Estonian health professionals is the temporary nature of working abroad. Many health professionals work according to a shift system (on certain working days) and therefore find it easy to provide health-care services in neighbouring countries (such as Finland, Sweden, Norway) while continuing to work in Estonia. Some medical doctors provide services on weekdays in neighbouring foreign states and at weekends return to Estonia where their families live and work. Some health professionals provide services abroad (in hospitals of northern Finland or family doctor practices, for example) for periods ranging from some months up to a half year and then return to Estonia. It is known that recruitment agencies employ Estonian nurses to cover temporary workforce shortages in Norwegian facilities.

2.4 *Summary*

Currently, the Estonian health system is not dependent on health professionals who have gained their education and further medical practise in foreign states. The evidence available since 2002 shows a marginal inflow of health professionals from other countries.

The HCB registry shows that most foreign doctors come from neighbouring countries such as the Russian Federation and Finland (HCB 2008). Over the last six years the HCB has registered 95 foreign health professionals (doctors, dentists, nurses), about half of whom have moved from Estonia to another EU Member State at the end of the observation period. This shows clearly that an important share of inflowing doctors use Estonia as a platform for moving to another country – hoping that entry to the registry will facilitate registration in a more tempting EU country (HCB 2008).

The 2004 EU accession led to a temporary rise in migration to neighbouring EU countries among doctors and nurses. The international outflow of Estonian health professionals occurs mostly within the European Economic Area (EEA) or Switzerland; a few have migrated beyond. Finland is the main destination of health professional emigration. Some migrating professionals provide cross-border health-care services while others work simultaneously in both Estonia and a neighbouring country. Between 2004 and 2009, the HCB issued around 1500 certificates to medical doctors, dentists and nurses but not all have left Estonia (HCB unpublished data 2008). To date, more health professionals have left the health sector within Estonia than have emigrated.

In summary, Estonia can be characterized as a state that has a moderate outflow of professionals to foreign states. In 2008, the proportion of health professionals with certificates to work abroad represented 1.8% of practising medical doctors, 1.2% of practising nurses and 1.9% of practising dentists. In recent years, the willingness to emigrate has remained relatively stable in the three professions. There are signs that the situation may have begun to change in 2009 as the overall economic crisis influenced professionals' perceptions and, potentially, their migration behaviour (see also section 5). In 2009, certificates were issued to the highest numbers of nurses (134; 1.6%) and dentists (40; 3.4%) and the second highest number of medical doctors (106; 2.6%) since records began in 2004. It is difficult to say whether these developments show the beginning of a new trend or indeed whether they are attributable to the economic crisis. However, it is argued that the situation is worth monitoring.

3. Vignettes on health professional mobility

Latin American medical doctor moving to Estonia for training and work

This doctor had studied dental care and surgery in her homeland but, as it was very difficult to get work in the best private hospitals there, chose to study and work in Estonia. Young doctors in her homeland are less motivated to work in public hospitals as they offer lower salaries than private hospitals. This doctor considers Estonia to have a fairer health system and to offer better possibilities to enter the labour market. Coming from outside the EU, she was required to pass an exam in order to register as a medical doctor. Starting with a postgraduate medical training (residency) in the University of Tartu, since autumn 2006 she has worked as a resident in one of the biggest hospitals in Estonia. She passed a three-month language course and speaks fluent Estonian. After completing her residency in Estonia, she had no problems registering as a medical specialist. She intends to remain in Estonia after graduation because she is satisfied with the working conditions and the way of life.

Medical doctor from the Russian Federation, working and living in Estonia

This 33 year old male doctor graduated from Astrakhan State Medical Academy in the Russian Federation. He moved in 2005 – his mother is Estonian and the pull of his roots was so strong that he intends to spend the rest of his life in Estonia. His biggest challenge was to overcome the language barrier as he spoke almost no Estonian when he arrived. With the support of a private teacher and daily practise he is now able to speak Estonian.

Coming from a non-EU state, this doctor was required to pass an exam or to undertake six months adaptation in a health-care facility in Estonia. He chose the latter, working in a small (50 bed) hospital before registering as a surgeon. He decided to remain in the same hospital. This young doctor has made such a good impression that the hospital clinical director would not hesitate to recruit other foreign medical doctors.

This foreign surgeon is satisfied with the operation of the Estonian health sector. He considers it to be more transparent and to pay much larger salaries than the Russian Federation.

Estonian nurse commuting between Norway and Estonia

This young Estonian nurse graduated from health-care college with a nursing degree and a specialization in emergency care. She works as a specialist in emergency care where she is very highly qualified in comparison to many of her colleagues. Earning a high salary (in comparison to a nurse's average salary), in 2007 she decided for economic reasons to work in Norway too. Each month she works two weeks in Norway on a temporary contract providing nursing services in a nursing home which does not use her emergency nursing skills. The Norwegian employer pays the commuting costs. The nurse works in Estonia for the other two weeks of each month. There is a strong incentive to commute as she is paid more for two weeks in Norway than for two months in Estonia.

She has now been working in the two countries for two years but finds the arrangement exhausting and stressful for herself and her relatives. Her family is in Estonia and she does not know how long she will be able to continue with this arrangement.

Estonian doctor moving to Finland for secure employment conditions

The health sector workforce was relatively underpaid when Estonia joined the EU in 2004. At the same time there were hard and long-drawn-out salary negotiations between the government, hospital unions and the doctors' trade union.

Dr S is a young family physician who completed her residency in 2004. She had to choose between continuing to work in Estonia under strained budgets or to take up a stable position offering six times the salary in a hospital in Kotka, Finland. Like a number of younger Estonian doctors that year, she chose to continue her career abroad.

In 2008 she was still working as a family physician in Kotka. Doctors' salaries have risen substantially in Estonia over the intervening four years but medical doctors practising in Finland still earn considerably more. Dr S is satisfied with her salary, her personal life (she married a Finn) and the ever-expanding Estonian community in Kotka. She left Estonia after graduating from university and established her new life abroad. Currently she has no intention of moving back to Estonia.

4. Dynamics of enlargement

Relative isolation over the 50 years following the Second World War changed the pattern of both immigration and emigration that took place mostly within the USSR. The health ministry of the USSR offered some medical doctors and nurses the possibility of working in foreign states, mostly developing countries.

A special agreement between the USSR and Finland also enabled some doctors to work in Finland. However, there is a lack of statistical information for this period and no data are available to estimate the emigration phenomenon before 1991.

The state borders opened when Estonia became independent in 1991. This initiated the first wave of labour migration as medical doctors and nurses started to seek better working conditions in nearby countries, initially Finland. Estonia was not part of the EU during that period and therefore those seeking to work in European countries were required to pass both the specialty and the language examination in order to start practising. As a result, emigrants were primarily the most progressive younger doctors and nurses with foreign language skills. Many of these have now returned to Estonia (Kallaste et al. 2004).

The initial strong interest in migration, particularly among medical doctors, can be explained by the opening of new career opportunities, free movement of workers and the mutual recognition of diplomas (Aaviksoo et al. 2006, Kallaste et al. 2004). Analysis of the movement of health professionals over the period 2004–2008 indicates that migration intentions had stabilized. However, migration intentions among health professionals increased in 2009, possibly related to the economic crisis. This was an exception and it is too early to consider this a general trend.

It is arguable that the main motivational factor for doctors and nurses seeking to leave Estonia was the relatively low wage levels. In 2004, 283 doctors and 118 nurses wanted to emigrate – over three times more doctors than the average over the next four years. Intense salary negotiations were launched with the trade unions in 2004 but the results were unpredictable and contributed to uncertainty among health professionals. In the following year a wage agreement increased pay levels and produced significant reductions in the number of health professionals wishing to leave – 79 doctors and 89 nurses in 2005 (Aaviksoo et al 2006, HCB unpublished data 2008).

While the migration of health professionals is not to be underestimated, it has been less than was anticipated prior to EU accession. The 2003 migration survey predicted the departure of 5% of health professionals (Kallaste et al. 2004). However, after a relative peak in 2004, 1.8% of practising medical doctors, 1.0% of practising nurses and 1.4% of practising dentists showed migration intentions in 2005 (HCB unpublished data 2008).

The trend of health professionals returning to Estonia after 2004 is a less investigated topic. There are no statistics that affirm whether professionals return after practising abroad and the reasons for returning or staying are unclear because only unsystematized evidence is available.

5. Impacts on the Estonian health system

Health professional mobility's impact on health system performance has become an important feature of international health policy debate over the last few years, both within Europe and worldwide (Buchan 2008). As migration and health professional mobility become increasingly important for health systems and population health, these issues will require greater policy attention at the multilateral level (MacPherson et al. 2007). The migration of professionals, health-system impacts of international recruitment and related ethical concerns were also highlighted in the recent *Tallinn Charter: Health Systems for Health and Wealth* (WHO Regional Office for Europe 2008).

Only limited research has been carried out in Estonia (Kallaste et al. 2004 and section 8). The scant evidence available suggests that health professional mobility is not a major influencing factor but does have a limited impact on many fronts of the health system such as health financing, service delivery, training arrangements and overall policy and regulation. In general there is no proof that health workforce mobility alone affects service availability or waiting times. However, the inflow of medical doctors and dentists has had a positive impact in certain geographical regions of Estonia. Those few doctors and dentists arriving from the Russian Federation and Ukraine have reduced the lack of health professionals in north-eastern Estonia.

In media and policy debates the Estonian Medical Association and the Estonian Hospital Association have reported that the health professional labour shortage is caused mainly by emigration (Ministry of Social Affairs 2008b). While there are shortages of some specific types of professionals in certain regions, these are related to both domestic and international mobility and the small numbers of specialists in some specialties (such as thoracic surgery, pathology) in Estonia. Hence, the movement of only one or two specialists can affect the provision of health-care services in a particular area. As a result, smaller providers have been proactive in recruiting part-time specialists from bigger hospitals (Ministry of Social Affairs 2008b).

The outflow of health professionals has a negative impact on the efficiency of the education system and financing, especially when young graduates emigrate. One means of addressing the gaps in the health workforce caused by migration is to train more specialists. However, education cycles are rather long and so results can only be seen after several years (Kallaste et al. 2004). The migration of young doctors has launched a discussion on setting incentives to stay – for example, reclaiming training costs from graduate doctors or recruiting providers; mandatory service after graduation – but many of these could have unpredictable impacts on the health system.

Health workforce migration has exerted significant pressure on health system financing. Workforce costs have been particularly affected by the salary negotiations between the trade unions, health-care provider associations and the government. These began in 2004 and recent salary increases have been faster in the health and social sector than elsewhere (see section 8). Migration can be connected to these decision-making processes and further interaction is found between the issuing of certificates to work abroad and salary negotiations. The number of issued certificates has always increased at the time of state-level salary negotiations although that does not mean that all those who receive a certificate migrate. Likely some of these applications are intended to exert pressure on employers and the state during negotiations.

The financial crisis that began in 2008 has potential to influence migration trends in coming years but it is still too early for any sound evidence of this. In early 2009, the salaries of health professionals remained constant while average salaries in other sectors decreased (NIHD 2009). At the same time there was an increase in the number of requests for the certificates required to work abroad. In comparison to 2008, the number of certificates issued in 2009 increased by 34% for medical doctors, 38% for nurses and 74% for dentists (HCB unpublished data 2009). These sharp increases may have been caused by uncertainty about the future or influenced by health professionals' perceptions of changes taking place within the health-care sector in 2009 – this needs further research.

Estonia is a source country that currently does not suffer any significant loss of health professionals, therefore there is little impact on the health system. At the same time, health-care workforce migration has become an important part of policy and political discussions over the past years.

6. Relevance of cross-border health professional mobility

Cross-border health professional mobility has no major influence on the Estonian health workforce. Health professionals from foreign countries represent only 0.1%–0.2% of the active health workforce in the country (HCB unpublished data 2008).

Between 2004 and 2009 the emigration of Estonian health professionals was not as high as forecast in several studies. More important challenges are posed by the ageing of doctors and dentists and retaining qualified professionals working in the health-care sector.

6.1 *Distributional issues influencing composition of the health workforce*

Regional variations and specialties

Despite the financial crisis, there is no information on a potential increase in unemployment in Estonian health care (Ministry of Social Affairs 2008a & 2009). The current situation in the medical doctor labour market is best characterized by a limited shortage in specific specialties (family medicine, anaesthesia, psychiatry, pathology and gynaecology) (see also section 5) and geographical regions (especially rural areas). Currently, a key problem is the lack of family doctors in small border municipalities and some small islands where family physicians from neighbouring areas often substitute for their colleagues. One proposal to address this problem involves cooperation between the University of Tartu and county governments in order that family doctors carrying out their residencies may be channelled temporarily to underserved rural areas.

It is difficult to recruit enough nurses in rural areas. Also, the nursing shortage has been increased by a relatively high number of nurses leaving the health sector (Ministry of Social Affairs 2008).

Attrition: registered health professionals exiting the health sector

The health professionals who move to other Member States are having less impact than the number of registered medical doctors and nurses who do not provide health-care services. Between 2004 and 2008, the number of doctors and nurses wishing to migrate showed a tendency to decrease. However, the number of doctors working outside the health-care sector appears to be increasing. In 2008, 20% of registered doctors and 23% of registered nurses worked outside the health-care sector (see also Tables 9.3 and 9.5). These health professionals usually find employment in pharmaceutical companies, government ministries and their agencies or other employment sectors (HCB 2008).

Ageing of health professionals

Estonian medical doctors are characterized by a high mean age (49.7 years) and a high number of women (74%) (HCB unpublished data 2008). Specialized doctors with the highest mean ages are internists (mean age 56); neurologists (55); and gynaecologists, oncologists and pathologists (54 for all). The ageing of Estonian health professionals is a very serious concern. The HCB registry indicates that 26% of doctors, 23% of dentists and 8% of nurses are 60 years or older. Most of them may retire in the near future although many medical doctors (79%) and nurses (59%) of retirement age continue to provide services (HCB unpublished data 2008), thereby reducing the shortages in some geographical areas.

6.2 *Educational system*

In Estonia, the education of health professionals is coordinated centrally with a state budget for training health professionals. The Ministry of Education and Research sets admission quotas for publicly funded state-commissioned student places. These are based on proposals by the Ministry of Social Affairs and agreed by the university, medical colleges and professional associations.

In addition, there are both state-commissioned and private student places for which students pay tuition fees. These students have the right to apply for any publicly funded places that become available during the study period. Private student places constitute 10% of all student places at the University of Tartu and the two health-care colleges.

Each year, 15 to 17 foreign students are accepted for undergraduate studies in medicine – 11% of all commissioned student places. Of these foreign students, 80% come from Finland. The University provides the first year's study in English but the rest of the training is in Estonian. Medical or dental training is followed by a three to five year residency. All residency programmes (postgraduate medical training programmes) are fully state-financed from the budget of the Ministry of Social Affairs (Parliament of Estonia 1995a & 1995b). Foreign students tend to leave after graduation from the basic training in medicine as postgraduate training may be more easily accessible in their native countries. Residency places in Estonia are limited to 90% of undergraduate training places and there is fierce competition.

Nursing education is provided mainly in Estonian and no foreign students have undertaken nursing studies since 1998. One health-care college provides some curricula in Russian in the first year and intensive Estonian language courses in north-eastern Estonia where residents are principally Russian-speaking.

Statistics from health-care colleges show that 80% of graduate nurses start work within their specialties. Unfortunately, there is a lack of further information on their career paths – for example, time spent in initial posts, intention to leave the health sector or migrate. There is no up-to-date official survey of the migration rate among Estonian health graduates. It would be appropriate to conduct such a survey in order to estimate the true figure.

In conclusion, the Estonian health education system has not been attractive to foreign students. However, health professional training in Estonia meets EU directives and fosters the outflow of Estonian health professionals to other Member States. This is especially popular among resident doctors who often complete part of their studies abroad (mostly in Finland).

6.3 *Implications of cross-border mobility*

The annual trends in health professional mobility to Estonia show insignificant inflows of doctors, nurses and dentists. However, those few doctors and dentists from the Russian Federation and Ukraine who remained working in Estonia are important for ensuring the sustainability of service provision in the hospitals of some underserved geographical areas (the islands and north-eastern Estonia). As in other Organisation for Economic Co-operation and Development (OECD) countries, foreign-trained doctors in Estonia have mainly contributed to filling service gaps in rural areas (Dumont et al. 2008).

Emigration of Estonian health professionals since EU accession has not been as high as anticipated. The ageing of medical doctors, nurses and dentists and the relatively high number of health professionals exiting the health sector pose greater challenges for workforce sustainability.

7. Factors influencing health professional mobility

In 2003, Estonian health sector professionals were surveyed on their willingness to work abroad. Results showed that about half would like to work abroad, either permanently or temporarily, and around 5% had definite plans to move. The regression models showed that migration intention depends on the usual sociodemographic and economic variables such as age, sex, marital status, home region, job security and dissatisfaction with current wages. The main reasons for wanting to work abroad were the expectation of higher salaries and better working conditions; the main obstacle was leaving family and home in Estonia (Kallaste et al. 2004).

The number of nurses willing to work abroad decreased between 2004 and 2006. The survey also revealed that the preferred duration of stay had changed over these two years – those with a definite plan to move abroad had decreased from 5.2% to 2.4%. The share of nurses willing to find seasonal jobs abroad had increased from 24.7% in 2003 to 47.9% in 2005 (Aaviksoo et al. 2006).

Although salary was continually cited as the main reason to emigrate, its relative share as a motivating factor decreased. Professionals' disappointment with the health-care system diminished and the opportunity to gain work experience was mentioned as a more important goal than it was in the earlier survey (Aaviksoo et al. 2006).

The highest willingness to move abroad was seen in medical doctors aged 30–39, followed by younger medical doctors and nurses in the 20–29 age group (Fig. 9.1). It appears that younger nurses are motivated to move abroad by

Fig.9.1 *Health professionals intending to migrate from Estonia, cumulative numbers, 2004–2008*

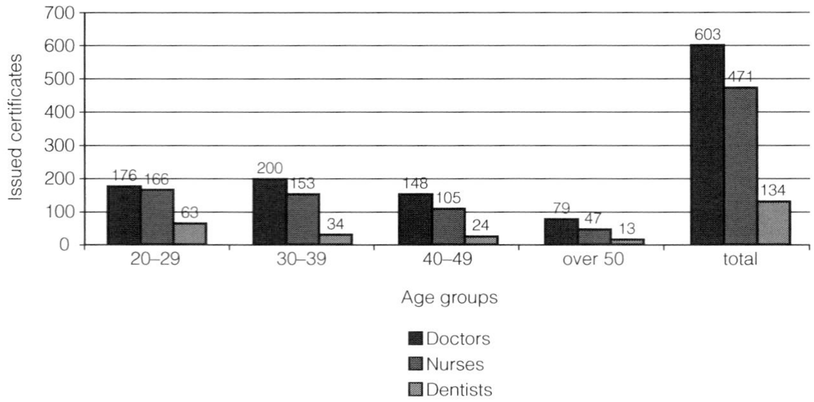

Source: HCB unpublished data 2008 & 2009.

higher salaries and their living situation since younger people tend not to have started families (HCB 2008, Kallaste et al. 2004).

8. Policy, regulation and interventions

Estonia has no specific policy on health professional mobility. Approved by the government in 2008, the *National Health Plan 2009–2020* includes some targets for human resources for health. However, the migration of health professionals is not mentioned in this or in other related programmes. Hence, the mobility of the health workforce is an underdeveloped policy issue in Estonia.

Health migration has been the subject of several studies (Aavikso et al. 2006, Estonian Migration Foundation 2006, Kallaste et al. 2004) and of media debate but there are no specific policies or programmes at governmental level. Migration policies make no distinction between general migration and health migration – both are based on the same principles and follow the same regulations. Managed migration means migration as provided by law – registration of the foreign labour-force (how many people and from which country), equal treatment and sufficient information concerning rights and obligations (Estonian Migration Foundation 2006).

The absence of any formal policy on health professional mobility and migration topics also means that the government does not actively recruit health professionals from other countries. All immigrants in the health sector have acted of their own volition or been recruited by hospitals and other providers.

Estonia has launched several long-term health programmes aiming to find the best solutions to problems and to promote health at both state and local levels. During the last decade, there has been more discussion of access, efficiency and quality problems in health care and quality has become the keyword (Estonian Migration Foundation 2006).

The temporary movements of young health professionals who practise in other countries are another important aspect of migration. Motivation schemes for prompting the return of these doctors and nurses need additional focus from individual providers as well as the articulation of overall policy to balance the practise of other countries and providers that actively recruit from Estonia.

Salary increases for health professionals have been the only, albeit very effective, instrument used to reduce emigration over recent years. On 1 January 2005, a minimum salary level agreement came into force between health professionals (medical doctors and nurses), trade unions, health-care provider associations and the state. It is highly likely that this has had a retention effect on health professional mobility (HCB 2008). A further agreement was signed in January 2006 to provide additional annual increases of minimum income in 2006, 2007 and 2008. There have been no subsequent salary negotiations at state level; specific salary levels are decided and defined at individual provider levels.

Health professionals who provide outpatient and inpatient care in hospitals are usually salaried employees. As the salary agreement extends to all practising doctors and nurses, there is no minimum salary difference between the hospitals and the ambulatory sector. However, many high-level providers of health-care services in certain designated hospitals pay higher hourly wages than the established minimum.

Health-care providers are either private entities (family medicine) or under public ownership but working under private legislation (hospitals). The Ministry of Social Affairs and, more recently, the NIHD monitor the financial status of providers and overall salary levels using statistical accounts and by facilitating an annual salary survey. The data mainly reflect average base salaries (Table 9.9) (NIHD 2008).

The national gross average income in Estonia has increased twice over the last six years; the salaries of health professionals have increased more frequently (2.5–2.8 times). This has been the outcome of a policy prioritizing health professionals, further supported by additional revenues in the health insurance system during the period of economic growth (EHIF 2009).

However, the economic crisis has led to reductions in overall salaries and raised the unemployment rate in 2008 and 2009. Latest data from the first quarter of 2009 show a continuous increase in the salaries of medical doctors (reaching up

Table 9.9 *Average monthly gross salaries (€) of health personnel in Estonia, 2002–2008*

	2002	2004	2006	2008	Increase between 2002 and 2008
Medical doctor	625	818	1126	1609	157%
Nurse	296	364	526	855	188%
Nursing assistant[1]	182	219	302	494	171%
Country-averaged monthly salary	366	431	549	788	115%

Source: NIHD 2009b. *Note*: nursing assistant education is based on practical training in the workplace or completion of a one-year course at health college.

to 2.2 times the country's average salary) but a slight decrease in the salaries of nurses and nursing assistants. The base salary has also increased but the shares of performance and bonus payments have decreased considerably (NIHD 2009). Overall, the health sector has seen smaller salary decreases and lower levels of unemployment than other economic sectors.

Dentists and their services are not covered by the salary agreement but dentists' salaries have been higher than those of other health professionals. The Estonian Health Insurance Fund (EHIF) purchases dental care for children but adult dental care is not included in the benefit package (except monetary subsidies for the elderly). Patients in Estonia make direct payments to providers who are free to set their own price levels. Providers have become less interested in applying for EHIF contracts as prices in dental care have risen and there has been increasing demand for (more profitable) adult dental care since economic growth began in 2004 (Koppel et al. 2008).

8.1 *Workforce planning and development*

Although there is no general migration policy for health professionals in Estonia, health professional mobility has been taken into account in the planning process led by the Ministry of Social Affairs in order to inform the Ministry of Education and Research and the training institutions (Ministry of Social Affairs 2008).

The continuous planning and monitoring of health professionals takes place at state level. This includes analysis of the dynamics of how many professionals have migrated and how many are working outside the health sector. Moreover, the Ministry of Social Affairs has financed several studies to map the outflow readiness of health professionals and their satisfaction with the working environment in Estonia (Aavikso et al. 2006; Kallaste et al. 2004).

The current health workforce planning model was developed by the Ministry of Social Affairs in 2005. It aims to improve human resource planning in the health-care system and to calculate the annual demand for training. The model takes account of the age profile of health professionals, migration, existing hospital network and planned capability for providing health-care services. A remarkable increase in the annual intakes of new medical students (from 110 to 140), medical residents (from 110 to 120) and general nurses (from 260 to 300) resulted from the planning model from 2005 to 2008.

The Ministry of Social Affairs considers 30 doctors and 80 nurses per 100 inhabitants to be the optimal rate for the next 10 to 15 years and is planning to continue funding annual admissions of 130 to 140 new medical students, 120 to 125 new medical residents and 300 general nurses (Ministry of Social Affairs 2008). The efficiency of health workforce planning is affected by the availability of financial resources for education, the capacity of the schools and sufficient numbers of candidates for admission (Ministry of Social Affairs 2008).

The most underdeveloped issue in workforce planning is how to draw medical doctors and nurses working outside the sector back into the health system. This has been discussed in the Ministry of Social Affairs but no policy has been introduced. Moreover, the active recruitment practices of some Scandinavian countries makes it even more difficult for the government to plan the needs of the health workforce as migration is induced by the demand side abroad rather than the domestic supply side (Estonian Migration Foundation 2006).

8.2 Cross-border regulatory frameworks and interventions

Mutual recognition of diplomas in the European Community

Since accession to the EU, the diplomas of Estonian medical doctors, nurses, midwives and pharmacists have been treated in accordance with diplomas awarded by other Member States (European Parliament and Council of the European Union 2005). An automatic recognition procedure applies to diplomas that meet EU educational standards. The Health Services Organization Act requires those with "Soviet-time diplomas" to have at least three years working experience in their own country before they are entitled to work in another Member State (Parliament of Estonia 2001).

In Estonia, three main legal acts harmonize the sectoral directives of medical doctors, dentists, nurses responsible for general care, midwives and pharmacists. Coordination of training in all professions is regulated by the University of Tartu Act (Parliament of Estonia 1995); the Health Services Organization Act and the Medicinal Product Act cover the registration and recognition of diplomas (Parliament of Estonia 2001; Parliament of Estonia 2004).

The Health Services Organization Act states that the HCB (now the Health Board – HB) bears responsibility for checking and monitoring the qualifications of medical doctors, dentists, nurses and midwives and ensuring that they meet the requirements.

The HB registration procedure is regulated under the Health Services Organization Act and regulations of the Minister of Social Affairs. Registration is compulsory for the provision of health-care services and pharmacy services in Estonia. Registration is a one-time action with a fee of €64 (1000 Estonian kroon); EU and Estonian citizens have the same registration conditions (Koppel et al. 2008; Parliament of Estonia 2001).

In conclusion, the EU directive on the mutual recognition of qualifications (European Parliament and Council of the European Union 2005) has been fully implemented into Estonian law. Estonia has a relatively liberal system for recognition of EU diplomas based on EU qualifications (applicant must have a diploma issued in the EU) rather than citizenship. The HB has reported no significant problems with the recognition process and free movement of health professionals within the EU is ensured.

Third-country health professionals

The HB assesses the compliance of the qualifications of non-EU nationals and may require them to take aptitude tests or complete probation periods (probation period was applied until 2007). Registration takes around two months but, once registered and employed by an Estonian health-care provider, non-EU nationals have the same wage conditions and opportunities for professional and career development as Estonian medical doctors and nurses. Also, there are no differences in access to undergraduate and postgraduate medical training (Parliament of Estonia 2001).

8.3 Bilateral agreements

Estonia is not involved in any official bilateral agreements but an informal memorandum was signed between Estonian and Finnish medical associations in 2005. This memorandum provides an umbrella to facilitate the mobility of medical doctors in both directions, giving guidelines on working requirements and providing relevant information such as contact points or trade unions in both countries.

The Estonian Nurses Union has not reported any similar collaboration with foreign nursing associations. Indeed, the organization has publicly announced the avoidance of any cooperation with foreign recruitment companies because it considers such practices to be unethical (Ilves 2007).

9. Conclusion

Analysis of the movement of human resources in the health system over the 2004–2009 period indicates that 709 medical doctors, 605 nurses and 174 dentists applied for and obtained certification of their professional qualifications to allow them to work in another EU country. Approximately half of the health professionals with certification actually left Estonia. In 2008, the proportions of individuals with certification represented 1.8% of practising medical doctors, 1.2% of practising nurses and 1.9% of practising dentists. Data for 2009 show significant increases on the numbers of certificates issued to the three professions in 2008 (medical doctors +34%, nurses +38%, dentists +74%) (HB unpublished data 2010). The financial and economic crisis also affects the health sector and is likely to encourage emigration among health professionals. Scandinavian, especially Finnish, health-care institutions employ active recruitment practices – providing information and covering travel and language-learning costs. These may also increase the number of health professionals leaving Estonia in the near future.

Among different age cohorts the biggest desire to move abroad was seen in younger health professionals aged 20–29, followed by the 30–39 age group (HCB unpublished data 2008). This may be connected to the fact that younger people usually have not started families, as this can curtail the desire to emigrate (Kallaste et al. 2004). Furthermore, younger individuals often move abroad for professional development purposes. The five most popular destinations are Finland, the United Kingdom, Sweden, Germany and Norway. Analysis of specializations (based on certification information) shows that doctors with no specialization constitute the largest group of emigrants, followed by family doctors, anaesthetists, radiologists and general surgeons (HCB unpublished data 2008).

Although Estonia loses a moderate number of health professionals to other countries, medical doctors and nurses who choose to work outside the health-care sector pose a more significant problem to the sustainability of the system (HCB 2008). The combined effect of attrition, migration and retirement will inevitably reduce the number of medical doctors and nurses in the near future. The number of doctors meets current targets in the National Health Plan for 2020 but there is a clear lack of nurses. A doctor's education takes an average of 10 years and therefore it is virtually impossible to respond to short-term shortages by using the intake in training. However, health-care providers have the potential to retain workers through targeted measures such as higher salaries and improved working conditions. A similar approach is visible among nurses where adjustments to training alone (such as higher intakes; modifying the curricula of medical schools to suit modern health system needs) might not be sufficient.

Between EU accession in 2004 and the economic growth that continued until 2008, the health workforce saw favourable working conditions and income levels. Salaries for medical doctors and nurses increased faster than the overall average and reached reasonable levels in the country. This is likely to have limited health workforce outflows. However, the situation has changed since the second half of 2008 – the financial and economic crisis has exerted moderate pressure and produced changes in the health system, although it is still too early to draw final conclusions.

In summary, international migration alone is not the largest problem currently facing the Estonian health system but it does need to be monitored closely. The key issues related to medical doctors and nurses are ageing and working outside the health sector. Mechanisms and policies should be developed at country level to steer and incentivize the health workforce in the decentralized Estonian system in which many push and pull factors that affect health professionals rest with individual health-care providers.

References

Aaviksoo A et al. (2006). *Eesti õdede töökeskkond ja motivatsioonitegurid: mõju tervishoiutöötajate töömotivatsioonile, tulemuslikkusele, migratsioonile ning võimalikud poliitikavalikud* [*Working environment and motivation factors of nurses in Estonia: impact on working motivation, performance and migration of health-care professionals, possible political choices*]. Tallinn, PRAXIS Center for Policy Studies (http://www.praxis.ee/ index.php?id=311, accessed 3 June 2009).

Atun RA et al. (2006). Introducing a complex health innovation – primary health care reforms in Estonia (multimethods evaluation). *Health Policy*, 79(1):79–91.

Buchan J et al. (2006). *Health worker migration in the European Region: country case studies and policy implications.* Copenhagen, WHO Regional Office for Europe.

Buchan J (2008). *How can the migration of health service professionals be managed so as to reduce any negative effects on supply?* Copenhagen, WHO Regional Office for Europe on behalf of the European Observatory on Health Systems and Policies.

Dumont C et al. (2008). *International mobility of health professionals and health workforce management in Canada: myths and realities.* (OECD Health Working Paper No. 40) (http://www.oecd.org/dataoecd/7/59/41590427.pdf, accessed 22 November 2009).

EHIF (2009). *Annual Report 2008*. Tallinn, Estonian Health Insurance Fund (http://www.haigekassa.ee/eng/ehif/annual, accessed 4 December 2009).

Estonian Migration Foundation (2006). *Managed migration and the labour market – the health sector. Small scale study.* (http://www.migfond.ee/user_upload/sss_ii tervishoiusektor_eesti__01.07.06.doc, accessed 3 June 2009).

European Parliament and Council of the European Union (2005). Directive 2005/36/EC of the European Parliament and of the Council of 7 September 2005 on the recognition of professional qualifications. *Official Journal of the European Union*, 255(48):22–142.

Habicht T, Habicht J (2008). Estonia: "good practice" in expanding health care coverage. In: Gottret P et al. *Good practices in health financing: lessons from reforms in low- and middle-income countries*. Washington DC, World Bank.

HCB (2008). *Health-care workers migration intention and registration information*. Tallinn, Health Care Board. (http://www.terviseamet.ee/tervishoid/tervishoiutootaja-registreerimine/aruandlus.html, accessed 1 June 2009).

Ilves L (2007). Soome ootab Eesti meditsiiniõdesid [Finland expects Estonian nurses]. *Lääne Elu*, 22 March 2007 (http://www.le.ee/?a=uudised&h=2007/3/22, accessed 29 September 2010).

Kallaste E et al. (2004). *Migration intentions of health professionals: the case of Estonia*. Tallinn, PRAXIS Center for Policy Studies (http://www.praxis.ee/fileadmin/tarmo /Projektid/Too-ja_Sotsiaalpoliitika/ Tervishoiutootajate_migratsioon_Eestist/ 11_ labour_Migration.pdf, accessed 29 May 2009).

Koppel A et al. (2008). Estonia: Health system review. *Health Systems in Transition*, 10(1):1–230.

MacPherson D et al. (2007). Health and foreign policy: influences of migration and population mobility. *Bulletin of the World Health Organization*, 85(3):200–206.

Ministry of Social Affairs (2005). *Social sector in figures 2005*. Tallinn (http://213.184.49.171/eng/HtmlPages/social_sector_2005/$file/social_sector_2005.pdf, accessed 22 May 2009).

Ministry of Social Affairs (2006). *Social sector in figures 2006*. Tallinn (http://213.184.49.171/eng/HtmlPages/arvudes2006koosinglise/$file/arvudes2006koos%20inglise.pdf, accessed 22 May 2009).

Ministry of Social Affairs (2008a). *Health, labour and social sector in 2007*. Tallinn (http://www.sm.ee/fileadmin/meedia/Dokumendid/Sotsiaalvaldkond/inglisekeelsed/sotsmin_ENG_trykki_1_.pdf, accessed 22 May 2009).

Ministry of Social Affairs (2008b). *National Health Plan 2009–2020*. Tallinn (http://www.sm.ee/fileadmin/meedia/Dokumendid/ASO/RTA/National_ Health_Plan_2009_2020.pdf, accessed 22 May 2009).

Ministry of Social Affairs (2009). *Health, labour and social life in Estonia 2000– 2008*. Tallinn (http://www.sm.ee/meie/statistika.html, accessed 22 May 2009).

NIHD (2008). *Health-care statistics 1998–2005*. Tallinn, National Institute for Health Development (http://www.tai.ee/index.php?id=5840, accessed 22 May 2009).

NIHD (2009a). *Health-care statistics 2006–2009 (THT10)*. Tallinn, National Institute for Health Development (http://pxweb.ee/esf/pxweb2008/Dialog, accessed 22 May 2009).

NIHD (2009b). *Tervishoiutöötajate tunnipalk marts* [*Hourly wages of health-care workers in March 2009*]. Tallinn, National Institute for Health Development (http://www.tai.ee/?id=5625, 15 November 2009).

Parliament of Estonia (1995a). *Universities Act*. Tallinn (http://www.legaltext. ee/text/en/X60039K4.htm, accessed 1 June 2009).

Parliament of Estonia (1995b). *University of Tartu Act*. Tallinn (http://www. legaltext.ee/text/en/X70009K2.htm, accessed 1 June 2009).

Parliament of Estonia (2001) *Health Services Organization Act*. Tallinn (http:// www.legaltext.ee/text/en/X40058K6.htm, accessed 22 May 2009).

Parliament of Estonia (2004). *Medicinal Product Act*. Tallinn (http://www. legaltext.ee/et/andmebaas/paraframe.asp?loc=text&lk=et&sk=en&dok=X9000 9k2.htm&query=ravimiseadus&tyyp=X&ptyyp=RT&pg=1&fr=no, accessed 22 May 2009).

Rechel B et al. (eds.) (2006). *The health-care workforce in Europe: learning from experience*. Copenhagen, WHO Regional Ofice for Europe on behalf of the European Observatory on Health Systems and Policies.

WHO Regional Office for Europe (2008). *The Tallinn Charter: health systems for health and wealth*. Copenhagen (http://www.euro.who.int/document/E91438. pdf, accessed 30 September 2010).

Chapter 10

From melting pot to change lab central Europe: health workforce migration in Hungary

Edit Eke, Edmond Girasek, Miklós Szócska

1. Introduction

Health professional mobility affects Hungary in numerous ways. Between 2004 and 2009, about 7000 Hungarian medical doctors, nurses and dentists applied for certification to work abroad (Table 10.1); between 2004 and 2008, 2329 foreign medical doctors, nurses and dentists registered in the country (Tables 10.6–10.8). There are indications that the outflow of health professionals,[1] combined with other adverse factors affecting the health workforce, endangers the sustainability of the Hungarian health-care system even in the short term. A significant number of the professionals who are thinking about leaving are in their professional prime and their professional distribution further upsets shortage patterns in certain specialties. The need for strategies to retain health professionals and encourage their return has been discussed for years but, despite professional warnings and research evidence, the importance of the phenomenon is still neglected. Some measures were introduced by the government in June 2009 but as yet there is no comprehensive human resources for health strategy.

---

1 This study uses the term Hungarian health professional for individuals who were born in Hungary, are Hungarian citizens and undertook their basic medical training in Hungary. Native Hungarian minorities in the surrounding countries are considered separately.

In order to understand health workforce migration in Hungary, and throughout central Europe, various historical aspects should be taken into consideration. Hungary has suffered serious impacts from the geopolitical conflicts of the 20th century. These have produced long-lasting effects that can be identified in current mobility trends, for example, people of Hungarian origin migrating back to Hungary and the broad international migration network of Hungarian diasporas in other countries.

Various waves of migration have been triggered by specific historical turning points. The 1920 Treaty of Trianon following the First World War removed and reassigned two thirds of the country's territory and resulted in 3.3 million ethnic Hungarians living in neighbouring countries. The end of this war and the following recession generated the first major wave of Hungarians migrating to Hungary and outflows from the Carpathian Basin to various parts of the world.

Further major rounds of emigration occurred after the Second World War as a result of changing political circumstances. Thus, generations of migrating Hungarian intellectuals and health professionals became established in host countries and created networks of community support. This study will describe the migration trends of health professionals entering and leaving Hungary across three periods: (i) 1945–1989; (ii) 1990–2004; and (iii) 1 May 2004–31 December 2009. It covers the volumes and directions of these movements; the role of European Union (EU) accession; the impact and relevance of inflows and outflows in the heath system and its workforce; and the factors influencing mobile health professionals, as well as the policies and instruments which surround the issue of health professional mobility in Hungary.

Limitations of the study

There have been difficulties with the availability, quality and validity of data as well as gaps in data continuity over time. This is partly due to the lack of proper consistency in data collection methods and to data holders changing repeatedly. Furthermore, most relevant and good quality data are recent, concerning the time after EU accession. There is political commitment (several legal changes were introduced in 2007 and 2008 to establish the legal background) to aggregate all human resources for health data into one database, managed by a single public data holder – the Office of Health Authorisation and Administrative Procedures (OHAAP), under the Ministry of Health. All existing human resources for health data files, mainly professional registries, have been transferred to OHAAP. The other main official data sources are the Hungarian Central Statistical Office (issues the annual Statistical Yearbook of Hungary and the Yearbook of Health Statistics), the Hungarian Medical

Chamber (HMC) and the Hungarian Chamber of Nurses and Allied Health Personnel, as well as other professional organizations, academic institutes and medical universities.

It is important to note that there are discrepancies even in the officially available data; OHAAP data are used wherever possible. Written sources are complemented by findings from expert and stakeholder interviews conducted from November 2007 to September 2009 with representative organizations (HMC, Council of the Hungarian Paramedic Professionals,[2] Hungarian Resident Doctors Association[3]); provider institutions (Hungarian National Ambulance and Emergency Service, county and city hospitals) and academic institutions (Semmelweis University, University of Debrecen, University of Pécs).

There are problems of interpretation and harmonization with international equivalents of human resources for health categories. These mainly concern two major difficulties with the nursing professions. Firstly, the registry of allied health workers comprises 30 categories and, while several of these concern nursing, there is no separate, well-defined subcategory for nurses. There is no national consensus on how many and which categories of allied health workers include data on nurses. Thus, international databases often take the number of allied health workers to be the number of nurses in Hungary, resulting in a significant overestimation. Secondly, the registry of allied health workers followed professions and specialties, rather than individuals. Individuals were re-registered (with a new number) with each new qualification in the relevant category. The number of individuals can be derived, but with some difficulties. Changes in the vocational education of nurses and allied health workers have also complicated data registry. Adjustments to the registry of allied health workers are in process to ensure simple and clear identification of individuals. Altogether less valid and consistent data are available for nurses and characteristically only for some time periods.

This study's conclusions remain tentative due to the lack of data, systematic reviews and research. Also, there is only anecdotal evidence for some mobility issues. Even so, the study is a first of its kind in collecting and analysing the material that is available.

This case study will begin by presenting Hungary's mobility profile in terms of the inflows and outflows of health professionals. This will be followed by examination of the importance of EU accession and health professional mobility's impact on the Hungarian health system. Next, there will be a discussion of the relevance of mobility and of other factors that influence the health workforce.

---

2 *Magyar Egészségügyi Szakdolgozói Kamara.*

3 *Magyar Rezidens Szövetség.*

Finally, an explanation of the motivations behind health professionals' decisions to leave or stay in the country will be followed by a description of the policies and interventions aimed at tackling health professional mobility.

2. Mobility profile of Hungary

2.1 *Cross-border mobility patterns of health professionals*

Data on cross-border movements since May 2004 indicate that Hungary has become a source country principally for western EU Member States. The estimated magnitude of outflows exceeds the measurable magnitude of inflows on several occasions. This holds true for all main health professional cadres which show relatively stable mobility patterns since May 2004.

Outflows

There are no data on the actual number of health professionals leaving Hungary but data on intention to work abroad come from two main sources. All health professionals who are Hungarian citizens or have obtained their diploma in Hungary must apply to the OHAAP (established in 2004) for certification (verification) in order to be able to work abroad.[4] Applicants have to pay for the document(s), the procedure is time-consuming and the certifications have temporary validity in most European countries. These data therefore reflect a relatively strong determination among the applicants. The second source stems from research. In 2004, The Semmelweis University Health Services Management Training Centre (SU HSMTC) and the Hungarian Resident Doctors Association started a project on migration research that evolved into a complex and comprehensive study of human resources for health. This is an ongoing study in which more than 4000 medical students (1st and 6th course) and resident doctors have responded to a questionnaire on their future plans, including their intention to work abroad and motivational background.

The available data on cross-border movements since May 2004 indicate that Hungary has become a source country, primarily for western EU Member States and secondly to non-European countries, mainly the United States of America. The mobility patterns of all main groups of health professional show slightly changing dynamics but overall have remained stable since May 2004 (Table 10.1).

---

4 There are seven kinds of certificates. The most important verify: (i) conformity, e.g. qualifications obtained in Hungary meet EU educational requirements and guidelines; (ii) vested interests, e.g. applicants who qualified before diplomas became EU conformant are entitled to EU recognition of titles; (iii) respectability, e.g. applicant has not been found guilty of professional misconduct.

Table 10.1 Applications for certification, by health professional group,[a] 1 May 2004–31 December 2009

Year	Medical doctors	Nurses	Dentists	Pharmacists	Midwives	Other health professionals	All categories
2004 (May-Dec.)	906	137	137	32	4	24	1 240
2005	889	285	78	33	4	91	1 380
2006	721	136	120	36	4	131	1 148
2007	695	160	114	29	6	115	1 119
2008	803	179	142	59	12	162	1 357
2009	887	419	158	37	7	106	1 614
Total	**4 901**	**1 316**	**749**	**226**	**37**	**629**	**7 858**

Source: OHAAP 2009. Note: [a] all applicants, whether residing in Hungary or elsewhere.

Table 10.2 *Health professionals resident in Hungary as proportions of all health professionals applying for certification, 1 May 2004–31 December 2008*

Year	Medical doctors resident in Hungary (%)	All medical doctors (100%)	Nurses resident in Hungary (%)	All nurses (100%)	Dentists resident in Hungary (%)	All dentists (100%)
2004 (May-Dec.)	504 (56%)	906	105 (77%)	137	71 (52%)	137
2005	604 (68%)	889	239 (84%)	285	60 (77%)	78
2006	520 (72%)	721	113 (83%)	136	84 (70%)	120
2007	590 (85%)	695	127 (79%)	160	83 (73%)	114
2008	730 (91%)	803	153 (85%)	179	117 (82%)	142
Total	**2 948 (73%)**	**4 014**	**737 (82%)**	**897**	**415 (70%)**	**591**

Source: OHAAP 2009.

Table 10.2 shows that a relatively high proportion of applicants were already residing abroad at the time of application. These should not be considered fresh migrants but rather reflect emigrant health professionals needing *retrospective* certification, presumably requested by their employers following EU accession in 2004. This hypothesis is supported by the fact that the highest proportion of applicants not resident in Hungary occurred in the year of accession in all three professional groups. Applicants can be Hungarian or foreign citizens independently of country of residence. Those residing in Hungary at the time of application indicate fresh emigration intentions, retrospective applicants residing outside the country signal that emigration has already taken place. Between 2004 and 2008, a total of 1066 medical doctors, 160 nurses and 176 dentists who had received their diplomas in Hungary applied for certification while living abroad.

Medical doctors and dentists show more intention to work abroad than nurses. Between 2004 and 2008, the annual percentages of total stocks of the three professional groups (see Tables 10.6–10.8) applying for certification were between 2% and 2.7% of medical doctors, 2% and 2.6% of dentists and around 0.2% of nurses (OHAAP unpublished data 2009). The certification data also support the findings of attitude surveys (Eke et al. 2009, Kovácsné Tóth 2004, SU HSMTC unpublished data 2003–2010). Data on validation requests obtained from several countries' foreign registry offices at one time point, September 2007, also confirm the magnitude of outflows. Some 2000 Hungarian medical doctors were registered between May 2004 and September 2007 in nine European countries (SU HSMTC unpublished data 2003–2010).[5]

5 Based on the official list of co-authorities provided by the OHAAP, all EU country authorities responsible for the

Table 10.3 *Declared target countries among all health professionals applying for certification, 1 January 2009–31 December 2009*[2]

	Number	(%)
Total applicants	**1 614**	**100**
Target countries		
1. United Kingdom	499	30.9
2. Germany	284	17.6
3. Italy	147	9.1
4. Austria	146	9.0
5. France	103	6.4
6. Sweden	100	6.2
1-6	**1 279**	**79.2**
Other countries	335	20.8

Source: OHAAP unpublished data 2009.

In 2009, the most popular destination countries were the United Kingdom and Germany, followed by Italy and by neighbouring Austria (Table 10.3).

Male medical doctors and nurses show most interest in migrating but interest is equal among male and female dentists (OHAAP unpublished data 2009). Examination of the age profiles and backgrounds of medical doctors[6] seeking to leave the country indicates that most applications come from those aged 30–39, followed by those aged 40–49 (OHAAP unpublished data 2009). Between 2004 and 2006, intention to migrate was seen mainly in doctors with a specialization rather than those with a diploma of general medicine. This tendency has changed and since 2007 specialists have represented a slightly smaller proportion of applicants. However, total numbers from EU accession until 31 December 2009 show that more specialists intended to migrate (Table 10.4). These include relatively important numbers with specializations that are in high demand (Table 10.5).

Before 1989, some carefully selected health professionals were able to work in non-socialist countries for specified periods. However, working abroad for longer periods or on a permanent basis resulted in automatic (that is, administratively initiated) loss of Hungarian citizenship and classification as an illegal emigrant (dissident). Between 1970 and 1987, 740 medical doctors

registration of foreign medical doctors were contacted by post or e-mail and asked to supply data on annual numbers of Hungarian medical doctors registered and entitled to work from 1 May 2004 until the time of request. Belgium, Denmark, Finland, France, Germany, Ireland, Portugal, Sweden and the United Kingdom supplied data showing a total of 2065 Hungarian medical doctors in these countries in the indicated period. OHAAP issued around 2980 certifications for medical doctors (eight months in 2004, 2005, 2006, eight months in 2007) in the same period.

6 Data not available for nurses and dentists.

Table 10.4 *Diplomas held by medical doctors[a] applying for certification, 1 May 2004–31 December 2009*

Year	Total number of applicants	Applicants with general medical doctor diploma		Applicants with specialist diploma	
		N	%	N	%
2004 (May-Dec.)	504	156	31.0	348	60.0
2005	604	143	23.7	461	76.3
2006	520	210	40.4	310	59.6
2007	590	320	54.2	270	45.8
2008	730	368	50.4	362	49.6
2009	887	474	53.4	413	46.6
Total	**3 835**	**1 671**	**43.6**	**2 164**	**56.4**

Source: OHAAP 2009. *Note*: [a] all applicants, whether residing in Hungary or elsewhere.

Table 10.5 *Specialties of medical doctors[a] applying for certification, 1 January 2009–31 December 2009*

Total number of medical doctors	887
Specialties	413
• Anaesthetics and intensive therapy	54
• General practice	43
• Internal medicine	25
• Ophthalmology	20
• Radiology	17
• Neonatology and paediatrics	14
• Orthopaedics	12
Other	228
General medical doctors (no specialization yet)[b]	474

Source: OHAAP unpublished data 2009. *Note*: [a] all applicants, whether residing in Hungary or elsewhere; [b] includes some (probably very few) specialists who did not give their specialization – presumably because they did not want to work in those fields abroad.

and 163 dentists left Hungary (Balázs 2004 & 2009, OHAAP unpublished data 2009).

Inflows of health professionals

Since May 2004, foreign health professionals who want to work in Hungary have been required to apply to the OHAAP for recognition of their qualifications. From 1 January 2000 until that date, the HMC was mandated to verify the diplomas of medical doctors and dentists and to maintain a registry. Membership of the HMC was mandatory and a prerequisite of employment until April 2007 when the legal roles of the HMC were transferred to the OHAAP. Registration with the OHAAP is now mandatory and HMC membership is voluntary.

Missing data make it challenging to estimate the number and proportion of foreign professionals in the health workforce. Non-EU citizens need a visa and a work permit (only aggregated data exist) but these are no longer required for EU citizens. The inflows include foreign citizens who trained in Hungary and stayed to practise in the country. Their number is estimated to be relatively low but exact data are not available.

The largest group of immigrant health professionals comprises Hungarians immigrating to Hungary. These are discussed in more detail below. If this group is excluded then the overall number and proportion of foreign health professionals is estimated to be small, although the proportion of non-Hungarian immigrants has increased. It is important to note that OHAAP data indicate the citizenship but not the native language of applicants. Consequently, for example, a Romanian citizen who applies for diploma recognition may be a native Hungarian or a native Romanian.

Between 2004 and 2008, a total of 639 foreign medical doctors, 1585 foreign nurses and 82 foreign dentists registered to practise in Hungary (Tables 10.6–10.8). In 2008, the proportion of foreign health professionals represented 3.6%, 1.3% and 3.7% respectively of the total (stock) for each of the three categories. For all three groups, immigrant health professionals are relatively younger and include a higher proportion of males than total stocks (OHAAP unpublished data 2009).

Table 10.6 *Foreign newly registered and all newly registered medical doctors (inflows); and foreign active and all active medical doctors (stock) in Hungary, 1 May 2004–31 December 2008*

Year	New registrations		Active medical doctors (stock)	
	All medical doctors	**Foreign medical doctors (%)**	**All medical doctors**	**Foreign medical doctors (%)**
2004 (May–Dec.)	1 124	154 (13.7%)	32 516	916 (2.8%)
2005	1 151	179 (15.6%)	33 017	1 067 (3.2%)
2006	1 069	148 (13.8%)	33 521	1 159 (3.4%)
2007	1 005	113 (11.2%)	33 105	1 207 (3.7%)
2008	960	45 (4.7%)	33 350	1 199 (3.6%)
Total	**5 309**	**639 (12.0%)**	**NA**	**NA**

Source: OHAAP unpublished data 2009.

Table 10.7 *Foreign newly registered and all newly registered nurses (inflows); and foreign active and all active nurses (stock) in Hungary, 1 May 2004–30 June 2009*

Year	New registrations		Active nurses (stock)	
	All nurses, n	Foreign nurses, n (%)	All nurses, n	Foreign nurses, n (%)
2004 (May–Dec.)	12 084	439 (3.6%)	97 498	919 (0.9%)
2005	9 888	420 (4.3%)	104 190	1 218 (1.2%)
2006	21 311	341 (1.6%)	110 592	1 366 (1.2%)
2007	7 984	195 (2.4%)	96 537	1 349 (1.4%)
2008	7 855	190 (2.4%)	91 537	1 217 (1.3%)
2009 (Jan–June)	1 937	23 (1.2%)	83 108	1 080 (1.3%)
Total	**61 059**	**1 608 (2.6%)**	**NA**	**NA**

Source: OHAAP unpublished data 2009.

Table 10.8 *Foreign newly registered and all newly registered dentists (inflows); and foreign active and all active dentists (stock) in Hungary, 1 May 2004–31 December 2008*

Year	New registrations		Active dentists	
	All dentists	Foreign dentists, n (%)	All dentists	Foreign dentists, n (%)
2004 (May–Dec.)	170	12 (7.0%)	5 247	150 (2.9%)
2005	163	21 (12.9%)	5 347	169 (3.2%)
2006	173	12 (6.9%)	5 442	171 (3.1%)
2007	192	19 (9.9%)	5 522	187 (3.4%)
2008	185	18 (9.7%)	5 513	203 (3.7%)
Total	**883**	**82 (9.3%)**	**NA**	**NA**

Source: OHAAP unpublished data 2009.

Particular mention should be made of the significant inflows of Hungarians immigrating to Hungary. The country is surrounded by neighbours that have significant Hungarian minorities – mainly Romania, Slovakia, Serbia, Ukraine and Austria.[7] Health professionals of Hungarian origin but holding foreign citizenship arrived in significant numbers, principally from Transylvania (Romania) but also from the countries of the former Yugoslavia, and peaked in

7 The last available data on the numbers of Hungarians in neighbouring countries were published on the web site of the Government Office for Hungarian Minorities Abroad (http://www.hhrf.org/htmh/en/), abolished in 2006. "According to the results of the censuses held around the millennium in each country in the Carpathian Basin, there are approximately 2.5 million Hungarians living in the neighbouring countries to Hungary. The most recent official figures regarding the number of Hungarians in the neighbouring countries are: Romania: 1,431,807 (2002); Slovakia: 520,528 (2001); Serbia and Montenegro (that time): 293,299 (2002); Ukraine: 156,600 (2001); Austria: 40,583 (2001); Croatia: 16,595 (2001); Slovenia: 6,243 (2002)."

1990. Generally, Hungarians living in the surrounding countries have not been considered to be foreigners; many Hungarian citizens in Hungary have roots in these countries or cross-border family relationships. Migration networks work effectively in such cases (see vignettes). Integration of these professionals may have been problematic at times but obviously there was no language barrier. These doctors and nurses have tended to settle in the north east of the country close to the Romanian, Slovakian and Ukrainian borders. Some are likely to have moved on to other countries after a short period of stay although no valid data are available.

Data are available on the inflows of medical doctors and dentists among the Hungarians moving to Hungary. Two main peaks can be observed. The first and most important was connected to the political changes of 1989–1990; the second followed Hungary's accession to the EU on 1 May 2004 (Balázs 2004 & 2009, OHAAP unpublished data 2009, Tables 10.9 & 10.10). Their distribution by specialties is not known but it appears that the first wave (1297 doctors, 290 dentists) included many specialists. The second wave (755 doctors and 107 dentists) comprised mainly younger medical doctors with newly obtained medical diplomas who moved to Hungary to start their residencies – first 26-month period of postgraduate medical training as resident doctor (Balázs 2004, 2005b & 2009). Tables 10.9 and 10.10 indicate the two four-year peaks within a twenty-year period (1988–2007) that accounted for the major part of the Hungarians immigrating to Hungary phenomenon.

Table 10.9 *Inflows of medical doctors of Hungarian descent, 1958–2008*

Time periods	Number of medical doctors	%
1958–2008	3 481	100
1988–1992	1 297	39.5
2003–2007	755	21.7
1988–2007	2 563	73.6

Sources: Balázs 2004 & 2009, OHAAP unpublished data 2009.

Table 10.10 *Inflows of dentists of Hungarian descent, 1972–2008[a]*

Time periods	Number of dentists	%
1972–2008	647	100
1988–1992	290	44.8
2003–2007	107	16.5
1988–2007	505	78.0

Sources: Balázs 2004 & 2009, OHAAP unpublished data 2009. *Note*: [a] no significant immigration of Hungarian dentists before 1972.

Data on Hungarians immigrating to Hungary also indicate that some movements took place during the Communist era and before EU accession. Hungary was a target country for immigration from other socialist countries; scholarship programmes among socialist countries were common and resulted in foreign professionals settling in the country and marrying Hungarian citizens. Many students, mainly from Africa and Cuba, studied at Hungarian medical schools but the difficulties of acquiring sufficient knowledge of Hungarian to undertake the same studies as native Hungarians increased the length of their training to as long as 10 years. It appears that substantial numbers of these students stayed to settle and work in Hungary after graduation but their precise numbers and motivation patterns are not known.

2.2 Summary

It seems that more is known about the inflows of health professionals from abroad than about outflows of Hungarian health professionals. Foreign health professionals who intend to work in Hungary can be accounted for as they must request certification from the OHAAP; data on outflows merely indicate (at best) a strong determination to work abroad. Still, these imperfect data indicate that Hungary is a source country rather than a destination. In 2008, the number of inflowing doctors (OHAAP recognized 64 foreign medical diplomas) was far lower than the estimated outflow (730 Hungarian-resident medical doctors requested certificates). Moreover, the apparently moderate share (about 2.5% per year since 2004) of medical doctors applying for certification amounts to almost 4000 medical doctors who applied for certification and potentially left the country between 2004 and 2009. Data from European countries' registry offices indicate that 2065 medical doctors from Hungary were registered abroad between 2004 and 2007.

3. Vignettes on health professional mobility

Hungarians immigrating to Hungary

PL is 50 years old and was born Hungarian in Brasov, Romania. He graduated in medicine at the University of Medicine and Pharmacy of Targu Mures, Romania.[8] He worked as a resident doctor in different specialties in hospital until November 1988 and within general practice until February 1989. PL married a Hungarian citizen and easily obtained work in the traumatology department of a county hospital in Hungary. He became a traumatologist in 1993. Since October 1996 PL has had permanent employment in the Medical Technology Department of a major pharmaceutical

---

8 This university provides theoretical training in Hungarian. Practical training is in either Romanian or Hungarian, depending on the native language of the patient.

company. Between 1997 and 2008 he also practised as a contracting physician (entrepreneurial contract) covering weekend shifts in traumatology.

KM is 29 years old, born Hungarian in Targu Mures, Romania and graduated in medicine at the University of Medicine and Pharmacy of Targu Mures Faculty of Medicine in 2004. Her husband, GZS, is also Hungarian and graduated from the same university. He was already working as a resident doctor in traumatology in Hungary when she started her residency in the rheumatology department of the same county hospital in 2005. They decided to move to Hungary while at university and a relative helped them to find work. Their main motivations were the option to choose their specialty, to use their native language at work and financial considerations (better salaries). They know many colleagues with similar backgrounds who work in Hungary.[9] GZS reports that most of his contemporaries live and work in Hungary. In the future, they are considering working in a western European country for some years but eventually want to live with KM's family in Hungary. KM has helped several acquaintances and a family member (from Transylvania, Romania) to find work in Hungary. Currently at home with her first child, KM's gross monthly salary is 100 000 forints (around €357). GZS earns a gross monthly salary of 110 000 forints (around €392) as he is close to his traumatology specialization exam. The couple applied for and obtained Hungarian citizenship within a year.[10]

Country of establishment changed, with long-term plans to stay abroad

ZSSZ graduated in medicine in Hungary in 2001 and became a general practitioner in 2009, at the age of 33. He worked in Hungary in the pharmaceutical industry for two years and as a general practitioner for six years, with more than one workplace at any one time. He migrated to England while his partner stayed in Hungary. Employed by a recruiting firm, he works as a resident medical officer in a private health-care provider's hospital on a contract running from January 2009 until the end of 2010. He usually goes home during leave as work cycles comprise two weeks work, one week leave; two weeks work, two weeks leave. He plans to stay in England for one to two years and has settled much better than expected.

In late 2007, several factors led ZSSZ to consider working abroad – working conditions, patient pathways that were impossible to follow, patient humiliation and constantly changing rules in Hungarian health care. The latest health reforms triggered his decision. In 2008, he began looking for work abroad mainly in Norway, Spain and other

9 Theoretically, it is possible to commute between Hungary and Romania along the eastern border but this is not common among health-care professionals. Conversely, there is strong anecdotal (but little scientific) evidence of Hungarian health professionals commuting daily/weekly across the western border in order to work in Austria.

10 Hungarian professionals from Romania who decide to work and settle in Hungary typically apply for Hungarian citizenship. This can run in tandem with their Romanian citizenship.

southern European countries. He registered on recruitment firm web sites but found his current job via a Hungarian acquaintance working in England who needed a partner to work in shifts. ZSSZ managed to obtain a contract and move within four weeks. He increasingly considers permanent work abroad but wants to visit other countries too. He wonders why he stayed so long at home in the hope that things would change and why the Hungarian health system has not collapsed yet. He shares his experiences and recommends his employer to acquaintances who ask for advice. Many friends already work abroad. His average net salary is £3300 for a three-week cycle, plus accommodation, meals and phone calls home and in England.

GE graduated in medicine in Hungary in 2004, aged 24. She started her residency in neurology in Budapest. Her first preference was neurosurgery but, as the only female applicant, she believes she stood no chance. She worked in Hungary for 18 months, 3 of which were spent in Finland on a Leonardo scholarship. Her partner, whom she already knew, is Finnish. Originally GE did not want to work abroad, but the contrast between her experiences at home and the stay in Finland made her decide to look for work there. She moved one year after deciding to leave. She began studying Finnish in Hungary and continued intensively for six months in Finland, from October 2006.

After one month probation, GE became a neurosurgery resident in Finland and was able to conduct research work in parallel. She has had very good experiences with the tutorial system; the supportive, helpful attitude of doctor colleagues ("you are treated like a slave, like a no-one as a resident in Hungary"); the well-organized health-care system; the transparency and the good official salary. She earns five times more than in Hungary and can double this with four duties per month (residents and medical doctors in Hungary often work more than five duties per month, payment is poor and residents are often unpaid). She sees a clear career pathway, both professionally and financially. This contrasts with Hungary where options are often determined by social/family networks. GE's mother is a practising medical doctor: "I saw the system and decided I did not to want to make my living out of informal payment".

GE is currently working on her PhD at Yale University in the United States of America. This opportunity arose through her Finnish workplace and she plans to return to Finland and continue her residency to become a neurosurgeon. One day she hopes to return and work in Hungary. She is not happy that she had to leave but would need many changes in the Hungarian health system before she would consider returning. These include a change of approach toward residents and junior doctors; changes to the rigid hierarchical system; transparent career pathways; the settlement of payment issues; cessation of the informal payment system and equal opportunities independent of gender, family and social relationships.

4. Dynamics of enlargement

EU accession has had an impact on health professional mobility to and from Hungary and has increased the importance and relevance of the issue, especially outflows of Hungarian health professionals. It is likely that health professional emigration (outflow) has increased since accession although precise evaluation is difficult as there are no available data on actual outflows. However, OHAAP data since May 2004 give a good comprehensive picture and reflect a strong intention to work abroad. Unfortunately, data on outflows between 1989 and May 2004 are entirely missing.

For Hungary and its surrounding countries, EU accession has not only opened the labour market for health professionals but also has led to deeper societal changes in perceptions and expectations. In turn, these influence migration patterns. The Hungarian health sector has faced important developments in recent years involving continuous and rapidly changing reform processes; radical financial restrictions; a resulting lack of transparency and consistency; and uncertainty. The population has experienced changes in the structure, range, quality and availability of health services, with many aspects raising serious questions regarding equity. For the health workforce, the unstable environment has meant deteriorating working conditions, social status and safety, as well as inadequate financial rewards.

Many observers have noted particularly that the general situation and options for the professional and career development of young professionals at the start of their careers have been worsening (Hodgson 2009). Again, there is no hard evidence as there has been no systematic research. On the other hand, expectations are rising. Since 1989, new generations of doctors, highly qualified nurses and other well-trained health professionals have emerged. Foreign languages are a prerequisite for university/college diplomas and these graduates are aware of the value of their qualifications. Unwilling to accept the system's traditional hierarchical structure and poor working conditions (including low salaries and informal payments), they are exploring alternative and more attractive professional and employment options. This was described by one of the health professionals interviewed for this study and echoed by others:

> *many young professionals are escaping from the Hungarian health-care system. They see the option to work abroad as a potential solution in which they do not have to leave their profession and can work in much better conditions, both professionally and elsewhere.*

At 4%–12%, the total migration potential[11] of Hungarians is generally low (Hárs et al. 2004). However, research by the SU HSMTC suggests that it is considerably higher among medical students and resident medical doctors – ranging between 60% and 72% with overall migration activity of 10%–20% (individuals who intend to work abroad and take active steps to do so) (Eke et al. 2009). The apparent contradiction between the research data on migration intention and OHAAP data on certification applications can be explained by several assumptions. Research data based on voluntary self-administered questionnaires reflect a less determined commitment than actual application to OHAAP. Medical students are still outside the labour market and may have idealistic pictures of their future but these are young ambitious individuals who speak foreign languages and have the option to enter the European labour market. Moreover, current medical training provides possibilities to obtain (EU-funded) scholarships and spend one or more semesters at medical university in another EU country, resulting in direct professional experience of other health systems. These are real and natural options for these young people who are aware of their opportunities and the value of a medical diploma in Europe.

The high total migration potential can also reflect the unfavourable changes in the Hungarian health system and especially the decreasing prestige of the Hungarian medical professions over the last years (whereas experiences abroad are highly regarded). The strong total migration potential among medical students and resident doctors can be interpreted as the result of a paradigm change in how new generations regard their position in society and options in the EU labour market, as well as a pathological phenomenon of the Hungarian health system and the career options it offers.

5. Impacts on the Hungarian health system

Currently, there is no available evaluation of how health professional mobility impacts on the health system and its functions[12] in Hungary (Girasek et al. 2009). However, it is estimated to have a significant impact on service delivery.

5.1 *Service delivery*

The inflow of health professionals of Hungarian origin between 1989 and 1992 is considered to have been crucial in maintaining the balance and sustainability of service delivery (Balázs 2004, 2005a & 2009). Immigrating Hungarian health professionals could find work easily and faced no language barriers; most

---

11 Total migration potential is a composite indicator containing all instances of intention to work abroad, short- or long-term, or to emigrate. The indicator is based on population surveys (Hárs Á et al. (2004).

12 For more information on health systems, their functions and objectives see WHO 2000.

of the 1297 medical doctors (Table 10.9) came from Romania (70% primary care; 54% specialist care) and Ukraine (16% primary care; 15% specialist care). Their geographical distribution in adult and mixed primary-care practices[13] indicates that they settled in the areas least favoured by domestic health professionals. These northern and eastern counties of Hungary have the lowest gross domestic product (GDP) but are close to the immigrants' countries of origin. The highest densities of immigrating Hungarian doctors in primary paediatric care and specialist care are found in Budapest and Pest counties, followed by the northern and eastern counties (Balázs 2004, 2005b & 2009). Domestic professionals favour the urban counties but cities still offer more job opportunities in paediatric and specialist care.

Before 1989, emigration from Hungary was treated as a criminal act. There are data on the volume of medical doctor outflows but the phenomenon was neither discussed nor analysed. In the years after 1989, there is likely to have been significant emigration but no valid data are available. Outflows since EU accession can be followed and data show a net outflow. The negative effects are openly discussed and some legal steps have been taken to prevent the outflow of young doctors (see section 5.2). Furthermore, the notable geographical inequalities in health professional distribution and health workforce shortages in rural and remote areas are likely to be exacerbated by health professional mobility. Specialists represent a significant proportion of outflows after May 2004 (OHAAP unpublished data 2009) (Table 10.4) and shortages are particularly important in specialties that can create major bottlenecks in health service delivery (including general practice, anaesthetics and intensive therapy, radiology). Outflows can have a crucial impact on small but vital diagnostic specialties (such as pathology) which have only a small number of resident posts. Hence, service delivery may be seriously affected by the potential loss of a few pathologists, even if a low absolute number, for example in a geographical region in which the only pathologist is emigrating.

5.2 *Resource creation and stewardship*

Currently there is no official strategy to attract foreign health professionals to Hungary. However, it is noteworthy that the idea of Hungarians immigrating to Hungary was informally encouraged among medical doctors and dentists between 1989 and 1991. Since EU accession, health professional mobility has made its way onto the political agenda via two (non-binding) policy documents. More concretely, measures to improve retention were introduced in 2009 through a new system of postgraduate medical training (see section

13 Hungary has three types of primary-care practice: (i) adult; (ii) paediatric; (iii) mixed. All have mandatory service delivery tasks. General practitioners can be either entrepreneurs (more than 90%) or state employees.

8.2). Presumably this was in response to increasing concerns over the migration of Hungarian health professionals, mainly medical doctors.

Professional mobility and (mainly) outflows are reported to impact on health service delivery and responsiveness and have exacerbated the deterioration of human resources for health over recent years (see also section 6). In combination with other factors, shortages of health professionals impact in varying degrees according to the level of care, specialty or geographical distribution. In tacit acknowledgement of these difficulties, health-care policy has been formulated as a direct reaction by seeking to introduce legal restrictions on migration and through ongoing efforts to try to limit outflows. Unfortunately, the lack of any comprehensive systematic research or impact assessment makes it difficult to measure the direct impact of migration.

6. Relevance of cross-border health professional mobility

In order to understand health professional mobility's role in the Hungarian health system, mobility must be seen in the context of wider health workforce issues. These include regional misbalances in personnel distribution; ageing of the health workforce; staff shortages in nursing and certain medical specialties; cuts in education capacity; attrition of health professionals to other economic sectors; and reforms leading to reductions in staff levels. In addition, the health system faces extra pressures caused by the underdeveloped social and complementary care sectors. Each of these issues affects the supply of and/ or demand for the health workforce and potentially may be aggravated by Hungarian health professionals leaving the country.

6.1 *Composition of the health workforce*

There are significant shortages and distributional imbalances in many regions of the country and in certain specialties, although to varying degrees. The distribution of human resources for health is uneven between the levels, forms and types of health care, cadres and specialties. There is a striking discrepancy between the expressed objectives of health policy and this uneven distribution. For example, strengthening of the role of primary care is a top priority but is not reflected in distribution of the health workforce. There are no incentives to manage and rectify the imbalances.

Levels of care

The Hungarian health system is centred on inpatients and the workforce distribution generally reflects the system's focus on, and cultural preferences for, medical and inpatient care. The need to shift towards outpatient and primary care is widely accepted and a declared policy priority but the speed, methods and justifications offered for structural change have raised strong doubts and objections. Moreover, the health system is challenged further by insufficient and inadequate funding and management of social care (for example, for individuals/families in crisis situations), support services (for example, home and residential care for elderly people) and complementary treatment facilities (for example, rehabilitation).

Geographical disparities

There are significant geographical inequalities in the distribution of health professionals – by region; level and type of care; profession and specialty; and living standards (Fig. 10.1). Medical doctors and dentists prefer to work in cities (especially in and around university cities) and more developed regions. There are shortages of health professionals in rural and remote areas and these may worsen as the health workforce emigrates. Primary health-care posts have been vacant for years (sometimes for as long as two decades) in some parts of the country. Locums have ensured the provision of some degree of functional service in these mainly rural and remote areas.

Fig.10.1 *Registered and active medical doctors per 10 000 population by geographical units, 2006[14]*

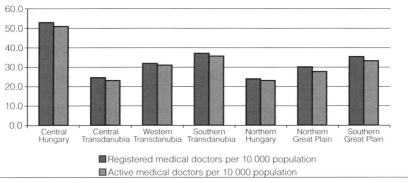

■ Registered medical doctors per 10 000 population
■ Active medical doctors per 10 000 population

Source: Hungarian Central Statistical Office 2007.

Shortages among specialists and nurses

Most doctors, particularly specialists, are concentrated in the capital and the main cities. Conversely, more than half of the current nursing vacancies are in Budapest.

The available official database provides data on several aspects of projected jobs and vacancies, including geographical distribution, but there are no further

---

14 Active medical doctors have active employment and fulfil the requirement of continuous medical education. Their entitlement to work is renewed regularly (every five years). The Hungarian medical and nursing professions have two types of registries: (i) Basic – one-off automatic entry on graduation; (ii) Active (operational) – for active professionals only, individuals apply for registration that must be renewed periodically (fulfilling requirements).

groupings according to most specializations. Also, the approved/projected number of staff posts does not reflect actual local demand and need according to the health status, morbidity and mortality rates of the population.[15]

Shortages concern medical specialties such as primary care, anaesthetics and intensive therapy, radiology and oxyology,[16] but many others are also understaffed. For example, specialists in paediatrics and neurology argue that recent trends indicate critical shortages, even in the short run. Lack of sufficient medical staff has already caused one paediatric department to close.

While nurses appear to be less interested in emigrating (Table 10.1), shortages of nurses and other allied health professionals are more serious in many areas. Understaffing is due mainly to low salaries, poor working conditions, heavy workloads and insufficient qualified personnel. These problems are particularly apparent in the capital city and several of the experts interviewed suggested that this is because better paid employment opportunities are available elsewhere. Many nursing directors report that even a small increase in salary is enough to make nurses leave to work in supermarkets or shopping centres. Work opportunities are more limited in the countryside but it is increasingly challenging to maintain supplies of nurses there too. Moreover, nursing services are supported by a relatively high proportion of allied health personnel who continue working after retirement age. Health leaders are warning that new legislation to ban this practice will aggravate undersupply.

6.2 Factors influencing size and composition of the health workforce

Educational system

Changes in vocational nurse education have contributed to nursing shortages. Before 1993, primary-school leavers (aged 14 years) could enrol on either a three-year programme of basic nursing education or a four-year course to train as a nurse, thereby gaining a secondary school vocational nursing certificate (giving access to higher education and university). Those entering three-year full-time training now must be at least 18 years old and require a secondary school certificate. The change has raised the average age of entry to the labour market from 17/18 to 22 years. In addition, recent transformations of the vocational education system have led to the closure of many institutions and

---

15 Historically, the distribution, volume, structure, etc. of health facilities (including the numbers and composition of the health workforce) were influenced less by objective considerations and more by political intentions and power. This inherited health system basically defines human resources for health patterns. Several attempts to restructure and reorganize the system on a professional and functional basis, and many changes, have not addressed workforce issues comprehensively. Only a few studies have explored human resources for health needs according to the listed factors; financial constraints and political influences have made it difficult to implement their recommendations.

16 Oxyology (emergency medicine) is a separate specialty in Hungary. Oxyologists generally work in emergency and intensive care units and as specialists in the Hungarian National Ambulance and Emergency Service.

drastically reduced training capacities. Experts[17] agree that this is currently the most serious bottleneck of health workforce supply.

In medical education, more than 1000 degrees were awarded annually between 1976 and 1982. However, numbers have not exceeded 1000 per year since 1988 and have fallen below 800 since 1996 (Balázs 2009). One unresolved issue is the lack of regulation to deal with the integration of medical doctors returning from abroad with a foreign basic medical education or specialization.

Retirement and demographics

Shortages can be expected as the older generation of physicians retires (Balázs 2009). The age pyramid of active physicians shows increases in older age groups, with variations by specialties and geographical areas, but is especially apparent in family medicine, radiology and rheumatology. The tendency has been increasing since the early 1990s and the supply of medical doctors does not balance the wastage rate. The situation is similar for allied health personnel, especially in nursing. At present, many medical doctors and nurses work after retirement age and contribute to the sustainability of health care.

Health professionals leaving or returning to the profession

Although this phenomenon is considered to be important in several health professions (especially among medical doctors and nurses), there are no valid data on the numbers of drop-outs during training or after a period working in health care, or on changes of career after graduation. Pharmaceutical companies are the most important alternative employers of medical doctors.

Data from the Hungarian Central Statistical Office (2008) show that there were 35 763 registered medical doctors and 32 202 active medical doctors in Hungary in 2007. Theoretically, comparison of these figures should provide an estimate of the number of leavers, including those who emigrate. However, this does not allow discrimination between types of attrition (Balázs 2003). Similarly, there are no data on health professionals who return to the health labour market, including those who re-enter the system after working abroad.

The health workforce has been significantly affected by ongoing health system transformations since April 2007, including a huge cut in the number of hospital beds (concerning about 10% of the hospital sector) over a period of a few months. Figures from the Ministry of Health and estimates in the press indicate that around 6000 people (1100 medical doctors; 4500 allied health personnel, mainly nurses) lost their jobs but confirmed numbers and the actual proportion of loss for the sector are not currently available (Világgazdaság 2007). A mobility

---

17 Interviews with and information released (at conferences, in the press) by nurse leaders, including Zoltán Balogh, President of the Hungarian Chamber of Nurses and Allied Health Personnel.

programme was set up to retain redundant health professionals within their professions and support (guide) their redistribution with financial incentives (Ministry of Health 2006a).[18] The scheme failed as fewer than 30 individuals applied. It is estimated that most of those who lost their jobs, mainly allied health personnel, left the health sector or found work abroad.

7. Factors influencing health professional mobility

7.1 *Intentions to migrate among medical students and resident doctors*

Following a 2003 pre-test, in 2004 the SU HSMTC research project began to collect data (Eke et al. 2006, 2008 & 2009) on professional expectations through voluntary questionnaires, individually structured interviews and focus groups. Target groups were medical students (1st and 6th year) and resident doctors (general medical doctors and dentists) studying in Hungarian at one of the four Hungarian medical university schools. Each annual cohort comprised 600–700 individuals. Several human resources for health issues were explored including the intention to migrate; the motivations behind these intentions; and aspects such as the planned period of stay and intentions to return. Databases were created, analysed and evaluated with the Statistical Package for the Social Sciences (SPSS); the research is ongoing. research project.

Between 2004 and 2008, 3815 questionnaires were completed (1975 by resident doctors, 1840 by medical doctors). On average, 60%–70% of resident doctors were contacted in this period, with a response rate of over 95%, producing the following results.

- Migration potential in these groups is between 60% and 70% (average range) with a migration activity[19] of around 10% (average range). This reached a maximum of 20% in some groups of resident doctors (particularly noticeable in 2006). Among different medical specialists in training, general practitioners show relatively lower migration potential (40%) in comparison to their peers in anaesthetics and intensive therapy or radiology (75%), for example.

- The main target destination regions (ranking first, second and third preferences) were English-speaking EU countries, followed by German-speaking EU countries and Nordic countries.

The main motivating factors indicated that two distinct approaches were used when considering whether to migrate or whether to stay in Hungary.

18

19 Taken active steps to be able to work and find employment abroad.

Those considering migration cited rather rational motivations such as salary, quality of life, the situation of the Hungarian health system and the working environment. Those preferring to remain in Hungary cited rather emotional influences such as family and friends. Moreover, respondents were asked about their perceptions of six dimensions in their target country (social prestige, career/research/professional opportunities, working conditions, standard of living). The results showed that all six aspects were perceived to be better, or significantly better, abroad. The survey also examined respondents' planned duration of work abroad and intentions to return. The results for resident doctors in 2008 are shown in Figs. 10. 2 and 10. 3.

The survey findings give valuable information to inform health policy-makers designing interventions to limit outflow and enhance return. The career expectations of young doctors should be noted particularly since they are

Fig. 10.2 *Reasons to emigrate among resident doctors intending to work abroad, 2008*

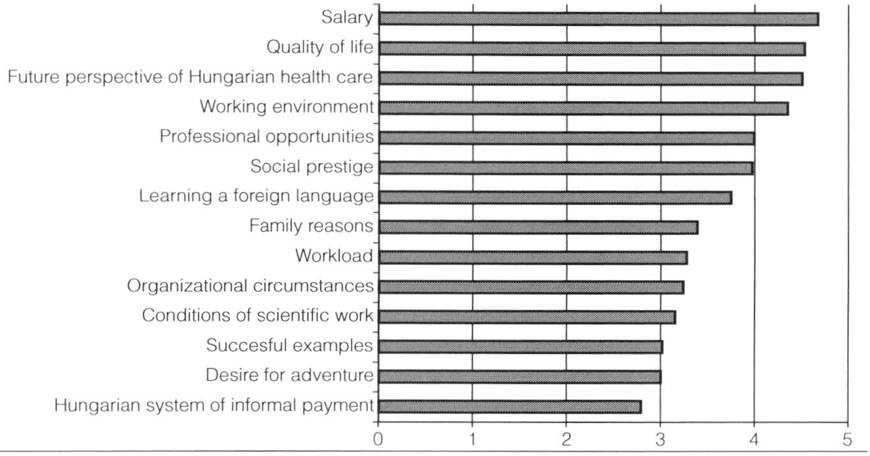

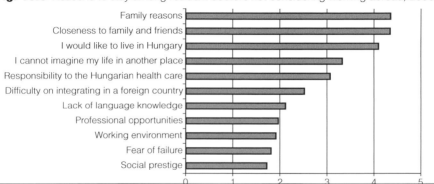

Source: Eke et al. 2009. *Note*: n = 441; Likert scale (5 = decisive influence, 1 = no influence at all).

Fig. 10.3 *Reasons to stay among resident doctors not considering working abroad, 2008*

Source: Eke et al. 2009. *Note*: n = 441; Likert scale (5 = decisive influence, 1 = no influence at all); graph shows 11 of the 17 most important reasons.

more mobile and better informed about career prospects in other countries. New generations of resident doctors often have the opportunity to spend time abroad during their training and have direct experience of other health systems.

7.2 *Intentions to migrate among nurses*

A survey of 226 students undertaking a Bachelor of Science degree in nursing was carried out between November and December 2003. This showed that 58% of the students planned to work abroad and 21% had taken active steps to do so. Their main motivations for thinking about migrating were: learning a new language (80%), career development (43%), increasing professional knowledge (57%) (Kovacsné Tóth 2004 & 2007).

Nurses make fewer applications to work abroad but their migration has potentially greater impact, given the critical shortage of nurses (OHAAP unpublished data 2009). Policy-makers should be vigilant of this situation.

7.3 *Mobility of Hungarian medical doctors immigrating to Hungary*

Until the 1980s, individuals starting their medical career in Romania could not choose freely between work options. Young medical doctors of Hungarian origin were typically compulsorily assigned to regions populated by Romanians. The aim was to enhance assimilation of the Hungarian minority while ensuring health-care provision in underserved areas. A research team explored these outplacement practises among new medical graduates of the University of Medicine and Pharmacy of Tirgu Mures between 1972 and 1989. In this period, medical doctors of Hungarian nationality were generally assigned to some of Romania's most remote and underdeveloped regions across the Carpathian Mountains.

Intended emigration among this group of mobile health professionals appears to have been motivated by dissatisfaction with their condition in the home system, including (no order indicated): the complicated, difficult postgraduate training system; limited options to obtain medical specialization; low remuneration; lack of individual freedom; and discriminatory practices whereby Hungarian-national medical doctors were placed in difficult areas. Migration to Hungary was therefore an escape route for this group (Balázs & Zoltán 2009).

8. Policy, regulation and interventions

8.1 *Prior to EU accession*

Bilateral agreements with some (such as Norwegian and Swedish) governments were in place before EU accession but no information on their implementation is available. Moreover, medical doctors and dentists with Hungarian nationality could enter the Hungarian labour market relatively easily between 1989 and May 1991. Emigrating mainly from the Carpathian Basin, registration required the preliminary endorsement of the Minister of Health. However, the procedure changed and became more complicated. From May 1991, all foreign medical doctors and dentists (including those with Hungarian nationality) have been required to pass an exam in order to obtain registration, a process initiated by the potential workplace (Balázs 2003 & 2005b, Balázs & Zoltán 2009).

8.2 Policies and policy development on health professional mobility

The importance and scale of the problem of health professional mobility has finally been acknowledged, particularly for outflows. However, no comprehensive strategy is yet in place. Policy measures aimed to limit outflow are isolated steps rather than integrated parts of any health-care reform process.

Government actions have mainly concentrated along two lines – policy papers and attempts to restrict migration. In recent years, the Ministry of Health has led the development of two policy papers focussed mainly on problem analysis and soft interventions. Both included sections on health professional mobility. The 2004 Green Paper (Ministry of Health 2004) discussed migration in a short, general manner without considering its potential management; the 2006 White Paper (Ministry of Health 2006b) went into greater detail and outlined policy options to handle migration. Both papers produced recommendations based on analysis and discussions but no actual action plan or strategy was attached or elaborated. They were never published officially and no action was taken due to political changes and lack of political support.

The second focus is on attempts to restrict migration. The political stakes of managing the human resources for health crisis have increased gradually over the last five years. There has been growing awareness of the problem but interventions so far have concentrated on attempts to limit migration through administrative measures without damaging the principles of free movement of labour. A new system of postgraduate medical training was introduced by government decree in 2009, presumably in response to increasing concern over the migration of Hungarian health professionals, mainly medical doctors (Government of the Republic of Hungary 2009). Under the previous system, all residents were central state employees contracted by the universities for the first 26 months of their training. The new system authorizes health-care institutions to apply directly to the Ministry of Health for resident places, according their needs, but no more than 10% of these places can be at the universities. Related finance is allocated according to the number of resident places. Residents contract with the institutions at the start of their residencies, having accepted the conditions for support of their training. These include the length of service required following qualification as a specialist. The Ministry of Health steers young medical doctors into identified shortage specialties (defined by committee) by increasing the remuneration by 50%.

There has been a clear improvement in monitoring as it has been possible to track health professional mobility since EU accession. OHAAP bears responsibility for delivering qualification certificates to those wishing to work abroad and for assessing the qualifications of foreigners wishing to work in Hungary. It now has the conditions in which to develop a comprehensive and regularly updated database on human resources for health.

Local interventions

Some policy interventions exist to attract and retain health professionals at local level. For years, local government authorities have collaborated with health-care organizations to offer incentives in rural areas where under-supply of health professionals is a long-running problem. Municipalities, local authorities and managers of health-care organizations try to give local answers to health workforce problems as they are most exposed to problems of service sustainability and staff availability. These efforts mainly remain local, individual and non-coordinated actions as potential employers offer career plans for health professionals to settle in their constituency. Many health-care institutions offer higher salaries and financial compensations to attract and retain specialists in the most critical fields such as anaesthetics and pathology. Support for accommodation is the most common non-financial incentive. It should be noted that recent initiatives have aimed to coordinate efforts and elaborate a comprehensive approach at county and regional levels.

Specific interventions

It is important to note the relatively new phenomenon of providing medical education to foreign professionals – Hungarian medical universities have offered programmes in German since 1983 and in English since 1987. These courses are increasingly popular mainly among students from the Middle East, Nordic countries, Germany and the United States of America.[20] Some graduates stay and work in Hungary. Since 2000, universities have been required to provide data on the number of medical students graduating in a foreign language for inclusion in the registry – medical degrees have been awarded to 1853 foreign students and 6186 Hungarian students; 259 foreign students and 1182

---

20 Semmelweis University (SU) established a branch in Germany in March 2008. Students study in German and obtain an SU degree (http://english.sote.hu/opening-ceremony-in-hamburg.html, accessed 15 December 2010).

Hungarian students have qualified as dentists. The foreign-language medical degrees show that Hungary attracts foreign students (a source of income for the universities). The medical training system is evaluated to be of a high level and Hungary has become an exporter of medical diplomas.

8.3 *Political force field of human resources for health*

Common experiences, new research and public actions by professional organizations have contributed to a recent increase in public awareness of the health workforce crisis in Hungary. Ministry of Health representatives say that human resources for health issues are considered critical. The issue is constantly on the agenda but it is not known what, if any, interventions are planned.

Growing media attention and public concern over access to services and their quality, safety and sustainability is increasing political pressure. Hopefully, this will create the momentum for more coordinated interventions.

9. Conclusion

The magnitude and character of international health professional mobility is among the most important of the human resources for health challenges in Hungary. Since EU accession, the country has experienced a significant loss of health professionals, mainly medical doctors. Negative net migration is worsened by the age profile, specialties and skill-mix of leavers. Health experts and the media warn that outflows are threatening the sustainability of the health-care system, even in the short run. Furthermore, the ageing population and health workforce (the latter at a more rapid pace) are influencing the quality and safety of services and the principles of equal access to health care in the country. Changes in the educational system also deepen the problem as insufficient numbers of health professionals are being produced.

The current magnitude of health professionals' intentions to migrate is a severe pathological symptom of the Hungarian system. Presumably, this has resulted mostly as a consequence of the adverse effects of health reforms, health policy interventions and economic restrictions. The human resources for health crisis can be managed effectively only if the root causes that motivate people to pursue their careers abroad are addressed comprehensively and pragmatically and followed up with a consistently elaborated action set.

References

Balázs P (2003). Migráció a magyar orvostársadalomban, és az 1989-es rendszerváltozás hatása [Migration in the Hungarian medical community]. *Egészségügyi Gazdasági Szemle*, 41(4):5–12.

Balázs P (2004). Az orvoslétszám tervezhetőségének problémái [Problems in the planning of medical doctor numbers]. *Informatika és Menedzsment az Egészségügyben (IME)*, 3(1):9–13.

Balázs P (2005a). Hazai és külföldi orvosok területi elhelyezkedése az alapellátásban [Domestic and foreign medical doctors in primary care]. *Medicus Universalis*, 38(2):75–80.

Balázs P (2005b). Migrációs hatások leképeződése a magyar orvostársadalomban [Migration effects in the Hungarian medical community]. *Informatika és Menedzsment az Egészségügyben (IME)*, 4(2):5–10.

Balázs P (2009). Nemzetközi migrációs hatások és belső tényezők Magyarország orvosi munkaerő-gazdálkodásban [International migration effects and intrinsic factors in the Hungarian medical labour market]. *Egészségügyi Gazdasági Szemle*, 47(4):12–20.

Balázs P, Zoltán Á (2009). Marosvásárhelyi orvosok a magyarországi orvosi karban. [Medical doctors from Targu Mures in the Hungarian medical community]. *Epidemiológia*, 6(2):95-110.

Eke E et al. (2006). Challenges for the public health policy by the European Union extension to the east. View on possible future development. International symposium: Economic and Sociopolitical Perspectives for Health Services in Central Europe (HealthRegio Project), Vienna, 27–28 February 2006.

Eke E et al. (2008). Research data on migration of Hungarian medical doctors. Analysis and evaluation. In: Moore J et al. (eds.) *National health workforce: the growth of challenging trends*. Paris, Centre de Sociologie et de Démographie Médicales.

Eke E et al. (2009). Migráció a magyar orvosok körében [Migration among Hungarian medical doctors]. *Statisztikai Szemle*, 87(7–8):795–827.

Girasek E et al. (2009). The potential impact of physicians' emigration on the Hungarian healthcare system. *International Symposium on the Performance of a National Health Workforce: How to assess it? How to strengthen it? Neuchatel, 14–16 October 2009.*

Government of the Republic of Hungary (2009). 122/2009 (VI. 12.) Korm. rendelet az egészségügyi felsőfokú szakirányú szakképzési rendszerről [Government Decree 122/2009 on higher health postgraduate training system].

Magyar Közlöny [*Hungarian Official Journal*], 2009/79 (http://www.complex. hu/jr/gen/hjegy_ doc.cgi?docid=A0900122.KOR, accessed 2 February 2011).

Hárs Á et al. (2004). The labour market and migration: threat or opportunity? The likely migration of Hungarian labour to the European Union. In: *Social Report 2004*. Budapest, TÁRKI.

Hodgson R (2009). The doctors are out. *The Budapest Times*, 15 November 2009 (http://www.budapesttimes.hu/index.php?option=com_content&task=v iew&id=13468&Itemid=27, accessed 15 December 2010).

Hungarian Central Statistical Office (2007). *Yearbook of Health Statistics 2006*. Budapest.

Hungarian Central Statistical Office (2008). *Yearbook of Health Statistics 2007*. Budapest.

Ministry of Health (2004). *Vitaanyag az egészségügyi dolgozók helyzetéről* [*Consultation document on the situation of health-care workers*]. Budapest.

Ministry of Health (2006a). Mobilitás Program – Áttelepülési támogatás az egészségügyi reform kapcsán érintett intézmények közalkalmazotti dolgozói számára

[Mobility Programme – Relocation assistance for public employees affected by the health-care reform]. Budapest (http://www.eum.hu/archivum/palyazatok/ mobilitas-program, accessed 15 December 2010).

Ministry of Health (2006b). *Human resource strategy for health* [*Az egészségügy human erőforrás stratégiája*]. Budapest.

OHAAP (2009). *Statisztikai archivum* [Statistical archive]. (http://www.eekh. hu/index.php? option=com content&task=view&id=109&Itemid=1, accessed 2 February 2011).

Világgazdaság (2007). Ismeretlen 1500 orvos sorsa [Fate of 1500 medical doctors is unknown]. *Gazdaság*, 20 July 2007 (http://vg.hu/gazdasag/ismeretlen-1500-orvos-sorsa-181423, accessed 1 February 2011).

WHO (2000). How well do health systems perform? In: *The world health report 2000 – Health systems: improving performance*. Geneva (http://www.who.int/ whr/2000/ en/whr00_ch2_en.pdf, accessed 21 October 2010).

Chapter 11

Definition of a source country: the case of Lithuania

Žilvinas Padaiga, Martynas Pukas, Liudvika Starkienė

1. Introduction

This study presents a definition of a source country from a Lithuanian perspective, examining health professional mobility and its impact on the national health system. This includes recent trends in relation to migration policies, cross-border mobility, influencing factors and other international and national interventions.

Health professional mobility began with Lithuanian independence but it was only after European Union (EU) accession that politicians started discussions on its possible negative consequences for the effective functioning of the national health system and initiated planning processes at governmental/ regional/local levels to determine the future supply and requirement of health professionals in Lithuania. EU accession has not produced the anticipated potentially serious increases in the outflow of health professionals. However, Lithuania is best defined as a source country and in that context it is essential to address concerns regarding the sustainability of human resources for health.

Lithuania is improving the workforce planning infrastructure step by step but still remains far short of achieving adequate information about the stocks, flows and effects of incentive schemes. Despite the lack of accurate emigration data in Lithuania, the findings of this study show that health professionals are leaving the country – attracted by better working conditions, better quality of life, higher prestige and higher pay. The domestic health workforce outflows have not led to the development of explicit policies to attract a foreign workforce to supplement the domestic stock of health professionals. The Ministry of Health has rather concentrated on reforming the health sector in order to retain and motivate Lithuanian health professionals to practise in Lithuania. However, the lack of success in reforming processes is usually caused by a lack of balance between process and product, and a failure of coordination between planners, policy-makers and other stakeholders.

Limitations of the study

Data on mobility have been collected from several sources – databases or registries of the Ministry of Health, Institute of Hygiene Health Information Centre, State Patient Fund of Lithuania, State Health Care Accreditation Agency, Lithuanian Dental Chamber, Statistics Lithuania, Ministry of Social Security and Labour, Migration Department and Residents Register Service. However, no one database or registry can provide all the necessary information in a timely manner. Incomplete information in terms of collected data indicators (for example the number of professionals, full-time equivalents, licences; distribution by region, age, gender or services performed by specialty; migration) and the inability to link these databases limits data validity and its usefulness. Complete information on migration in Lithuania remains difficult, if not impossible, to obtain without a more comprehensive registry (Table 11.1).

2. Mobility profile of Lithuania

The limited data available indicate that EU accession did not produce the anticipated outflows and the numbers and proportions of health professionals leaving the country remain low. The reasons for this are not clear but most likely include improved working conditions (enabled by EU structural funds for the health-care system), increasing salaries and more competition in destination countries.

At the current rate of migration, Lithuania's health system is not dependent on foreign health professionals.[1] Migration management and related policies remain relatively new and still lack political attention. Also, low levels of migration give more time to react adequately to the current situation in health human resources. However, vigilance is required as Lithuania is dependent on the health workforce situation in wealthier EU and European Economic Area (EEA) countries that actively recruit foreign health professionals (Ireland, Norway and the United Kingdom, for example).

---

1 This study defines a foreign health professional as a person other than a national of the Republic of Lithuania, whether a foreign national or a stateless person.

Table 11.1 *Data sources for information on human resources for health in Lithuania*

Data source	Institute of Hygiene Health Information Centre	Licence Registry at State Health Care Accreditation Agency	State Patient Fund
Available since	1993	1999	1999
Annual reports	Yes	No	No
Updating frequency	Annually	Every 5 years	Daily
Professions	Physicians, dentists, nurses, public health specialists, pharmacists	Physicians, dentists, nurses, pharmacists	Physicians and dentists holding contracts with SPF
Number of professionals	Yes	No	Special calculations required
Number of full-time equivalents	Yes	No	No
Number of licences	No	Yes	No
Distribution by gender	No	Yes	Special calculations required
Distribution by age	No	Yes	Special calculations required
Distribution by specialty	Yes	Yes	No
Distribution by regions	Yes	No	No
Distribution by services performed	No	No	Special calculations required
Mortality, retirement, migration	No	No	No

2.1 *Outflows*

Statistical data on the emigration of Lithuanian health professionals is available only from 2004 when the Ministry of Health started to issue certificates of good standing (CGSs) for health professionals wishing to practise abroad. The number of certificates issued does not reflect the real migratory flows as the holders may choose not to leave the country or may leave only on a short-term basis. During the first year of EU membership, 2.7% (357) of all Lithuanian medical doctors obtained certificates. That number almost halved to 1.4% (186) in 2005–2006[2] and fell to 0.9% (132) in 2009. Nurses show a different pattern – 0.4% (107) of all Lithuanian nurses were issued with certificates in 2004–2005, with relative increases to 0.7% (166) in 2005–2006

---

2 1 May 2005–30 April 2006.

and 1.1% (267) in 2009. Dentists show fluctuating numbers – 3.6% (81) of all Lithuanian dentists were issued with certificates during the first year of EU membership. These numbers fell to 1.7% (42) in 2005–2006 but rose to 3.1% (72) in 2009 (see section 4 on migration dynamics) (Ministry of Health unpublished data 2009, Pukas 2008).

2.2 Inflows

Ministry of Health data on inflows indicate that only 10 basic medical degrees, 12 medical specialty degrees, 10 nursing degrees and 11 dentistry degrees from countries outside the EEA (Armenia, Belarus, Russian Federation, Ukraine, Uzbekistan) were accredited between 2005 and 2008. Three dentistry degrees (in Norway and Poland) were recognized under Directive 2005/36/EC (European Parliament and Council of the European Union 2005). Thus, the percentages of foreign health professionals remain very low in comparison to the numbers of Lithuanian health professionals – the total economically active health workforce in 2008 comprised 13 403 medical doctors, 24 908 nurses and 2287 dentists.

Stock data on foreign health professionals are more problematic. The authorized Lithuanian authorities that collect and manage information on medical doctors and nurses (State Health Care Accreditation Agency), dentists (Lithuanian Dental Chamber) and pharmacists (State Medicines Control Agency) have neither data on their foreign-national members nor data by nationality on the numbers of licences issued. The only data available are the number of work permits issued to foreign nationals (Table 11.2). However, it should be noted that every person with an accredited degree does not necessarily apply for or obtain a work permit.

Table 11.2 *Work permits issued to foreign health professionals in Lithuania, 2005–2008*

	2005	2006	2007	2008	Total
Medical doctors	1	3	-	11	15
Nurses[a]	1	-	-	5	6
Dentists	1	-	1	-	2

Source: Lithuanian Labour Exchange unpublished data 2009. *Note*: [a] includes those with lower qualification.

The main medical specialties of those granted work permits between 2005 and 2008 were surgery (3), psychotherapy (2) and ophthalmology (4). Most (5) of the nurses held the lower qualification. Lithuanian Labour Exchange data, which are mostly similar to Ministry of Health data, show that the stock of foreign health professionals was mainly pooled from third countries (Belarus,

China, Israel, Lebanon, Pakistan, Russian Federation, Syrian Arab Republic, Ukraine); only three came from EEA countries (Latvia, Norway).

3. Vignettes on health professional mobility

Ophthalmologist migrating to join spouse

In 1992, Dr Sigita and her two children emigrated to Luxembourg to join her architect husband who had emigrated in 1991, the year that Lithuania became independent.

Having been a practising ophthalmologist at a Vilnius hospital, Sigita began language courses in French, Luxembourgish and German (Luxembourg's three official languages) before starting any procedures for diploma recognition. The languages were not the only requirement to begin medical practice in one of the smallest EU countries. It took more than five years for Sigita to be licensed as an ophthalmologist and granted a work permit. The establishment of a private practice was another challenge – not only the high cost but also the difficulty of attracting patients. Despite all the challenges and barriers, Sigita is now a well-known ophthalmologist in Luxembourg, has Luxembourg nationality, runs a business and is trusted by local and by French, German and Belgian patients. After investing so much in her training, business and settlement, it is unlikely that she and her family will ever return to Lithuania.

Permanent migration?

As a young and promising anaesthetist/intensive care specialist in one of Vilnius's largest hospitals, Dr Tomas decided to gain experience as a locum anaesthetist in a British hospital during his summer holidays in 2004. The initial one-month contract was extended to two months before he was offered an extension of up to six months. Family reasons (for example: the problem of adapting to a new country; career opportunities for his wife) made it difficult to decide to leave Lithuania. Nevertheless, the pull factors won. In an interview, Tomas rejected his colleagues' opinion that the main instigating factors for emigration are better revenues and living conditions. These factors surely played a role in the decision process but he was strongly incentivized by curiosity and the possibility of gaining experience as a specialist and working in the National Health Service (NHS).

After a few years abroad, Tomas is now well-integrated into the BHR University Hospitals NHS Trust, one of the biggest United Kingdom health-care organizations. His family is happy and he has no intention of returning to Lithuania in the near future.

Nurses emigrating in search of better conditions

January 2008 was difficult for the Lithuanian nursing community as nurses from different Lithuanian regions emigrated to Bergen, Norway. Regina, Lina, Regina, Jane, Ilona and Vilma were unanimous in identifying the main push factors: low salaries, inadequate working conditions, heavy workloads, inappropriate attitudes among hospital managers, possible job loss due to the ongoing restructuring/optimization process in the health sector. Most of the nurses had never practised abroad. One had tried (unsuccessfully) to settle in Ireland but she found Norway more attractive because of the flexible legal system for the settlement of foreign health-care specialists. Ireland requires perfect language skills, certification and a registration period of about one year; in Norway, nursing specialists need only basic language skills.

While it is natural for specialists to migrate within the enlarged EU, increasingly this process is supported intensively by special agencies, offering well-paid jobs and better living conditions in Norway. In this case a job is available after just two weeks of an intensive language course. Within a market offering "special discounts", it is not surprising that the nurses interviewed declared that they see no prospect of returning to practise in their homeland.

Dr Marijus, newly graduated emigrant

International mobility of health-care specialists does not depend on age. Dr. Marijus emigrated from Lithuania in 2004, just after graduating as a dentist from Kaunas University of Medicine. Working in the United Kingdom, his intention is to open a clinic as there is a bigger market and fewer bureaucratic barriers than in Lithuania. In addition, he feels that the United Kingdom offers many opportunities, not only to achieve better revenues but also to develop his professional skills. His wish is to acquire as much training and experience as possible and to use it eventually in Lithuania, although this may not happen soon.

---

4. Dynamics of enlargement

The absence of data hinders comparison of mobility before and after EU accession but a 2008 study compared Lithuanian and foreign data sources to determine health professional migration following EU accession (Pukas 2008). Currently, there is no simple and valid scheme to verify the employment status of those holding CGSs in order to determine whether or not they have migrated and, if so, to which destination country. However, comparison of different data sources revealed that 342 of the 543 medical doctors with CGSs were listed on foreign registries and 187 had no contract with the State Patient Fund. Both are indicators of being employed abroad and of having left Lithuania. Almost half (140) of the 273 nurses with certificates and 90 of the 123 dentists with certificates were listed on foreign registries. This suggests that Lithuanian health professionals who apply for CGSs have rather serious migration intentions. The main destination country for Lithuanian medical doctors, nurses and dentists proved to be the United Kingdom, followed by Scandinavian countries. The actual numbers of Lithuanian health professionals working abroad are likely to be even higher as the foreign registry data reflect only the most important target countries.

Data on CGSs (1 May 2004–30 April 2006) from the Ministry of Health (543 medical doctors, 273 nurses, 123 dentists) were used to compare emigration intentions with actual emigration. The mechanism for checking the real migratory flows was complex and time-consuming. Where information was available online (Austria, Belgium, France, Germany, Ireland, Italy, the Netherlands and United Kingdom for medical doctors; Germany, Ireland and United Kingdom for nurses and dentists) or upon request (Denmark, Norway and Sweden), the names and surnames of certification holders were checked in the registries of other EEA countries in order to confirm whether they actually practised abroad. The personal data of medical doctors were also checked in the database of the State Patient Fund to determine whether the professional continued to practise in Lithuania. The data produced by the two methods were then compared. Only the registries' analysis was available for nurses and dentists since these professionals do not have contracts with the State Patient Fund.

For medical doctors with certification it was found that 35.0% (125) in the 2004–2005 period[3] and 33.3% (62) in the 2005–2006 period[4] either had no contracts with the State Patient Fund or their contracts had expired. Research of the foreign registries found that 67.5% (241) of certificate holders in 2004–2005 and 54.3% (101) in 2005–2006 were registered abroad. During both periods, the largest proportions were registered in the United Kingdom (103 and 65), Denmark (38 and 11), Sweden (30 and 8), France (17 and 1) and Norway (10 and 4) (Fig. 11.1).

Of the 273 Lithuanian nurses with certificates, 140 were listed on foreign registries. In the 2004–2005 and 2005–2006 periods, the largest proportions of nurses with certificates were registered in the United Kingdom (25 and 45), Ireland (14 and 14) and Scandinavian countries (17 and 9) (Fig. 11.2).

Dentists appeared to have a greater propensity to emigrate – 90 of the 123 dentists with CGSs were listed on foreign registries. During both periods, the

---

3 1 May 2004–30 April 2005.

4 1 May 2005–30 April 2006.

Fig. 11.1 *Proportion of Lithuanian medical doctors registered in destination countries, 1 May 2004–30 April 2005 and 1 May 2005–30 April 2006*

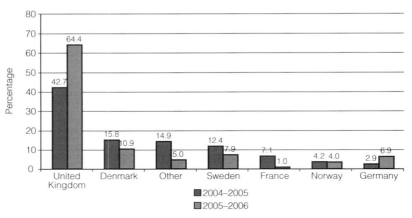

Source: Pukas 2008.

Fig. 11.2 *Proportion of Lithuanian nurses registered in destination countries, 1 May 2004– 30 April 2005 and 1 May 2005–30 April 2006*

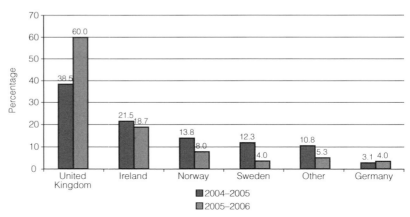

Source: Pukas 2008.

largest proportions of dentists were registered in the United Kingdom (46 and 27), Norway (5), Denmark (4) and other countries (4) (Fig. 11.3).

Comparison of domestic and foreign data sources showed that about 60% of medical doctors, 50% of nurses and 70% of dentists with CGSs were listed on foreign registries. The findings may suggest that Lithuanian health professionals applying for CGSs have rather serious migration intentions.

Fig. 11.3 *Proportion of Lithuanian dentists registered in destination countries, 1 May 2004–30 April 2005 and 1 May 2005–30 April 2006*

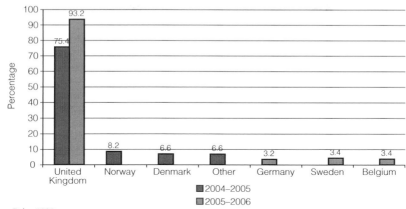

Source: Pukas 2008.

5. Impacts on the Lithuanian health system

Health professional migration's impact on health system performance has become an important feature of the international health policy debate in both Europe and worldwide. This highlights the potentially negative impacts of the emigration of health workers from low-income countries – including staff shortages; lower morale among remaining staff; and reduced quality and quantity of, and access to, services (Dumont & Zurn 2007). As a source country, this is particularly relevant to Lithuania because international mobility impacts on the Lithuanian health system.

Data from the Lithuanian Labour Exchange (2009) show an unmet demand for medical doctors, dentists and nurses; any of these medical professionals have a very high chance of employment. However, this does not necessarily indicate an overall shortage of these specialists in the whole country. A study by the Institute of Labour and Social Research (2006) found that the health-care and pharmacy sectors (except nursing) experience the biggest problems filling available vacancies (Table 11.3). For example, demand for psychiatrists was 24 times higher than supply; demand for other medical doctors was 3–10 times higher. Recruitment of neurologists or surgeons took an average of seven months. These delays underline the need for prompt action.

A study on health professional mobility revealed that gynaecologists, paediatricians, anaesthetists, surgeons, internists, doctors of laboratory medicine, general practitioners and medical doctors with basic medical training migrated most often in 2004–2006 (Pukas 2008). It is conceivable that the magnitude of vacant positions might have adverse consequences for health service delivery, especially when the mobility of the particular specialists is taken

Table 11.3 *Specialist posts with highest number of vacancies in Lithuania*

Specialist	Average time to fill vacancies (days)	Number of registered vacancies	Number of registered unemployed	Demand/supply ratio (number of registered vacancies/ number of registered unemployed)
Internist	90	204	130	1.6
Surgeon	204	77	3	25.7
Psychiatrist	152	72	3	24.0
Anaesthetist	139	50	5	10.0
Ophthalmologist	111	41	1	41.0
Neurologist	238	32	3	10.7
Medical doctor of physical medicine and rehabilitation	133	24	3	8.0
Gynaecologist	146	20	6	3.3

Source: Institute of Labour and Social Research 2006.

into account. However, no special studies have been carried out to examine health professional migration's impact on the number of services provided.

One of the main challenges for the future is the establishment of a comprehensive system of health workforce planning. So far, there has been no consistent and long-term policy in this area, especially one that takes account of mobility factors (see section 8). There are no specific regulations or other types of governmental or nongovernmental barriers to regulate health professional migration in Lithuania. It is also important to note that (unlike other EU and EEA countries such as Ireland, Norway, United Kingdom) Lithuania has neither proactive recruitment policies for foreign health professionals nor any national or regional plans to offer temporary contracts to health professionals from foreign countries.

There has been no specific research to evaluate how health professional migration affects population health status via health service delivery at institutional or system level. However, the State Patient Fund aimed to gain an impression of the possible implications of health professional outflow by evaluating 59 senior general practices – those in which over 50% of the listed population is over 50 years of age (Fig. 11.4). After evaluating the number of visits per year by size of practice, it was observed that general practitioners could not increase the number of services if the list size exceeded 1650 patients. There was no increase in the average of 5000 total visits per year even when the practice reached 2000 patients, the maximum figure recommended by the Ministry of Health. It is not simple to decrease the maximum recommended practice size;

Fig. 11.4 *Annual visits to general practitioners in 59 practices with senior populations (more than 50% aged over 50), 2006*

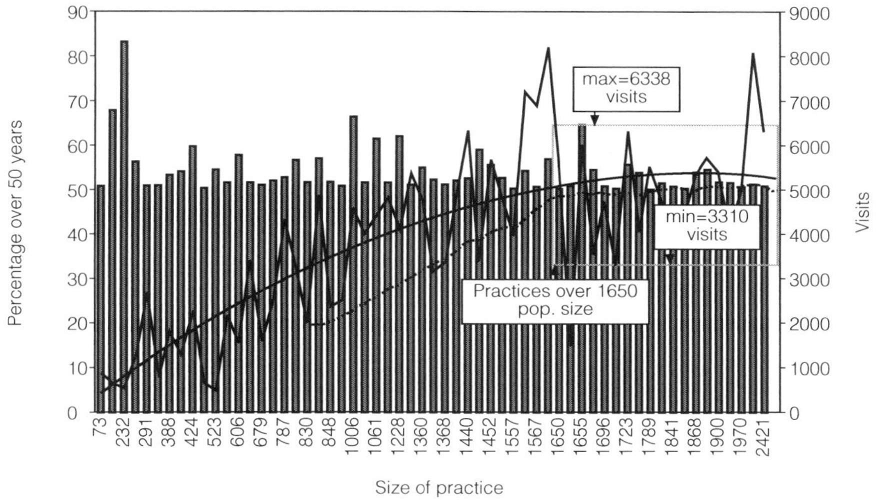

Source: State Patient Fund unpublished data 2006.

better to count the additional workforce required. Also, if general practitioners migrate (it is among the specialties at risk), those remaining would have limited capacity to provide all the services needed. Of course, it is not clear how and when such a situation would result in a deterioration in population health but these findings show the saturation point of health providers and indicate health professional mobility's potentially detrimental impact on the accessibility and quality of health services.

6. Relevance of cross-border health professional mobility

This section examines health professional mobility in the broader context of the Lithuanian system in order to understand its relative importance in comparison to other human resource issues that determine the size and composition of the health workforce. Overall, Lithuania appears to have a balanced situation with relatively low mobility rates and changes in the educational system allowing universities to increase the intake of students. However, this could change if the unfavourable economic context encourages health professionals to seek employment abroad.

6.1 *Distributional issues influencing composition of the health workforce*

The current situation in Lithuania can be described as one of maldistribution in the health professional stock (see Table 11.4). Women comprise a larger

Table 11.4 *Health professional stock and distribution in Lithuania, 2007*

Indicators	Total number (year)	Range (lowest and highest figures across districts/regions)	EU-27 average 2007
Medical doctors	13 729[a]	-	-
Medical doctors per 100 000 population	407.8[a]	Highest: Kaunas city (693.8) Lowest: Alytus district (51.5)	315.22
General practitioners per 100 000 population	77.5[2]	-	96.7
Medical doctors by specialties per 100 000 population	136.2[b]	-	106.1
Medical doctors working in hospital sector (%)	42.2%[b]	-	-
Medical doctors working in private sector (%)	Full-time: 8.2% Part-time: 22.9[a]	Number working in private practice is 2.8 times higher in urban areas	-
Total number of nurses	24 804[a] (almost half are general practice nurses)	-	-
Nurses per 100 0000 population	736.8[a]	Highest: Kliap□da city (1404.8) Lowest: Alytus district (189.9)	741.8
Nurses working in hospital sector (%)	58.8[b]	-	-
Nurses working in private sector (%)	-	-	-
Total number of dentists	2395[a]	-	-
Dentists per 100 000 population	71.1[a]	Highest: Kaunas city (125.1) Lowest: Joniškis district (19.9)	62.3
Dentists working in private sector (%)	Full-time: 49.2%. Part-time: 73.8%[a]	Number working in private practice is 2.6 times higher in urban areas	-
General practitioner–specialist ratio	1:7.4[a]	Highest: Vilnius county (1:10.7) Lowest: Telšiai county (1:3.4)	-
Doctor–nurse ratio	1:1.8[a]	Highest: Taurag□ county (1:2.9) Lowest: Vilnius county (1:1.3)	-
Anaesthetist–surgeon ratio	1:1.8[a]	-	-
Surgeon–surgical nurse ratio	1:2.5[a]	-	-
Hospital nurse–community nurse ratio	1:2.9[a]	-	-
Hospital–ambulatory sector ratio (doctors)	46.89%: 40.88%[a]	-	-
Hospital–ambulatory sector ratio (nurses)	58.96%: 32.76%[a]	-	-

Sources: [a] Institute of Hygiene Health Information Centre 2009; [b] WHO 2009.

proportion of the health workforce, a share that has remained relatively constant for several years. In 2008, almost 70% of medical doctors, 85% of dentists and 99% of nurses were women (Institute of Hygiene Health Information Centre 2009). This could have a negative impact on the active health workforce and health service delivery as female physicians tend to work fewer hours per week.

In 2008, the percentages of medical doctors (72%), nurses (60%) and dentists (53%) working in urban areas appeared relatively balanced as these districts contained 70% of the total population (Statistics Lithuania 2009). The geographical distribution of medical doctors has significant differences, for example – the number of medical doctors per 10 000 population ranged from a high of 80.9 in Kaunas city to a low of only 39.8 in Šiauliai city in 2008 (Fig. 11.5). However, there have been no attempts to relieve the imbalances (in either geographical distribution or specialties) by recruiting international health professionals.

Despite the ongoing structural reforms that aim to strengthen primary care in private settings, only a small proportion of medical doctors practise privately. Dentists are the exception as most have practised privately since the 1990s.

Fig. 11.5 *Number of medical doctors per 10 000 population, by administrative region, 2008*

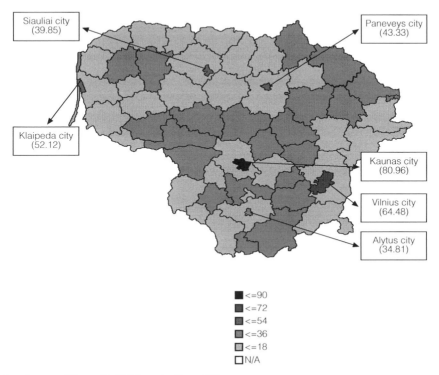

Source: Institute of Hygiene Health Information Centre 2009.

6.2 *Educational system*

During the 1990s, the number of places for medical studies was reduced by almost 50% (about 200–250 medical students per year). Following independence, in 2002 the number of study places was increased to 400 in response to the first research results on health workforce planning. Admission numbers have continued to grow over the past years and generally reflect the needs of the health system. It remains difficult to set admission levels as the intakes need to account for emigration of health professionals, early departures from the profession and retirement, all of which are difficult to quantify or even estimate (see below and section 2). Lithuania lacks official statistics on attrition rates but cohort studies performed at Kaunas University of Medicine indicate that 17.3% of medical students failed to finish their studies (Lovkyte 2004). Drop-out rates were lower in other study programmes.

Lithuanian universities are public and education is state financed, partly state financed (students pay about €300 out-of-pocket per year) and privately financed (students pay full costs of the programme, about €7500 and €8000 per year for medicine and dentistry respectively), depending on the enrolment limits and average admission grades. Basic educational information is provided in Table 11.5.

Table 11.5 *Educational institutions and students, by health profession, 2008*

	First-year students	Universities	Total students	Graduates (basic medical training)	Graduates (residency programme)
Medicine	490	2	3 321	322	556
Nursing	201	3	894	272	-
Dentistry	172	2	802	141	52
Pharmacy	115	1	713	150	-

Sources: Ministry of Education and Science 2009; Institute of Hygiene Health Information Centre 2009.

Considerable proportions of foreign students study biomedical sciences in Lithuania and their numbers are increasing every year. Kaunas University of Medicine (2009) data show 304 undergraduate students (studying medicine, odontology, pharmacy and public health – Masters in Public Health only) from 36 countries, representing about 5%–6% of all Lithuanian student stock in these fields. Most come from Israel (108), Lebanon (72), India (20), United Kingdom (11), Pakistan (10), Sweden (9), Poland (9) and France (8) but other source countries include Australia, Brazil, China, Estonia, Finland, Ireland, Kazakhstan, Malaysia, Nigeria, Republic of Korea and Sri Lanka.

6.3 *Leaving the system: retirement and attrition*

It is difficult to gather data on the number of health professionals who retire each year because Statistics Lithuania does not collect the relevant information on retirement by specialty or profession. The age structure of health professionals in Lithuania has not changed substantially over the last 10 years – 18.5% of medical doctors, 10.9% of dentists and 13.3% nurses were aged 55–64 years; and 9.8% of medical doctors, 5.3% of dentists and 1.9% of nurses were 65 and over (Institute of Hygiene Health Information Centre 2009). The percentage of medical doctors aged over 60 also varies by specialty. A high percentage of health professionals nearing, or over, the retirement age indicates that these specialists might leave their profession soon (Fig. 11.6).

The official retirement age is 60 years for women and 62.5 years for men. However, health professionals tend to continue working beyond these official retirement ages due to unfavourable retirement policies such as low pensions and fewer social privileges (Government of the Republic of Lithuania 1994*)*.

It is difficult to compare the health workforce outflows due to migration and attrition. Cohort studies of medical (Lovkyte 2004) and dentistry (Zakaite 2006) graduates of Kaunas University of Medicine were undertaken in order to analyse exits from the profession. These found that 73.5% of medical graduates held licences and only 61.6% were practising medicine in Lithuania. Among dentistry graduates, 90.8% were licensed and 82.7% were practising. However, the reasons for dropping out were not determined and losses could be due (for

Fig. 11.6 *Percentage of medical doctors older than 60 years, 2009*

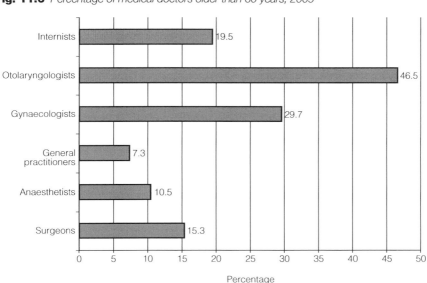

Source: State Healthcare Accreditation Agency (unpublished data), 2009.

example) to career shifts to other medical professions (such as pharmaceuticals); emigration; leaving the health workforce altogether; retirement; or even death.

6.4 *What does cross-border mobility mean for Lithuania?*

Lithuania has relatively low mobility rates and therefore appears to be relatively immune from the effects of cross-border mobility. Also, examination of the current health workforce stock indicates that there is no need to import health professionals. However, the unfavourable economic situation prevailing at the time of writing may significantly accelerate outflow rates. It is unlikely that this would be remedied by an inflow of professionals from EU-15 countries, shortages are more likely to be met by professionals from countries of the former Soviet Union (see also section 2).

The recent change in the educational system that allows universities to accept students paying the full cost of a study programme ensures higher numbers of students than the required need, thus compensating for any possible loss due to migration. Also, universities are marketing their programmes abroad in order to generate income from foreign students. It is difficult to say whether foreign students tend to leave the country after graduation or tend to settle in Lithuania and establish families. It is likely that the most outstanding students are being offered positions in university hospitals.

7. Factors influencing health professional mobility

Most efforts to stop the outflow of health professionals from Lithuania are aimed at improving the instigating factors by reforming the health-care system (see section 8). Intentions to leave Lithuania were examined by surveying medical doctors and medical residents in 2002 (Stankunas et al. 2004), pharmacists in 2004 (Smigelskas et al. 2007) and nurses in 2007 (Matuleviciute 2007). Table 11.6 summarizes their findings on the main factors influencing the migration intentions of Lithuanian health professionals.

8. Policy, regulation and interventions

8.1 *Policies and policy development on health professional mobility*

National-level policy interventions in Lithuania aim to target the main reasons for migration described in the previous section but no specific national policy has been adopted as yet. The policies are in line with the general migration policy adopted in 2007 (Government of the Republic of Lithuania 2007).

Table 11.6 *Factors influencing mobility of Lithuanian health professionals*

Instigating factors	Low salaries, long working hours, perceived low prestige, unsatisfactory working conditions
Activating factors	Personal: better quality of life, desire for a life change, previous habitation or professional training abroad Job-related: better professional opportunities, continuous professional training, better working conditions and working environment, relatives abroad, professional and social recognition
Facilitating factors	Very active recruitment agencies (e.g. Norway, United Kingdom). Attractive induction schemes – free language courses, social programmes, fewer barriers to start private practice, less bureaucracy
Mitigating factors	Separation from family, language skills, settling down with family in a destination country

Sources: Stankunas et al. 2004; Smigelskas et al. 2007; Matuleviciute 2007.

This aims to develop long-term economic migration control measures, such as regulating the economic factors that contribute to migration (better working conditions, social guarantees, higher salaries).

A government-approved health-care reform was implemented in two stages (2003–2005 and 2006–2008). This contributed to significant changes in working conditions as well as better distribution of the services and duties of health professionals (Government of the Republic of Lithuania 2003 & 2006). While not an explicit retention policy to moderate migration, the medical community (mainly medical doctors' and nurses' associations) had been pressing the Ministry of Health not only to restructure health-care institutions and improve infrastructure but also to increase salaries. In 2005, the Ministry of Health and the medical associations signed a memorandum on salary increases (20% annually for medical doctors and nurses in 2005–2008). This is likely to have had a positive influence on the high rates of drop-out from medical studies, attrition to other better paid professions and emigration rates.

Incentive schemes to promote deployment in remote areas are widely used to address regional maldistribution. Medical doctors who practise in rural areas receive financial bonuses and some hospitals offer free accommodation and transportation services. The ongoing reform made use of financial support from EU structural funds (2004–2006) – €19.7 million were assigned to modernize and develop the cardiology services infrastructure in the south-east region of Lithuania and €21.7million to modernize and develop the public health-care infrastructure – renovating most hospitals and supplying new medical equipment; and supporting improvement to general practitioner and primary health-care facilities. Moreover, some €268 million have been assigned to ensure available and high-quality essential health-care services for the period 2007–2013.

Further implementation aims to improve financial and non-financial incentives but the global economic crisis has raised some barriers against reaching the anticipated goals of the reform and may produce a different overall impact than that originally intended.

8.2 *Workforce planning and development*

Medical health workforce planning began in 2000, nursing workforce planning began only in 2006 and evaluation of need and long-term planning for dentists, pharmacists and public health professionals is still being developed. There is no explicit health human resource policy in terms of professional mobility. Also, the Lithuanian health-care system is rather independent of foreign health professionals and so they have little impact on the planning process.

In 2003, the Minister of Health approved the Strategic Planning of Health Human Resources in Lithuania in 2003–2020 programme. This was updated in 2005 to include new objectives aimed at integrating health human resources planning within overall health sector reform. The main strategic objectives of the policy are to:

- examine changes in health human resources at national, county and district level;

- enable health human resources planning by specialty at county and district levels based on population projections, mortality and morbidity trends and health-care reform objectives;

- develop a model for planning health human resources supply and demand based on health-care reform;

- develop projections of health human resources supply and demand by specialty.

This does not include some aspects of health human resources policy – production, management and regulation are covered in other strategic programmes. Currently, there is no unified register of health professionals but this could offer an effective managerial tool for achieving the objectives. More information about the institutions responsible for human resources for health is presented in Table 11.7.

8.3 *Cross-border regulatory frameworks and interventions*

EU Directive 2005/36/EC (European Parliament and Council of the European Union 2005) on the mutual recognition of qualifications is fully transposed into Lithuanian law. The Ministry of Social Security and Labour is responsible

Table 11.7 *Main national stakeholders involved in planning, production, management and regulation of health professionals in Lithuania*

Organization	Functions
Ministry of Health	Coordination and regulation; planning, management, regulation of human resources for health; sets minimum training requirements
Ministry of Education and Science	Coordination and regulation; determines student enrolment numbers and sets minimum training requirements; evaluates quality of training
Ministry of Finance	Finances education of health professionals and health-care system
National Board of Health	Advises parliament and government on long-term trends and human resources for health planning
Kaunas University of Medicine, Vilnius University, Klaipėda University and six colleges	Training health professionals; research on human resources for health
Institute of Hygiene Health Information Centre	Collection and processing of statistical information for human resources for health planning
State Health Care Accreditation Agency (under the Ministry of Health)	Regulation body maintaining registers of physicians and nurses
State Medicines Control Agency (under the Ministry of Health)	Regulation body maintaining register of pharmacists
Lithuanian Dental Chamber	Regulation body maintaining register of dentists
State Patient Fund	Collection of data on contracted physicians
Professional associations	Represent members' interests; set ethical standards; establish clinical guidelines

for coordinating the recognition of degrees and certifying professional qualifications acquired in the EEA. The Ministry of Health is a competent institution responsible for the recognition of degrees and proving the professional qualifications of medical doctors, nurses, dentists and pharmacists. Lithuania has a very liberal system for recognition of diplomas and does not impose any hurdles for migrant health professionals whose qualifications comply with the requirements laid down in the directive. The only condition is that an applicant should know enough of the Lithuanian language to enable them to work as a health-care specialist.

The Minister of Health approves two commissions for the recognition of qualifications obtained in non-EEA countries and applicable to all third-country health professionals. One commission covers medical doctors and dentists (Government of the Republic of Lithuania 2009a); the other covers general practice nurses and midwives (Government of the Republic of

Lithuania 2009b). Applicants seeking recognition of their diplomas submit an application form and accompanying documents to the Minister of Health who directs all the documentation to the commissions for consideration. It should be noted that the relevant commission makes a recommendation thirty days after receiving all the necessary documents and advises whether or not a qualification corresponds to requirements. The Minister of Health uses this advice as the basis for a final decision.

No specific and/or potential cross-border policy interventions are imposed at local or national level and Lithuania has no bilateral agreements on health professional mobility.

8.4 *Political force field of regulating and managing health professional mobility*

Lithuania still has no specific national policy to manage or regulate health professional mobility. Nevertheless, the issue of emigration, geographical maldistribution, health service quality and accessibility is included in various political documents, such as the working programmes of political parties and government ministries (Health; Education and Science; Social Security and Labour); resolutions of the National Board of Health and of health professional associations (Lithuanian Medical Association, Organization of Lithuanian Nursing Specialists, Lithuanian Dental Chamber, etc.) and other strategic documents. However, as yet there is no unified policy or strategy which could enable all the stakeholders to work together to achieve the strategic goals with a special emphasis on health professional resource planning.

9. Conclusion

As a source country, it is essential to consider concerns about the sustainability of human resources for health in Lithuania. The workforce planning infrastructure is improving but remains far short of holding relevant information about stocks, flows and the effects of incentive schemes. The Ministry of Health is the main stakeholder in this process of reforming the health sector with the intention of retaining and motivating health professionals to practise in Lithuania. However, the lack of success in reform processes is usually caused by a lack of balance between process and product and a failure of coordination between planners, policy-makers and other stakeholders.

The current situation in Lithuania is best described as limited shortages in some geographical regions and/or specialties. Health professional mobility is very sensitive to labour markets and can change scale and direction relatively quickly. Ongoing reforms since 2003 have focused on improving working conditions (pay, task distribution, infrastructure) for health professionals. It seems likely that the 2005–2008 salary increases in the Lithuanian health sector played a role in retaining health professionals. It can be assumed that health professional mobility may directly affect future health workforce stocks and population health outcomes if the net loss of Lithuanian health professionals is not redressed by foreign trained specialists. To date, comparatively few health professionals have emigrated but a well-managed migration policy is a prerequisite for avoiding a shortage of health professionals in the near future, particularly in those medical specialties that already experience recruitment problems.

Hopefully, successful implementation of the ongoing health sector reforms and careful planning will ensure that human resource policies, planning and practices are effective in maintaining the health workforce supply. However, Lithuania is heavily dependent on the situation in wealthier EU countries that actively recruit foreign health professionals. Increased health workforce migration is likely to see Lithuania recruit health professionals from countries of the former Soviet Union. This would continue a domino effect whereby a country replaces emigrating health professionals by importing a new workforce from abroad. Future developments remain hard to predict, not least in the global context of an uncertain economic outlook.

References

Dumont JC, Zurn P (2007). Immigrant health workers in OECD countries in the broader context of highly skilled migration. In: *International Migration Outlook 2007*. Paris, OECD Publishing.

Government of the Republic of Lithuania (1994). Valstybinių socialinio draudimo pensijų įstatymas (1994 m. liepos 18 d. Nr. I-549) [Law on State Social Insurance Pensions, 18 July 1994, No. I-549]. *Official Gazette*, 59-1153 (http://www3.lrs.lt/dokpaieska/ forma_e.htm, accessed 15 December 2010).

Government of the Republic of Lithuania (2003). 2003 m. kovo 18 d. Lietuvos Respublikos Vyriausybės nutarimas Nr. 335 ,,Dėl Sveikatos priežiūros įstaigų restruktūrizavimo strategijos patvirtinimo" [Resolution no. 335 of the Government of the Republic of Lithuania of 18 March 2003 On the Approval of the Strategy on the Restructuring of Health-Care Institutions]. *Official Gazette,* 28-1147 (http://www3.lrs.lt/ dokpaieska/forma_e.htm, accessed 15 December 2010).

Government of the Republic of Lithuania (2006). 2006 m. birželio 29 d. Lietuvos Respublikos Vyriausybės nutarimas Nr. 647 ,,Dėl Antrojo sveikatos priežiūros įstaigų restruktūrizavimo etapo strategijos patvirtinimo" [Resolution no. 647 of the Government of the Republic of Lithuania of 29 June 2006 On the Approval of the Stage II Strategy on the Restructuring of Health-Care Institutions]. *Official Gazette,* 74-2827 (http://www3.lrs.lt/dokpaieska/forma_e.htm, accessed 15 December 2010).

Government of the Republic of Lithuania (2007). 2007 m. balandžio 25 d. Lietuvos Respublikos Vyriausybės nutarimas Nr. 416 ,,Dėl Ekonominės migracijos reguliavimo strategijos ir jos įgyvendinimo priemonių 2007-2008 metų plano patvirtinimo" [Resolution No. 416 of the Government of the Republic of Lithuania of 25 April 2007 On the Approval of the Strategy on the Economic Migration Regulation and the Plan for Implementing Measures 2007-2008]. *Official Gazette*, 49-1897 (http://www3.lrs.lt/dokpaieska/forma_e.htm, accessed 15 December 2010).

Government of the Republic of Lithuania (2009a). 2009 m. sausio 22 d. Lietuvos Respublikos sveikatos apsaugos ministro įsakymas V-27 ,,Dėl Lietuvos Respublikos sveikatos apsaugos ministro 2000 m. spalio 26 d. įsakymo Nr. 577 "Dėl Gydytojų ir gydytojų odontologų profesinės kvalifikacijos vertinimo ir pripažinimo komisijos sudarymo ir jos nuostatų patvirtinimo" pakeitimo" [Order No. V-27 of the Minister of Health of the Republic of Lithuania of 22 January 2009 On Amending Order No. 577 of the Minister of Health of the Republic of Lithuania of 26 October 2000 On Approval of the Commission and its Regulations for Assessment and Recognition of Professional Qualifications of Doctors and Dental Practitioners]. *Official Gazette*, 12-495 (http://www3.lrs.lt/dokpaieska/forma_e.htm, accessed 15 December 2010).

Government of the Republic of Lithuania (2009b). 2009 m. sausio 22 d. Lietuvos Respublikos sveikatos apsaugos ministro įsakymas V-26 ,,Dėl Lietuvos Respublikos sveikatos apsaugos ministro 2001 m. kovo 26 d. įsakymo Nr. 192 "Dėl Užsienyje įgytos bendrosios praktikos slaugytojų ir akušerių profesinės kvalifikacijos vertinimo ir pripažinimo nuostatų tvirtinimo" pakeitimo [Order No. V-26 of the Minister of Health of the Republic of Lithuania of 22 January 2009 On Amending Order No. 192 of the Minister of Health of the Republic of Lithuania of 26 March 2001 On Approval of the Regulations for Assessment and Recognition of Professional Qualifications of General Care Nurses and Midwives, Acquired Abroad]. *Official Gazette*, 12-494 (http://www3.lrs.lt/dokpaieska/forma_e.htm, accessed 15 December 2010).

Institute of Hygiene Health Information Centre (2009). *Lithuanian health indicators information system.* Vilnius (http://www.lsic.lt/html/en/dpsen.htm, accessed 2 November 2010).

Institute of Labour and Social Research (2006). *Study of workforce demand and problems of filling in the vacancies. Report of the second stage of the study (2006).*

Vilnius   (http://www.ldb.lt/Informacija/Apie/Documents/ldv_2etapas.pdf, accessed 13 September 2010).

Kaunas University of Medicine (2009). *Facts and figures: statistics of International Relations and Study Centre.* Kaunas (http://trc.kmu.lt/en/degree-studies/general-info/facts-and-figures/, accessed 15 December 2010).

Lithuanian Labour Exchange (2009). *Barometer of employment possibilities.* Vilnius, Ministry of Social Security and Labour.

Lovkyte L (2004). *Planning of supply and requirements of physician human resources in Lithuania until 2015* [dissertation]. Kaunas, Kaunas University of Medicine.

Matuleviciute E (2007). *Nurses' intentions to work abroad* [thesis]. Kaunas, Kaunas University of Medicine.

Ministry of Education and Science (2009) *Trumpai apie bendrąjį priėmimą į Lietuvos aukštųjų mokyklų pagrindines ir vientisąsias studijas 2008 metas* [*Brief description of general admission to undergraduate and integrated studies in Lithuanian higher education institutions, universities and colleges, in 2008*]. Vilnius (http://www.lamabpo.lt/2008 priemimas.pdf, accessed 15 December 2010).

Pukas M (2008). *Lithuanian health-care professionals migration study* [thesis]. Kaunas, Kaunas University of Medicine.

Smigelskas K et al. (2007). Do Lithuanian pharmacists intend to migrate? *Journal of Ethnic and Migration Studies,* 33(3):501–509.

Stankunas M et al. (2004). The survey of Lithuanian physicians and medical residents regarding possible migration to the European Union [in Lithuanian]. *Medicina (Kaunas),* 40(1):68–74.

Statistics Lithuania (2009). Database of indicators. Vilnius (http://db1.stat.gov.lt/statbank/, accessed 15 December 2010).

WHO (2009). European health for all database [online database]. Copenhagen, WHO Regional Office for Europe.

Zakaite Z (2006). *Demand and supply projections for dentists* [thesis]. Kaunas, Kaunas University of Medicine.

Chapter 12

When the grass gets greener at home: Poland's changing incentives for health professional mobility

Marcin Kautsch, Katarzyna Czabanowska

1. Introduction

Though already commonplace in Poland, health workforce mobility escalated significantly on accession to the European Union (EU) in 2004 and the resulting disappearance of the barriers hindering health professionals seeking job placements abroad. Health professional mobility is not so large that it poses a significant threat to the health-care system in the short-term but it is a noticeable phenomenon. It is also suggested that the Polish educational system produces more health professionals than are lost in potential outflows to other states (Kaczmarczyk 2006). However, the number of medical personnel per capita in Poland is lower than the EU average (OECD 2008b).

Migrant health professionals' main destinations are the United Kingdom, Ireland, Germany and the Scandinavian countries. The main push factors for the Polish health workforce were financial. Only a limited number of health professionals choose Poland as their target country (barriers hinder such movements although language is less problematic for Slavic-speaking people). Those who do come are mostly from countries in which the gross domestic product (GDP) is lower than in Poland. Economic motivations may therefore prove to be key factors behind both inflows and outflows.

Until recently, health-sector salaries in Poland were relatively low – prompting immigration and discouraging the arrival of newcomers. Recent years have seen significant changes in migration patterns, probably largely caused by substantial increases in the income levels of health professionals (particularly medical doctors) in Poland. The growth in salaries was due to both protest actions by the professional group and increased funding in the health system – nominal expenditure on health care increased twofold in 1999–2008, with a relatively low inflation rate (OECD 2008b). The drop in emigration, especially among nurses, may also be due to unmet expectations related to professional experiences abroad (Greger 2004). Collected data point to differences in the migration patterns of medical doctors, dentists and of nurses, the two former groups being more mobile and having more positive experiences abroad. While not presenting a direct threat, it can be argued that health workforce emigration contributes to staff shortages in general and in certain specialties in the Polish health system. This issue has become even more important since the public purchaser of health services in Poland, the National Health Fund raised staffing requirements for health institutions that provide universally covered care (National Health Fund 2008).

Two key contextual factors should be borne in mind when examining migration in Poland and other central and eastern European (CEE) countries. Firstly, these countries represent relatively new democracies in comparison to those in the EU-15. Their cultural differences and legal limitations contribute to the fact that countries like Poland are still developing processes that are already well-established and standard in older EU Member States. This includes the free movement of professionals and patients. Secondly, it is important to note the increase in welfare levels over the last two decades and the political, social and economic changes in Europe. These are reflected by a 144% rise in Poland's GDP between 1990 and 2006, calculated by US$ PPP. This compares to 93% for the EU-12, excluding Luxembourg for which there are no available data (OECD 2008b).

This chapter begins by presenting Poland's mobility profile in terms of inflows and outflows of medical doctors, nurses and dentists. This will be followed by a discussion of the role of EU accession. An analysis of the impact and relevance of health professional mobility will be used to assess its weight in the system, not least when compared with other workforce issues. The final section will examine the policy context and measures/interventions aimed at managing health professional mobility.

Data sources and limitations of the study

This case study on health professional mobility to and from Poland is based on analysis of secondary databases using search engines on the Internet[1] as well as those of the World Health Organization (WHO), the Organisation for Economic Co-operation and Development (OECD) and Eurostat. Specific web pages of various professional EU and Polish organizations were accessed, including those of the Central Statistical Office (GUS), Ministry of Health, Polish Chamber of Physicians and Dentists and the Polish Chamber of Nurses and Midwives. Information sources include scientific articles, reports, statistics, grey literature and expert experience of the authors. The analysis of the scope of Polish health workforce migration is based on the numbers of professional qualification certificates issued by the Polish Chamber of Physicians and Dentists and the Chamber of Nurses and Midwives. Earlier research in the field used a similar methodology (Nosowska & Gorynski 2006).

García-Pérez et al. (2007) observed a lack of uniformity in registers and definitions in Poland. Having contacted several institutions and consulted several data sources the authors of the current study also found that data were often incomplete, unavailable, contradictory or inconsistent. It should be noted that it was not possible to obtain all the requested data as not all are being collected routinely. Additional information on the numbers of registered and practising medical doctors was obtained from the Polish Chamber of Physicians and Dentists. However, not all sections and not all cadres are covered with the same level of detail. The lack of data stems from the prevalent reporting modalities as well as the increasingly market-oriented health sector. For example, self-employed medical doctors are not subject to the same statistical registration as medical staff working in the public sector.

The increasing influence of market forces is reflected in the growing number of private health institutions and practices in the health system. These processes began in the mid 1990s and by 2006 67% of outpatient and 5% of hospital services were performed by private health institutions (GUS 2007a & 2007b). Moreover, Poles are making more use of services financed from private sources – in 2008 an estimated 36.8% of health-care spending was private (Komorowski & Hebda 2008). Private services are not registered by public statistics and therefore the data which describe the employment of health-care personnel, scope of the market and migration are elusive.

Such problems are not unique to research on migration. Experience proves that similar difficulties are encountered when analysing other aspects of the health system. For example, data sources on the numbers of hospitals and of hospital beds are rarely unanimous. In the absence of hard evidence, the authors have used information from their own experience of working with Polish health-care institutions.

---

1 Including Google scholar and metasearch of scientific databases.

Attempts to determine the magnitude and impact of migration are complicated by the fact that there are more than 300 000 registered nurses (having the legal capacity to discharge professional duties) in Poland but nurse organizations estimate that 200 000 actually work as nurses. Thus, an overestimated denominator contributes to inaccuracies when assessing magnitude. Conversely, the number of professional certifications issued is an indicator of health professionals' interest in working abroad, rather than actual emigration. The exact number of people who started working abroad following EU accession is not known (Ministry of Health 2009). In addition, emigrating nurses may find jobs related to care duties which require trained nurses but have different names and are not registered as nursing posts.

2. Mobility profile of Poland

2.1 *Outflows*

Poland's accession to the EU has had the greatest impact on the migration of Polish health professionals in recent years (Hajnosz 2004, Lesniowska 2005). Emigrating medical doctors are typically either in the prime of their careers (at 36–49 years old) or are very young and without specialization (Kudlicki 2006). Nosowska and Gorynski (2006) estimated that 3% of medical doctors, 3.6% of dentists and 1.2% of nurses considered emigrating in 2004. They concluded that health workforce outflows were not substantial but should not be disregarded if they continued at the same pace.

Although data on migration are not recorded, it is possible to determine emigration intentions based on the number of professional qualification certificates issued by professional chambers and associations such as the Polish Chamber of Physicians and Dentists and the Polish Chamber of Nurses and Midwives. These official documents certify professional qualifications and are a requirement for employment in the health sector of another country.

Official data show that more than 7000 medical doctors and 2000 dentists obtained certification of professional qualifications in 2005–2008, amounting to 6.1% and 6.7% respectively of certification holders in these two groups by the end of 2008 (Table 12.1). The data also show that the number of certification requests increased rapidly in the initial phase following accession but slowed from mid 2007.

The data presented in Table 12.2 reveal important differences between medical specialties. The majority of medical doctors applying for certification were anaesthetists and intensive care specialists; followed by thoracic surgeons and plastic surgeons. The fourth place was occupied by specialists in emergency

Table 12.1 *Practising medical doctors and dentists (stock) and certifications of professional qualifications issued in Poland, 2005–2008*

	Data as of:				
	30 June 2005	30 June 2006	30 June 2007	31 Dec. 2007	31 Dec. 2008
Medical doctors					
Registered medical doctors[a]	116 847	118 475	116 160	117 240	116 492
Certificates issued (cumulated)	3 579	5 114	6 237	6 724	7 138
Change on previous period (%)	-	(42.9)	(22.0)	(7.8)	(6.2)
Cumulated certificates as proportion of registered medical doctors (%)	(3.0)	(4.3)	(5.4)	(5.7)	(6.1)
Practising medical doctors in Poland (dated 31 December)	80 315	na	na	81 932	na
Dentists					
Registered dentists	30 283	31 089	30 405	30 605	30 873
Certificates issued (cumulated)	1 108	1 581	1 853	1 924	2 069
Change on previous period (%)	-	(42.7)	(17.2)	(3.8)	(7.5)
Cumulated certificates as proportion of dentists (%)	(3.7)	(5.1)	(6.1)	(6.3)	(6.7)
Practising dentists in Poland (dated 31 December)	12 188	na	na	13 304	na

Sources: GUS 2006a–2009a & 2006b–2009b, [a] Polish Chamber of Physicians and Dentists unpublished data 2008.
Note: na – no data available.

medicine. The ranking indicates that medical doctors with certain diagnostic or surgical specialties comprise the highest proportions of applicants. This may be because these groups have rather limited direct contact with patients and therefore do not need the degree of fluency in the target country language required for other non-surgical specialties. The lowest proportion of applications was recorded for medical doctors specializing in internal medicine (non-surgical specialties).

Although the certifications constitute a certain reference point, revealing intentions to emigrate, they should not be confused with actual mobility. Moreover, medical doctors have been leaving Poland without these documents. The Chair of the Polish Society of Anaesthesiology and Intensive Care estimates that until 2007 some 150 anaesthetists left Poland without certifications (Sikora 2007). However, the source does not explain how these individuals were employed abroad.

Table 12.2 *Certifications of professional qualifications by medical specialty, as at end 2008*

Specialty	Practising medical doctors	Certifications issued	Certifications issued as proportion of practising medical doctors %
Anaesthetics and intensive care	4 219	797	18.9
Thoracic surgery	222	36	16.2
Plastic surgery	160	25	15.6
Emergency medicine	538	71	13.2
Pathomorphology	497	59	11.9
Radiology and diagnostic imaging	2 136	233	10.9
Vascular surgery	282	29	10.3
Oral and maxillofacial surgery	90	9	10.0
Orthopaedics and traumatology of motor organ	2 473	248	10.0
Haematology	254	24	9.5
General surgery	5 594	482	8.6
Neurosurgery	433	37	8.6
Urology	1 089	77	7.1
Oncological radiotherapy	442	30	6.8
Paediatric surgery	738	48	6.5
Obstetrics and gynaecology	5 890	370	6.3
Gastroenterology	530	30	5.7
Transport medicine	108	6	5.6
Psychiatry	2 575	139	5.4
Internal medicine	14 709	746	5.1
Cardiology	2 385	121	5.1
Nuclear medicine	181	9	5.0
Clinical microbiology	68	3	4.4
Paediatric and adolescent psychiatry	215	9	4.2
Medical rehabilitation	1 298	53	4.1
Ophthalmology	2 963	115	3.9
Neurology	2 645	96	3.6
Paediatrics	6 364	221	3.5
Dermatology and venereology	1 642	55	3.4

Endocrinology	937	32	3.4
Otolaryngology	2 029	67	3.3
Allergology	1 024	33	3.2
Geriatrics	202	6	3.0
Lung disease	2 413	64	2.7
Communicable diseases	939	25	2.7
Nephrology	599	15	2.5
Rheumatology	1 503	36	2.4
Laboratory diagnostics	173	3	1.7
Occupational medicine	1 578	18	1.1
Public health	1 400	14	1.0
General practice	9 150	62	0.7
Clinical pharmacology	74	0	0
Clinical immunology	34	0	0
Clinical immunology	34	0	0
TOTAL	**82 795**	**4 553**	**5.5**

Specialty	Practising dentists	Certifications issued	Certifications issued as proportion of practising dentists %
Orthodontics	1 078	24	2.2
Oral surgery	729	8	1.1
TOTAL	**1 807**	**32**	**1.8**

Source: Ministry of Health 2009.

In comparison to medical doctors and dentists, relatively low number of nurses applied for certification. This may be because employers (e.g. long-term care providers) did not require such documents or because these nurses were employed to perform care activities that did not require professional qualifications.

It is impossible to determine the extent to which applications for certification can be translated into actual emigration numbers. Research conducted among health professionals indicates that before EU accession 35.2% of health professionals expressed the intention to emigrate but only 10.4% claimed that their intentions were definite (OECD 2008a). However, foreign data sources can provide valuable information on the numbers of Polish health professionals employed abroad as well as their destination countries.

Table 12.3 *Professionally certified nurses and midwives (stock) and certifications of professional qualifications issued in Poland, 2004–2006*

	1 May 2004 – 30 June 2005	1 May 2004 – 30 June 2006
Registered nurses and midwives	299 054	308 620
Certifications issued	3 204	5 912
Certifications issued as proportion of total nurses and midwives (%)	(1.1)	(1.9)
Estimate of certifications issued as proportion of number of practising nurses and midwives – simulation[a] (%)	*(1.6)*	*(3.0)*
Professionally registered nurses and midwives[b] (31 Dec)	206 977	NA

Sources: Ministry of Health, 2009, [b] GUS 2006a.
Note: [a] simulation calculated on the assumption that 200 000 nurses and midwives are practising.

Table 12.4 *Polish health professionals working in European countries, circa 2000*

Country of residence	Nurses	Medical doctors	Dentists	Pharmacists	Total
Austria	841	245	80	57	1223
Denmark	93	105	6	9	213
Finland	5	20			25
France	24	134	14		172
Greece	133	19			152
Hungary	13	11	13	4	41
Ireland	6	3			9
Luxembourg	3	4	1		8
Portugal		3			3
Spain	27	24			51
Sweden	475	678			1153
United Kingdom	263	282	42	31	618
Total	**1 883**	**1 528**	**156**	**101**	**3668**

Source: Dumont & Zurn 2007.

By around 2000, it is estimated that more than 3600 health professionals had emigrated from Poland to work in EU Member States (Table 12.4).

The particularly high figure for Austria demonstrates the fact that emigration to that country was much easier at the time. Also, the 2007 study did not obtain data from Germany. If these two points are disregarded, the main destination countries were Sweden, the United Kingdom and Denmark. Later research on migration patterns and outflow directions in subsequent years support these findings (Fig. 12.2).

García-Pérez et al. (2007) estimated that a total of approximately 3130 Polish medical doctors were registered in European Economic Area (EEA) countries around 2000. These estimates come relatively close to the total numbers presented in Table 12.5. Poland and other recent EU Member States (such as Malta, Romania, Hungary) show over 5% of medical professionals practising abroad (García-Pérez et al. 2007).

The numbers of Polish medical doctors newly registered in EU-15 Member States between 2000 and 2007 (Fig. 12.1) give a similar indication.

Fig.12.1 *New registrations of Polish medical doctors in EU-15, 2000–2007*

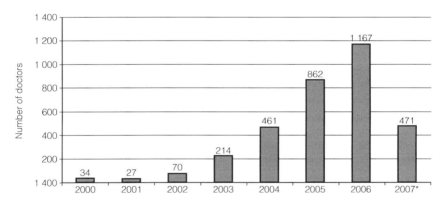

Source: Leśniowska 2007. *Note*: [a] data for 2007 only partially available. No data were available from Austria and Greece. Limited data were available from Germany (from 1 of 17 existing regional medical offices – *Landesärztekammer*), Ireland (registration of specialists not compulsory), Italy (26 of 69 regional medical offices – *Ordine Provinciale dei Medici Chirurghi e degli Odontoiatri*), Sweden (2004–2007 only), Spain (8 of 40 regional medical offices – *Colegio Oficial de Medicos*).

Despite the limitations in data availability, Fig. 12.1 indicates that relatively low numbers of medical doctors were registering in EU-15 countries between 2000 and 2002 – not exceeding 100 individuals. However, a surge in emigration began in 2003 and reached a peak in 2006. Data for 2007 do not cover the entire year but may point to a declining interest in emigration. It seems unlikely that the drop in registrations is caused by market saturation since there is still demand for health professionals in EU-15 countries. It is noticeable that emigration intensified rapidly after accession to the EU and subsided almost equally rapidly when health professional salaries in Poland began to increase in 2007 (see also Fig. 12.3). These data on new registrations in the EU-15 correspond well with the volume of certification applications (Table 12.2).

Total registrations for medical doctors indicate a change in the direction of outflows. Neighbouring Germany was preferred prior to accession but since then Great Britain has become the most popular destination, followed by Germany, Ireland and the less populated Scandinavian countries – Sweden and Denmark (Fig. 12.2). This may be explained by explicit immigration policies in these countries. Emigration to France is perhaps surprisingly low given that it is a large country and French is a popular language in Poland. Fig. 12.2 also confirms the steep rise in the number of medical doctors registering abroad in 2004–2007 (around 2800 registrations) in comparison to 2000–2003 (fewer than 500).

Fig.12.2 *Total registrations of Polish medical doctors in host countries, 2000–2007*

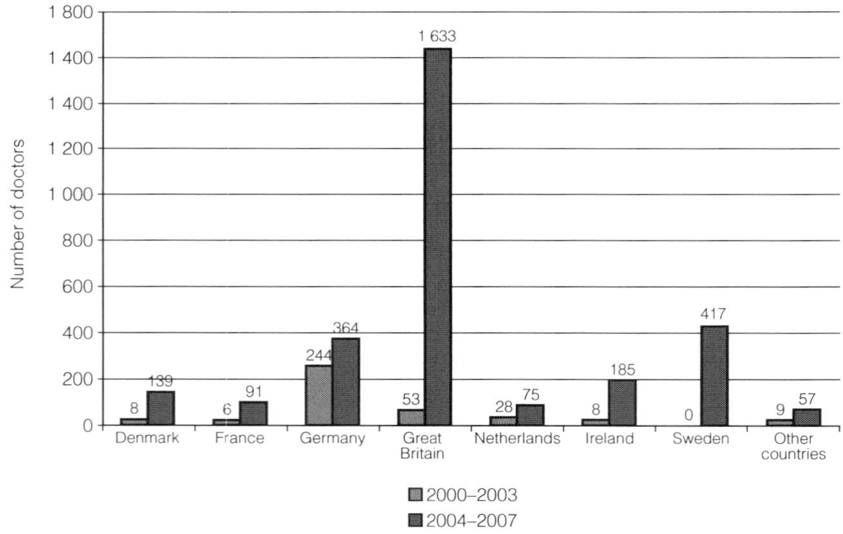

Source: Leśniowska 2007.

The limited data available on outmigration of health professionals from Poland do not allow identification of the age,[2] gender and specialties of the migrating workforce. This stems partly from deficiencies in the statistics currently available. However, it appears that younger specialists from Poland, having just gained their education and qualifications, are willing to migrate permanently to other European countries. Conversely, more senior medical doctors with long experience and families prefer short duties abroad rather than complete relocation (Gazeta.pl 2008).

---

2 Except data given by Kudlicki 2006 – see above.

It can be observed that some migratory movements are not permanent. Information from the Polish Chamber of Physicians and Dentists and the Polish Union of Anaesthesiology and Intensive Care suggests that most medical doctors who request certification work abroad for a set period (see section 3). In practice, an international employer often does not employ one person for a full contract but rather contracts with a group of four medical doctors. Each of these works for a three-month stretch in the year – as one doctor returns to Poland after three months, the next doctor arrives. Contracts limited to weekend work offer another form of international employment. Moreover, there are instances where medical doctors obtain certification but do not undertake any form of employment abroad. Conversely, some nurses emigrate to work abroad without applying for certifications (Ministry of Health 2009).

2.2 Inflows

The limited data available suggest that inflows of health professionals have been insignificant (Danielewicz et al. 2006). This is mostly due to the language barrier and the lack of a proactive recruitment policy – it can take up to 18 months to obtain a work permit and recognition of professional diplomas (Kicinger 2005). Around 2000, it is estimated that about 3% of all medical doctors and less than 1% of nurses working in Poland were foreign nationals (OECD 2008a, Zurn & Dumont 2008). Other estimates put the share of foreign medical doctors and of foreign dentists in 2009 to be less than 1% (Table 12.5). Ukraine is the main country of origin in terms of total registered medical doctors, inflows of medical doctors (41 between January and November 2009) and total dentists registered. Neighbouring Germany and Lithuania as well as the Russian Federation are also important source countries. Around 2000, Dumont and Zurn (2007) report that 1074 medical doctors from Ukraine and 486 from Lithuania were working in Poland. These numbers are in sharp contrast to recent data from the Polish Chamber of Physicians and Dentists (Table 12.6).

Table 12.6 shows the differences in numbers of foreign-trained, foreign-born and foreign-national medical doctors and dentists in 2009.

Table 12.6 shows the percentages of foreign-born and foreign-trained medical doctors to be between 2% and 3% of active medical stock. At the same time, health professionals who are not Polish nationals constitute 0.7% of total numbers. These two findings may indicate that Poland attracts individuals from the Polish community abroad (Polonia), especially from the countries of the former USSR. They may also imply that a relatively large number of Poles are educated abroad. Although numbers remain low, the 2009 inflows of newly registered foreign medical doctors (2.9%) and dentists (2.5%) were higher than the proportions of foreign medical doctors and dentists in the total and

Table 12.5 *Total numbers (stock) and new registrations (inflows) of foreign-national medical doctors and dentists in Poland, 2009*

Nationality	Medical doctors registered	Newly registered medical doctors (1 Jan–30 Nov)	Dentists registered	Newly registered dentists (1 Jan–30 Nov)
Bulgaria	13	1	8	0
Czech Republic	23	0	4	0
Germany	41	9	38	9
Lithuania	22	2	20	2
Russian Federation	48	5	9	2
Sweden	24	1	5	0
Ukraine	193	41	44	4
OTHER	411	32	88	20
TOTAL	**775**	**91**	**216**	**37**
Proportion of all medical doctors and dentists (%)	(0.6)	(2.7)	(0.6)	(3.0)

Source: Polish Chamber of Physicians and Dentists unpublished data 2009.

Note: includes only countries with more than 10 individuals in at least one category. Data from other countries is included in OTHER.

active stocks (below 1%). This may indicate foreign doctors' growing interest in working in the Polish health sector (as salaries have increased) but such a conclusion should be drawn with caution.

It should be noted that the data presented in Table 12.6 are substantially higher than data from the same source in Table 12.5. It was not possible to explain these differences although the causes could include double-counting; confusion between the three categories of foreign-trained, foreign-born and foreign; and possible mistakes in data collection/transcription. Once more this highlights the problems with obtaining accurate data. On the basis of the findings it is impossible to assess the number of specialists and whether they are employed in the private or public sectors or in outpatient or inpatient settings.

2.3 *Summary*

In Poland, the phenomenon of health professional migration generally means emigration. There are observable differences among professional groups – for

Table 12.6 *Total numbers (stock) and new registrations (inflows)[a] of foreign medical doctors and dentists among all registered and active medical doctors and dentists in Poland, 2009*

	Total	Professionally active	Newly registered
Medical doctors (stock)	132 638	120 663	3 430
Foreign-trained	2 868	2 547	74
Proportion of foreign-trained (%)	(2.2)	(2.1)	(2.2)
Foreign-born	3 887	3 040	119
Proportion of foreign-born (%)	(2.9)	(2.5)	(3.5)
Foreign-national	858	844	100
Proportion of foreign-national (%)	(0.6)	(0.7)	(2.9)
Dentists (stock)	36 633	32 038	1 230
Foreign-trained	1 068	963	17
Proportion of foreign-trained (%)	(2.9)	(3.0)	(1.4)
Foreign-born	957	675	27
Proportion of foreign-born (%)	(2.6)	(2.1)	(2.2)
Foreign-national	228	225	31
Proportion of foreign-national (%)	(0.6)	(0.7)	(2.5)

Source: Polish Chamber of Physicians and Dentists unpublished data 2009.

Note: [a] newly registered between 1 January and 30 November 2009.

example, medical doctors in certain specialties and nurses show less intention to emigrate. Emigration is falling from the peak that occurred after EU accession in 2004. Polish health professionals leave the country mainly for economic reasons but the recent change in salary levels (especially for medical doctors) has meant a declining interest in emigration. The data up to 2007 show that most health professionals emigrate to the United Kingdom, Germany and the Scandinavian countries. Moreover, the various mobility practices (including remigration, short-term work cycles, weekend work, rotas) make migration a mixed phenomenon.

3. Vignettes on health professional mobility[3]

Returnee

A is a midwife with a specialization in emergency nursing. Her 14 years in the profession include 18 months working abroad:

I decided to leave Poland and work abroad for three reasons: I wanted to obtain professional experience in a different country, generally the salaries of nurses were low in Poland and I wanted to master foreign language skills, in this case French. I was in a difficult financial situation, so when there was an opportunity I decided to try. I worked in a geriatric ward in France. The work that I was doing was not adequate to my professional competence and at first I felt that I was not developing at all. Professional career of a foreign nurse working abroad is very difficult and requires many years of effort. That is why I decided to come back to Poland; moreover my personal situation was a motivation. I wanted to get married.

Recruiter

A representative of a recruitment agency based in Poland gave this assessment:

The job placement division in our company has been in operation since 2003, recruiting staff (medical doctors) for the German market. At that time, we succeeded in placing a number of staff there. In 2003, mass emigration of doctors became a perceptible phenomenon which increased until 2006. I also know that clinical staff went to work in English-speaking countries and to Scandinavia, especially Sweden and Norway.

Since 2007, we have seen a very clear fall in the number of physicians leaving Poland for good; I can say that such migrations practically ceased to happen.

Generally speaking, there was only one main reason for emigration given by departing medical doctors, namely the level of compensation in Polish health care. Literally, only a handful of emigrants mentioned as inducing factors the opportunity for professional development or broadening their knowledge. Let me repeat, these were exceptions to the rule.

The strike wave that took place in Poland in 2006–2007 forced the management of health-care institutions to start paying much higher salaries to their clinical staff, especially to medical doctors. Since salaries in Poland's health-care sector rose so rapidly, interest in working abroad has all but disappeared. Such transfers simply became unprofitable.

On the other hand, since 2007 we have noted increasing numbers of returnees. Most people return from English-speaking countries, though it would be difficult for

---

3 All except the last vignette are based on private interviews carried out between May and August 2009.

me to estimate the scale of this trend. Among the reasons for coming home, medical doctors mention first of all the financial aspects, though certainly the cultural differences between Poland and the target countries induce the medical doctors to come back. If these are coupled with the problems in the workplace (unpleasant atmosphere or conflicts), doctors are additionally motivated to return.

Another reason to return is that medical doctors miss their families. Despite the relatively low prices of airplane tickets (and other means of transportation), sporadic weekend and/or holiday visits to Poland do not suffice in maintaining ties with family and friends. One may thus conclude that people find the separation from their relatives hard to bear, which induces return migration, or discourages medical doctors from leaving Poland, especially since local salaries have increased.

Migrants most often return home on completion of their probation period (six months), but in this instance I am not in a position to speculate about the scale of the phenomenon, either. There are sporadic cases of individuals who leave Poland a number of times in search of new job opportunities. If they do not like their job, they come back and seek other job placement opportunities abroad.

Daily commuter

Dr J lives in Poland but works and specializes in orthopaedics in Germany, driving 35km for his daily commute between home in Poland and work in Germany:

It is not a problem for me. I decided to work and upgrade my education abroad because in 2003 only a few lucky doctors managed to be enrolled for my favourite specialization. I like working in Germany, I have been well-received by my colleagues. My main problems were related to the language but it got easier with time.

I am not planning to practice in Poland after finishing my specialization due to the fact that the money I can earn abroad meets my financial expectations. Moreover, I would rather devote my free time to my family and rest instead of undertaking additional income-related activities.

Dentist practising at home and abroad[4]

Dr T is a dentist with a long professional experience. The owner of a private dental clinic in Lodz since 2003, she decided to travel abroad to increase her income. She leaves home at 5am to travel 300km to Krakow airport for a flight to Shannon, Ireland, and then on to Limerick. The trip takes eight hours. In spite of tiredness she sees her patients on the same day.

---

4 Based on Gazeta.pl 2008.

She has patients from several different countries because Polish doctors are highly respected in Ireland. Limerick is home to about 15 000 Poles (around a quarter of the population) and they need Polish doctors in different specialties with whom they can talk in their own language. Doctors are willing to provide services, even for a few days a month, as they can earn three times as much as in Poland. There is a shortage of specialists in Ireland and well-qualified Polish doctors are willing to cover the cost of travel and provide additional services on the island.

4. Dynamics of enlargement

Data from the Polish Chamber of Physicians and Dentists (see Table 12.1) show that 3% (3579) of Poland's 116 847 practising medical doctors collected the certifications required to seek job placements in other EU Member States within the first year of EU accession (data as of 30 June 2005). Over the following years, the proportion of certifications issued to practising medical doctors increased annually by an average of 1.2%. At the end of 2008, the proportion of total certifications issued reached 6.1% (Table 12.1). Data from the EU-15 show that new registrations of Polish medical doctors grew exponentially between 2000 and 2006 (Figs. 1 & 2).

Yet many health professionals do not leave permanently, as the vignettes show. Part-time jobs abroad are often treated as a means of earning extra money. Migration procedures were cumbersome before EU enlargement but accession and free movement appear to have made short-term stays and commuting between countries more common practices.

Undoubtedly, accession has had a great impact on the migration of Polish medical professionals. With the country's new status as an EU Member State, Polish citizens have the opportunity to exercise their newly acquired privileges (free movement of individuals and promotion of entrepreneurship). Given that the professional qualifications of health professionals are automatically recognized across borders, most legal barriers to working in other EU countries have disappeared.[5] This has opened up a host of entirely new opportunities to health professionals and brought about huge political and societal impacts (Ministry of Health 2009).

While political events made emigration possible, the substantial differences in compensation levels for health professionals in Poland and those in the EU-15 constituted another stimulus for migration. Until recently, financial considerations made Poland unattractive as a target country for foreign citizens. It can also be argued that accession and its effects on public expectations played

---

5 Of course, other barriers to migration remain. These include the cost of migration, language differences, finding employment, etc.

at least an indirect role in the social context of the 2006–2007 strikes that resulted in pay rises within the Polish health sector.

5. Impact on the Polish health system

It is difficult to evaluate the exact impact of health professional mobility. The absence of reports or studies makes it virtually impossible to establish a cause-and-effect link between the level of service delivery, the population's access to health services or the management of the system and migration. However, outmigration almost certainly exacerbates pre-existing workforce shortages not least in smaller hospitals and in certain medical specialties. Moreover, hospital managers appear to react to outmigration by proposing new contractual conditions to retain staff (see section 8).

Emigration contributes to staffing shortages that can be seen especially in small towns, county/poviat hospitals have problems employing adequate numbers of medical doctors.[6] Data collected by the Ministry of Health indicate shortages in almost all the professional groups studied. Table 12.7 compares the number of vacancies in the health workforce and registered unemployment in the professional groups.

Table 12.7 *Vacancies and registered unemployment in health professional groups, 2006*

Professional group	Vacancies	Registered unemployed	Vacancies per unemployed
Medical doctors	4 113	389	10.57
Dentists	86	103	0.83
Nurses	3 229	4 236	0.76
Midwives	312	690	0.45
TOTAL	**7 740**	**5 418**	**1.43**

Source: Ministry of Health 2009.

The fairly large number of unemployed nurses and midwives (with the concomitant strong demand for their services) may confirm the Polish Chamber of Nurses and Midwives' estimate that around 100 000 members of this group remain professionally inactive (see section 1 and Table 12.3). Conversely, unemployment among medical doctors was practically non-existent – with over ten vacancies for every unemployed person (Table 12.7). Those who did register as unemployed may have chosen to do so (for instance) in order to

---

6 Interview with chief executive officer of a county (general) hospital 5 May 2009.

retain their entitlements. Most vacancies were for posts in medical specialties.[7] These are presented in Table 12.8, including the data on certifications issued by the Polish Chamber of Physicians and Dentists and made available by the Ministry of Health upon special request.

Table 12.8 *Vacancies (2008) and numbers of certifications of professional qualifications issued (2004–2006 and 2008), by medical speciality*

Medical specialty	Vacancies (2008)	Certification holders as proportion of total registered medical doctors	
		May 2004–June 2006 %	As of 31 Dec 2008 %
Anaesthetics & intensive care	398	15.6	18.9
Internal medicine	312	1.4[a]	5.1
Emergency medicine	306	na	13.2
Paediatrics	230	na	3.5
General surgery	206	6.1	8.6
Psychiatry	170	na	5.4
Orthopaedics & traumatology of motor organ	125	7.4	10.0
Gynaecology and obstetrics	110	na	6.3

Sources: Ministry of Health 2009, Kaczmarczyk 2006. Notes: [a] as of 30 June 2005, na = no data available.

The data indicate that staffing shortages first affect the specialties in which relatively high proportions of medical doctors are applying for certification, particularly anaesthetics and intensive care as well as emergency medicine. Random data collection makes it impossible to perform statistical calculations to determine the likely migration rate of medical doctors by individual specialty. However, emigration of medical doctors contributes in some degree to staff shortages in the Polish health system. Although the present report does not consider allied health professional groups such as rehabilitation specialists or physiotherapists, shortages in these specialties are also being reported (Sikora 2007).

These findings should be kept in mind when considering the coverage of health professionals per population. Figures can be falsely reassuring – the number of health professionals with the right to practise may have remained remarkably stable over the last five years (Table 12.9) but this is due in part to emigrating individuals who remain on Polish registers.

---

7 Vacancies by voivodship/region are presented in Table 10. Explanation of the differences presented is beyond the scope of the present study.

Table 12.9 *Health professionals eligible to practise per 1000 population (2003–2007)*

	2003	2004	2005	2006	2007
Medical doctors	32.1	32.8	33.2	33.9	33.1
Dentists	8.6	8.9	9.0	9.2	9.3
Nurses	69.4	70.4	71.8	72.2	71.6
Midwives	8.5	8.5	8.6	8.7	8.6
Pharmacists	6.3	6.2	6.4	6.6	7.0

Sources: Ministry of Health Statistic Bulletins 2004–2008.

6. Relevance of cross-border health professional mobility

Health professional mobility has to be seen in the context of the relevant health system and its workforce. Migration to and from Poland are not the only influences on the size and characteristics of the health workforce. Other relevant health workforce issues include attrition, staffing shortages, waiting lists, regional distribution and medical education.

Attrition is a concern as dissatisfaction with working conditions and remuneration levels has led to major changes in the size and structure of the health workforce. These changes were already manifest in the 1990s as the numbers of medical doctors and nurses had decreased gradually during the previous decade (GUS 2000). Part of the observed decline in workforce numbers should be attributed to medical doctors moving into alternative careers – mostly as sales representatives of pharmaceutical companies but also as health-care managers (for local governments, public fundholders, health-care units) or within companies undertaking clinical trials. The extremely low salaries and limited opportunities to supplement income (unlike medical doctors) have contributed to the gradually waning interest in acquiring professional qualifications in nursing (Whitfield et al. 2002). It should also be noted that large Polish medical corporations currently looking for medical personnel are commissioning headhunting companies in the United Kingdom to recruit Polish returnees.[8]

The demand for, and availability of, health professionals varies by region of the country and by specialty (Table 12.10). This phenomenon is a continuing influence on individual institutions' capacity to provide services.

Given the financial constraints on public fundholders, waiting lists for medical services in Poland have become a more serious problem. Yet although commonplace in the public health system,[9] it is more striking that waiting lists

---

8 Interview with president of private medical company (service provider) in 2009.

9 Minister of Health (2005) addressed the problem of waiting lists on 26 September 2005, issuing a regulation on the medical criteria that health-care providers should use when placing patients on the waiting list for a given procedure.

Table 12.10 *Vacancies in public hospitals (full-time equivalents) by voivodship/region*

No	Voivodship (region)	Vacancies	
		Medical doctors	**Nurses**
1	Dolnośląskie	217	186
2	Kujawsko-Pomorskie	380	488
3	Lubelskie	500	389
4	Lubuskie	47	9
5	Łódzkie	247	211
6	Małopolskie	50	51
7	Mazowieckie	892	168
8	Opolskie	60	126
9	Podkarpackie	175	132
10	Podlaskie	193	119
11	Pomorskie	162	263
12	Śląskie	279	319
13	Świętokrzyskie	177	194
14	Warmińsko-Mazurskie	273	133
15	Wielkopolskie	196	216
16	Zachodniopomorskie	260	224
	TOTAL	**4 108**	**3 228**

Source: Sikora 2007.

and queues have also affected the private sector for some time. Individuals with private insurance or subscriptions for medical services (a bonus offered by some employers) have begun to experience problems accessing services (Pochrzęst 2008) and waiting lists for services paid out of pocket (a new practice in Poland) have become more common. This is due to a number of phenomena – an increasingly affluent society (more and more people can afford these services); emigration of medical doctors contributing to the limited workforce numbers; and private health service providers that are unwilling or unable to employ more staff (Kalbarczyk 2009). Hence, the shortage of personnel is a problem for both public and private providers. Problems with the supply of specialists are starting to affect even large institutions but are of most concern for health-care units (mostly in hospitals) in smaller towns and in rural areas.

While not presenting a direct threat, emigration of health professionals is likely to contribute to workforce shortages in the Polish health system. This issue has become more pertinent since the National Health Fund, the public purchaser of health services in Poland, raised staffing requirements for health institutions that provide universally covered care (National Health Fund 2008) but the Ministry of Health has not exercised its authority to increase the number of medical students – both nurses and doctors.

Local initiatives and effort led to the opening of a new medical school in Olsztyn (northern Poland) in 2008. As the first new medical faculty in Poland in over 40 years this leads to the conclusion that there is an absence of government-level action to increase the number of medical graduates. This should be seen in the context of the disparity between the medical workforce in Poland (22.8 per capita) and the OECD average (47.7) and between the number of medical graduates in Poland (6.1 per capita) and the OECD average (10.5) in 2006.

7. Factors influencing health professional mobility

Korczynska and Duszczyk (2005) report that up to 2004 there was an observed culmination of instigating factors that encouraged outflows and a lack of pull factors to attract potential immigrants to Poland. The main reasons for emigration were low salaries, difficult working conditions and limited possibilities for professional development. In later studies among final-year medical students, the main activating factors for leaving Poland were reported to be not only better income and career prospects but also greater prestige and better organization of work (Jośko et al. 2007).

Health professionals have cited low incomes, limited opportunities for professional development and poor working conditions among the reasons for emigration (Sikora 2007). Until recently there were significant differences between salaries in Poland and in the destination countries (Maniak & Nowak-Lewandowska 2004) but these differences have been decreasing. The highest and the lowest annual salaries of different categories of medical staff are shown in Fig. 12.3. It should be noted that these do not include medical doctors' private practice income as this remains difficult to determine. The method by which the Ministry of Health collates data precludes calculation of the average salaries of health professionals but it is clear that present compensation levels can be relatively high, even in comparison with other countries.

Fig.12.3 *Annual minimum and maximum salaries of public- and private-sector health professionals and the country average salary in Poland, January 2008*

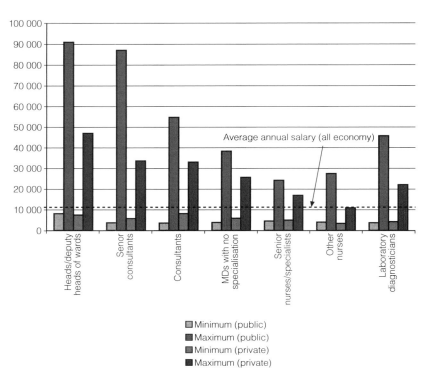

Source: Kalinowski 2008 *Note:* €1 = 3.62 Polish zloty.

Given that the other main motivating factors (possibilities of professional development or access to modern technologies) have not changed significantly in recent years, it appears that the increase in health professional salary levels in Poland is a major reason for the falling interest in migration, especially among medical doctors. This assertion is supported by the observed drop in emigration after salary levels increased. This has caused serious problems for agencies seeking to recruit enough medical staff to work abroad (see section 3).

In 2003, Greger carried out a survey of nurses employed in various health-care units in Poland. This revealed that lack of knowledge about the outside world can be a mitigating factor that hinders mobility among nurses. Many nurses who emigrate are making their first visit abroad and often experience culture shock and embarrassment due to communication problems: "Many migrants do end up coming home before the end of their contract, feeling very frustrated and looking for somebody to blame" (Greger 2004). Also, it can be difficult to adjust to the new working conditions as nurses in Poland have less autonomy than their peers in most EU-15 Member States.

8. Policy, regulation and interventions

8.1 *Mutual recognition of diplomas and bilateral agreements*

Adoption of Directive 2005/36/EC (European Parliament and Council of the European Union 2005) resulted in twelve sectoral directives (20 October 2007) that contributed to improving the transparency of qualifications and competences and facilitated mobility between countries throughout Europe. As a result, European countries such as Ireland, the Netherlands, Spain and the United Kingdom opened their markets to Polish health professionals (Korczynska & Duszczyk 2005, Riga 2007). Poland and the destination countries entered into bilateral agreements to recruit staff for a fixed period of time and provide cultural adaptation support. During the Polish Prime Minister's official visit to the Netherlands in 2001 the Dutch Prime Minister declared that "After Poland enters the European Union Poles should have access to the Dutch labour market" (Republic of Poland 2001). The Netherlands was the first country to make such a commitment and the EU-PHARE Polish-Dutch Twinning Project on Mutual Recognition of Qualifications for Medical Professions started a few years later.

8.2 *National-level policy development and interventions*

The authors' experience suggests that no proactive health policies and no coherent concept of operation for the national health system have been formulated at state level. Health policy concerning the health workforce and mobility has not been well-developed and government activities are limited only to general declarations about the need to keep health professionals at home.

Market mechanisms of compensation levels, demand levels and exchange rates determine the behaviour of health professionals by influencing whether they perceive working abroad as an attractive or unattractive option. However, various state interventions may indirectly have influenced the change in the Polish health workforce's emigration patterns – although these were rather more emergency fire-fighting initiatives rather than coherent and/or sufficient long-term policies. For example, although academic facilities increased the number of enrolled medical students in 2005 there has been only a small increase in the financial subsidy for medical universities (Lesniowska 2006).

Other interventions before EU accession aimed to reduce employment levels in health care. The main policy tool was state reimbursement of the redundancy payments made by public health-care institutions. There are no comprehensive data on the level of spending for this purpose but it is estimated at the level of around 293 million Polish zloty[10] in 1999–2005 (Ministry of Health 2003).

---

10 Exchange rate fluctuations during the six-year period allow only a very rough conversion – around €73 million.

In parallel, a 2001 regulation raised the salaries of all fully contracted health professionals in public health-care institutions by 203 Polish zloty (about €56) per month – whatever their positions, years of work experience, qualifications or implications for their health-care institutions. It was never made clear how the pay rise was to be paid and, while attractive for working staff, the initiative left numerous health-care institutions in debt.

Another initiative was preferred loans. Health professionals who decided to leave the public sector and start their own health provision businesses could apply for loans to help them start their enterprises. Mainly a response to the poor employment situation in Poland, these efforts have indirectly contributed to reducing the emigration of the Polish health workforce by giving financial, career-related and entrepreneurial incentives that may impact on the way in which domestic opportunities of professional development are viewed.

State intervention could be also observed in the recruitment of new candidates for health and health-related studies. Based on the prognosis of needs for graduates in given studies, the health minister determined the quotas for candidates in public and private higher education (Supreme Chamber of Nurses and Midwives 2008). At postgraduate level, the health minister issued the list of priority specializations. This was decided following discussion on patient access to specialist doctors in Poland and resulted in higher pay for medical doctors undertaking specialist training in the priority areas. In 2009, an intern in a non-priority specialization received 3170 Polish zloty (around €708)[11] during the first two years and 3458 Polish zloty (around €773) thereafter. A contemporary in a priority specialization received 3602 Polish zloty (around €805) and 3890 Polish zloty (around €869) respectively.

8.3 *Specific interventions and managerial tools*

In order to meet the increased financial expectations of medical staff who might otherwise change employer or emigrate, managers of health-care units are offering changes in employment status – from full-time employment contracts to fee-for-service self-employment agreements (with smaller obligatory insurance contributions). It is likely that expectation of higher salaries will result in organizational changes such as employing less-qualified staff to take over some simpler or administrative tasks and recruiting personnel in other countries (taking account of the language difficulties).

Historically, doctors in Poland have worked long hours of overtime but the necessity of adapting to the EU working time directive (European Parliament and Council of the European Union 2003) means that only self-employed

---

11 Exchange rate as at 1 July 2009 (http://www.pekaobh.pl/u235/navi/34413, accessed 26 January 2010).

doctors can increase their working hours (see section 1). In conjunction with staff shortages, these changes have encouraged medical doctors to move to contract employment (Sikora 2009).

8.4 *Political force field of health professional mobility*

For a number of years, Poland's health-care system has attracted harsh criticism from its users, each subsequent survey confirming the populace's low opinion (Czapiński & Panek 2009). The system's responsiveness has never been rated particularly highly and a lack of respect for patients' rights, their dignity and autonomy is all too common (Kautsch 2009). However, the system is likely to improve as it becomes more market oriented. Private health-care providers that offer services in the framework of universal health insurance have no political support from the public authorities but largely achieve patient satisfaction. Also, growing competition among private health providers may result in better quality services and attention to patient's needs.

9. Conclusion

When drawing a conclusion from the collected data it should be noted that there is varying information from some sources. This may be due to differences in the definitions of health professionals or registration formats noticed by García-Pérez et al. (2007).

The present study shows that Polish health professionals were emigrating to EU Member States even before formal accession but the phenomenon escalated significantly in 2004 following the disappearance of the barriers that had made it difficult for health professionals to seek job placements abroad. However, emigration fell almost equally rapidly as compensation levels for health professionals in Poland began to increase in 2007.

The findings of this study show differences in the migration patterns of the different health professions. Medical doctors and dentists are characterized by greater willingness to migrate and more positive experiences; nurses often encounter problems securing suitable employment (often taking positions beneath their professional qualification levels). From mid 2005 to the end of 2008, 6.1% of all practising medical doctors and 6.7% of all practising dentists had been issued with professional qualification certifications; 3% of practising nurses obtained certifications between mid 2004 and mid 2006. The apparent lower emigration levels among nurses may be due in part to their profession having less autonomy in Poland than in other, mostly EU-15, Member States. Also, emigrating nurses do not appear in statistics if they seek employment in (for example) long-term care facilities that do not require certification of qualifications. Emigrating doctors and nurses have moved mostly to the United Kingdom, Ireland, Germany and the Scandinavian countries.

Health professional mobility has contributed to a certain degree to the increasing number of vacancies in the Polish health sector – the highest numbers of vacancies are seen for anaesthetists and internists (though the latter is the most numerous professional group) and the specialist groups with the highest numbers of certification applications are anaesthetists, followed by medical doctors of diagnostic and surgical specialties.

Health professional mobility is a relatively new phenomenon that has not yet been studied sufficiently. However, it may be argued that recent migration patterns are not likely to constitute a lasting problem. Health professionals have been returning to Poland since 2007, attracted by salary increases resulting from attrition and migration; increased demand for medical services; and changing currency exchange rates. In the absence of well-considered retention policies and state measures, such market forces encourage health professionals who are considering emigration to stay at home and emigrants to return.

References

Czapiński J, Panek T (eds.) (2009). *Social diagnosis 2009. The subjective quality and objective conditions of life in Poland.* Warsaw, The Council for Social Monitoring (http://www.diagnoza.com/data/report/report_2009.pdf, accessed 1 December 2010).

Danielewicz R et al. (2006). Country report – Poland. In: Buchan J, Perfilieva G (eds.). *Health worker migration in the European Region: country case studies and policy implications.* Copenhagen, Division of Country Support, WHO Regional Office for Europe.

Dumont J-C, Zurn P (2007). Immigrant health workers in OECD countries in the broader context of highly skilled migration. In: *International Migration Outlook 2007.* Paris, Organisation for Economic Co-operation and Development.

European Parliament and Council of the European Union (2003). Directive 2003/88/EC of the European Parliament and of the Council of 4 November 2003 concerning certain aspects of the organisation of working time. *Official Journal of the European Union*, 46:9–18.

European Parliament and Council of the European Union (2005). Directive 2005/36/EC of the European Parliament and of the Council of 7 September

2005 on the recognition of professional qualifications. *Official Journal of the European Union*, 255(48):22–142.

García-Pérez MA et al. (2007). Physicians' migration in Europe: an overview of the current situation. *BMC Health Services Research*, 7:201 (http://www. biomedcentral.com/ 1472-6963/7/201, accessed 1 December 2010).

Gazeta.pl (2008). *Polscy lekarze wybierają Irlandię na dodatkowe dyżury* [Polish doctors choose Ireland for addtitional duty hours]. *Gazeta.pl Wiadomości*, 20 September 2008 (http://wiadomosci.gazeta.pl/Wiadomosci/10,88721,57155 55,Polscy_lekarze_wybieraja Irlandie_na_dodatkowe_dyzury.html, accessed 1 December 2010).

Greger J (2004). Poland. In: Van Eyck K (ed.). *Women and international migration in the health sector. Final report of Public Services International's participatory action research 2003*. Ferney Voltaire, Public Services International.

GUS (2000). *Concise Statistical Yearbook of Poland 2000*. Warsaw, Central Statistical Office.

GUS (2006a). *Concise Statistical Yearbook of Poland, 2006*. Warsaw, Central Statistical Office.

GUS (2006b). *Statistical Yearbook of the Republic of Poland 2006*. Warsaw, Central Statistical Office.

GUS (2007a). *Concise Statistical Yearbook of Poland, 2007*. Warsaw, Central Statistical Office.

GUS (2007b). *Statistical Yearbook of the Republic of Poland 2007*. Warsaw, Central Statistical Office.

GUS (2008a). *Concise Statistical Yearbook of Poland, 2008*. Warsaw, Central Statistical Office.

GUS (2008b). *Statistical Yearbook of the Republic of Poland 2008*. Warsaw, Central Statistical Office.

GUS (2009a). *Concise Statistical Yearbook of Poland, 2009*. Warsaw, Central Statistical Office.

GUS (2009b). *Statistical Yearbook of the Republic of Poland 2009*. Warsaw, Central Statistical Office.

Hajnosz I (2004). *Odpływ lekarzy* [The ebb of physicians]. *Gazeta Wyborcza*, 26 February 2004.

Jośko J et al. (2007). *Ojczyzna czy obczyzna? Plany zawodowe studentów Śląskiej Akademii Medycznej* [Home or exile? Professional plans of the Silesian Medical Academy students]. *Problemy Higieny i Epidemiologii* [Problems of Hygiene and Epidemiology], 88(1):20–23.

Kaczmarczyk P (2006). *Highly skilled migration from Poland and other CEE countries – myths and reality.* Warsaw, Center for International Relations (Reports & Analyses 17/06).

Kalbarczyk P (2009). Insurance group as the long-term business partner. *International Medical Business Forum MedMarket Conference, Warsaw, 21–22 April 2009.*

Kalinowski P (2008). *Wyszarpnięte pensje* [Grabbed away salaries]. *Medical Tribune,* 3/2008.

Kautsch M (2009). Podejście do potrzeb pacjenta w publicznych zakładach opieki zdrowotnej w Polsce [An approach to patient's needs in public health-care institutions in Poland]. In: Rudawska I, Soboń M (eds.). *Przedsiębiorstwo i klient w gospodarce opartej na usługach* [An enterprise and a client in service-based economy]. Warsaw, Difin.

Kicinger A (2005). *Between Polish interests and the EU influence – Polish migration policy development 1989–2004.* Warsaw, Central European Forum for Migration Research (CEFMR Working Paper 9/2005).

Komorowski S, Hebda M (2008). Woczekiwaniu na inwestora – rynek prywatnych usług medycznych w pierwszej fazie rozwoju [Waiting for an investor – the market of private medical services in the first phase of its development], *Forum Biznesu Medycznego MedMarket* [*Medical Business Forum*], Warsaw, 5 June 2008.

Korczyńska J, Duszczyk M (2005). *Zapotrzebowanie na prace obcokrajowcow w Polsce. Proba analizy i wniosków dla polityki migracyjnej* [*Demand for work of the foreigners in Poland. A trial analysis and conclusion for the migration policy in Poland*]. Warsaw, Instytut Spraw Publicznych, Krajowa Izba Gospodarcza [Institute of Public Affairs, National Chamber of Commerce].

Kudlicki L (2006). *Nowa Wielka Emigracja* [New great emigration]. *Bezpieczeństwo Narodowe [Quarterly of the National Security Bureau of Poland],* I-2006(1):90–110.

Leśniowska J (2005). Problem Migracji Polskij Kadry Medycznej [Problem of the migration of Polish medical personnel]. *Polityka Społeczna [Social Policy],* 4/2005.

Leśniowska J (2007). Migration patterns of Polish doctors within the EU. *Eurohealth,* 13(4):7–8.

Maniak G, Nowak-Lewandowska R (2006). Wybrane aspekty emigracji zarobkowych i ich konsekwencje dla rynku pracy w Polsce po 1 maja 2004 roku [Selected aspects of financial gain from emigration and its impact on the labour market in Poland after 1 May 2004]. *Presentation at the Third Assembly of Economy Chairs, Międzyzdroje, 5–7 June 2006.*

Minister of Health (2005). *Rozporządzenie Ministra Zdrowia z dnia 26 września 2005 r. w sprawie kryteriów medycznych, jakimi powinni kierować się świadczeniodawcy, umieszczając świadczeniobiorców na listach oczekujących na udzielenie świadczenia opieki zdrowotnej* [*Regulation of the Minister of Health dated 26 September 2005 on the medical criteria that health-care providers should use when placing patients on the waiting list for a given procedure*]. National Health Fund (Dz.U.05.200.1661).

Ministry of Health (2003). *Ocena realizacji programów działań osłonowych i restrukturyzacji w ochronie zdrowia* [Assessment of support programmes and restructuring in health care]. Warsaw.

Ministry of Health. *Statistic Bulletins 2004–2008.* (http://www.csioz.gov.pl/biuletyn.htm, accessed 1 December 2009).

Ministry of Health (2009). *Migracje polskich lekarzy, pielęgniarek i położnych po przystąpieniu Polski do Unii /Raport z realizacji programu w 2006r.* [*Migration of Polish physicians, nurses and midwives after joining European Union. Report on the realization of the programme in 2006* (http://www.mz.gov.pl/wwwmz/index?mr=&ms=&ml=pl& mi=565&mx=0&ma=7876, accessed 18 April 2009).

National Health Fund (2008). *Zarządzenie Nr 93/2008/DSOZ Prezesa Narodowego Funduszu Zdrowia z dnia 22 października 2008 r. w sprawie określenia warunków zawierania i realizacji umów w rodzaju: leczenie szpitalne* [Ruling number 93/2008/ of the President of the National Health Fund from 22nd October 2008 on contracting hospital services (http://www.nfz.gov.pl/new/index.php?katnr=3&dzialnr=12& artnr=3493&b=1, accessed 12 November 2009).

Nosowska KT, Gorynski P (2006). *Migracja personelu medycznego do pracy za granica w okresie pierwszego roku po przystapieniu Polski do Unii Europejskiej.* [Migration of medical personnel to work abroad during the first year of joining European Union] *Problemy Higieny in Epidemiologii* [*Problems of Hygiene and Epidemiology*] 87(1):55–60.

OECD (2008a). *International migration outlook 2008*. Paris, Organisation for Economic Co-operation and Development.

OECD (2008b). OECD health data 2008: statistics and indicators for 30 countries, (December 2008 second Internet update). Paris, OECD Publishing.

Pochrzęst A (2008). *Leczysz się prywatnie? To poczekaj do czwartku* [Do you go to a private doctor? Then wait till Thursday]. *Gazeta Stołeczna*, 23 September 2008.

Republic of Poland (2001). Materials and documents: speeches and addresses. *Chronicle,* No.8–9/2001 (http://www.msz.gov.pl/files/file_library/31/010809_332.doc, accessed 10 December 2009.

Riga A (2007). *Dutch health and social care: international labour mobility*. Maastricht, Comparative European Social Research and Theory (http://cesrt.hszuyd.nl /files/RESEARCH%20THEMES/Social%20work%20practice/DutchHealthSocCare_Riga%20website%20versie.pdf, accessed 6 November 2009).

Sikora D (2007). Szpitalom *brakuje młodych lekarzy i specjalistów* [Hospitals lack young doctors and specialists]. *Gazeta Prawna* [Legal Newspaper], 18 January 2007.

Sikora D (2009). *Aby obejść przepisy o czasie pracy szpitale zatrudniają lekarzy na zlecenie* [Hospitals commission doctors to go around the regulations on the working hours]. *Dziennik Gazeta Prawna* [Legal Newspaper Daily], 2 October 2009.

Supreme Chamber of Nurses and Midwives (2008). *Analiza poziomu wykształcenia zarejestrowanych pielęgniarek i położnych* [*Analysis of the educational level of registered nurses and midwives*]. Warsaw, Naczelna Rada Pielęgniarek i Położnych.

Whitfield M et al. (2002). *A TFR Report – A preliminary analysis of hospital cost and activity data*. School of Health and Related Research, University of Sheffield (Scharr, Report Series No. 4).

Zurn P, Dumont J-C (2008). *Health workforce and international migration: can New Zealand compete?* Paris, Organisation for Economic Co-operation and Development (OECD Health Working Paper No. 33).

Chapter 13

Emigration of health professionals as an emergent challenge? Romania's accession to the European Union

Adriana Galan, Victor Olsavszky, Cristian Vladescu

1. Introduction

Romania is predominantly a source country for health professionals and health professional mobility represents an emergent challenge for policy-makers. This situation is the result of European Union (EU) accession in 2007 and (probably even more importantly) other dynamics related to demographics and poor planning and management of the health workforce.

In 2006, the mass media raised concern by predicting "massive" emigration of medical doctors and nurses that would jeopardize the proper operation of the health system. The scale of emigration in 2007 was indeed high – 1421 medical doctors left in that year. This affected the most economically deprived area (North-East Region) of Romania more than other regions but the overall phenomenon was not as dramatic as expected in 2008 and 2009 and showed no signs of jeopardizing the health system. Yet by the end of 2009 the economic crisis had begun to impact deeply on Romanian society, including the health system. Moreover, some additional disincentives for health professionals were introduced in 2010, including a 25% salary decrease and reductions in staff. Thus, developments concerning the domestic workforce combined with the emigration of health professionals to become a critical concern.

The verification certificates issued by the Ministry of Health and the certificates of good standing (CGSs) issued by the Romanian College of Physicians (RCP) provide some data but Romania has no accurate information on international inflows and outflows of health professionals. This is particularly true for nurses. A good monitoring system that integrates the existing data sources for health professional mobility is essential to support decision-making and policy responses in the country.

To date, there is no human resources policy document on health professionals in Romania. Some elements are scattered throughout other sectoral health strategies but an effective health workforce strategy has been lacking and some of the measures undertaken to retain health professionals in rural and remote areas have not proved effective.

Limitations of the study

There is no monitoring system on health professional mobility. Data on inflows and outflows and on the mobility of health professionals within the country are extremely scarce and of poor quality, with low levels of accuracy and completeness. Overall, data on medical doctors are perceived to be of better quality and accuracy than those on nurses and midwives. However, some fragmented data sources offer a rough estimate of the mobility phenomenon (see Table 13.1).

Existing data do not allow any comparison of temporary and permanent health professional migration. The data on verification certificates issued by the Ministry of Health provide an overall annual estimate of intentions to leave and have been collected since 2007. However, they are not an accurate measure of

Table 13.1 *Main data sources and data holders on health professional mobility in Romania*

Data holder	Type of data
Ministry of Health and its subordinate institution, the National Centre for Organising and Ensuring the Health Information System (NCOEHIS)	National registry of medical doctors and dentists Number of requests for diploma recognition certificates
RCP	National registry of practising medical doctors
Romanian College of Dental Practitioners	National registry of practising dentists
Order of Nurses and Midwives (OAMMR)	National registry of practising nurses and midwives
National Institute of Statistics	Labour force survey
Ministry of Labour, Family and Social Protection	Data on temporary work contracts mediated through its accredited structures

emigration because not all applicants go on to migrate. In 2007, EU accession induced many applications from medical doctors already working abroad and seeking to comply with their new status as EU citizens. The data presented in this case study show that only 1421 of the 4990 medical doctors who requested verification certificates in 2007 actually emigrated – less than a third (28.4%) (Dragomiristeanu et al. 2008, Ministry of Health 2008).

2. Mobility profile of Romania

Although not fully supported by reliable information, it appears that outflows of Romanian health professionals have been increasing since EU accession in January 2007. This section assesses the cross-border mobility patterns of health professionals at national and regional levels, taking account of inflows and outflows. There are significant regional variations – the most economically deprived region of Romania is more affected by emigrating medical doctors than other regions. The extent of nurse emigration is underestimated by the existing data sources which are of insufficient quality and do not cover all nurses leaving the country. It may be that the data on nurses are of lesser quality partly because the government considers the exodus of medical doctors to be more problematic for the health system.

No data are available on the mobility of dentists – whether to, from or within the country. Nearly all dentists are private providers who earn considerably higher incomes than other medical doctors, therefore it is likely that they prefer to work in Romania. The media have not reported any warning signals concerning significant migration flows among dentists.

2.1 *Outflows*

Since 2007, all medical doctors (including dentists), nurses and midwives applying to the Ministry of Health have been issued with certificates of diploma recognition based on a preliminary verification.

Medical doctors

Official data on diploma verification applications indicate that about 10% of active medical doctors had the intention to leave the country in 2007. In the two years following this accession year, the total number of applications showed clear signs of decreasing.

Table 13.2 *Practising medical doctors applying for diploma verification to work in EU Member States, 2007–2009*

	Medical doctors applying for diploma verification	
	Total	% of practising medical doctors
2007	4 990	10.2
2008 and (Jan–May) 2009	2 683	a

Source: Ministry of Health unpublished data 2009. *Note*: ª cannot be calculated because it includes only the period January–May 2009.

Most data related to the mobility of medical doctors can be retrieved only from specific studies. In 2008, the RCP carried out an emigration study of all practising medical doctors (Dragomiristeanu et al. 2008). The outmigration rate was calculated based on the number of CGSs issued by each district branch of the RCP. It should be noted that destination countries request CGSs for registering procedures and therefore they indicate only the intention to leave and not actual emigration. Nevertheless, they are considered to be better proxies than the verification certificates.

About 3% (1421) of the total number of practising medical doctors left Romania in 2007 and more than 90% of these requested CGSs for EU Member States (Dragomiristeanu et al. 2008). The highest proportion of applications came from medical doctors in Iasi district in the North-East Region, the most economically deprived area in Romania (Table 13.3). The most common medical specialties of applicants were family medicine, intensive care and psychiatry.

France, Germany, Italy and the United Kingdom appear to be the favoured destination countries – a finding supported by the high numbers reported from these destination countries. Data from the French medical chamber[1] show that 1000 Romanian medical doctors registered in France between January 2007 and July 2008 (CNOM 2009). The German medical chamber[2] reported 927 foreign medical doctors from Romania (Federal Physicians Chamber 2009) and the British General Medical Council (GMC) had 671 new registrants from Romania between 2003 and 2008 (see Table 8.4). In 2009, the European Migration Network Italy reported that 555 Romanian doctors were registered with the Italian Medical Association (EMN 2009).

---

1 *l'Ordre des Médecins.*

2 *Bundesaerztekammer.*

Table 13.3 Romanian regions and declared destination countries of medical doctors applying for CGSs, 2007

Region	Practising medical doctors	CGS applicant medical doctors		Declared destination countries in order of popularity
		Total	%	
North-East	6 407	321	5.0	UK, France, Germany, Italy, Belgium, Denmark, Australia, Israel, Sweden, Portugal, USA, Netherlands, Spain, Ireland
Iasi district[a]	2 021	256	12.7	Belgium, France, Denmark, Germany, UK, Australia, Israel, Italy, Sweden, Portugal, USA, Netherlands, Spain
South-East	4 414	65	1.5	France, Germany, Italy, UK, Netherlands, Canada, Pakistan, Sweden, Belgium, Australia
South-Muntenia	5 112	45	0.9	France, UK, Italy, Norway, Belgium, Ireland
South-West Oltenia	4 402	48	1.1	France, UK, Italy, Germany, Canada, Sweden, Middle East
West	5 501	184	3.3	UK, France, Germany, Hungary, Italy, Switzerland, Sweden, Ireland, Netherlands, Norway, Canada, USA, Spain
North-West	6 413	170	2.7	France, UK, Germany, Ireland, Finland, Spain, Canada, Italy, Ireland, Sweden, Austria, Belgium, Netherlands
Centre	5 461	88	1.6	UK, Italy, France, Germany, Ireland, Netherlands, Ireland, USA, Belgium, Luxembourg
Bucharest-Ilfov	12 720	500	3.9	
Bucharest[b]	12 481	494	3.9	South Africa, Australia, Belgium, Canada, Cyprus, Denmark, Switzerland, France, Germany, Greece, Ireland, Israel, Italy, Luxembourg, UK, Monaco, Norway, Netherlands, Portugal, USA, Slovakia, Spain, Sweden
ROMANIA	**50 430**	**1 421**	**2.8**	

Source: Dragomiristeanu et al. 2008. Note: [a] Iasi district is part of the North-East Region; [b] Bucharest is part of Bucharest-Ilfov region.

Updated data from the RCP show that 1252 medical doctors requested CGSs in 2008. Similar to 2007 (Table 13.3), most of the certificates were issued in Bucharest (448) and Iaşi (184). Overall migration intentions remained stable between the two years and showed only a slight fall – from 1421 to 1252 (RCP 2009).

Prior to accession, the NCOEHIS carried out another special study concerning the emigration of health professionals. The data (Pertache & Ursuleanu 2006) show that 360 Romanian medical doctors left the country in 2004. Most (76%) had been working in hospitals in Romania and only 6% were family doctors, in contrast with the high numbers of family doctors in 2007. However, this is only a rough estimation that probably underestimates the phenomenon.

Unofficial data show substantial increases in requests for verification certificates in 2010 – with applications averaging over 300 per month. In a recent interview, the Minister of Health acknowledged that the emigration phenomenon of doctors and nurses is rising and most likely will continue in the next 10 to 15 years. He admitted that over 9000 doctors have requested verification certificates since 2007 (Realitatea.net 2010).

Nurses and midwives

Almost nothing is known about the extent of nurse and midwife emigration because not all EU countries request a verification certificate. Consequently, even the number of certificates issued by the Ministry of Health and the OAMMR provide only rough estimates of the intention to leave; a considerably higher number could be leaving the country. The official data that are available cover nurses and midwives together. These show that 2896 nurses and midwives applied for diploma verification in 2007 – 3.4% of the workforce (Table 13.4). The total number of applications appeared to fall in subsequent years – similar to what was observed among medical doctors (Table 13.2).

A Ministry of Health study carried out in 2005 shows that 1652 Romanian nurses were working abroad that year (1.9% of all practising nurses) and that 82% of all nurses who emigrated were hospital nurses (Pertache & Ursuleanu 2006).

Since the exact extent of emigration is not known, the intention to emigrate and subjective appreciation of the phenomenon have been used as proxy indicators. The University of Medicine and Pharmacy "Victor Babeş" carried out a study on a national representative sample. This revealed that most nurses (25%) who intend to migrate usually live in the more deprived areas, such as the North-East Region (Olsavszky 2008). The OAMMR reports that about 5000 nurses have chosen to work abroad since 2007. For instance, the general manager of

Table 13.4 *Applications for diploma verification from nurses and midwives applying to work in EU Member States, 2007–2009*

	Total applicants	% of all nurses/midwives[a]
2007	2896	3.4
2008	1977 (issued 1813)	1.6
Jan–April 2009	612 (issued 172)	[b]

Sources: Ministry of Health unpublished data 2009, [a] WHO 2009. *Note*: [b] data on number of certificates available for only part of 2009.

the University Hospital, one of the biggest hospitals in Bucharest, reported that 80–100 of its nurses had been recorded as leaving the country to work abroad – about 10% of the hospital's nurses (Informaţia Medicală 2009).

Generally, nurses and midwives who intend to emigrate are aged 26–35, come from urban areas, have specialized in general medicine and graduated from private nursing college. Nevertheless, over half of all Romanian nurses do not want to migrate (Olsavszky 2008).

Data from other countries provides additional information on actual emigration. Italy's acute nursing shortage has made it an attractive destination country – the diplomas of 2420 Romanian nurses were recognized in 2005 alone (Chaloff 2008). Data from Germany show 606 nurses of Romanian nationality working there in 2008 (Federal Employment Agency 2009). Data from the United Kingdom show 493 newly registered Romanian trained nurses/midwives between 2003 and 2008 (see Table 8.5). The data from destination countries indicate that the scale of outmigration is considerably higher than that suggested by the data on diploma verifications (Table 13.4).

2.2 Inflows

Medical doctors

Table 13.5 summarizes the general immigration phenomenon after 2000. There are almost no data on foreign medical doctors working in Romania but it is likely that the constant high numbers of immigrants from the Republic of Moldova include medical doctors and nurses. It is widely known that Moldovan medical doctors move to Romania to specialize in non-clinical fields (such as epidemiology and public health) as in Moldova the training periods for these specialties are too short for EU recognition. Indeed, the new EU rules for diploma recognition make it unlikely that high numbers of non-EU medical doctors will have arrived in Romania since 2007, although some may arrive to obtain their university training.

Table 13.5 *Immigrants (permanent settlers) by country of origin, 2000–2005*

Country	2000	2001	2002	2003	2004	2005	2006	2007
Austria	84	68	81	69	90	76	75	126
Canada	60	93	131	181	175	153	187	271
China	-	-	-	-	-	1	362	375
France	110	101	80	83	101	117	125	184
Germany	227	207	224	231	296	238	252	423
Hungary	173	111	62	56	68	74	103	249
Iraq	-	-	2	2	-	1	121	129
Iran	-	-	2	-	-	7	120	139
Israel	57	101	108	148	185	134	156	239
Italy	70	81	91	112	163	216	313	844
Republic of Moldova	**9 146**	**8 682**	**5 214**	**1 881**	**1 254**	**1 917**	**4 349**	**4 019**
Syrian Arab Republic	-	-	15	11	14	13	151	228
Turkey	-	-	35	17	22	33	273	522
USA	161	191	227	235	259	311	292	466
Other	2 200	1 398	1 044	1 315	1 470	1 050	731	1 199

Source: National Institute of Statistics 2008b.

Nurses

The Ministry of Education, Research and Innovation is responsible for clearing the diplomas of foreign-trained nurses but there are no available data on the number of incoming nurses.

3. Vignettes on health professional mobility

Romanian nurse ready to emigrate again

MS was a chief medical nurse on a plastic surgery ward. She was recruited by a Cypriot who studied medicine and completed specialization training in Romania. MS was contracted to work in Cyprus for a five-year fixed term and obliged to return to her country of origin (Romania) when the contract ended. Working in a private, small-scale clinic that specialized in aesthetics service provision, she had clear responsibilities ranging from operating room preparation to the provision of post-surgical care. She had only two patients under supervision per day.

On returning to a hospital in Romania, MS found a much more complex pathology in the wards in comparison, with at least 25 patients per day under her supervision. In Cyprus she had received €1500 per month plus accommodation; in Romania she received only €500, after 29 years of practice. MS noted that facilities had improved during her absence and that the medical equipment in Romania was equal to that in Cyprus. However, taking account of all the advantages in Cyprus (financial incentives and workload), she is ready to accept a new job offer there (Informația Medicală 2009).

Emigrant Romanian doctor who might consider returning

Dr OB lives and works in Switzerland as a senior scientific expert in a pharmaceutical company, with a motivational salary and excellent working conditions. He has worked in several European countries, the United States of America and Brazil. In Romania he worked as an assistant professor at the University of Medicine and Pharmacy of Iasi.

Initially, he left Romania for only three months to work at the Max-Delbrück Centre for Molecular Medicine in Berlin. A German colleague and friend helped him to develop his career from postdoctoral fellow to senior scientist in the field of cardiovascular pathophysiology. He was motivated to work longer in Berlin by the solid infrastructure that helped him to develop his own research.

He would consider returning to Romania only if offered a position suited to his wide experience and professional aspirations. His elderly parents are another reason to return (Revista Medica 2008).

4. Dynamics of enlargement

Before 1990, there was an overall lack of transparency in all statistical information. Emigration was generally unknown as Romanians were not allowed to travel, with very few exceptions and especially not to western Europe or North America. Consequently, there are no data available to estimate the emigration scale before 1990. A study to investigate emigration patterns before 1990 (Zaman & Sandu 2004) showed that historical links and associated cultural ties played a role in explaining migration pathways. For instance, before 1990 some ethnic groups (Germans, Hungarians, Jews) were allowed to emigrate following political agreements with their respective governments (Table 13.6).

After 1990, the majority of Romanians who emigrated were highly educated, including medical doctors (Zaman & Sandu 2004). In 1985, 13.6% of the total number of highly educated emigrants were medical doctors/pharmacists (most

Table 13.6 *Emigration trends among population with higher education in Romania, by ethnic group, 1989–2000*

Period	Total	Romanians	Germans	Hungarians	Jews	Others
1980–1989	34 410	12 634	14 761	4 829	1 450	736
%	100	36.7	42.9	14.0	4.2	2.2
1990–2000	36 117	23 509	8 012	3 866	294	436
%	100	65.1	22.2	10.7	0.8	1.2

Source: Zaman & Sandu 2004.

likely ethnic Jews and Germans) but in 2000 the proportion declined to 9.9% (Galan 2006) (Table 13.7). This relatively small percentage within the total number of emigrants can be explained in part by the requirement for medical doctors to fulfil appropriate registration and licensing requirements in their destination countries before starting employment. Licensing procedures were frequently viewed as lengthy, complex and costly processes and some emigrants preferred to repeat their training at a medical university in the destination country (especially the United States of America and Canada) rather than undergo the licensing procedures (Galan 2006). The same study highlighted that Germany was the main recipient country for highly educated Romanian emigrants prior to 2000.

Romanians who emigrated before 1990 were usually permanent settlers[3] who joined their families abroad as there was no temporary emigration. In 2002,

Table 13.7 *Emigration trends among highly educated population in Romania, by profession, 1985–2000*

Year	All highly educated emigrants	Engineers/ architects (%)	Medical doctors/ pharmacists (%)	Economists (%)	Other (%)
1985	3 132	39.3	13.6	8.2	38.8
1987	3 756	39.4	13.4	7.9	39.4
1989	4 318	41.7	15.7	7.5	35.2
1991	2 782	54.3	12.4	7.9	25.3
1993	1 752	66.3	15.8	10.7	7.2
1995	4 218	49.9	11.7	16.3	22.2
1997	3 497	52.1	12.2	16.8	18.9
1999	2 450	65.9	12.3	16.8	5.1
2000	3 384	52.9	9.9	16.8	20.4

Source: Zaman & Sandu 2004.

---

3 Legally admitted immigrants expected to settle permanently in the destination country (Stilwell et al. 2003).

Romania was granted the right to free movement of people in the Schengen Area. This began an important outflow of Romanians (most likely including health professionals) leaving for temporary work in Italy (50%), Spain (24%), Germany (5%) and Hungary (4%) (UNFPA 2007). Another study estimated that the temporary emigration rate was between 10% and 28% of the total population after 2002 (Sandu 2006); the proportions of emigrating health professionals are unknown.

An Organisation for Economic Co-operation and Development (OECD) study shows that about 10% (5180) of the total number of medical doctors and 5% (4440) of nurses trained in Romania worked in any of the OECD countries during 2000–2005 (Simoens & Hurst 2006). These percentages were higher for Romanians than for citizens of any other former communist countries – Hungary: 7.2% medical doctors, 2.4% nurses; Bulgaria: 6.2% medical doctors, 2.6% nurses; Poland: 5.8% medical doctors, 4.6% nurses.

Italy's acute nursing shortage has made it an attractive destination country for Romanian nurses both before and after EU accession. One OECD study (Chaloff 2008) shows that 3864 non-EU nurses were recognized in Italy in 2005, 62.6% (2420) of whom were from Romania. According to the Italian Nursing Association (IPASVI), 34 000 foreign nurses were registered by late 2008 (around 10% of its total membership). Romania was the most important source country with 8497 nurses, representing 25% of foreign registered nurses in Italy (see also section 2).[4]

After accession in 2007, Romanian medical doctors became one of the most numerous cohorts of foreign medical doctors working in France. In 2008 they represented 40% of the foreign medical doctors registered with the French medical chamber according to its president, Michel Legmann (Le Télégramme. com 2009). In 2009, Romanian medical doctors were second only to Belgians as the largest nationality of foreign medical doctors in France.

By comparing the emigration figures for medical doctors in 2004 (360) with the numbers of CGSs issued in 2007 (1421) and 2008 (1252), it can be argued that EU accession facilitated medical doctors' decisions to work abroad (Dragomiristeanu et al. 2008, Pertache & Ursuleanu 2006). However, mobility is no new phenomenon as a considerable number of medical doctors and nurses were leaving before 2007 (Simoens & Hurst 2006).

5. Impacts on the Romanian health system

In Romania, there is little evidence that health workforce mobility impacts

---

4 Data presented in Chapter 6.

on the four functions of a health system set out in the World Health Report 2000 – (i) service delivery, (ii) resource generation, (iii) financing and (iv) stewardship. A report by the Presidential Commission for Romanian Public Health Policies Analysis and Development (Vladescu et al. 2008a) analysed some implications of the poor management of health human resources within the Romanian health system. This study found that primary care is confronted with a health professional deficit. Given that family medicine is one of the most demanded specialties in some EU countries (France, for example), it is most likely that problems of access to primary care services will increase even further if the emigration of family doctors continues and/or increases.

One possible effect of medical doctor migration is long-term scarcity of some specialties and skills at hospital level. This is especially true in the underprivileged regions of Romania. Even when the Ministry of Health advertises job vacancies for missing specialties, the lack of retention mechanisms means that the posts continue to remain unoccupied.

Increasing emigration of medical doctors and nurses in 2010 is jeopardizing the proper running of many facilities, especially the small municipal hospitals. For example, the municipal hospital in Corabia (Olt district) is facing a very difficult situation, both financially and in human resources. The high migration rate among medical doctors has led to this hospital becoming a temporary stop for specialists seeking to work in the big university or district hospitals (Corabia.ro 2008).

The big district hospitals are also experiencing difficulties. For instance, the district hospital in Piatra Neamt (Neamt district) has 183 vacancies (12% of total staff), 35 of which are for medical doctors. The emigration problem is compounded by the government-imposed block on all new recruitment in the public system that was introduced in January 2010. The hospital is barely able to ensure provision of the emergency teams necessary to secure emergency care (Evenimentul 2010).

Analysis of the health status of the population reveals that Romania has some of the poorest health indicators among EU countries (Vladescu et al. 2008a). A mix of specific indicators for developed countries (e.g. high mortality from cardiovascular disease, increasing incidence of cancer) and specific indicators for developing countries (including the re-emergence of some communicable diseases such as tuberculosis and sexually transmitted infections) can be seen in morbidity and mortality data. While there is not sufficient evidence that health professional mobility is impacting on health status, it may be that the disparities in health between rural and urban areas are influenced by the real shortages in the coverage of health professionals in rural areas.

6. Relevance of cross-border health professional mobility

For the Romanian health system, health professional emigration seems to be as problematic as the internal disparities. One important issue is the yearly waste of human resources, despite the country's low density of health professionals compared with other EU countries. This is not due to emigration alone.

6.1 *Distributional issues influencing composition of the health workforce*

Shortages and geographical inequalities of medical doctors and specialists

Data from 2007 indicate that Romania had 224 registered medical doctors per 100 000 inhabitants, significantly lower than the EU average (Table 13.8). A similar situation can be observed for nurses.

Table 13.8 *Health professionals per 100 000 inhabitants, Romania and EU, 2000–2007*

Year	Medical doctors		Family doctors[a]	Dentists		Nurses	
	RO	EU	RO	RO	EU	RO	EU
2000	204	307	51	37	56	402	671
2002	210	316	52	41	57	418	699
2004	222	321	53	46	58	400	726
2006	217	321	54	49	60	397	746
2007	224	322	54	54	na	na	na

Source: WHO 2009. *Note*: [a] Ministry of Health 2008, no comparable EU data for family doctors; na – not available.

The stable rates in the numbers of health professionals shown in Table 13.8 are hiding large inequalities in geographical coverage and medical specialties. Most health professionals (especially medical doctors) are concentrated in the big university cities (Fig. 13.1) and in the most economically developed regions. In 2005, the number of inhabitants per medical doctor was more than five times higher in rural areas than in urban areas (Table 13.9).

The situation related to primary care professionals is also alarming. An NCOEHIS study (Pertache & Ursuleanu 2006) revealed a critical situation concerning coverage of the rural population as well as large disparities between the administrative regions of Romania – 98 rural localities had no family doctor in 2005 while no urban locality faced such a problem (Tables 13.10 and 13.11). This situation has resulted from the lack of good incentives to attract medical doctors to rural and/or deprived areas and the absence of retention mechanisms for existing rural health personnel.

Fig. 13.1 *Density of medical doctors in the six most important university cities and average density in Romania, 2005*

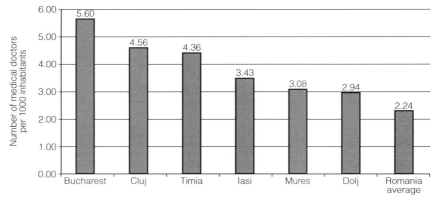

Source: National Institute of Statistics 2006.

Table 13.9 *Coverage of medical doctors by development regions and residence in Romania, 2005*

Region	Inhabitants per medical doctor			Medical doctors per 100 000 population		
	Region	Urban	Rural	Region	Urban	Rural
National average	450	278	1 768	222.2	358.3	56.6
North-East	564	286	2 778	177.2	349.6	43.9
South-East	655	426	1 982	152.6	234.5	50.5
South	773	430	1 773	127.3	232.4	56.4
South-West	514	295	1 536	194.6	339.2	65.1
West	367	260	1 316	272.4	384.5	75.9
North-West	407	240	1 770	245.9	415.5	56.5
Centre	465	313	1 732	214.9	319.5	57.7
Bucharest-Ilfov	203	188	972	492.5	532.8	102.9

Source: Pertache & Ursuleanu 2006.

Table 13.10 *Health professionals at primary health-care level in Romania, 2005*

	No. family doctors	Total population	No. enrolled on a family doctor list	No. of nurses	No. of localities with nofamily doctor
Total	10 595	21 624 689	19 226 642	13 770	98
Urban	6094	11 880 347	11 294 464	7 370	0
Rural	4501	9 744 342	7 932 178	6 400	98

Source: Pertache & Ursuleanu 2006.

The geographical coverage of medical specialties is also imbalanced. NCOEHIS data from 2007 indicate that important specialties are missing in some districts, including infectious diseases, anatomical pathology, gastroenterology, haematology, nephrology and urology. Cardiology and neurology are underrepresented in some districts, usually in the least privileged regions. These shortages imply that even small-scale emigration of specialists from these districts is likely to have profoundly negative impacts on the health system and on service delivery.

Since 1990, several health system reforms in Romania have prioritized primary health care. In late 1994, changes in the provision and payment of general practitioner services were introduced in 8 pilot districts (of a total of 40 districts), covering 4 million people. Payment moved from fixed salary to a combination of age-adjusted capitation, fees for service and bonuses related to difficult conditions of practice and professional rank. The experiment showed that differences in access between rural and urban areas persisted as the limited financial incentives were not sufficient to attract more medical doctors to rural areas (Jenkins et al. 1995).

In 2009, the Ministry of Health and the National Health Insurance Fund introduced incentives for medical doctors working in remote areas. These include an increased allowance for working in "isolated" areas or full reimbursement of activities for medical doctors with over 2500 subscribed patients. Despite this, certain regions still have insufficient health professional cover and the incentives have not proven effective to date.

Shortages and geographical inequalities in the nursing workforce

Changing educational systems for nurses over time and a poor reporting system make it difficult to calculate the real stock of nurses in Romania. In 2005, the registry for nurses and midwives was implemented in each district health authority. This was expected to show an increase in the total number of reported nurses as it included the private nursing school sector. However, the total nursing stock actually decreased, from 86 833 nurses in 2004 to 80 804 in 2005 and 85 785 in 2006 (WHO 2009). These fluctuations may have been due to different reporting systems and the flows of nurses who chose to work abroad even before EU accession. It is noteworthy that the Ministry of Health reported 113 368 registered nurses in 2006, almost 30 000 more than on the HFA database.

The OAMMR estimates that there are about 35 000 graduates per year from all public universities and private nursing colleges. Yet, while a large number of graduates finish nursing school, the reported density of nurses per 100 000 inhabitants in Romania is lower than the EU average. It can be concluded that not all graduates go on to work in the health system. There is a huge discrepancy between the Ministry of Health estimate of planned numbers in the health system, about 2000 new nurses per year, and the OAMMR estimate of 35 000 nursing graduates per year. This allows for the production of nurses for export.

There are geographical disparities in nurse coverage too. Table 13.11 presents these inequalities between administrative regions.

6.2 Factors influencing size and composition of the health workforce

Educational system

In the last 10 years the number of applicants to the medical universities has decreased constantly from 7 to 8 candidates per place to only 0.9 candidates per place at the University of Medicine and Pharmacy "Carol Davila" in Bucharest. Likely explanations include the lengthy specialist training for medical doctors and the new opportunities offered by the labour markets in Romania and in the EU. The gender mix of graduates is about 60% women and 40% men. There is no *numerus clausus* in place and each university decides how many students to admit. On average, each year 3700 students graduate and there are approximately 1400 specialist training places in 52 specialities (Vladescu et al. 2008a & 2008b).

The European Credit Transfer and Accumulation System is fully implemented. Since EU accession, medical students who obtain their licences in Romania are able to go elsewhere for their specialization. Since 2007, a few Romanian students have enrolled on specialization programmes in France. It is likely that more will follow them in the coming years but too soon to estimate how many will return to Romania to practise.

Since 1990, nurses have been trained exclusively in nursing colleges (following the abolition of nursing high schools). In compliance with EU accession requirements, university degree courses were introduced for nurses in 2003 but there were limited possibilities for practising nurses to upgrade their academic qualifications. Recent plans aim to develop masters programmes for nurses who graduated during the first Bologna cycle. Despite these accession requirements, Law 307/2004 (Official Monitor 2004b) allowed private nursing colleges to provide non-degree training programmes and gave existing students the chance to finalize their studies. After 2007, the private colleges enrolled no new students. Nevertheless, following pressure from nursing college owners, in 2008 Romania obtained EU permission to continue nurse training in colleges and for these diplomas to be recognized at EU level.

Table 13.11 *Primary health professional coverage by administrative regions and by urban/rural area in Romania, 2005*

Development region	Inhabitants per medical doctor	Patients per family doctor list (average)	Inhabitants per nurse	Inhabitants per community nurse	Localities with no family doctor
Total	**2 041**	**1 815**	**1 571**	**45 240**	**98**
North-East	2 324	2 031	1 636	27 259	15
South-East	2 320	2 019	1 666	34 294	15
South-Muntenia	2 180	1 874	1 521	61 678	15
South-West Oltenia	1 863	1 613	1 305	24 278	4
West	1 657	1 561	1 502	87 748	11
North-West	1 976	1 914	1 321	85 544	19
Centre	1 814	1 669	1 744	97 326	19
Bucharest-Ilfov	1 657	1 462	2 049	76 151	0
Urban	**1 950**	**1 853**	**1 612**	**111 031**	**0**
North-East	2 020	1 965	1 570	135 036	0
South-East	2 221	2 028	1 717	686 70	0
South-Muntenia	2 095	1 904	1 550	694 58	0
South-West Oltenia	1 957	1 868	1 710	219 212	0
West	1 643	1 672	1 449	72 205	0
North-West	1 864	1 900	1 341	484 611	0
Centre	1 749	1 670	1 743	302 996	0
Bucharest-Ilfov	2 071	1 855	2 046	90 862	0
Rural	**2 165**	**1 762**	**1 523**	**26 265**	**98**
North-East	2 626	2 096	1 691	16 913	15
South-East	2 455	2 005	1 606	21 116	15
South-Muntenia	2 244	1 851	1502	57 101	15
South-West Oltenia	1 785	1 401	1 183	13 449	4
West	1 681	1 363	1 605	140 593	11
North-West	2 122	1 734	1 391	44 261	19
Centre	1 920	1 666	1 745	48 357	19
Bucharest-Ilfov	2 463	1 860	2 073	29 914	0

Source: Pertache & Ursuleanu 2006.

Retirement

Law 19/2000 (Official Monitor 2000) and the relevant amendments concerning the public pension system, set the standard retirement ages for all professions at 60 years for females and 65 years for males. In addition, the RCP issued decision 4 (Official Monitor 2008a) that all medical doctors can continue their activity up to the age of 65 years. This applies to both sexes but is conditional upon obtaining a yearly authorization from the RCP. Family doctors living and practising in rural areas can continue working up to the age of 70 but also require annual authorizations. This has been accepted by all the competent bodies and there are no incentives for early retirement for medical doctors.

A similar decision is in place for female nurses who may work up to 65 years of age (Official Monitor 2008b). Male and female nurses aged over 65 can practise only in the private system, with annual authorization from the OAMMR.

Demographics

Data from the NCOEHIS reveal that 27% of all medical doctors (including dentists) in 2007 were in the 45–55 age group and likely to retire within the next 10–15 years. This compares with 21% of medical doctors aged 25–35 (Table 13.12). If this trend continues there will be a dramatic decline in the number of medical (especially family) doctors in the next decade.

The majority of the stock of medical doctors is female (67%). Maternity leave creates temporary exits from the health system, mainly before the age

Table 13.12 *Medical doctors in Romania, by age group and sex, 2007*

Age group	Males		Females		Total	
	No.	%	No.	%	No.	%
25–30	1 714	9.4	3 555	9.3	5 269	9.3
31–34	2 010	11.0	4 966	13.0	6 976	12.3
35–39	2 501	13.7	6 315	16.5	8 816	15.6
40–44	1 939	10.6	5 035	13.2	6 974	12.3
45–49	1 554	8.5	4 220	11.0	5 774	10.2
50–54	2 992	16.4	6 692	17.5	9 684	17.1
55–59	1 464	8.0	4 068	10.6	5 532	9.8
60–64	1 455	8.0	1 896	4.9	3 351	5.9
65+	2 627	14.4	1 524	4.0	4 151	7.3
TOTAL	**18 256**		**38 271**		**56 527**	

Source: National Institute of Statistics 2008a.

of 40, and can contribute to temporary declines in the total active stock. This needs to be considered within workforce planning.

People leaving the health sector – attrition

Health professionals are estimated to leave the health system at an annual rate of between 10% and 30%. This includes the emigrating workforce, personnel who leave the health system to become health representatives of different companies and others who move into research or shift to another domain of activity. Other exits are due to retirement or death (Vladescu et al. 2008a).

6.3 *What does cross-border mobility mean for Romania?*

Although Romania appears to be a source rather than a destination country, the current scale of emigration seems to be less significant than the internal disparities described. In the short-term, Romania appears to have low dependence on foreign medical doctors and nurses. However, if cross-border mobility is not managed properly and the country continues to lose important volumes of health professionals to emigration, it is possible that the sustainability of the system will be at risk.

The analysis shows that the South and South-East Regions have the worst coverage of health professionals. The North-East Region has the lowest coverage of medical doctors in rural areas (Table 13.11) and the highest emigration rate (Table 13.3) which can negatively impact service delivery in rural areas (Dragomiristeanu et al. 2008). Emigration from the university cities of Bucharest, Iasi and Cluj is less problematic as there is better coverage of medical doctors. However, emigration might have a severe negative impact in rural areas.

Overall, the high annual loss of active health professionals is one of the major health workforce issues in Romania. While there are various reasons for leaving, the total loss is estimated at between 10% and 30%. This wastage calls for decision-makers' attention and should be addressed by a coherent retention strategy.

7. Factors influencing health professional mobility

There are several main reasons for the emigration of the Romanian health workforce: lower salaries than in other non-health professions (for instance law, IT, banking); unsatisfactory social status; lack of performance recognition; limited career development opportunities; and wide discrepancies between the levels of competence and working conditions (equipment; access to consumables, drugs and modern diagnosis tests).

Since 1990, the inadequate working conditions, lack of sufficient incentives and poor career development mechanisms have generated a disappointed health workforce and a high percentage of health professionals who wish to emigrate, particularly the young. After two decades of continuous reforms in the health system the social status of medical doctors and other health professionals has not improved significantly.

Globally, a decent average income for a medical doctor is considered to be about three times the average national income (Lewis 2000). In 2008, specialist doctors in Romania earned 1.5–2 times the average income (Vladescu et al. 2008a). Young resident medical doctors receive about €200 per month, about one third of a specialist doctor's income. This partly explains why young medical doctors are the most willing to work abroad.

The National Employment Agency (EURES) mediates work contracts for Romanian medical doctors going abroad. EURES analysed the average salary of emigrant health professionals in their destination countries. This showed that the official salary of a medical doctor in Romania is between €400 and €800 per month but as much as four times higher in Germany or Switzerland, at €1200 and €3000 respectively (Ministry of Labour, Family and Social Protection *2007, 2008 & 2009*).

In 2007, the monthly income of nurses was about €364, lower than the national income average for the health sector (National Institute of Statistics 2008b).

7.1 *Instigating factors*

A representative sample of medical doctors working in Romania was surveyed to investigate the major influences behind their potential intentions to leave the country (RCP 2007). The main reasons for choosing to work abroad were the low level of wages (55%) and poor working conditions (40%) in Romania. The study also investigated reasons for dissatisfaction with daily professional activities. These were shown to be the lack of resources (especially modern medical equipment) and limited career opportunities.

The Federation of Solidarity for Health (2007) trade union surveyed 600 nurses and midwives in three districts of Romania (Galati, Calarasi, Prahova) by age group, sex and type of employer. Of these respondents, 65% expressed a wish to work abroad for a higher salary. As in other studies, about 40% of the respondents complained about working conditions; 50% mentioned lack of motivation, a proxy for low wages. When asked about the management of the health system, 45.3% of respondents were unhappy with current health reform implementation and 52% complained about the low level of health system financing and poor administration of funds.

7.2 *Activating factors*

The Federation of Solidarity for Health (2007) survey emphasized that 86% of respondents declared that the successful careers of colleagues working abroad had influenced their intention to move to another country.

Another potentially important factor is that many Romanian medical doctors travel or study abroad (especially for postgraduate educational programmes such as masters degrees or for specialization) and have a better understanding of foreign health systems. It can be assumed that a proportion of these people would like to continue working in the countries in which they have studied.

7.3 *Facilitating factors*

Accession gave Romania the right to free mobility of people within the EU. Several EU Member States (such as France, Germany, the United Kingdom) have active recruitment policies that target Romania, amongst others. Job vacancies in these countries are advertised intensively in the mass media and in public places (such as metro stations) and applications can be sent to recruitment companies in any country via the Internet. In France, many Romanian medical doctors apply to web-based companies such as L'Association pour la Recherche et L'Installation de Médecins Européens (ARIME).[5] This not-for-profit organization attracts foreign medical doctors by offering free transport to France and French language training; a settlement bonus, support for the compulsory enrolment with the l'Ordre des Médecins, counselling and general support. The company also organizes medical doctor recruitment days in Bucharest. Private Romanian and foreign recruitment companies also mediate work contracts abroad.

Romanian medical doctors are also attracted to work in non-EU countries such as the United States and Canada. Emigration to these countries is facilitated by good systems of selection and integration policies for immigrants. Also, the Romanian diasporas in these countries play a key role in attracting highly educated immigrants.

7.4 *Mitigating factors*

Family concerns may deter individuals from migrating – the desire to keep

5 http://www.arime.fr/index.php?lang=uk, accessed 18 January 2010.

the family together, care for elderly parents, maintain links with friends or to preserve national customs.

The recent global economic crisis may prevent emigration as migrants may encounter hostile social environments in receiving countries. This is based on anecdotal evidence that includes the opinion of returnees from foreign countries, not necessarily health professionals.

8. Policy, regulation and interventions

To date, the Ministry of Health has not adopted a comprehensive health workforce policy. However, some elements of a human resources strategy can be observed in some health strategies of other sectors.

Since 1990, health human resources policy-making has seen the arrival of actors other than the Ministry of Health and the Ministry of Education, Research and Innovation. The most important of these are the National Health Insurance Fund, NCP, Romanian College of Dental Practitioners, Romanian College of Pharmacists, OAMMR and the trade union Sanitas.

Prior to EU accession, the RCP asked the Ministry of Health to prepare a strategy for health workforce planning and development. This was to consider the high emigration rate expected after 2007, especially among younger medical doctors. However, the process of drafting a national strategy has been delayed as it has not been seen as a priority and there have been several changes of health minister.

8.1 *Workforce planning and development*

The national public health strategy (Ministry of Health 2004) explicitly mentions the need for health workforce planning mechanisms but no such mechanisms have been put into practice. Existing planning is based solely on a relatively constant number of medical positions in the public sector. Each year, the district health directorates report their estimated needs for each specialty for a five-year period based on new inflows to, and exits from, each specialty. Decisions to increase/decrease the number of trainees in any particular specialty are taken on an ad-hoc basis.

Similar procedures apply for nurses as the Ministry of Health approves the number of posts at hospital level. The number of nursing students admitted to the university colleges is strictly regulated by the Ministry of Education, Research and Innovation but the number of students entering other nursing schools is not controlled. The oversupply of nurses described above should be regarded as a consequence of the lack of monitoring and planning mechanisms.

Recent legislation and policies for regulating the health professions have been governed mainly by EU harmonization requirements for mutual recognition of diplomas. Policies have targeted mainly training; upgrading educational and training facilities; and retraining of some health professionals (such as nurses who graduated in the early 1990s).

Workforce and education policy decisions concerning health professionals have been modified frequently in the last decade. However, these modifications have not been transparent, coherent or supported by evidence and have rarely been followed up by concrete action (Vladescu 1999).

A new government was appointed in December 2008 following the general election. The new Minister of Health announced that one priority is the development of a specific health policy for rural areas in order to improve rural populations' access to health services. In 2009, new incentives were introduced for health professionals working in rural areas but so far they have proved ineffective.

8.2 Cross-border regulatory frameworks and interventions

Mutual recognition of diplomas in the European Community

Law 200/2004 (Official monitor 2004a) with further revisions (Official monitor 2008a) is fully transposing European Directive 2005/36/EC (European Parliament and Council of the European Union 2005) for the recognition of professional qualifications in the EU. The Ministry of Education, Research and Innovation is the national coordinator for the supervision of all sectors involved with diploma recognition. Verification certificates are required for all medical doctors (including dentists), nurses and midwives who started their basic training before accession (January 2007). They will not be necessary for students who started their training after 2007 (graduating in 2013). The RCP also issues the CGS that confirms that a medical doctor has been effectively and lawfully engaged in actual medical practice for at least three consecutive years during the last five years.

The Ministry of Labour, Family and Social Protection reports that Romanian citizens face some restrictions on accessing the labour markets in 10 of the 26 EU Member States – Austria, Belgium, France, Germany, Ireland, Italy, Luxembourg, Malta, the Netherlands and the United Kingdom. Bilateral discussions and agreements between the respective health ministries and professional bodies ensure that Romanian medical doctors and nurses can work in all EU countries, despite these restrictions. No particular problems have been reported concerning diploma recognition and access to the European health labour market.

Third-country health professionals

Article 370 of the health reform law (Official Monitor 2006) entitles the following foreign citizens to practise as a medical doctor in Romania.

a. Any citizen of an EU Member State, SEE country[6] or Switzerland who has graduated from a medical university in their country of origin.

b. Any citizen of a third country having permanent settler status in Romania and a diploma recognized by Romania or any EU Member State; or having documents issued by any EU Member State that prove a professional experience of at least three years in the medical field.

Article 1 of Law 307/2004 (Official Monitor 2004b), stipulates similar provisions for nurses and midwives.

8.3 *Political force field of regulating and managing health professional mobility*

The Ministry of Health continues to be the main centre of power for direct and indirect control of the number of medical doctors, dentists, nurses and other health professionals. Direct control consists of approving the number of posts and types of specialty within public health units. Indirect control is exerted by issuing common regulations with the professional associations in order to ensure better geographical distribution.

The Romanian Constitution holds that parliament should have a key position in the elaboration of health policies and legislation. In reality, legislative initiatives from parliament have been strongly influenced by the Ministry of Health and the National Health Insurance Fund. However, parliament introduced successive changes during the drafting period of the legislation related to nurses such that the final law did not meet EU accession requirements. The OAMMR attributes this to lobbying by the private nursing school owners (Olsavszky 2008). It was only after accession negotiations ended that the law was changed in order to meet EU requirements.

Sanitas is the main trade union for nurses and midwives. Affiliated to the National Trade Union Confederation, it works continuously for higher incomes in the health sector but is less successful in influencing the development of a workforce policy.

---

6 Albania, Bosnia & Herzegovina, Bulgaria, Croatia, Greece, Montenegro, Republic of Moldova, Romania, Serbia, Slovenia, the former Yugoslav Republic of Macedonia, Turkey.

9. Conclusion

The results of this case study highlight the Ministry of Health's limited capacity for planning, training and managing human resources for health in Romania. Currently, there is no comprehensive health workforce policy and the issue appears to have low political priority. Clearly there is a waste of human resources (medical doctors and nurses), with large annual losses due not only to cross-border mobility but also to attrition, over-production of nurses and internal disparities in geographical coverage by medical doctors and specialists. Inadequate working conditions, a lack of reasonable incentives and an unsatisfactory career development system have generated a disappointed health workforce. This includes a high percentage of health professionals who wish to work abroad, especially among the younger age groups. For the Romanian health system, the outflow of health professionals in the context of the economic crisis appears to be as problematic as the internal disparities or the poor management of health human resources.

It can be said that Romania faced a brain drain of researchers at the beginning of the 1990s. Since 2007, it has faced an exodus of health professionals and the globalization of Europe has produced a high demand for medical doctors. . Romanian medical doctors are beginning to hold top positions within other EU health systems but the majority are still requested to work in remote areas in EU countries.

Romania is largely a source country but it holds more information about medical doctor outflows than about nurses who leave. This may be because the government considers the emigration of medical doctors to be a bigger loss for the health system. Even the data on the nursing stock are based on rough estimates and lack accuracy and quality. Evidence from other EU countries shows that thousands of Romanian medical doctors and (especially) nurses have migrated. Hence, it is vital that Romania develops: (i) a good monitoring and control system for cross-border mobility and other factors related to entries and exits from the health workforce; and (ii) better tools to manage the inflows and outflows of health professionals and minimize any losses for the national health system.

References

Chaloff J (2008). *Mismatches in the formal sector, expansion of the informal sector: immigration of health professionals to Italy*. Paris, Organisation for Economic Co-operation and Development (OECD Health Working Papers No. 34).

CNOM (2009). *Atlas de la démographie médicale 2009. Situation au 1ᵉʳ janvier 2009.* Paris, Conseil National de l'Ordre des Médecins.

Corabia.ro (2008). Spitalele din județ, la limita autorizării sanitare [District hospitals ready to lose their practice authorization]. *Corabia.ro,* 21 March 2008 (http://www.corabia.ro/site/stire-2-spitalul-orasenesc-corabia-la-limita-autorizarii-sanitare.html, accessed 15 November 2010).

Dragomiristeanu A et al. (2008). Migratia medicilor din Romania [The migration of medical doctors from Romania]. *Revista Medica*, 17 March 2008 (http://www.medicalnet.ro/content/view/498/31/, accessed 28 June 2009).

EMN (2009). *Politiche migratorie, lavoratori qualificati, settore sanitario [Migratory policies, qualified workers, health sector].* Rome, European Migration Network Italy (First Report EMN Italy).

European Parliament and Council of the European Union (2005). Directive 2005/36/EC of the European Parliament and of the Council of 7 September 2005 on the recognition of professional qualifications. *Official Journal of the European Union*, 255(48): 22–142.

Evenimentul (2010). Salariile mizere alungă medicii din țară. Spitale pustii [Poor salaries are pushing the doctors out of Romania. Empty hospitals]. *Evenimentul*, 19 August 2010 (http://www.evenimentul.ro/articol/spitale-pustii.html, accessed 15 November 2010).

Federal Employment Agency (2009). *Statistik Beschäftigung.* Bonn (http://www.pub.arbeitsagentur.de/hst/services/statistik/detail/b.html?call=l, accessed 22 June 2009).

Federal Physicians Chamber (2009). *Ärztestatistik.* Berlin (http://www.bundesaerztekammer.de/page.asp?his=0.3, accessed 22 June 2009).

Federation of Solidarity for Health (2007). *Calitatea vietii profesionale si tendinta de a munci in strainatate a profesionistilor din sanatate [The quality of professional life of health professionals and their tendency to work abroad].* Bucharest (http://www.solidaritatea-sanitara.ro/en/sociological-studies.html, accessed 8 December 2010).

Galan A (2006). Health worker migration in selected CEE countries – Romania, Czech Republic, Serbia and Croatia. In: *Health worker migration flows in Europe: overview and case studies in selected CEE countries – Romania, Czech Republic, Serbia and Croatia.* Geneva, International Labour Office (ILO Working Paper No. 245).

Informația Medicală (2009). Migratia medicilor [Medical doctors' migration]. *Informația Medicală*, 19 February 2009 (http://www.informatiamedicala.ro/stiri-medicale/Migratia-medicilor-239.html, accessed 15 November 2010).

Jenkins S et al. (1995). *Evaluation of the health reform in eight pilot districts in Romania.* London, Institute for Health Sector Development.

Lewis M (2000). *Who is paying for health care in eastern Europe and central Asia?* Washington, International Bank for Reconstruction and Development/The World Bank.

Ministry of Health (2004). *National public health strategy.* Bucharest.

Ministry of Health (2009). *Statistical Yearbook 2008.* Bucharest

Ministry of Labour, Family and Social Protection (2007). *Quarterly Statistical Bulletin,* no.*1 (57)/2007.*

Ministry of Labour, Family and Social Protection (2008). *Quarterly Statistical Bulletin,* no.*1 (61)/2008.*

Ministry of Labour, Family and Social Protection (2009). *Quarterly Statistical Bulletin,* no.*1 (65)/2009.*

National Institute of Statistics (2008a). *Health units activity 2007.* Bucharest.

National Institute of Statistics (2008b). *Statistical yearbook 2008.* Bucharest.

Official Monitor (2000). *Law 19/2000 related to the public pension system and other social insurance rights.* (No. 140/01.04.2000).

Official Monitor (2004a). *Law 307/2004 related to the practise of the medical nurse and midwife professions as well as the organization and functioning of the Order of Medical Nurses and Midwives in Romania.* (No. 578/30.06.2004).

Official Monitor (2004b). *Law 200/2004 related to the recognition of diplomas and professional training for the regulated professions in Romania.* (No. 500/03.06.2004)

Official Monitor (2006). *Law 95/2006 related to the health reform.* (No. 372/28.04.2006).

Official Monitor (2008a). *Law 117/2008 changing and adding Law 200/2004.* (No. 410/02.06.2008)

Official Monitor (2008b). *Emergency Ordinance 144/2008 related to the practise of the medical nurse and midwife professions as well as the organization and functioning of the Order of Medical Nurses and Midwives in Romania.* (No. 785/24.11.2008)

Olsavszky V (2008). *The role of human resources in health system reform, particularly during the transition period; the nurses.* Timişoara, University of Medicine and Pharmacy "Victor Babeş".

Pertache I, Ursuleanu D (2006). *Population coverage with health personnel at primary care level.* Bucharest, National Centre for Organising and Ensuring the Health Information System.

Realitatea.net (2010). Ministrul Sănătăţii: Migraţia medicilor va continua în următorii 15–20 de ani [Minister of Health: MDs' migration will continue for the next 15–20 years]. *Realitatea.net*, 12 August 2010 (http://www.realitatea. net /ministrul-sanatatii-migratia-medicilor-va-continua-in-urmatorii-15-20-de-ani_729148.html, accessed 15 November 2010).

RCP (2009). *Migratie medici* [*MDs' migration*]. Press release 18 February 2009. Bucharest, Romanian College of Physicians (http://cmr.ro/content/view/672/11/, accessed 9 March 2010).

Revista Medica (2008). As accepta o pozitie in Romania potrivit experientei si aspiratiilor mele profesionale [I would accept a job position in Romania according to my professional experience and expectations]. *Revista Medica*, 27 February 2008 (http://www.medicalnet.ro/content/view/475/88/, accessed 15 November 2010).

Sandu D (2006). *Living abroad on a temporary basis. The economic migration of Romanians: 1990–2006.* Bucharest, Open Society Foundation.

Simoens S, Hurst J (2006). *The supply of physician services in OECD countries.* Paris, Organisation for Economic Co-operation and Development (OECD Health Working Papers No. 21).

Stilwell B et al. (2003). Developing evidence-based ethical policies on the migration of health workers: conceptual and practical challenges. *Human Resources for Health*, 1(1):8.

Le Télégramme.com (2009). *Démographie médicale. Un sombre diagnostic.* Morlaix (http://www.letelegramme.com/ig/generales/france-monde/france/demographie-medicale-un-sombre-diagnostic-09-09-2009-542187.php, accessed 8 November 2009).

UNFPA (2007). *Populaţia şi dezvoltarea României – prognoze şi posibile soluţii* [*Population and development of Romania – forecasts and possible solutions*]. (Informative Bulletin no. 3/2007), United Nations Population Fund, Romania (ftp://ftp.unfpa.ro/unfpa/NewsletterPD3.pdf, accessed 8 December 2010).

Vladescu C (1999). *Health system policy reform in Romania – a critical analysis.* Bucharest, InfoMedica.

Vladescu C et al. (2008a). *Report of the Presidential Commission for Romanian Public Health Policies Analysis and Development.* Bucharest (http://www. presidency.ro/?lang=ro, accessed 22 June 2009).

Vladescu C et al. (2008b). Romania: Health system review. *Health Systems in Transition*, 10(3):90-94.

WHO (2009). European health for all database. Copenhagen, WHO Regional Office for Europe (http://data.euro.who.int/hfadb/, accessed 22 June 2009).

Zaman G, Sandu S (2004). Flows and non-EU Europe – Romania. In: *The brain-drain – emigration flows for qualified scientists project. Maastricht* (http:// www.merit.unimaas.nl/braindrain/Part5.Flows_and_non-EU%20Europe-Romania.pdf, accessed 22 June 2009.

Chapter 14

Mobility of European human resources: how to keep the Slovak health-care system healthy?

Kvetoslava Beňušová, Miloslava Kováčová, Marián Nagy, Matthias Wismar

1. Introduction

Before the division of Czechoslovakia, a forty-year period of political and economic isolation (1948–1989) had closed the foreign borders. This resulted in minimal migration and a legal obligation to work that resulted in a surplus of health personnel. Within Czechoslovakia, Slovakia was self-sufficient in terms of the structure and quality of the health workforce – there were sufficient quantities of qualified health professionals and continuous increases in the numbers graduating from medical faculties and secondary medical schools.

The opening of borders in 1989 and EU accession in 2004 have affected this formerly stable and self-sufficient system that sustained and produced Slovak human resources for health. Harmonization of education and increasingly automatized processes for the mutual recognition of qualifications have removed most administrative barriers to successful competition and the migration of health professionals in the European Union (EU) market. Various data sources suggest that thousands of Slovak health professionals are now working in other EU Member States.

Slovakia has become a source country for health professionals and now faces the challenge of increasing the attraction of the domestic labour market in order to respond adequately to the Slovak population's need for high-quality and safe health care. These developments have produced a need for better documentation and analysis of the free movement of health professionals in order to better regulate human resources for health in Slovakia. This has moved up the national political agenda and the Slovak government has implemented various interventions for better management of the cross-border mobility of health professionals. However, it should be noted that health professional mobility is not the only health workforce issue that needs to be addressed in order to regain self-sufficiency.

This study starts by presenting the mobility profile for Slovakia, focusing on medical doctors, nurses and dental doctors. This is followed by an analysis of the accession process and how health professional mobility impacts on the Slovak health system and a discussion of the relevance of health professional mobility vis-à-vis other workforce issues. The last section covers policy and regulation and draws attention to recently implemented interventions that should help to manage health professional mobility.

Limitations of the study

Little information, knowledge or evidence is available on the cross-border mobility of health workers over the past 20 years. There have been no long-term systematic investigations concerning Slovakia and only occasional surveys and studies are available (see references below).

In general, there are wide variations in the estimates of Slovak nationals working abroad – especially in EU Member States. The Slovak authorities have practically no detailed information on, or comprehensive evaluations of, the exact extent and structure of labour emigration flows nor of their impacts on the country's labour market. This makes it necessary to rely on data from the domestic Labour Force Survey or information from other countries (Divinský 2007).

The Ministry of Health is an important source of data that can shed some light on health professional mobility. This ministry issues confirmation of the equivalence in education for health professionals who obtained their medical education in Slovakia or in the former Czechoslovakia, whose training started before accession to the EU in May 2004. However, an application for equivalence certification data indicates an intention to work in another country rather than actual migration.

Between 2004 and 2008 there was a strong discontinuity in reporting data. Adoption of the Slovak health system reform acts in 2004 led to some competences moving from state authorities to other levels and authorities. The professional organizations were given responsibility for collecting data but national coordination was not ensured. Data were unavailable for certain periods, thereby interrupting the reporting of some mandatory statistics on health professionals. The National Health Information Centre (NHIC)[1] collects and processes data on health professionals; the Ministry of Health's coordinating role in this has been reinforced since 2008 (Government of the Slovak Republic 2004a).

Other potential data sources were of limited use for this study. The Slovak Medical Chamber issues confirmations of professional integrity to medical doctors seeking to migrate. Professional organizations collect data on the documents issued for potential emigration but do not provide information on the number of applicants who actually leave the country. Registration with the relevant chambers is a prerequisite for performance of a health profession but these registers are currently being elaborated and updated. Faculties of medicine and other faculties responsible for health professional education register the total numbers of students admitted and graduates but do not differentiate between Slovaks and foreign nationals. The Foreign Police department records data on total immigration but does not identify occupational groups.

It is not only data on migration of health professionals that are lacking. There is also no follow-up of those working outside their professions but within Slovakia.

Given the data limitations, this study is based on analysis and information from the Ministry of Health and the NHIC; information from the managers of health-care facilities, professional organizations and trade unions; and other available studies and published information cited in the text.

2. Mobility profile of Slovakia

Notwithstanding the unavailability of some key data and limitations in the data that are available, it is possible to conclude that the estimated outflows of health professionals are not matched by any equivalent inflows from other countries for the period between May 2004 and December 2009. In fact, the health workforce contains a minimal proportion of foreign nationals.

2.1 *Outflows*

General labour migration is an important topic for Slovakia. At the end of 2006, the most reliable data on labour migrants from Slovakia ranged from 180 000 to 230 000 people (Divinský 2007, Divinský & Popjaková 2007, Katuščák 2006, Reichová et al. 2006). Thus, in 2006, the share of Slovak

---

1 National Institute of Health Informatics and Statistics until 2006.

nationals working in the EU reached about 8%–10% of the total stock of employed persons, 7%–9% of the total economically active population and 5%–6% of the total working age population (the reference basis for the Labour Force Survey) in Slovakia (Divinský 2007, Hajnovičová 2006). The proportion of health-care professionals within these migrants was not determined.

The Slovak population's main destination countries are Austria, the United Kingdom, the Czech Republic and Germany, as well as Ireland, Hungary and Italy. Austria became the main destination country originally for political reasons as the 1968 emigration wave of Slovak citizens that travelled through Austria created personal relationships and social networks. The attraction now is economic (Divinský 2007). A common history as a single state dating back to 1918 means that the Czech Republic remains the second most popular destination country for temporary or permanent emigrants from Slovakia. This is reinforced by the similarity of the Slovak and Czech languages (requiring no translation in everyday life), similar social conditions, close cultural ties and geographical proximity (Divinský 2007).

Medical professionals working in Slovakia in 2007 comprised 34 040 active nurses, 16 201 active medical doctors and 2697 active dental doctors (NHIC unpublished data 2009). Ministry of Health data indicate that the equivalency of education confirmations required to perform a health profession in EU Member States were issued to 3741 health professionals between 1 May 2004 and 30 April 2007 – 1780 nurses, 1377 medical doctors, 194 physiotherapists, 164 pharmacists, 109 dental doctors, 77 midwives, 27 radiology assistants and 13 paramedics (Beňušová 2007). These confirmation holders were surveyed on their motivations to practise in another Member State (Fig. 14.1). The most popular intended destination countries for these Slovakian health professionals were Austria, the Czech Republic, the United Kingdom and Germany. Most nurses (40.9%, 728) declared an intention to migrate to Austria; most medical doctors chose Germany (21.8%, 300) or the United Kingdom (17.1%, 235) (Beňušová 2007).

The demographic composition of these health professionals with equivalence confirmations shows that the most common age group (43.8%) is 30 years and below (Beňušová 2007). Graduates and young health professionals express greater interest in emigration. Medical doctors and nurses show no differences in their motivation for migration, regardless of age and place of origin (Beňušová 2007). Graduates of medical and pharmaceutical faculties show a tendency to permanent migration (Reichová et al. 2006).

In addition to domestic sources, European Commission (2007) statistics provide information on the recognition of Slovakian qualifications for the performance

Fig.14.1 *Health professionals with equivalence confirmations, by declared destination country, 1 May 2004–30 April 2007*

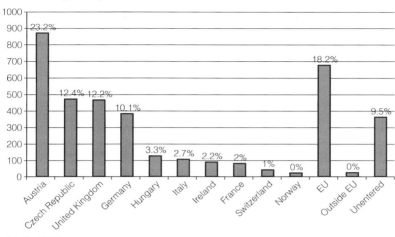

Source: Beňušová 2007.

Fig. 14.2 *Age groups of health professionals with equivalence confirmations, 1 May 2004–30 April 2007*

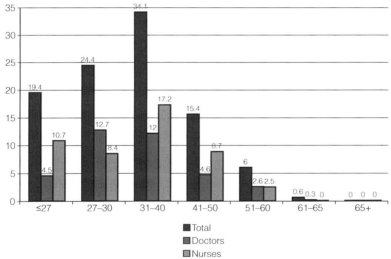

Source: Beňušová 2007.

of certain medical professions in EU Member States between January 2005 and December 2006. Over a period of two years, other EU Member States granted recognition to a total of 3243 health professionals including 2640 nurses,[2] 348 medical doctors, 129 pharmacists, 65 dental doctors[3] and 61 midwives.

2 Delay in data delivery means that these numbers exclude Germany, France and three traditional destination countries – Austria, United Kingdom and Italy (2005). There is reason to believe that the data from other Member States show even higher numbers of nurses with recognized qualifications from Slovakia.

3 Historically, dental doctors in Slovakia have been university-qualified health professionals in the field of oral health and health care.

Ministry of Health data on issued licences to practise medicine appear to underestimate the true magnitude of health professionals leaving to work in the EU. This is seen in a comparison of the Ministry of Health data (1 May 2004–30 April 2007) and the European Commission data on the approved qualifications of health professionals in individual Member States (January 2005–December 2006). This demonstrates that Member States automatically accept Slovakian diplomas for some health professions without seeking Ministry of Health affirmation of equivalence in accordance with EU minimum guidelines. For example, 2640 nurses from Slovakia were registered as qualified in other EU Member States (even this number is an underestimate) between January 2005 and December 2006 but the Ministry of Health was requested to assess the equivalence of only 1780 cases over an even longer period (May 2004–April 2007).

Since the EU statistics do not include data from the large traditional target countries (such as Germany, Austria and the United Kingdom) it may be assumed that substantially more health professionals than the 3243 reported are likely to have left Slovakia between January 2005 and December 2006. National data from these three countries show that 503 Slovak medical doctors and 180 Slovak nurses were working in Germany in 2008 (see Chapter 5); some 2600 Slovak nurses applied for diploma validation in Austria between 2003 and 2008 (see Chapter 1); and 381 Slovak medical doctors and 208 Slovak nurses registered on the General Medical Council (GMC) and Nursing and Midwifery Council (NMC) registers in the United Kingdom in 2003–2008 (see Chapter 8).

Between 1 May 2004 and 31 March 2009 the Slovak Health University issued a total of 311 equivalence confirmations of specialization for medical doctors. The most numerous specialties were anaesthetics and intensive medicine, surgery, gynaecology and obstetrics, radiology, internal medicine and neurology (Ministry of Health unpublished data 2009). In the authors' experience, shortages in Slovak hospitals primarily concern these specializations. Table 14.1 compares the annual average numbers of issued confirmations with the annual numbers of specialists graduating. It should be noted that the equivalence data are likely to be underestimates as not all specialists planning to leave Slovakia request these documents.

2.2 Inflows and stocks of foreign health professionals

There are no data on the inflows of foreign health professionals between 1 May 2004 and 31 December 2008. However, stock data provide a good indication that inflows were minimal. Data are available for 2007 only but these show

Table 14.1 *Increase/decrease in numbers of medical doctors in Slovakia by selected specializations*

Specialization	Issued confirmations 1 May 2004–30 April 2009		Average number of graduates/year (2004–2008)
	Total	Average/year	
Anaesthetics and intensive medicine	65	13	29
Surgery	49	10	25
Gynaecology and obstetrics	26	5	22
Radiology	22	4.5	17
Internal medicine	19	4	14
Neurology	11	2	12

Source: Ministry of Health unpublished data 2009.

that foreign health professionals comprised less than 1% of the total number of medical doctors, dental doctors, nurses and midwives. Of the 125 foreign medical doctors (Table 14.2), 68 (54%) came from EU countries and 57 (46%) came from third countries. The most important countries of origin were the Czech Republic (27); Ukraine (19); Islamic Republic of Iran and Poland (7 from each); Afghanistan, Bulgaria and the Russian Federation (6 from each) (NHIC unpublished data 2009).

Table 14.2 *Foreign-national medical doctors working in Slovakia, 2007*

	Foreign-national medical doctors	%	All medical doctors
All medical doctors	**125**	**0.7**	**16 999**
- male	77	1.1	7 317
- female	48	0.5	9 682
Active medical doctors	**119**	**0.7**	**16 201**
- male	75	1.1	7 004
- female	44	0.5	9 197

Source: NHIC unpublished data 2009.

The percentage of foreign dental doctors in the Slovak workforce is similarly marginal (Table 14.3). Among only 18 foreign dental doctors, 4 were from Germany, 3 from Ukraine and 2 from the Russian Federation.

Table 14.3 *Foreign-national dental doctors working in Slovakia, 2007*

	Foreign-national dental doctors	%	All dental doctors
All dental doctors	18	0.7	**2 744**
- male	8	0.8	1 066
- female	10	0.6	1 678
Active dental doctors	17	0.6	**2 697**
- male	8	0.8	1 045
- female	9	0.5	1 652

Source: NHIC unpublished data 2009.

The share of foreign nurses within the total nursing workforce (Table 14.4) is even smaller than the shares of foreign medical doctors and dental doctors. Most foreign nurses and midwives (16) were from the European Economic Area (EEA) countries and Switzerland.

Table 14.4 *Foreign-national nurses working in Slovakia, 2007*

	Foreign-national nurses	%	All nurses
All nurses	27	0.1	**34 040**
- male	0	0.0	590
- female	27	0.1	33 450

Source: NHIC unpublished data 2009.

2.3 Conclusion

Despite the limitations of existing outflow data and the lack of inflow data, it is possible to say that outflows of qualified health professionals are not balanced by inflows, whether from EU Member States or from third countries. A total of 3741 health professionals emigrated between 1 May 2004 and 30 April 2007, an annual average of 1247 (Beňušová 2007); yet only 171 foreign health professionals were working in Slovakia in 2007. The data on how many foreign health professionals moved to Slovakia following EU accession are not yet available. However, the proportions of foreign health professionals working in 2007 show that they fall far short of the thousands of Slovak medical doctors and nurses who obtained confirmations of equivalence from the Ministry of Health and/or approval of their qualifications in individual Member States. As the outflow of Slovak health professionals is not compensated by inflows of foreign health professionals, it is necessary to make up for the loss by training new staff.

3. Vignettes on health professional mobility[4]

Slovak nurse and family emigrated to Austria

Elena is a 45 year old general nurse of Slovak nationality who qualified in the territory of Slovakia. She graduated from secondary health school in 1984 and then worked for 20 years in anaesthetics and intensive medicine, surgery, dialysis departments in a district and a regional hospital and later in a general practitioner's facility in a regional capital city in Slovakia. Divorced and the mother of one child, Elena also provides financial support to her parents – one has a disability; the other has retired. She responded to an advert placed by an Austrian agency recruiting experienced nurses in geriatric hospital care and was employed immediately. Having worked in Austria for two years she applied for official confirmation that her qualification was in conformity with EU directives. She intended to register with the Austrian Medical Chamber in order to obtain health and social insurance that would ensure social and health security for all her family in Austria. Elena's education alone did not qualify for automatic recognition but her long-term practice qualified her to be recognized as a fully qualified nurse under Article 23 of Directive 2005/36/ES. Those who can provide proof of adequate practice in the Slovak Republic have no problem acquiring recognition of their qualifications but do not always apply for confirmation of equivalence as Austria recognizes their qualifications directly as an EU Member State.

Slovak nurse with higher education: difficulties with diploma recognition

Jozef is a Slovak citizen who was born in eastern Slovakia the 1970s. He completed the higher education course in nursing at the secondary health school in 1998, before accession to the EU. Having qualified, he worked as a general nurse in the internal medicine department of the regional hospital in his home town. However, an overload of work resulted from changes in the hospital's human resource policy (1 nurse: 50 patients: 1 shift) and drove him to seek work abroad. He applied to the Ministry of Health for equivalence confirmation with the intention of working in Ireland. He hoped for more "humane" working conditions and greater appreciation based on the higher professional qualification he had obtained in Slovakia. The Ministry of Health issued confirmation of the equivalence in education according to acquired rights. This entitles the holder to claim automatic and unconditional recognition in all EU Member States. However, the Irish Nursing Board requested confirmation of the authenticity of his English language education, mailed directly from the Ministry of Health rather than the applicant. The Ministry of Health satisfied this unusual request in order to accommodate the applicant and his qualification was recognized in 2006–2007.

---

4 From interviews in May and June 2009.

> ### *Emigrant medical doctor, neurosurgery specialist: difficulties with diploma recognition*
>
> Anna is a 36 year old Slovak medical doctor. In 2006 she obtained a specialized diploma in neurosurgery in the Slovak Republic, a document eligible for automatic recognition under amendment C of Directive 93/16/EHS. She worked full-time as a neurosurgeon in the hospital in a regional capital city in Slovakia with the intention of joining her husband who had opened a private neurology practice in Germany. Having established contact with a prospective employer, in 2009 she applied for recognition of her neurosurgery diploma. The German Chamber of Physicians questioned her diploma under a new directive that came into effect at this time. Anna was asked to confirm the equivalence of education according to Article 25 of Directive 2005/36/ES, despite the fact that her document was directly cited in an amendment (5.1.2 and 5.1.3). She sought help from her competent authority – the Slovak health ministry. The ministry sent an explanatory letter to the German Chamber of Physicians and Anna's qualification was recognized.

4. Dynamics of enlargement

Labour emigration from Slovakia has increased dramatically over the past few years. Between 2000 and 2006, the number of Slovak nationals working abroad increased from 49 300 to 168 800 (Divinský 2007).

Slovakia was self-sufficient in health professionals before 1989 but is now facing significant outflows. Exact figures are not available but Ministry of Health data on issued confirmations for practising medicine abroad, as well as European Commission data on approved qualifications of health-care professionals in individual Member States, show an annual estimated average of 1 500 Slovak health professionals leaving to work in European countries. This represents half of the annual average production of graduates from secondary health schools and universities in the observed health professions in Slovakia (Table 14.6 in section 5). Even if all these health professionals returned immediately to Slovakia, the ageing of existing health-care providers (approaching retirement age) and overall ageing of the population (increasing demand for health care) means that there would not be enough health professionals to provide full cover in all the health services.

Ministry of Health data indicate that Slovak health professionals do not need confirmations of equivalency of their education as before. The numbers of medical doctors, dental doctors and nurses asking for confirmation of equivalency of their education in accordance with EU regulations peaked between 2004 and 2006 but since then have tended to decrease (Table 14.5). Some of these reductions may be due to the new dynamics of migration as

Table 14.5 Applications for equivalency of education confirmations for medical doctors, dental doctors and nurses: numbers issued and refused, 2004–2009

Year	Medical doctors		Dental doctors		Nurses	
	Confirmations issued	Applications refused	Confirmations issued	Applications refused	Confirmations issued	Applications refused
2004[a]	442	5	22	12	306	139
2005	594	6	30	10	504	228
2006	376	4	30	2	425	138
2007	267	2	27	4	204	87
2008	250	1	18	1	183	81
2009 [b]	217	1	16	1	146	81
Total	**2146**	**19**	**143**	**30**	**1768**[b]	**754**

Sources: Ministry of Health 2006a–2009a; [b] Ministry of Health unpublished data 2009. *Note:* [a] 1 May–31 December 2004.

Slovak health professionals do not need proof of equivalence to work in other EU countries. European Commission (2007) data indicate that EU Member States have become accustomed to Slovak health professionals' qualifications and foreign employers do not always require equivalence confirmations. Slovak citizens living abroad thus benefit directly from the free movement of persons gained with EU accession while it becomes more difficult for Slovak authorities to gain true estimates of outflows.

Migration trends among Slovak health professionals are likely to slow without any government intervention or coordination. The global financial crisis and its impact on all EU Member States in 2009 and 2010 means that health professionals who lose their jobs abroad are likely to return home. However, it would be premature to draw any conclusions on the number of returning health professionals as the relevant data are not yet available.

5. Impacts on health systems

Since accession, the outflow of qualified health professionals from the Slovak health system has become a significant social phenomenon with serious consequences.

Table 14.6 shows the weight of the annual average number of equivalence confirmations issued by the Ministry of Health proportional to the annual average number of graduates in a health profession (column F). Initially, it appears that Slovakia is producing sufficient numbers of health professionals proportional to its population (column C). However, columns E–G give a clear indication of emigration's potential impact on the health workforce in Slovakia.

Issued confirmations show only migration intentions and health professionals are likely to emigrate without requesting confirmation of equivalence but, when migration is factored in, Table 6 highlights that the Slovak system is at risk of producing too few new health professionals. Column G shows that this is a concern for all main categories of health professionals but particularly for nurses. Medical assistants were established as a new profession in 2001 with the intention of compensating for the undersupply of new nurses.

The President of the Chamber of Dental Doctors reports that approximately half of the newly graduated young dental doctors at the two Slovak dental medical faculties (Ministry of Education unpublished data 2009) emigrate for work abroad every year, mostly to the Czech Republic and the United Kingdom. This leads to shortages in smaller communities and cities particularly (Divinský 2007, SME.sk 2007a). There have been similar sizeable shortages of medical doctors, mainly general practitioners, and nurses in Slovakia (Divinský 2007). Thousands have emigrated to the Czech Republic, Austria, Germany,

Table 14.6 *Overview of inflows to and (potential) outflows from the Slovak health workforce, by selected indicators*

Health profession	Graduates per year (annual average) 2004–2007	Graduates per 100 000 population (annual average)	WHO average of graduates per 100 000 (2003) [a]	Issued confirmations for other EU Member States (annual average) 1 May 2004–1 May 2007 [b]	Production of graduates vs. migration intentions (B–E)	Graduates per 100 000 population (annual average) after deduction of issued confirmations	Reaching retirement age (annual average)
A	B	C	D	E	F	G	H
Medical doctors	500[c]	10	10	375	125	2	229[d]
Dental doctors	54[c]	1	2	25	29	0.5	118[d]
Pharmacists	163[e]	2	3	31	132	1.6	N/A
Nurses	176[f]	4	31	329	-153	- 2.8	231[g]
Midwives	5[f]+32[g]	0.7	3	18	19	0.3	N/A
Physiotherapists	79[f]	1.5	N/A	48	31	0.6	N/A
Medical assistants (assistant nurses)	1167[f]	22	N/A	0	1167	22	Currently irrelevant (new designation)
Other	500[f]	10	N/A	7	493	9	N/A

Sources: [a] WHO Country Office, Slovakia; [b] Health Education Department of the Ministry of Health unpublished data 2007; [c] Institute of Information and Education Prognosis unpublished data 2009; [d] Health Education Department of the Ministry of Health unpublished data 2005; [e] NHIC 2006a & 2007a; [f] NHIC 2007a & 2008a; [g] Health Education Department of the Ministry of Health unpublished data 2007; NHIC 2006a, 2007a & 2008a.

the United Kingdom and Ireland, driven by factors such as low salaries and unfinished reforms. The Association of Slovak Hospitals reports that approximately 2000 medical doctors are needed at present and estimates that around 100 health professionals are leaving Slovakia every month (Divinský 2007, SME.sk 2007b).

Planning must take account of health workforce outflows as they increase the total expenditure on health professional education. A sufficient number of graduates must be available in order to ensure replacement of these losses, requiring more graduates than educational institutions are able to offer. Ministry of Health analysis shows that one medical student in Slovakia costs approximately €33 000 per year of the university medicine curriculum. Expenditures on further specialization training in general medicine are approximately €8000 per year, a total of €26 000 for three years and three months of training (Beňušová 2008). At present, these expenditures are covered by employers and the state. Emigration results in destination countries acquiring highly qualified workforces without the associated education costs; Slovakia loses both human resources and the costs invested in expert education. Further possible negative consequences of emigration include decreases in labour productivity and the country becoming less attractive for foreign investors (Reichová et al. 2006).

The many factors influencing migration require simultaneous action on several levels to influence the behaviour of health professionals. Current unfavourable demographic trends (Government of the Slovak Republic 2009) in Slovakia and a lack of qualified specialists impact on the availability and quality of health care in different regions. They also pose a potential danger to the continuity of health-care provision (including prevention), particularly in some parts of the system such as ambulatory health care, public health, emergency medical care and mental health care.

6. Relevance of cross-border health professional mobility

The previous sections have demonstrated that the magnitude and impact of health professional mobiliy is an important issue for the health workforce and health systems in Slovakia. However, it is not the only workforce issue that the country is currently facing.

Low incomes are considered to be one of the main reasons why health professionals leave the country or their professions. Larger health facilities have particular difficulty retaining sufficient health personnel and decreasing levels of staff place a higher burden on remaining personnel, entailing the risk of burn-out. Ageing and retirement also diminish a workforce that is reported to be producing too few new graduates to compensate for internal and migratory outflows (Buchan et al. 2007).

6.1 *Education system*

The universities are not meeting the increased requirements of the health-care system by producing sufficient numbers of health professionals – particularly nurses, midwives, physiotherapists, radiological assistants and paramedics. Too few candidates are being admitted due to low population growth and low interest in joining these physically and mentally demanding professions which carry large workloads and risks. Currently, there is no *numerus clausus* in place.

Slovakia faces the challenge of increasing the productivity of the education system without damaging educational quality. Secondary health schools and universities must to be able to meet the staffing needs to provide available, systematic, professional and quality health care for all citizens. This will need to take account of both the changing number of Slovak health professionals and current demographic developments. There is some possibility of admitting foreign citizens from developing countries to medical studies in Slovakia but it is vital to recognize that the basic medical training in third countries is very often not compatible with the EU's minimum educational standards that apply in Slovakia. Also, foreign citizens who complete the medical study programme and obtain EU-recognized qualifications may not stay to work in Slovakia.

For Slovakia, the loss of the migrating health workforce implies increased total expenditures on education if there are to be sufficient human resources. The same level and quality of education is needed in order to ensure patient safety and protection within the provision of health-care. This must be taken into account in planning as it requires more graduates than present educational capacities allow. Demographic trends in Slovakia indicate declining numbers of secondary school graduates and therefore fewer potential candidates for the medical and nursing professions.

The challenge to produce adequate numbers of health professionals takes place within the context of a rapidly and radically changing educational and training system. The professional training of nurses, midwives, physiotherapists, paramedics and radiology assistants was transferred from secondary schools to universities in 1992. University training for medical doctors, dental doctors and pharmacists was modified and curricula were accredited to harmonize fully with European guidelines. This ensured automatic recognition of qualifications in EU Member States as well as better regulation of these professions. Universities became legal entities and self-governing institutions under the Ministry of Education; only one is operated by the Ministry of Health. Overall, the total number of admitted candidates and graduates does not balance the numbers leaving the system on retirement.

6.2 *Employment perspectives*

Unemployment among graduates of health-related studies is not a factor that influences emigrating Slovak health professionals. In 2007, there were 372 unemployed secondary-school graduates of health-related studies – 1.9% of the total number of unemployed graduates of secondary schools (19 134 persons in 2007) and a negligible proportion of the total number of unemployed people (245 253) in Slovakia (Herich 2009). In 2006, there were 86 unemployed university graduates in academic health-related studies including general medicine, dental medicine, pharmacy, nursing, midwifery and physiotherapy. These represented 3.1% of all unemployed university graduates (2771) and a negligible proportion of all unemployed people (273 437) in Slovakia (Zvalová et al 2007).

Secondary health schools collect employment data on their graduates that provides other valuable information. For example, despite career prospects that are already good, factors such as higher pay and better working conditions provide incentives for graduates to take higher education courses in health studies in order to improve their salaries further or to work abroad. The latter means that Slovakia does not receive the returns from this investment in education. This was confirmed by a study conducted on a sample of health professionals, including recent graduates, leaving Slovakia to work abroad in 2004–2008 (Beňušová 2007).

6.3 *Retirement and demographics*

Based on Ministry of Health data, the Ministry of Education's *Operational Programme Education* reveals that more than 40% of those working in the dental profession fall into the retirement or pre-retirement age category. The situation is similar for specialist doctors – including pathologists, paramedics, general practitioners (for adults as well as for children and adolescents), anaesthetists and psychiatrists – and for nurses, midwives and psychologists (Ministry of Education 2007).

Table 14.7 shows the numbers of medical doctors, dental doctors and nurses approaching retirement age. In 2007, ageing of the health workforce meant that those aged over 50 made up 45% (8230) of the total stock (18 219) of medical doctors and 62% (1769) of the total stock (2862) of dental doctors. Nurses aged over 40 comprised 53.48% (18 206) of the 34 040 total stock (NHIC 2008b).

Table 14.7 *Medical doctors, dental doctors and nurses approaching retirement (natural persons), 2004–2007*

Medical doctors	Total	age 50+	
	natural p.	natural p.	%
2004	16 707	6 798	40.69
2005	16 318	7 132	43.71
2006	17 040	7 585	44.51
2007	18 219	8 230	45.17
Dental doctors	**Total**	**age 50+**	
	natural p.	natural p.	%
2004	2 870	1 571	54.74
2005	2 919	1 667	57.11
2006	2 714	1 637	60.32
2007	2 862	1 769	61.81
Nurses	**Total**	**age 40+**	
	natural p.	natural p.	%
2004	34 007	16 797	49.39
2005	32 319	16 579	51.30
2006	32 568	17 247	52.96
2007	34 040	18 206	53.48

Sources: NHIC 2005, 2006b, 2007b & 2008b.

The legal retirement age is 62 years (Government of the Slovak Republic 2003). Shortages in the health workforce and the necessity to attract more candidates present an argument for special consideration of the retirement policy for these demanding professions. Some of the health professional organizations argue that the health professions could be made more attractive by allowing their members to retire earlier or through tax cuts.

Slovakia faces major public policy challenges from slowing workforce growth, workforce ageing and the economic burden that demographic ageing will impose on those of productive age (Šikula et al. 2008).

7. Factors influencing health professional mobility

Beňušová (2007) found that admission to education and changes in the system or quality of education did not play a significant role in health professionals' decisions to emigrate. Like the rest of the population, health professionals are motivated to migrate by the prospect of improving their own economic status (to "make money") and that of their family ("helping to solve financial and housing issues of a family") (Reichová et al. 2006).

Reichová and colleagues found the most significant migration intentions in the group of pharmaceutical and medical graduates (8 out of 10 respondents). These graduates associate employment abroad with professional specialization and tend to leave their professions much less than graduates in other professions (Reichová et al. 2006). Analysis of the length of stay abroad shows that medical faculty graduates show a tendency to permanent emigration – almost every one of those seeking to work abroad was considering permanent migration (Reichová et al. 2006).

Nurses mention the improvement of language skills as an incentive for emigration. Medical doctors cite discontent with medical supplies and technical equipment in their workplace and "low social status". Nurses also mention these two factors but reverse their order of importance (Beňušová 2007). Nurses aged 41–50 years consider excessive workload to be an important factor (Beňušová 2007). "Earning money" is a motivating factor not only to leave the country (Beňušová 2007) but also to leave the health sector.

These survey results correspond with the findings of managers of health-care facilities, trade unions and professional organizations. Health professionals' more pronounced tendency towards permanent labour migration (Reichová et al. 2006) should be taken as a warning signal that the current Slovak health system is not attractive for workers and relevant policies are required to improve this situation.

8. Policy, regulation and interventions

8.1 *Policies and policy development related to health professional mobility*

The main objective of policies on health professional mobility is to retain health professionals through better remuneration; improved social recognition, working conditions and education; and the reconstruction of hospital infrastructures. The election of a new government in 2006 brought about policy change and a move to follow health-sector priorities, including an employment policy based on a process of collective negotiations (Government of the Slovak Republic 1991 & 2001). One of the main priorities for health policy is to stabilize and restore self-sufficiency in the health workforce in the country.

Policies on human resources for health are based on priorities identified in the *Details of the Government Manifesto for the Health Sector* published in 2006

(Ministry of Health 2006b). Government goals for building human resource capacity in the 2006–2010 period are explicitly indicated in the elaborated document through which, pursuant to Articles 5 and 25, the government aims to improve the (financial and moral) evaluation of work and the social position of health workers by:

a. introducing amendments to the Labour Code and to the Act on Remuneration of Employees in Execution of Work of Public Interest;

b. implementing a system of moral evaluation of individuals, working groups and health-care facilities;

c. amending all minimum education standards for health workers and communication skills training;

d. making information on ethical committees of self-governing regions and of health-care facilities accessible to the general public;

e. developing health education in order to ensure appropriate numbers of qualified experts for all health professions;

f. implementing motivation and stabilization measures in order to ensure the required number and structure of qualified health workers; and

g. supporting and implementing innovations in the continuing medical education of health workers.

The goals specified under c, e and g should be achieved by utilizing resources from both the European Regional Development Fund (ERDF) and the European Social Fund (ESF). These are available to the Slovak Republic until 2013 (Ministry of Health 2006b).

In cooperation with the European Observatory on Health Systems and Policies, in June 2007 the Ministry of Health held a policy dialogue – Planning on Human Resources for Health in Slovakia. The objective was to support policy development by analysing opportunities and strategies for new approaches to planning and new policies of human resources in health to address challenges for the health workforce (Buchan et al. 2007).

Spending on health is only 5.26% of the gross domestic product (GDP). Such a limited level is a major stumbling block for health workforce policies and for fair competitive remuneration conditions for health professionals in Slovakia. In 1996 the government committed to the establishment of a remuneration system that would guarantee doctors salary levels comparable with other sectors. However, the lack of financial resources meant that this objective could not be met (Buchan et al. 2007).

Interventions

Over recent years, the Slovak government has implemented various interventions to manage health professional mobility. The measures reflect the concerns described in previous sections and focus on the modernization of health-care facilities, retention of specialized medical doctors and increasing remuneration levels.

Slovakia has embarked on a programme to make health facilities more attractive for patients and the health workforce by reducing inequalities in the distribution of resources and technical capacities. Funded by the ESF's Operational Programme: Education and the ERDF's Operational Programme Health, €250 million is being invested in the modernization of Slovak health organizations between 2007 and 2013. This should help to reduce emigration motivated by outdated or inadequate equipment in many large health-care facilities (Ministry of Education 2007, Ministry of Health 2007b).

According to Ministry of Health data, €125 million were allocated for 24 health-care facility projects across Slovakia and 2 technical assistance projects (enabling Ministry of Health to implement the Operational Programme Health) during the three years (2007–2009) in which the Operational Programme Health allowance was implemented. By 31 December 2009 24 of these projects were in the executing phase. Only 5.01% of the allocated resources have been used so far and so the effect of the supported interventions is not yet markedly evident. However, publicly available reports indicate that this 5.01% has produced 11 720.57 m^2 of reconstructed and equipped space for the provision of health care in general and specialized hospitals and 660 m^2 for ambulatory care facilities in Slovakia (Ministry of Health 2010). It will not be possible to evaluate the impacts on Slovak health professional migration until the modernization of the Slovak health-care facilities is complete.

The Operational Programme: Education intervention focuses on the retention of specialist medical doctors, aiming to balance the regional differences in available workforce capacities in Slovakia and EU Member States. Specialized training is funded on condition that the enrolled medical doctors work in Slovakia for a specified period of time after successful completion of their studies. Those who fail to meet this obligation must repay their EU grant so that funding may be used for another specialist. The programme was implemented in 2008, with resources amounting to €35.6 million for 2007–2013. However, no official data are available on the numbers of specialized doctors trained under the scheme (Ministry of Education 2007).

In the three years of implementation (2007–2009), the Operational Programme: Education has assigned €12.5 million of the €35.6 million allocated to Slovakia

(Ministry of Health 2009b) from the ESF (Ministry of Health 2008b). Five of the fourteen Operational Programme Education projects implemented had been completed by 31 December 2009.

Financial support from the 2008 pilot call initially funded three months of a doctor's specialized training – this was completed by 110 specialist doctors (Ministry of Health 2009b). The regions of Nitra, Žilina, Trenčín, Košice and Prešov participated in the projects and benefitted from the training of additional specialized health professionals including general practitioners, dental doctors, anaesthetists, clinical oncologists, clinical immunologists and allergologists (Ministry of Health 2009b). Doctors funded in this way were contracted to remain and practise in the territory of the relevant Slovak self-governing region for at least one year after completion of their specialization or face sanctions (Ministry of Health 2008c).

Following successful evaluation of the pilot project for medical doctors in November 2008, the Ministry of Health announced that the self-governing regions (excluding Bratislava) could apply for financial support for specialized training for all health professionals, not just selected medical specializations. The training period was extended from 3 months to a maximum of 36 months (Ministry of Health 2008d) and the contractual period for remaining and practising in the relevant Slovak region was increased (depending on the length of the financial support) to a maximum of five years. All the eligible self-governing regions have implemented projects based on the second Operational Programme Education (Ministry of Health 2009b) but information on the number of experts trained was not available at the time of writing – the expected deadline is January 2012.

Another important intervention was the increase in salary levels for health professionals. The gradual increase of health insurance resources has created conditions for an increase in the salaries of health professionals. These were backed up by political decisions (Government of the Slovak Republic 2006, Ministry of Health 2006b] and strikes among the health workforce.[5] These were called by the medical trade union (April–May 2006) in order to secure its demands before the untimely parliamentary elections in June 2006. The main requests included an immediate adequate salary increase for doctors and other health professionals and increases in health insurance resources. These requests were also supported by other professional associations and health professionals from several large and smaller hospitals.

---

5 Recorded in various media reports (Spravy.pravda.sk 2006a & 2006b, Topky.sk 2006, SME.sk 2006, Loz.sk 2006).

Fig. 14.3 *Comparison of average monthly salaries of medical doctors and nurses and average monthly salary in Slovakia (€), 2005–2009*

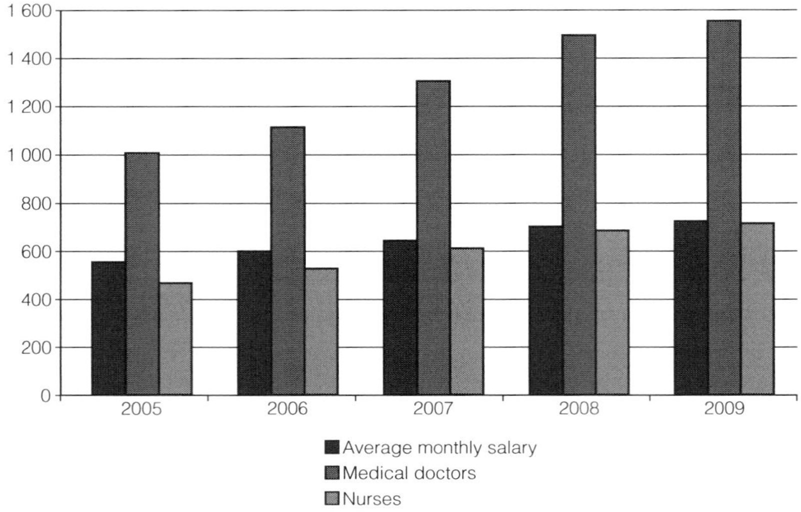

Source: NHIC unpublished data 2009.

The average monthly salary of medical doctors was 181.6% of the average monthly salary in Slovakia in 2005 but had risen to 214.7% by 2009. Nurses' average salary was 84.6% of the average monthly salary in 2005 and 98.8% in 2009. Between 2005 and 2009, the average monthly salaries of medical doctors and nurses had increased by 53.5% and 51.7%, respectively. It is possible that improved salaries were a factor in reducing applications for equivalence confirmations – an indication that fewer health professionals may be intending to emigrate.

The economic crisis will have an impact on the resources available for further improvement of health professionals' working conditions and therefore other retention options such as non-financial incentives and housing support will be investigated. The impact on emigration or the return of health professionals has yet to be evaluated.

One approach that has not been explored is the export of health services. The low prices and comparatively high quality of some health services in Slovakia have the potential to attract patients from abroad. Treatments such as dental services, cosmetic surgery and balneal services should be promoted in other countries and will provide domestic work opportunities for health professionals.

8.2 *Workforce planning and development*

Human resource policy (including planning) falls under the competencies of health-care facilities. It is partially influenced by funders of health-care facilities and trade unions, with the Ministry of Health holding a legislative and monitoring role. In legislative procedures the government collaborates with and is advised by professional organizations and trade unions in the health sector (Ministry of Health 2006b). Tripartite negotiations also cover human resources in health (Government of the Slovak Republic 2007a) but Slovakia has few experts on this subject. This results in a lack of planning and management skills to address issues such as the lack of team work, communication problems and the absence of continuing education programmes for human resource management in health-care facilities.

Slovakia has no formal human resources planning mechanism. Universities fall under the responsibility of the Ministry of Education but have autonomy to determine their own numbers of medical students. Minimum staffing levels are not mandatorily defined at hospital level. Further medical education (specializations and certifications following university degrees) in the system is characterized by a high number of specialties (219). Continuing professional education is mandatory in Slovakia but must be self-financed by health professionals or by their employers. There is a lack of health management training – nearly 25% of hospital managers have had no specific managerial training (Buchan et al. 2007).

A six-month training twinning project was held in 2008. The objective of Improvement of Working Time Organisation in the Health Sector was to improve the quality and effectiveness of health services through the development of human resources in the health sector and to improve the managerial skills of hospital managers (Ministry of Health 2008e). A national project for training health professionals in effective communication is being prepared for consideration. Other projects are being prepared at national, regional or local levels concerning the sustainability of health professional education and early identification of burn-out syndrome.

8.3 *Regulatory frameworks*

Despite very low inflows of foreign health professionals Slovakia has implemented the European frameworks for mutual recognition. The frameworks offer two possibilities for the status of migrant health professionals from EU Member States.

1. **Visitor** – a person who practises occasionally and on a temporary basis (maximum 30 days per calendar year). Subject to notification to the Ministry of Health, in accordance with Act No. 578/2004 Coll., paragraph 30 (Government of the Slovak Republic 2004a) which is a transposition of

Articles 5–9 of Directive 2005/36/EC on the recognition of professional qualifications (European Commission 2007).

2. **Settled (established) person** – based on the recognition of professional qualification for professional purposes pursuant to Directive 2005/36/EC on the recognition of professional qualifications (European Commission 2007). Two ministries share the competences: (i) Ministry of Education issues confirmations on the recognition of pre-graduate education; and (ii) Ministry of Health issues confirmations on the recognition of diplomas on specializations and certificates.

This process applies the EU principles and rules of the automatic recognition of qualification, including acquired rights, as well as the recognition based on a general recognition system, including the application of compensation mechanisms (Government of the Slovak Republic 2007a).

Foreign nationals from third countries are not entitled to practise under "temporary provision of services". In addition to recognition of professional qualification, third-country nationals require a residency permit issued by the Ministry of Interior and a work permit issued by the Ministry of Labour, Social Affairs and Family in order to practise.

International bilateral agreements on the recognition of professional qualifications signed by Slovakia apply only for academic purposes. These include training, exchanges of experts, participation in international events organized in other contracting countries and cooperation between health organizations. The Ministry of Health has concluded no bilateral contracts on health professional mobility and there are no existing valid contracts on this subject.

9. Conclusion

International studies have identified that human resources, including professionals and expert capacities, play a crucial role in the success of health systems in terms of their outputs, services and impacts. This study has identified Slovakia as a source country for health professional mobility, losing considerable numbers of qualified health professionals to other EU countries. Between May 2004 and April 2007, some 3700 Slovak health professionals applied for equivalence confirmations to work in another EU country. However, other data sources indicate that this is an underestimate of emigrants as Slovak health professionals, especially nurses, do not necessarily need equivalence documents for employment abroad. Slovakia is now facing the challenge of staff shortages, underproduction of health professionals and a looming demographic trend.

Stabilization and re-establishment of the self-sufficiency of the health workforce is one of the main priorities for health policy in the country.

This analysis of health professional mobility in Slovakia indicates the need to concentrate on implementing: (i) a system of data collection covering regular inflows and outflows of health professionals, including different specialties; and (ii) regular surveys of motivation for labour migration and for maintaining health professionals' medical practice in order to establish whether retention measures are effective. In addition, systematic research on demographic and sociological data should be implemented to monitor other factors that influence the size and composition of the workforce. Appropriate training and the increase of technical capacities to ensure better research and monitoring should also be considered.

There is also a need to enhance short-, mid- and long-term planning at both regional and national level. Employers should be supported in their efforts to retain existing workforces and even to attract those who have left – better remuneration for nurses and other highly qualified staff in health organizations is an issue that needs to be addressed. In addition, emigrant health professionals working abroad should be recruited to return to work in Slovakia. Overall, governance, planning and analysis of human resources for health need to be strengthened. A core set of priorities should be identified in order to design an action plan on human resources for health for Slovakia.

References

Beňušová K (2007). *Vplyv smerníc Európskej únie na reguláciu zdravotníckeho povolania sestra v Slovenskej republike* [*Impact of EU directives on regulation of the nursing profession*]. [Thesis]. Trnava University in Trnava, Faculty of Health and Social Work, Department of Nursing, Physiotherapy and Clinical Disciplines.

Beňušová K (2008). Právo etablovania zdravotníckeho pracovníka na území iného členského štátu [Right of establishment for medical professional in another Member State]. *Prezentácia Ministerstva zdravotníctva Slovenskej republiky publikovaná na Medzinárodnom seminári o migrácii pracovnej sily v zdravotníctve, 19.-20. jún 2008, Bratislava* [*Report of Ministry of Health of the Slovak Republic at the International Seminar on Migration of the Health Workforce, Bratislava, 19–20 June 2008*].

Buchan J et al. (2007). Policy dialogue: Human resources for health in Slovakia: the way forward. *European Observatory on Health Systems and Policies Policy Dialogue on Planning of Human Resources for Health in Slovakia. Bratislava, 18–19 June 2007.*

Divinský B (2007). *Labour market – migration nexus in Slovakia: time to act in a comprehensive way.* Bratislava, International Organization for Migration, 2007.

Divinský B, Popjaková D (2007). *Koľko Slovákov pracuje v zahraničí (jeden expertný odhad)* [*How many Slovaks are working abroad? (an expert estimate)*] Bratislava, International Organization for Migration.

European Commision (2007). *Implementation of the Directive 2005/36/EC on the Recognition of Professional Qualifications. Statistical summary of decisions of recognition of qualifications covered by the sectoral system of recognition.* Brussels, Directorate-General Internal Market and Services, Knowledge-based Economy, Regulated professions (MARKT D/17123/2007-EN).

Government of the Slovak Republic (1991). Zákon NR SR č. 2/1991 Zb. o kolektívnom vyjednávaní v znení neskorších predpisov [Act No. 2/1991 Coll. on collective bargaining, as amended]. *Collection of Laws,* No.1/1991. (http://www.zbierka.sk/zz/predpisy/default. aspx?CiastkaID=2143, accessed 13 February 2011).

Government of the Slovak Republic (2001). Zákon NR SR č. 311/2001 Z.z. Zákonník práce v znení neskorších predpisov [Act No. 311/2001 Coll. Labour Code, as amended]. Collection *of Laws*, No.130/ 2001 (http://www.zbierka.sk/ zz/predpisy/default.aspx?CiastkaID=3593, accessed 13 February 2011).

Government of the Slovak Republic (2003). Zákon NR SR č. 461/2003 Z.z. o sociálnom poistení v znení neskorších predpisov [Act No 461/2003 Coll. on social insurance, as amended]. *Collection of Laws*, No.200/2003 (http://www. zbierka.sk/zz/predpisy/default.aspx?CiastkaID =4185, accessed 13 February 2011).

Government of the Slovak Republic (2004a). Zákon NR SR č. 578/2004 Z.z. o poskytovateľoch zdravotnej starostlivosti, zdravotníckych pracovníkoch, stavovských organizáciách v zdravotníctve a o zmene a doplnení niektorých zákonov v znení neskorších predpisov [Act No. 578/2004 Coll. on health-care providers, health professionals and professional organizations in the health service, and amending and supplementing certain acts, as amended by later regulations]. *Collection of Laws*, No.245/ 2004 (http://www.zbierka.sk/zz/ predpisy/default.aspx? CiastkaID=4484, accessed 13 February 2011).

Government of the Slovak Republic (2004b). Zákon NR SR č. 576/2004 Z.z. o zdravotnej starostlivosti, službách súvisiacich s poskytovaním zdravotnej starostlivosti a o zmene a doplnení niektorých zákonov v znení neskorších predpisov [Act No 576/2004 Coll. on health care and healthcare-related services, and amending and supplementing certain acts, as amended by later regulations]. *Collection of Laws*, No.243/2004 (http://www.zbierka.sk/zz/predpisy/default.aspx?CiastkaID=4482, accessed 13 February 2011).

Government of the Slovak Republic (2006) *Programové vyhlásenie vlády Slovenskej republiky 2006* [*Manifesto of the Government of the Slovak Republic 2006*]. Bratislava.

Government of the Slovak Republic (2007a). Zákon NR SR č. 103/2007 Z.z. o trojstranných konzultáciách na celoštátnej úrovni a o zmene a doplnení niektorých zákonov (zákon o tripartite) [Act No. 103/2007 Coll. on tripartite consultations at the national level and on amending and supplementing certain acts (Tripartite Act)]. *Collection of Laws*, No.57/2007. (http://www.zbierka.sk/zz/predpisy/default.aspx?CiastkaID=5243, accessed 13 February 2011).

Government of the Slovak Republic (2007b). Zákon NR SR č. 293/2007 Z.z. o uznávaní odborných kvalifikácií v platnom znení [Act No. 293/2007 Coll. on recognition of professional qualifications]. *Collection of Laws*, No.133/ 2007 (http://www.zbierka.sk/zz/predpisy/ default.aspx?CiastkaID=25559, accessed 13 February 2011).

Government of the Slovak Republic (2009). *Správa o zdravotnom stave obyvateľstva za roky 2006–2008* [Report on the health situation of Slovak citizens 2006–2008]. Bratislava (http://www.rokovania.sk/Rokovanie.aspx/BodRokovaniaDetail?idMaterial=8893, accessed 16 July 2009.

Government of the Slovak Republic (2010). Nariadenie vlády SR č. 296/2010 Z.z. o odbornej spôsobilosti na výkon zdravotníckeho povolania, spôsobe ďalšieho vzdelávania zdravotníckych pracovníkov, sústave špecializačných odborov a sústave certifikovaných pracovných činností [Regulation of the Government of the Slovak Republic 296/2010 Coll. on professional qualifications of health professionals, on further education of health professionals' specializations and certified procedures]. *Collection of Laws*, No.112/2010 (http://www.zbierka.sk/zz/predpisy/default.aspx?CiastkaID=26227, accessed 13 February 2011).

Hajnovičová V (2006). *Vývoj zamestnanosti v Slovenskej republike v období 1995–2005* [*Employment trends in the Slovak Republic 1995–2005*]. Bratislava Prognostický ústav SAV [Institute for Forecasting, Slovak Academy of Sciences].

Herich J (2009). Uplatnenie absolventov stredných škôl v praxi. Sezónny cyklus 2007/2008 [The application of secondary school graduates in practice. Seasonal cycle of 2007/2008]. In: *Koncepcia odborného vzdelávania a prípravy žiakov na výkon povolania a odborných činností v zdravotníctve do roku 2013* [*The concept of vocational education and training students to practise and professional activities in health care by 2013*]. Bratislava, Institute of Information and Prognoses of Education (http://www.uips.sk/sub/uips.sk/images/JH/ UplatnenieA08_prezent_1.xls, accessed 16 July 2009).

Katuščák B (2006). *Nadnárodná migrácia za prácou zo Slovenska do EÚ (vývoj, stav, trendy)* [*Transnational labour migration from Slovakia to the EU (evolution, status, trends)*]. Bratislava, Ústredie práce, sociálnych vecí a rodiny [Central Office of Labour, Social Affairs and Family].

Loz.sk (2006). Lekárske odborové združenie. Štrajk. [Medical trade association. Strike]. *Loz.sk*, 5 June 2006 (http://www.loz.sk/strajk.html, accessed 21 December 2009).

Ministry of Education (2007). *Operačný program Vzdelávanie, Ministerstvo školstva Slovenskej republiky NSRF SR 2007–2013* [*Operational Programme Education. NSRF SR 2007–2013*] Bratislava (http://opv.health-sf.sk/zakladne-dokumenty/operacny-program-vzdelavanie-zd, accessed 16 July 2009).

Ministry of Health (2006a). *Annual Report of the Ministry of Health of the Slovak Republic for 2005.* Bratislava (http://www.health.gov.sk/?dalsie-materialy&sprava=vyrocne-spravy-mzsr), accessed 1 December 2010.

Ministry of Health (2006b). *Rozpracovanie programového vyhlásenia vlády na podmienky rezortu zdravotníctva* [*Details of the government manifesto for the health sector*]. Bratislava (http://www2.health.gov.sk/redsys/rsi.nsf/0/ed6ef554f023b81fc12572 130038b115/$FILE/ PVV_SR_cast_zdravotnictvo.rtf, accessed 16 July 2009).

Ministry of Health (2007a). *Annual report of the Ministry of Health of the Slovak Republic for 2006.* Bratislava (http://www.health.gov.sk/?dalsie-materialy&sprava=vyrocne-spravy-mzsr), accessed 1 December 2010.

Ministry of Health of the Slovak Republic (2007b). *Operačný program Zdravotníctvo NSRF SR, 2007–2013* [*Operational Programme Health. NSRF SR, 2007–2013*] Bratislava (http://opz.health-sf.sk/operacny-program-dravotnictvo/co-je-opz, accessed 13 February 2011).

Ministry of Health (2008a). *Annual report of the Ministry of Health of the Slovak Republic for 2007.* Bratislava (http://www.health.gov.sk/? dalsie-materialy&sprava=vyrocne-spravy-mzsr, accessed 01/12/2010.

Ministry of Health (2008b). *Leták zameraný na opatrenie 2.2 OPV, rok 2008* [*Leaflet designed to measure 2.2 OPV, 2008*]. Bratislava (http://opv.health-sf.sk/rok-2008, accessed 12 August 2010).

Ministry of Health (2008c). Prílohy k výzve. Ministerstvo zdravotníctva Slovenskej republiky vyhlasuje výzvu na predkladanie žiadostí o NFP. Archív výziev Operačného programu Vzdelávanie. [Annex No. 20 to Call: Model treaty on the promotion of specialized training of health workers from the Operational Programme Education]. In: *Archív výziev Operačného programu Vzdelávanie* [*Operational Programme Education Archive*]. Bratislava (http://opv.health-sf.sk/archiv-vyziev-2008/mz-sr-vyhlasuje-vyzvu-na-predkladanie-ziadosti-o-nfp-o-nfp, accessed 12 August 2010).

Ministry of Health (2008d). Archív výziev Operačného programu Vzdelávanie [Archives of challenges Operational Programme Education]. Bratislava (http://opv.health-sf.sk/archiv- vyziev-2008/vyzva-v-ramci-opatrenia-22-opv-zamerana-na-doplnenie-systemu-zdravotnictva-o-kvalifikovanych-odbornikov, accessed 12 August 2010).

Ministry of Health (2008e). Informácia o projektoch financovaných z prostriedkov Prechodného fondu v rezorte Ministerstva zdravotníctva SR v rokoch 2006 – 2009. Zlepšenie organizácie pracovného času v zdravotníctve [Information on projects funded by the Transition Fund in the Ministry of Health in 2006–2009. Improving the organization of working time in health care]. Bratislava (http://www2.health.gov.sk/redsys/rsi.nsf/0/F73C917426276C39C125765 B003A87E1?OpenDocument, accessed 13 February 2011) (Project SK/2005/017 - 464.05.02).

Ministry of Health (2009a). *Annual report of the Ministry of Health of the Slovak Republic for 2008.* Bratislava (http://www.health.gov.sk/?dalsie-materialy&sprava= vyrocne-spravy-mzsr, accessed 1 December 2010).

Ministry of Health (2009b). *Spravodajca opatrenia 2.2 operačného programu Vzdelávanie* [*Rapporteur measure 2.2 Operational Programme Education*]. Bratislava, European Programmes and Projects Section, Ministry of Health of the Slovak Republic (http://opv.health-sf.sk/rok-2009, accessed 12 August 2010).

Ministry of Health (2010). *Zhodnotenie implementácie Operačného programu Zdravotníctvo k 31.12 2009 (záverečná správa)* [*Evaluation of the implementation of the Operational Programme Health, 31.12.2009 (Final Report)*]. Bratislava, Consulting Associates Ltd. Bratislava for the Ministry of Health of the Slovak Republic (http://opz.health-sf.sk/hodnotiace-spravy/zhodnotenie-implementacie-operacneho-programu-zdravotnictvo, accessed 12 August 2010).

NHIC (2005). *Health statistics yearbook of the Slovak Republic 2004.* Bratislava, National Health Information Centre.

NHIC (2006a). *Health yearbook of the Slovak Republic 2005, First edition.* Bratislava, National Health Information Centre.

NHIC (2006b). *Health statistics yearbook of the Slovak Republic 2005.* Bratislava, National Health Information Centre.

NHIC (2007a). *Health yearbook of the Slovak Republic 2006, First edition.* Bratislava, National Health Information Centre.

NHIC (2007b). *Health statistics yearbook of the Slovak Republic 2006.* Bratislava, National Health Information Centre.

NHIC (2008a). *Health yearbook of the Slovak Republic 2007, First edition.* Bratislava, National Health Information Centre.

NHIC (2008b). *Health statistics yearbook of the Slovak Republic 2007.* Bratislava, National Health Information Centre.

Reichová D et al. (2006). *Sprístupnenie trhov práce vo vybraných krajinách EÚ a vývojové trendy na trhu práce v SR* [*Opening of labour markets in selected EU Member States and development trends of the labour market in the Slovak Republic*]. Bratislava, Institute for Labour and Family Research (Research Project No. 2118-2006).

Šikula M et al. (2008). *Dlhodobá vízia slovenskej spoločnosti* [*Long-term vision for Slovak society*]. Bratislava, Economic Institute of the Slovak Academy of Sciences.

SME.sk (2006). Komora sestier podporuje lekársky štrajk [Chamber of nurses supports medical strike]. *SME.sk*, 10 April 2006 (http://www.sme.sk/c/2670214/komora-sestier-poSME.skdporuje-lekarsky-strajk.html, accessed 13 February 2011).

SME.sk (2007a). V obciach a malých mestečkách už zubára takmer nenájdete [In villages and small towns almost cannot find a dental doctor now]. *SME.sk*, 12 February 2007 (http://www.sme.sk/c/3142963/v-obciach-a-malych-mesteckach-uz-zubara-takmer-nenajdete.html, accessed 15 February 2011).

SME.sk (2007b). Hrozí nám nedostatok lekárov [We risk a shortage of doctors]. *SME*, 19 February 2007 (http://dennik.sme.sk/c/3153649/hrozi-nam-nedostatok-lekarov.html, accessed 15 February 2011).

Spravy.prada.sk (2006a). Nemocnice podporujú LOZ, nie všetky však vstúpia do štrajku [Hospitals support medical trade union, but not all join the strike]. *Spravy.prada.sk*, 4 April 2006   http://spravy.pravda.sk/sk_domace.asp?r=sk_domace&c=A060404_143751_sk_domace_p23, accessed 13 February 2011).

Spravy.prada.sk (2006b). Lekári nevylučujú ostrý štrajk [Doctors do not preclude a sharp strike]. *Spravy.prada.sk*, 20 March 2006 (http://spravy.pravda.sk/lekari-nevylucuju-ostry-strajk-dnb-/sk_domace.asp?c=A060320_183014_sk_domace_p12, accessed 13 February 2011).

Topky.sk (2006). Zdravotníci vyšli do ulíc [Health professionals took to the streets]. *Topky.sk*, 13 April 2006 (http://www.topky.sk/cl/10/110348/ Zdravotnici-vysli-do-ulic?from=bleskovky, accessed 13 February 2011).

Zvalová M et al. (2007). *Uplatnenie absolventov vysokých škôl v praxi. 1. etapa. Zamestnateľnosť a zamestnanosť absolventov vysokých škôl [Application of graduates in practice. Stage 1. Employability and employment of graduates]*. Bratislava, Oddelenie analýz a prognóz vysokých škôl, Ústav informácií a prognóz školstva [Department of Analyses and Forecasts of Higher Education, Institute of Information and Prognoses of Education]. (http://www.uips.sk/sub/uips.sk/ images/MK/Studie/Uplatnenie_pre_tlac.pdf, accessed 12 August 2010).

Chapter 15

Addressing shortages in the health workforce: Slovenia's reliance on foreign health professionals, current developments and policy responses

Tit Albreht

1. Introduction

For several decades Slovenia has been an attractive destination country for medical doctors and dentists from countries of the former Yugoslavia such as Bosnia and Herzegovina, Croatia and Serbia. Three main factors triggered considerable inflows to Slovenia: (i) a chronic shortage of health professionals; (ii) the numerous opportunities for medical and dental graduates that resulted from these shortages; and (iii) an expanding health-care sector at a time of significant limitations in several other republics of the former Yugoslavia.

Slovenia still relies to a large extent on foreign health professionals. In 2008, 21.8% of all active medical doctors and 22.7% of all dentists were foreign trained. Overall, about 80% of all immigrant medical doctors and dentists in Slovenia come from three countries in the area – Croatia; Bosnia and Herzegovina; and Serbia. There are few data on the inflows and outflows of nurses but the limited evidence available suggests that they have lower levels of mobility than medical doctors and dentists.

Slovenia has lacked a sound and long-term human resource policy for health care with which to address shortages and other health workforce management and development issues in a coherent manner. However, over the last five to ten years there have been several attempts to make the workforce self-sufficient by educating sufficient numbers of health professionals within Slovenia. Training capacity was expanded by opening an additional medical faculty in Maribor in 2003 and four additional nursing schools between 2003 and 2008. These developments have not yet produced any significant effect on the inflows to Slovenia but this is likely to change when the additional domestic production has come on stream.

Data sources and limitations

The main source of data on medical doctors and dentists was the Register of Physicians (including medical doctors and dentists) held by the Medical Chamber of Slovenia (MCS). The MCS produces data on foreign medical doctors and dentists which, according to their definitions, include those who are foreign born, foreign nationals and foreign trained. The data show separate numbers for medical doctors and dentists as both professional groups are members of the MCS. Most of the data on foreign health professionals fall into the categories of foreign trained and foreign born, which include some Slovene nationals.

Registration data are complete, especially for third-country nationals who are obliged to comply with the requirements of the Ministry of Health's registration exam. In addition, all medical doctors and dentists practising anywhere in the health services (including public health) are required to obtain a licence to practise. Licensing is the responsiblity of the relevant professional chambers and the completeness of their data depends on the compliance of both individuals and providers.

An additional data source is the National Health Care Providers Database (NHCPD). All medical doctors, dentists and nurses are enrolled in the NHCPD on completion of the registration exam. The NHCPD therefore has relatively comprehensive coverage, missing only those doctors, dentists and nurses who do not pursue careers in their professional fields.

Most of the data on nurses were obtained through the NHCPD and through a provider survey. Overall, data on nurses were difficult to obtain as public authorization to keep a nursing and midwifery register was granted to the Nursing Chamber of Slovenia (NCS) only in 2008. This is currently in the verification phase and consequently there is only minimal information on foreign nurses based on reliable sources. Hence, for this study, a postal survey was used to enquire about foreign-trained nursing professionals in all hospitals and primary health-care centres in mid-October 2009. The findings are presented in section 2.

2. Mobility profile of Slovenia

2.1 *Inflows*

In view of the changing circumstances in surrounding countries, near and further away, Slovenia remains a destination country for health professionals from other former Yugoslavian states. Before independence in 1991, especially during the 1970s and 1980s, Slovenia offered possibilities for medical and dental graduates to start their careers quickly. By contrast, overproduction of medical and dental graduates in other republics of the former Yugoslavia delayed the start of their careers – requiring them to work mostly in unpaid posts during their internships and then to wait for paid training posts in most specialties. Thus, three countries (Bosnia and Herzegovina, Croatia, Serbia) became the source of 80% of immigrant medical doctors and dentists. This is clearly seen in the structure of foreign health professionals shown by country of origin (Tables 15.2, 15.3 & 15.4).

Expansion of the capacity of health-care providers caused sudden increases in demand for foreign health professionals that required significant immigration. These movements were first evaluated quantitatively by Albreht and Klazinga (2002). Based on previous projections (Kastelac & Schlamberger 1973, Kastelac et al. 1976, Ravnikar et al. 1986), and taking account of the specifics of the Slovene health-care system, there were estimates that 5200 medical doctors would be needed by 2000. The actual number in 2000 was about 4400 (National Institute of Public Health 2001).

Between 1992 and 1995, inflows virtually ceased and some health professionals returned to their countries of origin, mostly to Serbia but also to Croatia and Bosnia and Herzegovina. More importantly, political unrest prevented the movement of potential immigrant health professionals, especially from Croatia and Bosnia and Herzegovina, although these migration movements picked up quickly when the situation improved. These processes have not been thoroughly documented but are based on the observations of health-care managers of main hospitals and primary health-care centres.

The direction of flows reversed in 1995–1996 and immigration started again, stimulated by the much improved economic situation in Slovenia as well as uncertainties in the source countries. Immigrants were mostly from Bosnia and Herzegovina and Serbia; and from Croatia and the former Yugoslav Republic of Macedonia to a lesser degree. Today, these countries still comprise the highest shares among foreign health professionals in Slovenia. However, a more nuanced picture emerges when different groups of health professions are examined.

Medical doctors

Slovenia has relied and still relies to a considerable extent on foreign medical doctors. Since 2003, every fifth medical doctor practising in Slovenia has been foreign trained, usually in the neighbouring countries – increasing from 17.4% of all active medical doctors in 1992 to 22.5% in 2008 (Table 15.1). In absolute terms, numbers more than doubled from 608 in 1992 to 1497 in 2008.

Table 15.1 *Foreign-trained medical doctors within all active medical doctors in Slovenia, 1992 and 2003–2008*

	1992	2003	2004	2005	2006	2007	2008
Foreign-trained medical doctors	**608**	**1 225**	**1 293**	**1 335**	**1 407**	**1 450**	**1 497**
Foreign-trained medical doctors in all active medical doctors (%)	17.4	20.3	20.7	21.0	21.6	22.3	22.5
All active medical doctors	3 486	6 045	6 240	6 370	6 525	6 502	6 642

Source: MCS unpublished data 2009.

The largest shares of medical doctors have come from Croatia, followed by Bosnia and Herzegovina and Serbia. Table 15.2 presents foreign medical doctors by country of origin, nationality and place of training. Croatia has been the major source country of medical doctors for more than ten years and shows an increasing tendency. Conversely, the numbers of medical doctors from Bosnia and Herzegovina show a stabilizing trend from 1992.

Dentists

Generally, dentists show the same patterns of mobility as medical doctors and there are similarly high numbers of foreign dentists – 22.7% in 2008. However, the proportion of foreign medical doctors has increased over the last 16 years while the proportion of foreign dentists among all active dentists has decreased slightly since 1992 (Table 15.15 in annex).

Table 15.3 shows that most foreign dentists come from Croatia, followed by Serbia and Bosnia and Herzegovina. These findings are in line with the results on medical doctors.

Table 15.2 *Foreign-born, foreign-trained and foreign-national active medical doctors (stock) in Slovenia,1992, 2000 and 2003–2008*

Status	Country	1992	2000	2003	2004	2005	2006	2007	2008
Slovene citizens – foreign trained	Austria	9	15	17	21	21	21	21	21
	Bosnia & Herzegovina	3	5	6	6	6	6	6	6
	Croatia	76	107	117	119	122	123	123	125
	Hungary	4	9	9	9	10	10	10	10
	Italy	7	13	17	17	17	21	23	23
	Serbia	13	18	20	20	21	21	21	21
	Other[a]	2	2	4	4	4	4	4	4
	Total	**114**	**169**	**190**	**196**	**201**	**206**	**208**	**210**
Slovene citizens – foreign born	Argentina			2	2	3	5	6	6
	Austria	3	5	5	6	6	6	7	7
	Bosnia & Herzegovina	17	55	60	60	60	61	61	61
	Bulgaria	2	3	4	4	4	5	5	5
	Croatia	310	390	403	405	407	411	413	414
	Former Yugoslav Republic of Macedonia	9	14	18	18	18	19	19	19
	Hungary	9	12	13	13	14	14	14	14
	Italy	1	3	3	4	4	4	4	6
	Russian Federation	1	2	4	5	5	5	5	6
	Serbia	97	153	175	176	178	183	184	186
	Other[a]	7	14	20	21	21	21	21	21
	Total	**456**	**651**	**707**	**714**	**720**	**734**	**739**	**745**
Foreign nationals	Bulgaria			3	3	3	4	5	8
	Bosnia & Herzegovina	1	16	30	33	37	39	41	45
	Croatia	34	81	141	156	161	171	176	183
	Former Yugoslav Republic of Macedonia		2	17	19	20	25	27	31
	Germany			1	2	4	4	4	5
	Italy	1	4	6	6	7	9	11	12
	Russian Federation		4	5	5	6	7	7	7
	Serbia	1	20	50	67	75	102	119	134
	Serbia & Montenegro		14	63	72	73	73	73	73
	Slovakia			1	1	7	8	9	9
	Other[a]	1	6	11	19	21	25	31	34
	Total	**38**	**147**	**328**	**383**	**414**	**467**	**503**	**541**

Source: MCS unpublished data 2009. *Note*: [a] Countries with n<5 in 2008.

Table 15.3 *Foreign-born, foreign-trained and foreign-national active dentists in Slovenia, 1992, 2000 and 2003–2008*

Status	Country	1992	2000	2003	2004	2005	2006	2007	2008
Foreign trained	**Total**	**25**	**41**	**44**	**49**	**50**	**50**	**51**	**54**
	Bosnia and Herzegovina	1	3	3	3	3	3	3	4
	Croatia	20	31	34	39	40	40	41	42
	Hungary	1	3	3	3	3	3	3	3
	Other [a]	3	4	4	4	4	4	4	5
Foreign born	**Total**	**186**	**223**	**232**	**233**	**237**	**241**	**242**	**243**
	Bosnia and Herzegovina	7	19	20	20	20	20	20	20
	Croatia	111	127	133	134	138	139	139	140
	Former Yugoslav Republic of Macedonia	3	3	3	3	3	4	5	5
	Serbia	63	71	73	73	73	73	73	73
	Other [a]	2	3	3	3	3	5	5	5
Foreign national	**Total**	**12**	**29**	**44**	**53**	**62**	**69**	**75**	**84**
	Bulgaria		1	1	1	3	3	4	7
	Croatia	12	24	31	36	37	37	39	39
	Former Yugoslav Republic of Macedonia		2	2	3	7	9	9	11
	Serbia		2	10	13	15	20	22	25
	Other [a]	0	0	0	0	0	0	1	2

Source: MCS unpublished data 2009. *Note*: [a] Countries with n<= 3 in 2008

Nurses

Slovenia appears to be less reliant on foreign nurses than it is on foreign medical doctors and dentists – only 24 foreign nurses were registered on the NHCPD in 2009. However, the small number is also due to the fact that the NCS did not obtain the public authorization to keep a nursing and midwifery register until 2008. This study sought to augment this incomplete information base by carrying out a postal survey on foreign-trained nursing professionals in all hospitals and primary health-care centres in mid October 2009. Data were received from 39 of the 63 primary health-care centres (55% population coverage) and from 14 hospitals (50%), including the three biggest hospitals that comprise about 60% of all hospital beds. The findings are presented in Table 15.4. Data on yearly inflows are available but, unfortunately, it was not possible to compile representative stock data on nurses.

Table 15.4 *Countries of origin of foreign[a] nursing professionals in Slovenia, 1992, 2000 and 2005–2008*

	1992	2000	2005	2006	2007	2008	Total
Austria	0	0	0	4	0	0	**4**
Bosnia and Herzegovina	0	22	2	21	9	3	**57**
Canada	0	1	0	0	0	0	**1**
Croatia	3	20	0	6	4	8	**41**
Former Yugoslav Republic of Macedonia	0	12	0	3	1	1	**17**
Germany	0	3	1	2	1	2	**9**
Hungary	0	0	0	0	0	1	**1**
Ireland	0	1	0	0	0	0	**1**
Montenegro	0	4	0	0	0	1	**5**
Serbia	2	24	0	7	6	9	**48**
Switzerland	0	0	0	3	0	0	**3**
Ukraine	0	0	0	0	0	1	**1**
Total	**5**	**87**	**3**	**46**	**21**	**26**	**188**

Source: Survey of public providers of health care – primary health-care centres and hospitals, October 2009. *Note*: [a] Foreign nationals and foreign trained.

The findings suggest that the highest number of early inflows occured in 2000 from Serbia, Bosnia and Herzegovina, Croatia and the Former Yugoslav Republic of Macedonia. From 2005 to 2008, annual inflows of nurses ranged between 3 in 2005 and 46 in 2006. Overall, annual inflows vary on a relatively small scale, particularly in comparison with the inflows of medical doctors and dentists.

2.2 Outflows

There are no fully reliable data on the actual numbers of health professionals leaving Slovenia but it is possible to estimate the phenomenon from indications and proxy data. Overall, this suggests that outflows occur to a limited extent.

Currently, the loss of health professionals to other countries is not severe as the estimated numbers are rather low. The largest outflows of medical doctors occurred in 2002 and 2005 but still only around 1% of all medical doctors and dentists submitted requests for bona fide statements to the MCS in the period 1999–2007 (see Table 15.12 & Table 15.17 in annex). Data provided by other countries also indicate that Slovene medical doctors showed a low interest in emigration.

The same findings were reported for nurses. Nurses rarely studied abroad and so the mobility of this category of health professions would be minimal. The same would apply to pharmacists.

Box 15.1 *Registration regulations and procedures in Slovenia*

All health professionals are required to comply with the national registration regulations. Graduates of medical and other university-level health schools must pass a registration exam, normally taken after internship. This is organized by the Ministry of Health which issues certificates to successful candidates. Registration exams are a requirement for graduates who are third-country nationals (except citizens of countries of the former Yugoslavia who had completed their registration requirements anywhere on its territory prior to 25 June 1991)[1] but not for European Union (EU) citizens.

In addition, all medical doctors and dentists practising anywhere in the health services (including public health) are required to obtain a licence to practise. The responsibility for these licences lies with the MCS which is required to maintain a register of all medical doctors and dentists under the terms of the Medical Services Act (Republic of Slovenia 1999). Foreign nationals from third countries applying for licences in Slovenia are required to produce their registration details from the country of origin. These include their full programme of specialty training which is scrutinized by the specialty training commission of the MCS. The MCS has three options: (i) full recognition of the specialty training in the country of origin; (ii) part recognition of the specialty training in the country of origin; and (iii) imposition of additional requirements. The latter are clearly defined and candidates are required to meet these specifications or they will be refused approval of their specialty training in the country of origin.

Dentists are granted a licence after completing a one-year internship. Licences must be recertified every seven years, based on evaluation of continuing medical education. Nurses who passed the registration exam used to register with the Ministry of Health but since 2008 this ministry has empowered the NCS similarly to the respective medical and pharmacists chambers. However, it will take some time before the process of licensing is fully implemented.

---

3. Dynamics of EU enlargement

Given the deficits in the numbers of medical doctors and nurses in Slovenia it was hoped that health professionals from other EU accession countries would have greater interest in migrating, particularly from those countries with gross domestic products (GDPs) below 80% of the EU average. This has not materialized – there are individual cases of health professionals opting to

---

1 Date when Slovenia became independent.

enquire about the possibilities of employment in Slovenia but these have never reached significant dimensions (see Tables 15.2, 15.3 & 15.4).

Salaries and general incomes in Slovenia still lag behind those of Austria and Italy as well as some more distant Member States and are the most likely reason why citizens of other EU countries tend not to move to Slovenia. This is seen in their comparatively low numbers within all foreign practising medical doctors and dentists, especially in comparison to the numbers of the same categories of professionals migrating to Slovenia from third countries. However, there are growing numbers of EU nationals among all foreign medical doctors and dentists – their share has risen gradually from below 8% to roughly 20%. This is a result not only of a growth in the absolute number of health professionals from the EU but also to a decline in the number of health professionals from third countries.

There was some expectation that Slovene doctors, dentists and nurses would move to other (mainly old) EU Member States. Around 1% of all medical doctors and dentists have sought bona fide papers to seek employment in other EU Member States (see Table 15.12 & Table 15.17 in annex). Data from the destination countries[2] show a growth in the numbers of Slovene medical doctors emigrating to Austria (2003:4, 2007:10), Germany (2003:11, 2007:28), Italy (2003:0, 2007:6) and the United Kingdom (2003:8, 2007:19). Dentists moved only to Austria (2003:13, 2007:15) and Germany (2003:0, 2007:4); nurses moved only to Austria (2003:9, 2007:43). Overall, these numbers are in line with the numbers of Slovene health professionals who registered interest in practising abroad.

Overall, Slovene health professionals did not leave Slovenia in larger numbers after accession. Most of the emigrating health professionals went to neighbouring countries and the United Kingdom but never exceeded 1% of the total workforce in Slovenia. The proportions of nurses who emigrated were even lower.

4. Impacts on health systems

Given the share of foreign medical doctors and dentists among all practising health professionals in Slovenia, it is clear that foreign-trained and foreign-born doctors represent an important addition to the domestic health workforce. It was not possible to analyse the structure of foreign health professionals by region or at the provider level but the NHCPD shows a rather clear picture of foreign professionals taking up posts in certain underserved areas in north eastern Slovenia, especially at the primary care level. This conclusion cannot be

2 See Chapters 1, 5, 6 and 8.

substantiated by a structured analysis but may be drawn from the geographical distribution of immigrant health professionals. Typically, these are concentrated in the major clinical centres, in smaller regional hospitals and in primary care settings in demographically challenged areas.

Inflows of medical doctors, dentists and nurses were officially incorporated into the health reform proposed in 2003 (Keber et al. 2003). It is clear that Slovenia relies on incoming health professionals to a considerable extent for the continued functioning of its health-care system, both in terms of occupying all the available posts and in assuring good geographical distribution and physical access to health services.

5. Relevance of cross-border mobility

More than one fifth of currently licensed and practising medical doctors and dentists are either foreign citizens or foreign graduates, therefore cross-border mobility is an important contributor to the health workforce balance in Slovenia. The age structure of the immigrant medical doctors shows that most migrated to Slovenia prior to 1992. It is known that the number of foreign-trained, foreign-born and foreign-national medical doctors was already of considerable scale in 1992, because they were required to register with the MCS in order to obtain a valid licence to practise.

Immigration before 1992 was mainly driven by long waiting times for different career posts in other parts of Yugoslavia, while the later wave was of a new type,

Table 15.5 *Foreign-trained medical doctors and dentists among all active and practising medical doctors and dentists in Slovenia*

Foreign-trained	Sex	1992 %	2000 %	2003 %	2004 %	2005 %	2006 %	2007 %	2008 %
Medical doctors	Male	20.8	22.1	25.2	25.7	26.2	27.0	28.0	28.2
	Female	14.2	14.3	16.2	16.7	16.8	17.3	17.9	18.2
	Total	**17.4**	**17.8**	**20.3**	**20.7**	**21.0**	**21.6**	**22.3**	**22.5**
Dentists	Male	31.6	27.3	26.0	26.1	26.5	26.7	26.5	26.6
	Female	23.5	20.6	20.3	20.6	20.7	20.7	20.4	20.3
	Total	**26.6**	**23.1**	**22.5**	**22.7**	**22.9**	**23.0**	**22.7**	**22.7**
Total share of foreign medical doctors and dentists	Male	22.5	22.9	25.4	25.7	26.3	26.9	27.8	27.9
	Female	16.3	15.6	17.0	17.5	17.6	18.0	18.5	18.7
	Total	**19.2**	**18.8**	**20.7**	**21.1**	**21.3**	**21.8**	**22.4**	**22.6**

Source: MCS unpublished data 2009.

driven particularly by the career development and employment opportunities for medical doctors from other countries of the former Yugoslavia. These doctors sought to move from areas of chronic overproduction of medical doctors and dentists to start or base their careers in Slovenia.

The demographic structure of some key categories in Slovenia's health workforce is rather unfavourable as growing proportions of health professionals are over 55 years of age. In practical terms this means that 30% of all practising medical doctors, almost 40% of all practising dentists and around 25% of all practising registered nurses are due to retire over the next 10 years (National Institute of Public Health 2009). This is unlikely to cause a problem with the supply of nurses as several new nursing schools are already in operation and, given the duration of these courses, it is estimated that any shortages will be met within the next five to seven years.

5.1 *Educational system*

A *numerus clausus* is in place for all key categories of health professionals (medical doctors, dentists, nurses, pharmacists). First introduced in 1962 for Slovenia's only medical faculty, the *numerus clausus* is now defined separately and applied to each of the two medical faculties and all the other health science faculties in the country. The government is required to justify and obtain parliamentary approval for the *numerus clausus* every year. The numbers of new admissions to medical, dental and nursing studies (Table 15.6) and the numbers of graduates in these three studies (Table 15.7) are shown below.

Table 15.6 *New admissions to medical, dental and nursing studies in Slovenia, 2006–2008*

	2006	**2007**	**2008**
Medical students	333	305	298
Dentistry students	64	66	64
Nursing students	319	396	473

Sources: Health Statistics Annuals of the respective years. National Institute of Public Health of Slovenia.

Table 15.7 *Numbers graduating in medical, dental and nursing studies in Slovenia, 2005–2007*

	2005	**2006**	**2007**
Medical graduates	162	128	174
Dentistry graduates	33	42	42
Nursing graduates	154	192	204

Sources: Health Statistics Annuals of the respective years. National Institute of Public Health of Slovenia.

Slovenia imposes no costs for studying at any secondary- or tertiary-level education which is part of the network of national education providers. No official figures are available on attrition rates but, historically, attrition rates for health professional studies have rarely exceeded 5% (unpublished data from medical faculties and nursing schools 2009).

There are few foreign-national students in Slovenia. Official data for the 2007–2008[3] academic year show that the Faculty of Medicine, University of Ljubljana had 31 foreign-national students, less than 0.2% of a total of 1622 students. The Faculty of Pharmacy had 24 foreign-national students in a total of 930 (2.6%) and the Faculty of Health Sciences had 59 foreign students in a total of 1095 (5.4%).

For many years there were serious imbalances between the number of health professionals graduating from the different university programmes and the actual needs of the health system. Many efforts to overcome this situation resulted in the following developments:

- opening of a second medical faculty in Maribor;

- establishment of new nursing schools in Jesenice, Novo mesto, Celje, Slovenj Gradec and Murska Sobota (joining those in Ljubljana, Maribor and Izola);

- increasing uptakes in the two medical faculties – from 150 in the mid 1980s to 280 in recent years.

There have been substantial changes in the educational system for nurses, especially during the 1980s, and a number of structural changes are still ongoing. Until 1984 Slovenia followed a system of vocational and post-secondary education in nursing care. Vocational education consisted of a four-year course composed of about two years of general education (similar to that in high schools) and two years of practical training on the wards. Pupils who completed this programme would obtain the title of middle nurse. There was a similar programme of midwifery. Post-secondary education was established in two schools for nursing in Ljubljana and Maribor. Successful graduates of the two-year course gained the title of higher nurse, reflecting the school's status (Higher School for Nursing).

In 1984, a reform of studies brought significant changes to this system. Vocational training for all nursing professionals was integrated in a programme for health technicians. Midwifery at the secondary, vocational level was abolished as it was intended that nursing would be an integral service, including the tasks of these midwives. However, a special study programme – the gynaecological-obstetrical track – was established in the 1990s, effectively representing the

---

3 *Source*: http://www.uni-lj.si , accessed 5 July 2009.

»silent« return of midwifery as a separate professional group, this time at the tertiary educational level.

Post-secondary education experienced the most profound changes during the 1990s:

- introduction of a three-year post-secondary education in nursing – aiming to upgrade educational levels to achieve more competencies and greater responsibility and thus a better position in the system;

- gradual expansion of study programmes and establishment of new nursing schools in response to chronic shortages of nurses throughout the 1990s and 2000s.

EU regulation of nursing professionals reinforced this process. This also marked the clear distinction between nurses (graduates of nursing schools) and health technicians (graduates of vocational schools). These conformations affected nurse mobility from countries that had not yet reformed their nursing studies, namely Bosnia and Herzegovina and Serbia, as nurses with incomplete graduate education (non-compliant with the EU regulation on regulated health professionals) cannot apply for first time registration in Slovenia.

5.2. *Deficits of health professionals*

Slovenia has faced a deficit of health professionals over decades. In the 1920s and 1930s there was only one medical faculty in Ljubljana and this covered only the first three years of studies. A complete medical faculty was formed in 1945 but it was not until 2003 that a second medical school was established in Maribor. There were oscillating numbers of medical doctors and dentists in the 1960s and 1970s and intense expansion in the number and capacity of providers (especially primary health-care centres) in the 1970s and into the 1980s. All these changes occasionally exposed the fragility of human resource planning in Slovenia – the *numerus clausus* restricted the number of students admitted to medical, dental, nursing and pharmacy studies but the resulting number of graduates did not meet these growing needs. The most dramatic example was the sudden shortage of 300 medical doctors[4] that arose on completion of the University Medical Centre in Ljubljana in 1973. Medical doctors from other parts of Yugoslavia were invited to fill these gaps.

The failure to take account of the health systems's reliance on inflows of foreign health professionals was particularly important in the 1970s and in the early 1980s (Albreht 1999, Albreht & Klazinga 2002) as military conflicts in other countries of the former Yugoslavia halted the inflows of medical doctors,

---

4 Official estimate by the Secretariat for Health and Social Care (effectively Ministry of Health in Slovenia) – internal reports from 1973.

dentists and nurses almost instantly. These type of shortages continued on a smaller scale but were slightly obscured as the economic crisis of the 1980s required a slower pace of health-care growth. The problem was exacerbated by the new requirements for the registration of medical doctors and dentists from 1992 and, in the late 1990s and early 2000s, these deficits became evident in overt problems such as shortages of staff for on-call services and duties and difficulty filling general medical posts. In response a number of new schools were opened for medical doctors and nurses.

Annual decisions on the number of admissions were based mostly on the retrospective impression of needs. The health reform proposal of 2003 (Keber et al. 2003) indicated that there could be a need to import health professionals but no formal policy has been introduced. One study (Albreht 1999) shows an imminent deficit of medical doctors in the following 10 to 15 years. In addition, Svetina (2007) presents a 40-year curve showing a dissonance between the cycle of the number of students admitted and the needs for medical doctors and dentists. This shows a 12-year cycle which oscillates in the shape of a sinusoid curve.

5.3 *Demographic change*

Slovenia's health workforce faces another major challenge from a rapidly developing demographic transition. The rapid growth in the number of older people will affect all types of health professionals but is particularly important for nursing professionals and within chronic disease management. This will add to the existing pressures resulting from the changing pattern of hospital treatments. The average length of hospital stay has reduced by 40% since the early 1990s (National Institute of Public Health 1991–2009), resulting in patients leaving hospitals less fully recovered. In addition, there are shortages of nurses in certain fields such as care of the elderly, chronic disease and palliative care for patients with terminal illness (Filej et al. 2001, Zorec et al. 2001).

6. Factors influencing health professional mobility

6.1 *Inflows*

Higher salaries are the main reason why foreign health professionals move to Slovenia. In 2008, a specialist's average monthly salary was €1200 in Croatia (Metro-portal.hr 2008) and reached €750 in the Republic of Srpska in Bosnia and Herzegovina (Ekapija 2010). In 2009, a specialist's average salary was around €1000 per month in Serbia (Republic Institute for Health Insurance 2010). A specialist's net monthly salary is between €1600 and €3000 in Slovenia, resulting from the development of an increased gradient in the economic power of the former member countries of the Yugoslav federation over the last few years.

Anecdotal information and some reports from health-care providers indicate that two key issues caused foreign health professionals to leave employment in Slovenia. Firstly, personal circumstances – mainly difficulties with basic living arrangements such as moving to Slovenia and buying property. Secondly, incomes may be high in comparison to other countries of the former Yugoslavia but the remaining gradient in salaries between Slovenia and older EU Member States makes it likely that many ambitious career-oriented health professionals will move to those countries. Some may seek to stay in Slovenia only in order to obtain the right to free movement.

6.2 Outflows

Three main motivational factors appear to drive Slovene medical doctors to seek employment abroad. Firstly, the possibility of earning higher salaries. In 2009, gross annual salaries for medical doctors and dentists in Slovenia were between €50 000 and €70 000. This compares to €142 000 in Germany in 2007 (Krankenkassen Deutschland); €78 700–€147 000 in Austria in 2006 (OE24.at 2008) and €62 000 in Italy in 2000 (Barham & Bramley-Harker 2004). Secondly, the possibility of professional development in fields which either do not exist or are difficult to enter in Slovenia. Thirdly, specific research interests that can only be carried forward in the appropriate setting.

In the absence of any previous surveys on medical graduates' potential interest in moving to other countries, a self-administered questionnaire was applied for the purpose of this study. The survey was carried out among fifth-year students at the Faculty of Medicine of Maribor. Out of the 58 enrolled students, 45 participated in the survey (77.6%). Of these, 69% were females and the average age was 24 years. The most important reported drivers for working in another country were: having few possibilities to specialize in their preferred specialty (29%); the chance to earn more than in Slovenia (22%); and the desire to live and work in another country (22%). The three most preferred destination countries are all outside Europe – Australia, the United States and Canada. The United Kingdom was the most popular European country but was ranked fourth, with around 60% of Canada's score. Other countries of interest included Germany, Austria, Spain, Switzerland, Sweden and the Netherlands. The most important factors stimulating these decisions were the possibility to develop professionally, to specialize in a preferred specialty and to achieve higher salaries.

7. Policy, regulation and interventions

7.1 *Policies and policy development on health professional mobility*

Between 1990 and 2000 there was no active policy to attract health professionals to work in Slovenia, partly because of the general opinion that any shortages were only temporary. Growing shortages of medical doctors and nurses between 2000 and 2004 led the Ministry of Health to announce its intention to recruit foreign medical doctors, nurses and some other categories of health professionals. This never materialized, partly because of diverging views on this topic among the key actors (Ministry of Heath, Health Insurance Institute of Slovenia – HIIS, professional chambers) and partly because of insufficient interest among foreign health professionals. Since then, there has been no national strategy or policy to attract foreign health professionals or to establish incentives for working in Slovenia. There is less difficulty in securing adequate numbers of pharmacists as this faculty has anticipated prospective needs during the last 15 to 20 years.

As mentioned above, the different key actors hold rather divergent positions. The HIIS is the main financier of compulsory health insurance and thus (indirectly) the principal employer in Slovene health care. This organization is reserved about expanding the numbers of health professionals and is very conservative about increasing salaries in a system that is already facing overall medical inflation from challenges such as the financial crisis, demographic transition, the changing pattern of morbidity and new health technologies.

7.2 *Workforce planning and development*

Workforce planning in health care is implemented through the policies of the Ministry of Health, the respective professional chambers and, to some extent, the Ministry of Higher Education. The latter consults with other ministries on the proposed numbers of students admitted to different university studies and the *numerus clausus*. Policies of individual faculties may vary as they may identify certain deflections from these limitations imposed through the *numerus clausus*. Foreign nationals working in Slovenia have not always been properly accounted for within the planning process. In the early 1990s their input was minimized and led to underestimations of their contribution. A more consistent picture has been developed through different workforce studies, estimates and projections.

There have been several attempts to make Slovenia self-sufficient, the most important resulting from the realization that foreign health professionals would not be capable of overcoming all the deficits in Slovene health care (Albreht

2002 & 2005). This started intense activities to enlarge the capacity for health professional education in Slovenia in order to achieve self sufficiency.

Only two models have so far been used to forecast the supply and demand of health professionals: (i) demography of the population within an individual profession; and (ii) a simple equilibrium model that takes account of the present number of health professionals. Projections in the 1990s and early 2000s worked on the underlying assumptions that it was necessary only to replace those health professionals who were leaving health care through retirement, incapacity or by moving to a different profession.

Using demography of a given profession as the key determinant implies that the supply and demand for that profession are balanced and the needs for its services are well-covered. However, this is not substantiated in any study. Similarly, use of the equilibrium concept implies that numbers are balanced and that the system does not need to grow further.

7.3 *Mutual recognition of diplomas in the EU*

Directive 2005/36/EC on the mutual implementation of diplomas (European Parliament and Council of the European Union 2005) is fully implemented in Slovenia for citizens of EU Member States who qualified in their country of origin. The responsible authority is the Ministry of Labour, Family and Social Affairs. No significant problems have been reported to the Ministry of Health or to the respective professional chambers.

7.4 *Bilateral agreements*

The main bilateral agreement concerning health professional mobility was signed between the Socialist Federal Republic of Yugoslavia and the USSR (Government of the Socialist Federal Republic of Yugoslavia 1989). Together with the adoption of rules regarding the mutual recognition of degrees between the countries of the former Yugoslavia, this agreement ensures automatic recognition of the degrees of all graduates from the former USSR and from the area of the former Yugoslavia who graduated before 25 June 1991. However, once recognition has been formally established, health professionals must complete the licensing procedure of the MCS or the relevant professional chamber.

The main aim of this bilateral agreement was to enable health professionals to move freely between the countries and facilitate access to the wider labour market. This agreement will become less important and less relevant as the system becomes dominated more and more by new generations of health professionals who will be subject to the same requirements as any third-country national.

7.5 *Third-country health professionals*

Candidates from third countries without a bilateral agreement face a lengthy administrative procedure. This requires them to state clearly their professional interests and accept any additional educational, practical and technical requirements, which are often time-consuming. While the degree itself may have been recognized, the MCS may prescribe in specific detail which part of the previous training cannot be recognized. Recognition of these degrees is handled by the Ministry of Higher Education (administration) and the respective faculties (academic criteria and evaluation) but issuing of a licence depends solely on the evaluation of a candidate's previous training and actual professional capacity.

7.6 *Specific interventions and managerial tools*

There are no specific interventions and/or managerial tools in place to manage health professional mobility. On occasions, individual providers (e.g. hospitals and primary health-care centres) actively search for available health professionals.

8. Political force field of regulating and managing health professional mobility

The political force field regulating and managing health professional mobility is a reflection of the overall health professional regulatory system. Slovenia opted for a decentralized system by empowering independent professional associations – the chambers (*Zbornice*). These regulate all the affairs concerning the professional pathway of the regulated health professions except for the state registration exam for medical doctors and dentists. This remains the responsibility of the Ministry of Health.

Around 70% of all medical doctors, 45% of all dentists and 80% of all nurses still work in the public sector and therefore the regulation of the salary system is an important factor that can impact on the political force field. The setting is largely dependent on the formation of the government at any one time as Slovenia's political arena is rather fragmented. Given that the government is usually composed of four political parties with a range of political affiliations, a compromise is the usual outcome.

The MCS is interested in maintaining tight control over the registration and licensing criteria for any medical doctors or dentists wishing to pursue careers in active medical or dental service in Slovenia. It does not object to importing professionals but is reluctant to modify the recognition and certification procedures and criteria as suggested in the health reform proposal in 2003. The NCS is similarly keen to retain the rather restrictive policies as there have been uneven developments in the education of nursing professionals across south eastern Europe.

The Ministry of Health and the respective professional chambers influence the regulation and management of health professional mobility. The former determines the incentives for health professionals in terms of salaries; the latter act as licensing and, to some degree, registration authorities. Their preferences particularly affect third countries as they have autonomy in setting the rules for licensing and registration and therefore can significantly influence inflows from these countries. This is particularly relevant for Slovenia as the large majority of immigrating health professionals come from third countries.

It is likely that the Ministry of Health would favour larger inflows of foreign health professionals, given that there are serious current deficits in the key health professional groups – medical doctors, dentists and nurses. Yet, there is a rather restrictive policy on potential immigration from third countries which is defended on the grounds of maintaining good educational and training standards. This often results in rather lengthy procedures (6–12 months or more) during which candidates are unable to work in their profession and therefore require resources to cover that period. The effects are evidenced in the decline of interest among medical doctors from countries of origin that have been major sources.

9. Conclusion

Slovenia is a country that depends to a considerable degree on foreign medical doctors and dentists but has been more successful in securing adequate numbers of nursing professionals. In the past self-sufficiency was only achieved through flows of professionals within the former Yugoslavia. This was not properly recognized in the transition to independent state and in the first decade of its existence and has led to overt deficits.

With almost a quarter of all medical doctors and dentists coming from abroad, Slovenia is a destination country for health professionals from the area of the former Yugoslavia and elsewhere in the Balkans. A similar structure in the countries of origin of the immigrant population can be seen for nurses.

Slovenian health professionals have not yet moved to other countries in larger numbers. This is an encouraging trend but the reasons for it still need to be explored. There appears to be a significant proportion of medical students who are interested in moving to other countries if better professional and research opportunities arise. Most would move to non-European countries.

References

Albreht T (1999). Analiza profesionalne demografije zdravnikov in zobozdravnikov v Sloveniji 1986 do 1995 z ocenami za obdobje 1996 do 2010 [Analysis of physicians' and dentists' professional demography in Slovenia 1986 to 1995 with estimates for the period from 1996 to 2010]. *Zdravniski Vestnik*, 68(11):647–653.

Albreht T (2002). *Estimates of the needs for medical doctors in Slovenia for the period 2002–2020 based on the analysis of the demographic characteristics of the medical doctors' population*. Ljubljana, Institute of Public Health of the Republic of Slovenia.

Albreht T (2005). *Analysis of the coverage with nursing staff and evaluation of stepwise measures and projections up to the year 2033*. Ljubljana, Institute of Public Health of the Republic of Slovenia.

Albreht T, Klazinga N (2002). Health manpower planning in Slovenia: a policy analysis of the changes in roles of stakeholders and methodologies. *Journal of Health Politics, Policy and Law*, 27(6):1001–1022.

Barham L, Bramley-Harker E (2004). Comparing physicians' earnings: current knowledge and challenges – A report for the Department of Health. London, NERA Economic Consulting.

Ekapija (2010). Leading business portal of Serbia [website] (http://www.ekapija.com/website/sr, download October 2010).

European Parliament and Council of the European Union (2005). Directive 2005/36/EC of the European Parliament and of the Council of 7 September 2005 on the recognition of professional qualifications. *Official Journal of the European Union*, 255(48):22–142.

Filej B et al. (2001). Mednarodni projekt o količini in kakovosti v zdravstveni negi [International project on quantity and quality in nursing care]. *Obzor Zdrav Neg*, 35(5):175–179.

Government of the Socialist Federal Republic of Yugoslavia (1989). Law on the ratification of the agreement between the Federal Executive Council of the

Assembly of the Socialist Federal Republic of Yugoslavia and the Government of the Union of Soviet Socialist Republics on mutual recognition of documents of education and of academic degrees (in Slovene). *Official Gazette of the SFRY*, No. 10/89.

Institute of Public Health of the Republic of Slovenia (2001). *Health statistical annual 2000*. Ljubljana.

Kastelic I, Schlamberger K (1973). *Numeric shortcomings of health professionals in view of personnel quantitative norms (situation on 1.1.1972 and 1.1.1973)* [in Slovene]. Ljubljana, Zavod SR Slovenije za zdravstveno varstvo.

Kastelic I et al. (1976). *A possible increase in the number of health professionals in the SR of Slovenia from 1976 to 1980 with insights into the increases in the period 1970 to 1975* [in Slovene]. Ljubljana, Zdravstveno Varstvo.

Keber D et al. (2003). *Zdravstvena reforma: pravičnost, dostopnost, kakovost, učinkovitost: osnutek* [*Health reform: fairness, access, quality, efficiency: a draft*]. Ljubljana, Vlada Republike Slovenije, Ministrstvo za zdravje.

Krankenkassen Deutschland (2010). [website] (http://www.krankenkassen. de/, accessed October 2010).

Metro-portal.hr (2008). Komora traži 20.000 kuna plaće za liječnike specijaliste. *Metro-portal.hr*, 16 March 2008 (http://metro-portal.hr/vijesti/ hrvatska/komora-trazi-20-000-kuna-place-za-lijecnike-specijaliste, accessed at: 14 December 2009).

National Institute of Public Health (1991–1993). *Health statistics annuals 1990–1992*. Ljubljana.

National Institute of Public Health (2009). *Health statistics annual 2008*. Ljubljana.

OE24.at (2008). Ärzte beim Geldverdienen Spitze. *OE24.at*, 15 April 2008 (http://www.oe24.at/oesterreich/politik/ Aerzte_beim_ Geldverdienen_Spitze _293542.ece, accessed 14 December 2009).

Ravnikar B et al. (1986). *Planning of increase in the number of health professionals in SR of Slovenia by the year 2000 with adjustments of the needs and possibilities in education*. Ljubljana, Zdravstveno Varstvo.

Republic of Slovenia (1999). Medical Services Act. *Official Gazette of the Republic of Slovenia*, 98:14653-14661.

Republic Institute for Health Insurance (2010. Data and news [website] (www. rzzo.rs, download October 2010).

Svetina S (2007). *Letno število diplomantov medicine in načrtovanje vpisa* [Annual number of medical graduates and the planning of admissions to medical studies]. *Zdravniški vestnik*, 76(12):835–838.

Zorec M et al. (2001). Razvoj metodologije merjenja količine dela v zdravstveni negi v mednarodnem projektu [Development of methodology to measure quantity of the work in nursing care in an international project]. *Obzor Zdrav Neg*, 35(5):181–184.

Annex.

Table 15.8 *Numbers, specializations and percentages of foreign-trained newly registered medical doctors (flow data), 2003–2008*

	2003	2004	2005	2006	2007	2008
Foreign newly registered medical doctors (yearly inflows)	90	68	42	72	43	37
Foreign newly registered among all active foreign medical doctors (%)	7.3	5.3	3.1	5.1	2.9	2.5
All active medical doctors	6045	6240	6370	6525	6502	6642
All active foreign medical doctors (stock)	1226	1294	1336	1408	1451	1497
Specializations of newly-registered medical doctors:						
Anaesthesiology, reanimatology and perioperative intensive medicine	6	2	4	2	2	2
Abdominal surgery	0	0	0	0	0	0
Dermatovenerology	1	0	1	1	0	3
Family medicine	5	0	1	0	1	0
Physical and rehabilitation medicine	1	1	1	0	0	0
Gynaecology and obstetrics	2	1	2	0	0	0
Infectious diseases	0	0	1	0	0	1
Internal medicine	4	2	4	4	4	1
Public health	1	0	0	0	0	1
Clinical microbiology	1	0	2	1	0	0
Maxillofacial surgery	0	0	0	0	0	0
Occupational medicine and medicine of traffic and sports	2	0	0	0	0	1
Neurosurgery	1	0	0	0	0	0
Neurology	1	0	0	1	1	1
Neuropsychiatry	0	0	0	0	0	0
Nuclear medicine	1	0	0	0	0	0
Ophthalmology	1	2	1	3	0	0
Oncology with radiotherapy	0	0	0	0	0	1
Orthopaedic surgery	1	0	0	0	0	1
E.N.T.	1	1	2	0	0	0
Pathology	1	0	0	1	0	1
Paediatrics	3	2	1	1	2	0
Plastic, reconstructive and aesthetic surgery	0	0	0	0	0	0
Pneumology	1	0	0	1	0	0
Psychiatry	1	0	0	0	2	2
Radiology	1	1	0	0	2	0
Forensic medicine	0	0	0	0	0	0
General surgery	3	2	0	1	0	2
Transfusion medicine	0	1	0	0	0	0
Urology	1	0	1	2	0	0
General practice	50	53	21	54	29	20

Source: MCS unpublished data 2009.

Table 15.9 *Numbers and percentages of medical doctors returning to Slovenia after practising abroad, 2003–2008*

	2003	2004	2005	2006	2007	2008
All returning medical doctors	12	10	13	12	7	3
Returnees as proportion of all active medical doctors	0.2	0.2	0.2	0.2	0.1	0.1
All active medical doctors	6045	6240	6370	6525	6502	6642

Source: MCS unpublished data 2009.

Table 15.10 *Foreign-trained medical doctors working as medical doctors in Slovenia (stock), by specializations, 1992 and 2003–2008*

	1992	2003	2004	2005	2006	2007	2008
Foreign-trained medical doctors	**608**	**1225**	**1293**	**1335**	**1407**	**1450**	**1497**
Foreign-trained among all active medical doctors (%)	17.4	20.3	20.7	21.0	21.6	22.3	22.5
All active medical doctors	3486	6045	6240	6370	6525	6502	6642
Specializations of foreign-trained medical doctors:							
Anaesthetics, reanimatology and perioperative intensive medicine	41	79	81	85	87	89	91
Abdominal surgery		1	1	1	1	1	1
Dermatovenerology	6	17	17	18	19	19	22
Family medicine	84	135	135	136	136	137	137
Physical and rehabilitation medicine	21	33	34	35	35	35	35
Gynaecology and obstetrics	46	75	76	78	78	78	78
Infectious diseases	2	4	4	5	5	5	6
Internal medicine	54	87	89	93	97	101	102
Public health	7	13	13	13	13	13	14
Clinical microbiology	2	6	6	8	9	9	9
Maxillofacial surgery		2	2	2	2	2	2
Occupational medicine and medicine.of traffic and sports	46	61	61	61	61	61	62
Neurosurgery	1	4	4	4	4	4	4
Neurology	5	10	10	10	11	12	13
Neuropsychiatry	8	11	11	11	11	11	11
Nuclear medicine		1	1	1	1	1	1
Ophthalmology	11	27	29	30	33	33	33
Oncology with radiotherapy		0	0	0	0	0	1
Orthopaedic surgery	9	16	16	16	16	16	17
E.N.T.	13	21	22	24	24	24	24
Pathology	2	10	10	10	11	11	12
Paediatrics	47	74	76	77	78	80	80
Plastic, reconstructive and aesthetic surgery	2	2	2	2	2	2	2
Pneumology	1	4	4	4	5	5	5
Psychiatry	19	43	43	43	43	45	47
Radiology	27	40	41	41	41	43	43
Forensic medicine	3	4	4	4	4	4	4
General surgery	53	83	85	85	86	86	88
Transfusion medicine	4	8	9	9	9	9	9
Urology	6	11	11	12	14	14	14
General practice	88	343	396	417	471	500	529

Source: MCS unpublished data 2009.

Table 15.11 *Sex and mean age of foreign-trained medical doctors in comparison to all medical doctors in Slovenia, 1992 and 2003–2008*

	1992	2003	2004	2005	2006	2007	2008
Male	356	691	724	744	778	791	805
Female	252	535	570	592	630	660	692
Total – foreign-trained medical doctors	**608**	**1226**	**1294**	**1336**	**1408**	**1451**	**1497**
Male	1709	2737	2819	2839	2886	2820	2850
Female	1777	3308	3421	3531	3639	3682	3792
Total – all medical doctors	**3486**	**6045**	**6240**	**6370**	**6525**	**6502**	**6642**
Female foreign-trained medical doctors (%)	41.5	43.6	44.1	44.3	44.7	45.5	46.2
Female medical doctors (%)	50.9	54.7	54.8	55.4	55.8	56.6	57.1
Mean age – foreign-trained medical doctors	**44**	**49**	**50**	**51**	**51**	**52**	**52**
Male	45	52	52	53	53	54	55
Female	41	47	48	48	48	49	49

Source: MCS unpublished data 2009.

Table 15.12 *Medical doctors applying for diploma verification to work in EU Member States (including specializations), 2003–2008*

	2003	2004	2005	2006	2007	2008
Medical doctors applying for diploma verification	**29**	**29**	**40**	**47**	**51**	**65**
Applicants for verification among all medical doctors (%)	0.5	0.5	0.6	0.7	0.8	0.9
All active medical doctors	6045	6240	6370	6525	6502	6642

Source: MCS unpublished data 2009.

Table 15.13 *Foreign-trained newly registered dentists (including specializations), 2003–2008*

	2003	2004	2005	2006	2007	2008
Foreign-trained newly registered dentists	9	15	14	11	8	12
Foreign-trained newly registered among all active foreign-trained dentists (%)	2.8	4.5	4.0	3.1	2.2	3.2
All active dentists	1418	1472	1520	1562	1615	1676
All active foreign-trained dentists	319	334	348	359	367	380

Source: MCS unpublished data 2009.

Table 15.14 *Numbers and percentages of dentists returning to Slovenia after practising abroad, 2003–2008*

	2003	2004	2005	2006	2007	2008
All returning dentists	1	5	5	7	1	1
Returnees as proportion of all active dentists (%)	0.1	0.3	0.3	0.5	0.1	0.1
All active dentists	1418	1472	1520	1562	1615	1676

Source: MCS unpublished data 2009.

Table 15.15 *Foreign-trained dentists working as dentists in Slovenia (stock), 1992 and 2003–2008*

	1992	2003	2004	2005	2006	2007	2008
Foreign-trained dentists	223	320	335	349	360	368	380
Proportion of foreign-trained dentists among all active dentists (%)	26.6	22.6	22.8	22.9	23.1	22.8	22.7
All active dentists	839	1418	1472	1520	1562	1615	1676
Specializations of foreign-trained dentists:							
Maxillar and dental orthopaedics	8	16	17	18	18	18	18
Oral surgery		2	2	3	3	3	3
Child and preventative dentistry	2	6	6	6	6	6	6
Parodontology		0	0	0	0	1	1
Dental prosthetics	3	4	4	4	4	4	4
General dentists	207	288	302	314	325	332	345
Dental diseases and endodontics	3	4	4	4	4	4	3

Source: MCS unpublished data 2009.

Table 15.16 *Sex and mean age of foreign-trained dentists in comparison to all dentists in Slovenia, 2003–2008*

Sex	1992	2003	2004	2005	2006	2007	2008
Male	100	140	146	154	159	163	170
Female	123	179	188	194	200	204	210
Total – foreign-trained dentists	**223**	**319**	**334**	**348**	**359**	**367**	**380**
Male	316	538	560	581	596	616	640
Female	523	880	912	939	966	999	1036
Total – all dentists	**839**	**1418**	**1472**	**1520**	**1562**	**1615**	**1676**
Shares by sex							
Female foreign- trained dentists (%)	55.2	56.2	56.3	55.7	55.7	55.6	55.3
Female dentists (%)	62.3	62.1	61.9	61.8	61.8	61.9	61.8
Mean age – foreign-trained dentists	**42**	**50**	**50**	**51**	**51**	**52**	**52**
Male	42	50	51	51	52	52	53
Female	42	50	50	51	51	52	52

Source: MCS unpublished data 2009.

Table 15.17 *Dentists applying for diploma verification to work in EU Member States (including specializations), 2003–2008*

	2003	2004	2005	2006	2007	2008
Dentists applying for diploma verification	**4**	**7**	**9**	**10**	**13**	**18**
Applicants for verification among all dentists (%)	0.3	0.5	0.6	0.6	0.8	1.1
All active dentists	1418	1472	1520	1562	1615	1676

Source: MCS unpublished data 2009.

Part IV

Case studies from third countries having applied for EU membership

Chapter 16

Health professionals emigrating from Serbia: consequences of the geopolitical situation and economic downturn

Ivan M. Jekić, Annette Katrava, Maja Vučković-Krčmar

1. Introduction

The political, social and economic situation in Serbia has influenced health professional mobility since the 1960s. Serbia was a federal unit within the Socialist Federal Republic of Yugoslavia that broke apart in the 1990s. These events and the economic crisis from 1970 to 2001 resulted in approximately 400 000 Serbs leaving the country (Statistical Office of the Republic of Serbia 2002), including 30 000 highly educated persons who migrated primarily to western European countries (Djikanovich 2006).

In line with overall outflows, Serbia has been a source country for health professional mobility over the last 40 to 50 years. It is estimated that a total of 10 000 Serbian health professionals have moved to work abroad since 1960 (Grečić et al. 1998). Germany (28%) and Switzerland (15%) are the most popular destination countries for health professionals but neighbouring countries (predominantly Slovenia) are becoming more popular through their association with the European Union (EU), geographical vicinity, similar languages and cultures and established social networks (Grečić et al. 1998). Aside from Serbia's political and economic situation, health professional outflows are due to high salary differentials in comparison to more affluent western European countries; oversupply of medical doctors; ineffectiveness of the health system; unsatisfactory working conditions and ill-defined career development. Hence, cross-border outflows are the focus of this research.

Economic emigration to western European countries increased between the two world wars and especially after the Second World War but Yugoslav citizens did not emigrate in substantial numbers until the mid 1960s. The increasing economic crisis during the 1970s and 1980s also increased the outflows of highly educated people. Emigration from the region accelerated during the 1990s, precipitated by the drastic fall in living standards and soaring poverty that resulted from the civil wars (Pavlov et al. 2008).

In December 2009, Serbia's potential EU accession brought about three positive developments that may impact on health professional outflows from Serbia: (i) the EU Council decided that the Interim Agreement with the Republic of Serbia would be implemented as soon as possible; (ii) the first meeting of the Interim Committee under the EU-Serbia Interim Agreement was held in Belgrade, 2 March 2010; and (iii) since December 2009, citizens of Serbia no longer need to be in possession of a visa in order to travel to the 25 EU Member States and 3 non-EU countries that are part of the Schengen area.

The following sections will analyse the characteristics of health professional emigration from Serbia in an attempt to systematize the information, knowledge and evidence available. This will cover migration intentions, facilitating factors and constraints as well as workforce policies, including manpower planning at national level.

Data sources and limitations of the study

To date, there has been no in-depth analysis of the scale, directions and impacts of labour migration and particularly the emigration of health professionals from Serbia. Comprehensive insight into both the current situation and future perspectives faces some important limitations in terms of data availability and quality. This study used incomplete data from national services and data from destination countries and international organizations in the absence of any single authoritative source or indeed other adequate national statistical resources on health professional mobility.

The lack of robust data concerning health professional mobility may be associated with the general lack of registration of the health workforce which also hinders the monitoring of internal health workforce imbalances. It is also difficult to classify migrants according to the different countries of the former Yugoslavia as records relate to when it was a single country (Vuković 2005). Since data were neither representative nor of good quality, the information was complemented with expert interviews, grey literature and other available information to provide the most accurate picture possible. Furthermore, data on inflows into receiving countries are considered more reliable than data on outflows, not least because there is a widespread belief that, through error or omission, many countries underestimate the extent of outflows (Bach 2003).

The search strategy included interviewing a multitude of organizations and obtaining data from various sources. These include the health professional chambers and associations, the Institute of Public Health, Ministry of Health, selected large provider institutions, the Statistical Office and the National Employment Service. Information was fragmented and had to be gathered from the various data sources by special request.

Data on the current stock of health professionals are relatively reliable with some inconsistencies in reporting between and within the various organizations. No single authority documents health professional mobility and therefore this required a wider search for documentation on labour force mobility in national and international sources. This report includes the largest amount of available information to date._

2. Mobility profile of Serbia

National and international migration reports and studies, as well as interviews with representatives of organizations, were used to document the general situation of emigration and health professional mobility. The latter can be described within three significant time periods in Serbia: (i) 1960–1989; (ii) 1990–1999; and (iii) since 2000. Mobility within these time periods is described in the following paragraphs.

2.1 *Emigration patterns in former Yugoslavia (1960–1989)*[1]

Emigration to developed European countries did not become substantial until the mid 1960s but had increased even more by the end of that decade. Bilateral agreements and other documents indicate that 232 267 Yugoslav citizens worked mainly in Germany, Austria, Switzerland and France between 1965 and the end of 1992 (Grečić 1998). Emigration to western countries reached its peak in 1970 when 47 018 people from Serbia and Montenegro went to work abroad. The National Employment Service records that around 85 000 citizens found jobs without mediation of relevant services – 70 000 unskilled and semi-skilled and 15 000 highly skilled (Grečić 1998). The emigration of highly educated people became significant during the 1970s and accelerated with the economic crisis at the beginning of the 1980s (Grečić 1998). In contrast to

1 Neither research nor interviews produced any evidence of significant professional mobility among nurses between 1960 and 1989.

cross-ocean migration, which tended to be permanent, European migration was conditioned primarily by economic factors and was generally temporary.

Medical doctors have experienced a relatively open market in western European countries since the 1960s. The Serbian Medical Association (SMA) and medical doctors interviewed attribute this to the fact that Yugoslavian and Serbian medical school diplomas were recognized in a number of European countries in those years and these citizens did not require visas. The most popular destinations for health professionals, mostly medical doctors, were Germany (28%) and Switzerland (15%) (Djikanovich 2006). Thus, the former Yugoslavia held a specific position in postwar Europe and, unlike most other countries of eastern Europe, was one of the few that produced sufficient numbers of medical doctors and dentists. Motivations for working abroad were both economic and more pronounced professional reasons such as better career opportunities.[2]

During this period there was no organized system to monitor the mobility of Serbian medical doctors. Those seeking to work abroad obtained first contacts through colleagues and/or relatives already living or working in the destination country. Medical doctors would usually be accepted to work for a trial period under a temporary residence and work permit. Their superiors would apply for permanent permits following positive assessment of their professional skills and competence. The specialties in demand were anaesthetics, radiodiagnostics, pathology and different types of specialized surgical disciplines that lack trained medical doctors. Additionally, some medical doctors sought temporary work for one to six months.

Expensive education produced deficits in the numbers of dentists in the 1960s and 1970s in some European countries such as Switzerland and Germany. At that time, newly graduated dentists from Serbia/Yugoslavia were motivated to emigrate by economic concerns, low salaries, poor working conditions with no potential for professional development and no possibility of opening private practices.[3]

Emigration became regular in the early 1960s, mostly by word-of-mouth marketing, and became common among dentists from other central and eastern Europe (CEE) countries later in the decade. For example, in 1968 the Swiss Dental Association engaged a number of trained Czech dentists at 80% of the average salary of a Swiss assistant dentist, thereby effectively closing the market for trained dentists from the former Yugoslavia.[2]

---

2 Interviews with SMA representatives.
3 Interviews with dentists 2009.

2.2 *Emigration patterns in former Yugoslavia (1990–1999)[4]*

This decade was characterized by political instability and economic downturn as the former Yugoslavia dissolved in war circumstances. Serbia faced a new large wave of emigrants at the beginning of the 1990s. Research of the migration patterns (Kutlača & Grečić 2005) found that an estimated 30 000 university graduates left Serbia and Montenegro during the last decade of the 20th century.

The scale of medical doctors' emigration was affected significantly by the context of war in Serbia and was also of relevance in Croatia. Diplomas were not recognized, visas were difficult to obtain and, in the absence of a formal system, potential future employers placed rigorous criteria on applications. At the request of its members the SMA began issuing membership certificates, one of the indicators of migration and mobility. In 1993, the first year of crisis and sanctions, between 500 and 600 certificates were issued to SMA members. Therafter, 50–70 certificates were issued annually until 1999 when numbers increased to 250–300.[5]

With its significant oversupply of medical doctors, Serbia is an example of a country in which outward migration reduced unemployment pressures in the health profession.

2.3 *Health professional mobility since 2000[6]*

During the 1990s and into early 2000, the step-by-step disintegration of the former Yugoslavia was the main factor influencing migration waves. By the end of 2000, the Serbian government had entered into a phase of reform and general labour migration patterns changed. Emigration had been directed towards western Europe, especially Germany and other German-speaking countries but, in recent years, neighbouring countries have become more attractive for Serbian migrants. For example, Pavlov et al. (2008) noted that the Croatian authorities issued over 8000 work permits to Serbian citizens in 2008, as well as 2500 extensions.

Serbia is a potential candidate for EU membership. Since March 2002, the European Commission has reported regularly to the Council and the Parliament on the progress made by the countries of the western Balkans region. On 29 April 2008 Serbia and the EU signed a Stabilisation and Association Agreement and an Interim Agreement on trade and trade-related matters (Commission of the European Communities 2009). In addition, the following three positive developments (European Commission 2010) in Serbia's path to EU membership may impact on emigration.

---

4 Neither research nor interviews produced any evidence concerning the professional mobility of dentists and nurses between 1990 and 1999.

5 Interviews with SMA 2009.

6 Neither research nor interviews produced any evidence concerning the professional mobility of dentists.

1. On 7 December 2009, the Council of the EU decided that the Interim Agreement with the Republic of Serbia would be implemented as soon as possible. This provides for the establishment of a free trade area between the EU and Serbia and regulates some important aspects of economic life, notably in competition and state aid. It also guarantees that the EU market will remain open to virtually all Serbian products as it includes the trade concessions that the EU has granted to Serbia since 2000.

2. Since 19 December 2009, citizens of Serbia have not needed visas to travel to the 25 EU Member States and 3 non-EU countries that are part of the Schengen area. The abolition of the visa regime means that Serbian citizens can stay in these countries for up to 90 days within a six-month period for tourism or similar reasons. However, Serbian citizens still require a separate permit in order to work or attend school in EU Member States and therefore visa liberalization is likely to have little impact on outflows of health professionals who move for work reasons.

3. On 22 December 2009, Serbia submitted its application to become a candidate state for membership of the EU.

Medical doctors

The SMA reports that 130–170 certificates have been issued annually since 2000 and over 200 in 2008; a total of 1300 to 1700 certificates were issued over a ten-year period (2000–2010). However, this evidence can only be taken as approximation, since there are no data on specialty, regional distribution, country of destination or length of stay (permanent/temporary) and some medical doctors may have made repeated applications. The Clinical Centre of Serbia, employing approximately 1200 medical doctors, reports that 62 medical doctors left the country between 2003 and 2008 and only 4 came back.[7]

While general health professional emigration remains at relatively low levels there is time to raise awareness on the importance of addressing this issue at policy level. This should create an environment that facilitates migration for the benefit of professional development while preventing shortfalls in the health workforce (Pavlov et al. 2008).

Overproduction and the resulting unemployment of medical doctors in Serbia suggest the potential for increasing outflow rates. The age structure of emigrating health professionals is a particular concern as young professionals are most likely to seek professional opportunities abroad, leaving behind an increasingly ageing workforce.

---

7 Interview with Director of Human Resources.

Overall, interviews with key professional associations revealed three main characteristics influencing health professional mobility for Serbian medical doctors over the last decade. First, the EU market was relatively closed and filled with medical doctors from new Member States. Second, the processes for recognizing diplomas were complicated, costly and time-consuming – overseas countries in particular had complicated re-certification and licensing procedures. Third, successful migrants are mostly employed in lower professional positions in recipient countries.

Nurses

Most Serbian nursing categories are not recognized in the EU because they do not qualify for consideration under Directive 2005/36/EC (European Parliament and Council of the European Union 2005). Since most Serbian nurses do not hold a higher education degree, they migrate mostly to work in nursing homes for elderly people and rehabilitation centres.

Currently there is no professional authority that organizes and records the mobility of nurses in Serbia. Interviews with nursing associations revealed that the migration of nursing professionals has been neither significant nor systematic, in comparison to other CEE transitional countries. The Chamber of Nurses and Health Technicians of the Association of Health Workers of Serbia is the largest nursing association, having over 36 000 members. Since 2000, this association has issued an estimated 300 certificates to nursing professionals wishing to emigrate.[8] It reports the top destination countries to be Italy, the United Kingdom, Australia, Canada and Switzerland. Additionally, an interview with a representative of the largest university hospital in Serbia, employing an estimated 3000 nurses, reported that between 2003 and 2008 73 nurses left the country and only 8 returned to their positions.

There is no evidence that EU enlargement in 2004 and 2007 affected health professional mobility in Serbia. It should be noted that Serbian citizens are required to pass the recognition and equivalence assessment (nostrification) procedure whereas, according to the *acquis communautaire*, health professionals who are European citizens may use a general system for the recognition of higher education diplomas (Council of the European Communities 1989, European Parliament and Council of the European Union 2005).

---

8 Interviews with President of the Association of Health Workers of Serbia and of the Serbian Society of Nurses, Midwives and Technicians in 2009.

3. Vignettes on health professional mobility

Anaesthetist: emigrating, returning and commuting

Now aged 74, this qualified physician started an anaesthetics residency in a big general hospital in Belgrade in 1962. While still a resident, he joined the Yugoslav cardiothoracic surgery team going to Algeria in 1964. He spent 13 months there and achieved an impressive track record of anaesthesias – almost 200 for cardiac surgery and 100 for thoracic surgery.

In 1967, he was offered both a Von Humboldt stipendium from a German university hospital and a post in a private Swiss hospital. He accepted the latter, stayed in Switzerland for four and a half years and obtained a work permit. Thereafter, he became a senior consultant in a big regional hospital and an honorary senior consultant in a nearby university hospital. On the recommendation of two university professors, he became one of only two (at the time) foreign members of the Swiss Anaesthesia Association.

In 1971, he applied successfully for a newly established assistant professorship in a big university hospital in Belgrade. Having returned to the country he pursued a successful academic career until retiring as a full professor in 2001. In parallel, between 1972 and 2005, he regularly replaced his former Swiss colleagues once or twice a year for periods ranging from 15 days to up to 3 months. He worked in 10 Swiss cantons in 15 hospitals (small to large; private, public and university hospitals) in all three languages. His overall total of ten years of service entitled him to a Swiss pension.

Dentist: permanent emigrant

Now aged 74, this qualified dentist began work in Serbia in a dentistry practice that offered no possibility of career development or of starting a private practice. At that time, there were insufficient numbers of dentists in some European countries such as Switzerland and Germany. Established practices lacked trained assistants and advertised regularly in professional bulletins. The need was so great that 27 Swiss dental practices showed interest when this Serbian dentist submitted his application.

This dentist emigrated to Switzerland in 1962, starting work as an assistant dentist in a small city practice and changed practices over time to achieve better and better employment conditions. Two years after emigrating he was joined by his fiancée – also a dentist, with a promising career at Belgrade University School of Dentistry. They settled in Switzerland, married and after 15 years opened a successful private practice in which they worked until retirement. She also worked in paediatric dentistry in a university hospital in a large city. They raised their son and daughter in Switzerland and motivated other university peers to start their careers there.

Surgeon: emigrating and returning

Now aged 53, this surgeon was offered a German Academic Exchange Service (DAAD) stipendium to work as a resident in Ear Nose and Throat & Maxillofacial (ENT&MF) surgery in 1989. He spent a year in a number of German university hospitals and thereby established his first contacts.

He returned to the ENT&MF university hospital in Belgrade and took his specialty exam in 1990. In the 1990s, he explored the possibilities of working abroad. At that time diplomas from Serbia were no longer recognized but his were nostrified a few months before the start of the wars and the imposition of sanctions (1992). He went to Spain and began working as a general practitioner when his credentials were homologized in 1994. However, he returned to Belgrade following problems related to the nostrification of his surgical credentials.

Given his outstanding performance in his residency year and his academic track record, his German professors recommended him for a vacancy in a big university hospital in Norway in 2001. The Norwegian colleagues showed most interest in the letters of recommendation from the three German professors and the video tape of his surgeries. He was granted a three-month trial period after which a temporary licence was issued on the recommendation of his superiors. He worked an additional 3 months in 2003 and 12 months in 2004–2005. He was offered a permanent position as a head of department on a contract offering favourable financial conditions as well as provisions for his wife and children. However, he declined for reasons concerning the permanent adaptation of the family, the different culture and the prospect of improved conditions in the home country. He returned to Serbia and has proceeded with his surgical and academic career – becoming deputy director in 2001 and professor in 2009.

Surgeon: permanent emigrant?

In 2006, this 37 year old surgeon asked for unpaid leave of absence from the hospital that had employed him for the 11 years since he had completed his studies. Struggling with a monthly salary of less than €500 he had decided to provide consulting services to a national sports team in Serbia. His wife worked as a teacher but, with two young sons, they still could not earn enough to support the family in the Serbian social environment.

A sports club contact offered the opportunity to work as a medical doctor for an Olympic volleyball team in the Middle East. Having been educated abroad during elementary school and therefore fluent in English, he decided to accept. The job was well-paid in comparison to Serbian rates but in reality did not come close to meeting his actual expenses in the foreign country. In addition, living abroad for more than five months meant that he was separated from his core family when they needed him most.

> Professionally, he was out of clinical practice – not practising surgery as he worked with healthy young adults. He began to consider returning to Serbia but in 2009 was recommended for, and accepted, a permanent post as an orthopaedic surgeon in a Middle East hospital. He and his family are still living there.

4. Impacts on the Serbian health system

There is no direct evidence of how health professional mobility impacts on the four functions of the Serbian health system – financing, service delivery, resource generation and stewardship. Hence, it is not possible to evaluate the repercussions that health professional emigration have on the health of the population, the responsiveness of the system or financial protection from ill health. It is plausible that health professional emigration has some effects on service delivery, resource generation and financing, as presented below, but no evidence on its impact on the governance of the health system was identified.

Service delivery

It is difficult to evaluate whether migration has created or exacerbated any imbalances in the regional distribution of health professionals given the lack of research on the causality between health professional mobility and impacts on the Serbian health systems. However, it can be surmised that an indirect chain reaction arises from professional mobility impacting on service provision which in turn affects the distribution of specialist doctors in rural areas.

Both internal mobility and the emigration of particular categories of (specialized) doctors and nurses can affect the supply and availability of, and access to, certain services (increasing waiting times, for example). There are current concerns about the self-sufficiency of the system and the sustainability of service delivery in certain areas, particularly cardiovascular surgery, anaesthetics and radiology. The physician-to-population approach has been the prevailing method of manpower planning, involving negotiations about the concrete numbers for each specialty or field. The Ministry of Health is currently updating the Health Institution Network Plan that prescribes the number of beds and physicians by region for each type of health-care institution (primary, secondary and tertiary care) (Republic of Serbia 2006a). One of its aims is to address an over-concentration of staff in urban areas at the expense of poorer, more remote, under-served areas in which posts remain vacant.

Resource generation

Serbia produces more medical doctors than it can employ. Since 2002, the Ministry of Health has adopted and implemented a very restrictive policy to regulate the overproduction of health professionals. Transparent needs-based rules for obtaining specialization were established, resulting in future trends in declining numbers of trained specialists. However, the combined effect of this policy and the existing overproduction of graduates will remain one of the most important factors influencing whether young professionals decide to go abroad (Djikanovich 2006).

Given the oversupply of medical doctors nationwide, the scale of outflows does not present an immediate threat to the provision of clinical services although this may not be the case in certain specialty areas. Migration is a symptom of deeper problems in the Serbian health system, such as the challenges of retaining health professionals and of improving workforce planning to reduce oversupply. This requires greater attention to more general human resource practice and management in the health system.

Financing

It costs around US$ 300 000 to produce one highly skilled expert and takes at least ten years after formal graduation to create a single world expert. Hence, the direct losses from accelerated brain drain from Serbia and Montenegro are between US$ 9 billion and US$ 12 billion if calculated on the basis of the number of specialists leaving the country. The real (still hidden) financial losses are much higher even if measured only in lost profits and inadequate replacement of the experts lost (Kutlača & Grečić 2005).

Long-term migration may undermine the return on the country's investment in education and training. The reasons why health professionals migrate are not dissimilar to those that prompt moves from the public to the private sector: better pay, better prospects and better working conditions. Where there is sufficient demand in the private sector (for example, for pharmacists) professionals will often prefer to stay in their home country. The professions' desire to ensure that they meet international professional standards also assists migration.

5. Relevance of cross-border health professional mobility

This section will examine to what extent cross-border mobility (inflows and outflows) is relevant to the Serbian health workforce and system concerning other health workforce issues such as geographical distribution and demographic and other factors. Mobility in Serbia is asymmetrical, losing more health professionals than it attracts. It is estimated that approximately 10 000 Serbian health professionals are working abroad (Statistical Office of the Republic of Serbia 2002). This is a significant number but probably still an underestimate of the real phenomenon.

5.1 *Health workforce characteristics and developments*

The size of the Serbian health workforce has increased considerably over the last 20 years. In 2008, the public sector employed a total of 121 483 health professionals (Fig.16.1). This was a net increase of almost 45% on the 84 044 employed in 1988 (Fig. 16.2).

Fig. 16.1 *Public sector health workers in Serbia, 2008*

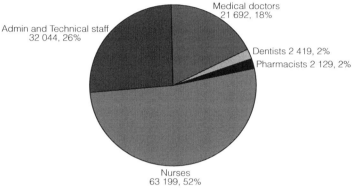

Source: Institute of Public Health of Serbia 2008. *Note:* n=121 483.

Fig. 16.2 *Public sector health workers in Serbia, 1988*

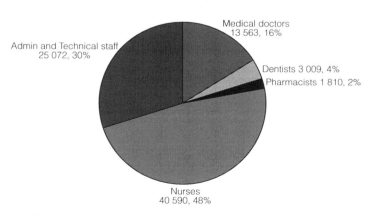

Source: Institute of Public Health of Serbia 1988. *Note:* n=84 044.

Comparison of categories of workers over a twenty-year period reveals that nurses and medical doctors increased in both number and proportion. The largest increase was in nursing staff numbers – 22 609 more (from 48% to 52% of the total); there were 8129 (16%–18%) more medical doctors. The numbers of administrative and technical staff decreased proportionately (30%–26%) although actual numbers increased by 6972. The proportion of pharmacists remained constant (2%) with a slight increase in numbers (319); both numbers and the proportion of dentists fell – by 590 and 2% respectively.

The following key issues are highlighted as current characteristics of the Serbian health-care workforce: (i) a high number of specialist doctors among medical doctors; and (ii) generally low motivation among hospital nurses due to low salaries and limited career prospects.

Just over half of all medical doctors currently work in the hospital sector and specialist doctors are distributed across all sectors, including primary care.

Over 75% of active medical doctors work in the public sector as specialists, while 10% are undergoing training in specialties. A further 15% are described as non-specialists located mainly in primary health-care facilities. There is a need to reassess this balance as well as that between specializations in the secondary and tertiary services.

Nurses in hospitals have low levels of motivation due to low wages and limited career advancement.[9] This requires a system of incentives to improve the quality of work and productivity. The above-mentioned intrinsic factors contribute to nurses emigating to other countries to seek employment.

Regional imbalances

Regional distribution of the health workforce is very important for a well-functioning system. There are considerable regional imbalances in Serbia's workforce, including the distribution of medical doctors and specialists but most markedly the regional distribution of nurses. Since information is scarce it is difficult to assess the relevance of internal health workforce distribution in Serbia and the extent to which migration may have created, exacerbated or improved any imbalances. However, data on the regional distribution of health professionals across the country are available (Table 16.1).

It can be observed that 21 692 medical doctors, 2419 dentists and 63 199 nurses were employed in the public sector in 2007 – 87 310 in total. In Belgrade, 28% of health professionals are concentrated in the capital city. Comparison to the national average for health professionals per 100 000 population shows that large urban centres with university and specialized hospitals have markedly higher numbers of medical doctors and nurses than more remote areas. At 397 per 100 000 population, Beogradski has a much higher density of medical doctors than the national average (289 per 100 000). Sremski shows the lowest density at 178 per 100 000 (Table 16.1).

---

9 Interviews with Nurses Association of Serbia 2009

Table 16.1 *Regional distribution of public health sector professionals in Serbia, 2007*

	Total population by 2002 census	Per 100 000 population			Total medical staff		
		Doctors	Dentists	Nurses	Doctors	Dentists	Nurses
SERBIA	7 498 001	289	32	843	21 692	2 419	63 199
Central Serbia	5 466 009	305	33	874	16 666	1 792	47 751
Northern Serbia - Vojvodina	2 031 992	247	31	760	5 026	627	15 448
Regions							
Severno Backi	200 140	202	25	718	405	50	1 438
Severno Banats.	165 881	207	26	765	344	43	1 269
Srednje Banats.	208 456	213	31	756	445	65	1 576
Zapadno Backi	214 011	214	26	694	459	56	1 486
Juzno Banatski	313 937	241	32	808	757	100	2 537
Juzno Backi	593 666	340	38	910	2 017	226	5 405
Sremski	335 901	178	26	517	599	87	1 737
Beogradski	1 576 124	397	34	1 117	6 259	538	17 610
Macvanski	329 625	204	22	670	671	72	2 209
Kolubarski	192 204	201	23	649	386	44	1 248
Podunavski	210 290	218	29	683	459	60	1 437
Sumadijski	298 778	327	31	793	977	93	2 369
Zlatiborski	313 396	232	28	826	727	87	2 589
Moravicki	224 772	229	31	688	514	69	1 547
Raski	291 230	259	37	723	753	109	2 105
Branicevski	200 503	229	25	807	460	51	1 619
Pomoravski	227 435	289	32	903	658	73	2 053
Rasinski	259 441	217	26	651	562	67	1 690
Borski	146 551	271	29	909	397	43	1 332
Zajecarski	137 561	304	25	927	418	34	1 275
Nisavski	381 757	439	53	1 026	1 675	202	3 916
Toplicki	102 075	264	35	776	269	36	792
Pirotski	105 654	261	38	756	276	40	799
Jablanicki	240 923	259	39	652	624	94	1 571
Pcinjski	227 690	255	35	698	581	80	1 590

Source: Institute of Public Health of Serbia 2007.

Geographical imbalances are more pronounced for nurses. Once again, Beogradski has the highest ratio at 1117 per 100 000 population against the national average of 843 per 100 000. Conversely, Sremski shows a density of only 517 nurses per 100 000 population, well below the national average and less than half of the ratio for Beogradski. This demonstrates the scale of geographical and urban/rural imbalances which are particularly pronounced in the distribution of nurses.

Educational system

About 1100 medical doctors graduate each year, roughly three times the number undergoing specialist training (Table 16.2). This arises because the Ministry of Health has established quotas for specializations but the medical faculties have not responded with the corresponding *numerus clausus*. These data indicate an oversupply of both medical doctors and specialists that creates unemployment and an incentive to emigrate.

Table 16.2 *Graduate medical doctors, dentists and pharmacists in Serbia, 1998–2005*

	1998	1999	2000	2001	2002	2003	2004	2005
Medical doctors	877	936	1 092	963	871	977	1 084	1180
Dentists	209	218	216	253	245	243	302	384
Pharmacists	183	238	259	262	270	243	310	369

Sources: Statistical Office of the Republic of Serbia 2001–2007.

The National Employment Service reports an increase in the number of unemployed health professionals since 2000. At the end of 2007, 1998 medical doctors, 966 dentists and 269 pharmacists were registered as unemployed (Statistical Office of the Republic of Serbia 2007). This may be attributed to the high number of new graduates.

Demographics

The Serbian health workforce can be characterized as predominately female. Nursing is predominantly a female profession (Djikanovic 2006) and the majority of the 63 199 nurses in Serbia are women (Institute of Public Health of Serbia 2007). Within the private and the public sector there is a total of 27 599 medical doctors, 57% (15 731) of whom are female. Belgrade has the largest number of female doctors (6447). Central West is the only region in Serbia with a higher proportion of male doctors (Table 16.3).

Retirement

The age profile of the medical workforce offers considerable scope for change

Table 16.3 *Male and female doctors per region in Serbia, 2008*

	Males	Females	Total	Females in total workforce (%)
Belgrade	3 573	6 447	10 020	64%
South East	2 554	3 520	6 074	58%
Central West	3 590	2 228	5 818	38%
Vojvodina	2 151	3 536	5 687	62%
Total Serbia	11 868	15 731	27 599	57%
Kosovo	288	431	719	60%

Source: Serbian Medical Chamber unpublished data 2008.

to address workforce outflows. In Serbia, full pension rights are obtained at 58 years for women and 63 for men. Among all medical doctors 17% are aged over 55 and a further 15% are over 50 (Statistical Office of the Republic of Serbia 2007); 23% of all specialist doctors are aged over 55. These doctors will become eligible for retirement in the next 10 years and, assuming that 20% retire, could release about 4000 current posts. Forecasts indicate that the public health system will require only 2000 of these posts. In addition over 10 000 medical doctors will graduate over the next 10 years, given the current capacity. Hence, 60% of these newly trained doctors will likely swell the already substantial cohort of unemployed doctors – currently about 2000–3500 per year (Cochrane & Crilly 2003).

Aiming to decrease the overall number of employees in the health sector, in 2005 and 2006 the Ministry of Health implemented early retirement schemes/ incentives based on the employee's years of service and age. These mostly targeted administrative and technical staff and have resulted in the rationalization of human resources for health. By 2007, 14 399 health professionals had left with severance packages – 9812 in November 2005 and 4587 in March 2006. No evidence is available on the implications for health workforce planning.

5.2 *What does cross-border mobility mean for Serbia?*

Serbia's difficulties with cross-border mobility and reform of the health system and the public sector are largely the result of long-term problems in planning and managing human resources. Health professional mobility is a symptom of Serbia's recent history, the economic downturn of the 1990s and a lack of attention to the complex and politically sensitive human resources agenda. Moreover, this migration is part of the broader dynamic of change and mobility within health-care labour markets and therefore should be addressed within wide-ranging policies. International mobility, internal migration and recruitment have complex dynamics covering the rights and choices of individuals; the motives and attitudes of health professionals; government approaches to managing, facilitating or attempting to limit the outflow or inflow of health professionals; and the intermediary role of recruitment agencies.

6. Factors influencing health professional mobility

In Serbia, health professional emigration is due to various factors including the high salary differential between Serbia and richer countries; the greater effectiveness of foreign health systems and their perceived better working conditions; and the destination countries' political and economic stability relative to Serbia.

The Serbian administration faces challenges common to transitional economies as social and economic inequalities have increased. The Statistical Office (2007) reports sustained high unemployment – 808 200 persons in September 2007, with 9% of the total population living below the poverty line. The average net monthly income is around €330.

In 2008, labour market conditions improved slightly as the employment rate rose to 53.3% and registered unemployment fell to 14.8%. These were 51.5% and 18.3% respectively in 2007. Nominal wages grew by 17.9% year-on-year in 2008. Yet, despite strong economic growth rates in recent years, unemployment remains at a relatively high level (Commission of the European Communities 2009). Around 2000 medical doctors in Serbia are already unemployed and over 1100 graduate each year. In April 2009, the National Employment Service in Serbia reported that approximately 7000 nurses, 2000 dentists and 1000 pharmacists were unemployed (National Employment Service 2009).

Instigating factors

Significant wage differentials between health professionals in Serbia and other countries are not easily bridged. For example, the average annual salary of a medical doctor is US$ 199 000 in the United States, US$ 11 532 in the Czech Republic and £94 000 in the United Kingdom; the OECD median is US$ 70 324 (Sigrid et al. 2006). In Serbia, the average annual salary of a health worker is US$ 8500 to US$ 9000 (Statistical Office of the Republic of Serbia 2009).

Other push factors can be concerns about political and economic instability, low professional satisfaction and poor working conditions. All the negative factors identified here have characterized the reality of life in Serbia intensively over the last two decades, peaking at the end of the 20th century.

Activating factors

Geographical proximity, shared language and customs and a common educational curriculum may affect the choice of destination country. The countries of the former Yugoslavia share the same language (Slovene and Macedonian are slightly different) and have had similar educational curricula.

The Serbian diaspora in destination countries and the success stories of colleagues who have emigrated for better career opportunities contribute to the decision-making process. Nurses consider personal reasons (including marriage in a foreign country) to be important and one of the main motives for moving.

Mitigating factors

Health professionals from Serbia who want to practise in another country often encounter higher requirements for qualifications, work permits and language competency. There are also complicated and demanding nostrification procedures, especially for the United States, the United Kingdom and the Scandinavian countries. These obstacles mean that emigration trends mainly will be among young Serbian medical doctors.[10]

7. Policy, regulation and interventions

Serbia is still experiencing the difficulties and limitations that most transition countries encounter when implementing reforms. This is due to:

- weak and unstable economies;

- lack of clear vision or common goals among health and finance ministries and the medical profession;

- insufficient experience of formulating policies in health economics, health insurance, quality assurance and modern management of human resources, or of a systemic approach to problems.

An explicit policy for human resource planning for health professional mobility was introduced in 2002 when the government adopted the *Health Policy of Serbia* (Ministry of Health 2002), identifying seven aims. Human resources for health was included as one of these aims under the heading "Improvement of the human resources for health care." In February 2003, the Ministry of Health adopted the *Health Strategy 2003 to 2015*, proposing a number of changes to health financing, essential health packages and the mandates of health institutions (Ministry of Health 2003). Human resource planning was not mentioned.

---

10 Interviews with SMA representatives and health professionals 2009.

Regional migration from less developed rural areas to city centres and possible shortages in certain rural communities could be an indicator for internal migration but this has had no systematic analysis. In the late 1980s, demographic changes and internal migration accentuated the need for more in-depth long-term health workforce planning. There appeared to be no need for labour market planning as the large numbers of unemployed health-care professionals guaranteed a steady inflow of professionals into the system. Unfortunately, systematic numeric and structural data were not recorded.

Articles 164–202 of the Serbian health-care law (Republic of Serbia 2005) set out the provisions by which health professionals practise their professions. However, the law does not include a policy framework for either human resource planning or health professional mobility. Continuing and/or increasing trends in unemployed medical doctors will require national-level mechanisms to register both the emigration and internal migration of health professionals (Wiskow 2006). Since 2009, the Serbian Medical Chamber has maintained a database for doctors in the private and public sector as part of its licensing and relicensing responsibilities.

A human resource strategy recommendation to the Ministry of Health (Cochrane & Crilly 2003) states that, in the medium term (five to ten years), the public health provider network requires 18 000 medical doctors overall. Of these, 12 600 would be specialists staffing secondary and tertiary care. The strategy included a proposal to reduce the total number of medical doctors by 11% but, six years later, Serbia was employing 25% more (20 000 in 2003; 25 000 in 2009). There are no projections of future demand for doctors at both national and regional levels and no evidence that a human resources strategy has been adopted and implemented.

7.1 *Planning methods*

Serbia has experienced various systems of medical manpower planning but the oversupply of medical doctors has persisted. In the period immediately following the Second World War medical doctors were appointed by ministerial decree. By the late 1950s there were no limits on the numbers of students accepted by medical faculties but a *numerus clausus* was adopted in the 1960s. Those decisions were mainly service- and facility-driven with a strong link between politics, health policy and manpower planning in health care.

The leading method of manpower planning in Serbia was similar to Slovenia's and was based on calculations involving the demographic data of various population groups. Norms for the required numbers of medical doctors were determined by simple physician/population ratios. The payer, then the state, played a decisive role in determining needs by means of the various administrative bodies. The schools of medicine filed annual proposals that matched their capacity with the Ministry of Health needs assessment but there was no link between the requirements for medical staff planning and the supply of training places (Albreht & Klazinga 2002).

The *Health Policy of Serbia* adopted in 2002 included improvement in the human resources for health care (Ministry of Health 2002). That same year, the Ministry of Health adopted and implemented a very restrictive policy to regulate the overproduction of specialist doctors. However, there is no link between the requirements for medical staff planning and the supply of training places.

7.2 National interventions

The new health system has maintained the regulatory role of the Ministry of Health and its intention to ensure equity, especially in universal access. At national level, new stakeholders have been introduced in the form of professional regulatory bodies. The Serbian Medical Chamber, Serbian Chamber of Dentists, Serbian Chamber of Pharmacists, Serbian Chamber of Biochemists and Serbian Chamber of Nurses and Health Technicians were established in 2006 and 2007, in addition to the existing Serbian Chamber of Health Care Institutions. These five new chambers of health professionals have the aim and purpose of contributing to continuous professional development, improved knowledge and skills and professional responsibility and accountability, by issuing licences to practise their profession and monitoring workforce stocks. The National Assembly of the Republic of Serbia founded the Health Council of Serbia in 2009 as a professional advisory body. Its responsibilities include advising on enrolment policies of medical faculties and schools and cooperating with relevant state institutions and other bodies in proposing rational enrolment policies for medical faculties and schools.

This research found that Serbia has signed several bilateral agreements related to mobility and outmigration with third countries. Job assignment is related to the health professionals employed in Serbia and who have been sent to work abroad by their employers for temporary work arrangements or post graduate education/research. So far, Serbia has a total of 27 concluded agreements and approved multilateral conventions for social insurance with Austria, Belgium, Bosnia and Herzegovina, Bulgaria, Croatia, Czech Republic, Denmark, Egypt, France, Germany, Hungary, Italy, Libya, Luxembourg, Montenegro, the Netherlands, Norway, Panama, Poland, Romania, Slovakia, Slovenia, Sweden, Switzerland, The Former Yugoslav Republic of Macedonia, Turkey and the United Kingdom (see annex).

8. Conclusion

Political developments, conflict and economic sanctions in the 1990s resulted in a significant deterioration of Serbia's economy and about 400 000 Serbs left the country, including 10 000 health professionals (Statistical Office of the Republic of Serbia 2002). The restructuring of the economy is now at a phase in which many jobs are bound to disappear as new ones are created and unemployment rates remain high.

Serbia inherited a medical workforce that was state-controlled between 1945 and 1991. Since then, the workforce has been characterized by a surplus of available health professionals, particularly medical doctors. There is a rising trend of unemployment in most branches of health care and at all levels of education but this is most apparent among medical doctors and dentists. The Ministry of Health reports that 200–300 young medical doctors and 800 nurses have been employed since 2006.[11] This represents the beginning of an employment up-trend.

In order to enrol for any kind of specialization, medical doctors are required to have two years of official working experience and it is estimated that around 2000 unemployed medical doctors (National Employment Service April 2009) were denied the opportunity to enrol for specialization. Therefore, it can be assumed that mostly young, newly graduated physicians will be the most likely to consider migration. Low salary levels are an additional push factor.

The findings of this study indicate that the oversupply of health workers should be addressed by reviewing the intake policies of the medical schools in Serbia and introducing needs-oriented planning of health worker education. National-level mechanisms are required to register professionals going abroad. Health professional associations strongly agree on the need for a national policy and coordinated health manpower planning. Workforce planning should be population and needs based in order to retain an appropriate skill-mix in the country (Djikanovich 2006). Medical human resource planning will remain an important topic for many years and a broader spectrum of stakeholders will produce negotiations that are more demanding and more in need of compromise. New approaches to manpower planning will also be required.

Within the phases of pre-accession and accession to the EU, it seems realistic to expect that Serbia will have even greater exposure to health professional mobility. This will increase as barriers to emigration decrease and while there are still significant differences in economic parameters and gaps to be filled in some EU Member States. Source countries that lose skilled health staff through outmigration may find that their health systems encounter difficulties such as

---

11 Interviews with Ministry of Health representatives in 2009.

staff shortages, lower morale among the remaining health-care staff and a reduced quality or quantity of health service provision. Nevertheless, the migration of health workers can also have positive aspects by assisting countries that have an oversupply of staff and offering a solution to staff shortages in destination countries. It can also allow individual health workers to improve their skills, career opportunities and standard of living (Buchan 2008). In Serbia, national health policies to monitor this process and mitigate the negative effects are still to be devised but it will be important to learn from the experiences of previous transition countries.

References

Albreht T, Klazinga N (2002). Health manpower planning in Slovenia: a policy analysis of the changes in roles of stakeholders and methodologies. *Journal of Health Politics, Policy and Law.* 27(6):1001–1022.

Bach S (2003). *International migration of health workers: labour and social issues.* Geneva, International Labour Office (ILO Working Paper 2009).

Buchan J (2008). *How can the migration of health service professionals be managed so as to reduce any negative effects on supply?* Copenhagen, WHO Regional Office for Europe on behalf of the European Observatory on Health Systems and Policies.

Cochrane D, Crilly T (2003). *Serbia and Montenegro: human resource strategy report, 2002.* Washington, World Bank.

Commission of the European Communities (2009). *Serbia 2009 progress report accompanying the communication from the Commission to the European Parliament and the Council. Enlargement strategy and main challenges 2009–2010.* Brussels (Commission Staff Working Document SEC(2009)1339).

Council of the European Communities (1989). Directive 89/48/EEC of 21 December 1988 on a general system for the recognition of higher-education diplomas awarded on completion of professional education and training of at least three years' duration. *Official Journal*, L019:16–23.

Djikanovich B (2006). Health worker migration in selected CEE countries: Serbia. In: Wiskow C (ed.). *Health worker migration flows in Europe: overview and case studies in selected CEE countries – Romania, Czech Republic, Serbia and Croatia.* Geneva, International Labour Office.

European Commission (2010). *Enlargement: Serbia* (http://ec.europa.eu/enlargement/ potential-candidates/serbia/relation/ index_en.htm, accessed 6 January 2011).

European Parliament and Council of the European Union (2005). Directive 2005/36/EC of the European Parliament and of the Council of 7 September 2005 on the recognition of professional qualifications. *Official Journal of the European Union*, 255(48): 22–142.

Grečić V et al. (1998). *Jugoslovenske spoljne migracije Savezno ministarstvo za rad, zdravstvo i socijalnu politiku* [*External migrations of Yugoslavia, Federal Ministry for Labour, Health and Social Policy*]. Belgrade, Institut za međunarodnu politiku i privredu, Savezni zavod za tržište rada i migracije [Institute for International Politics and Economy, Federal Institute for Labour Market and Migrations].

Institute of Public Health of Serbia (1988). *"Dr. Milan Jovanović Batut" Health Statistical Yearbook of Republic of Serbia*. Belgrade

Institute of Public Health of Serbia (2007). *"Dr. Milan Jovanović Batut" Health Statistical Yearbook of Republic of Serbia*. Belgrade

Institute of Public Health of Serbia (2008). *"Dr. Milan Jovanović Batut" Health Statistical Yearbook of Republic of Serbia*. Belgrade

Kutlača Đ, Grečić V (2005). *Brain drain and their impact on research and development system: case study of the Republic of Serbia, 2005.* http://www.diplomacy.bg.ac.yu, *accessed April 2009*

Ministry of Health of Serbia (2002). *Health policy of Serbia*. Belgrade.

Ministry of Health of Serbia (2003). *Health strategy 2003 to 2015*. Belgrade.

National Employment Service (2009). Monthly statistical bulletin: unemployment and employment in the Republic of Serbia, March and April 2009. Belgrade (http://www.nsz.gov.rs, accessed 10 February 2011).

Pavlov MT et al. (2008). *Migration and development: creating regional labour market and labour migrants circulation as response to regional market demands. Serbia.* Belgrade, Group 484 (http://www.grupa484.org.rs/files/Compendium%   20Labour%20Migration%20Conference%202008.pdf, accessed 15 November 2009).

Republic of Serbia (2005). The Law on Health Care and subsequent decree on the basis of article 47 of this law. *Official Gazette*, 28 November 2005 (RS 107/05).

Republic of Serbia (2006). Decree on the Health Institution Network Plan. *Official Gazette*, 19 May 2006 (RS 42/2006).

Sigrid D et al. (2006). *Health workers wages: an overview from selected countries. Evidence and information for policy.* Geneva, World Health Organization.

Statistical Office of the Republic of Serbia (2001). *Statistical yearbook of Serbia, 2001*. Belgrade.

Statistical Office of the Republic of Serbia (2002). *Statistical yearbook of Serbia, 2002*. Belgrade.

Statistical Office of the Republic of Serbia (2003). *Statistical yearbook of Serbia, 2003*. Belgrade.

Statistical Office of the Republic of Serbia (2004). *Statistical yearbook of Serbia, 2004*. Belgrade.

Statistical Office of the Republic of Serbia (2005). *Statistical yearbook of Serbia, 2005*. Belgrade.

Statistical Office of the Republic of Serbia (2006). *Statistical yearbook of Serbia, 2006*. Belgrade.

Statistical Office of the Republic of Serbia (2007). *Statistical yearbook of Serbia, 2007*. Belgrade.

Statistical Office of the Republic of Serbia (2009). Република Србија, Републички завод за статистику, Статистика зарада број 319 – год [Salaries per employee categories in Serbia, October 2009, 319–2009]. *LIX*, 25.11.2009.

Vuković D (2005). Migrations of the labour force from Serbia. *SEER SouthEast Europe Review for Labour and Social Affairs*, 04/2005:139–150 (www.ceeol. com, accessed 13 December 2010).

Wiskow C (2006). *Health worker migration flows in Europe: overview and case studies in selected CEE countries – Romania, Czech Republic, Serbia and Croatia*. Geneva, International Labour Office (ILO Working Paper 245).

Annex

Republic of Serbia: 27 bilateral agreements (concluded) and multilateral conventions (approved)

1. Austria – Agreement between Federal Republic of Yugoslavia and Republic of Austria on social insurance (*Official Gazette of FRY*, 1998. International agreements No. 7/98). New agreement 1 May 2002 (http://www.zso.gov.rs/english/medjunarodni-ugovori.htm, accessed 31 January 2011). Institute for Social Insurance, Republic of Serbia (http://www.neurope.eu/articles/Serbia-and-Switzerland-sign-agreement-on-social-insurance/103315.php accessed 31 January 2011).

2. Belgium – Convention on social insurance between Socialist Federal Republic of Yugoslavia and Kingdom of Belgium (*Official Gazette of FPRY*, 1956. International agreements No. 7/56; *Official Gazette of SFRY*, 1970. International agreements No. 34/70). New agreement signed July 2010 (http://www.ekapija.com/website/sr/page/330543_en, accessed 31 January 2011).

3. Bulgaria – Convention on social insurance between the Federal Republic of Yugoslavia and People's Republic of Bulgaria (*Official Gazette of FPRY*, 1959. International agreements No. 4/59). A new agreement is expected to come into power in 2011. Institute for Social Insurance, Republic of Serbia (http://www.zso.gov.rs/english/medjunarodni-ugovori.htm, accessed 31 January 2011).

4. Czech Republic – Convention on social insurance between the Federal People's Republic of Yugoslavia and Czechoslovakia since 1958. Since 1 December 2002 – Agreement between the Federal Republic of Yugoslavia and the Czech Republic on social insurance (*Official Gazette of SRY*, 2002. International agreements No. 7/02). Institute for Social Insurance, Republic of Serbia (http://www.zso.gov.rs/english/medjunarodni-ugovori.htm, accessed 31 January 2011).

5. Slovakia – social insurance agreement since 1958 (*Official Gazette of FPRY*, 1959. International agreements No. 1/59).

6. Denmark – Convention between Socialist Federal Republic of Yugoslavia and Kingdom of Denmark on social insurance (*Official Gazette of SFRY*, 1980. International agreements No. 5/80).

7. France – General Convention on social insurance between the French Republic and Federal Republic of Yugoslavia (*Official Gazette of FPRY*, 1951. International agreements No. 4/51. *Official Gazette of SFRY,* International agreements Nos.1/67 [1967], 17/71 [1971], 22/75 [1975], 7/77 [1977], 5/79 [1979] and 9/90 [1990]).

8. Italy – Convention on social insurance between the Federal People's Republic of Yugoslavia and the Republic of Italy (*Official Gazette of FPRY*, 1959. International agreements No.1/59).

9. Luxembourg – Agreement between Serbia and Montenegro and Grand Duchy of Luxembourg on social insurance. New agreement since 1 September 2005 (*Official Gazette of SaM* 2004, International Agreements No. 10/04.

10. Hungary – Agreement on social insurance since 1958. Official Gazette of SFRY – International agreements No. 33/75. Institute for Social Insurance, Republic of Serbia (http://www.zso.gov.rs/english/medjunarodni-ugovori.htm, accessed 31 January 2011). New agreement is in its final phase.

11. Netherlands – Convention on social insurance between Socialist Federal Republic of Yugoslavia and the Kingdom of the Netherlands (*Official Gazette of SFRY*, 1980. International agreements No.11/80).

12. Norway – Convention between Socialist Federal Republic of Yugoslavia and the Kingdom of Norway on social insurance (*Official Gazette of SFRY*, 1975. International agreements No. 22/75).

13. Poland – Convention on social insurance between Government of the Federal People's Republic of Yugoslavia and Government of the People's Republic of Poland (*Official Gazette of FPRY*, 1958. International agreements No. 9/58).

14. Germany – Agreement between Socialist Federal Republic of Yugoslavia and Federal Republic of Germany on social insurance (*Official Gazette of SFRY* – International agreements Nos. 9/69 [1969] and 4/76 [1976]).

15. Sweden – Convention between Socialist Federal Republic of Yugoslavia and the Kingdom of Sweden on social insurance (*Official Gazette of SFRY*, 1979. International agreements No.12/79).

16. Switzerland – Convention on social insurance between Socialist Federal Republic of Yugoslavia and the Swiss Confederation (*Official Gazette of SFRY*. International agreements Nos. 8/63 [1963] and 12/84 [1984]) New agreement signed October 2010 (http://www.neurope.eu/articles/Serbia-and-Switzerland-sign-agreement-on-social-insurance/103315.php, accessed 31 January 2011).

17. United Kingdom – Convention on social insurance between Federal People's Republic of Yugoslavia and the United Kingdom of Great Britain and Northern Ireland (*Official Gazette of FPRY*. International agreements Nos. 7/58 [1958] and 10/60 [1960]). Institute for Social Insurance, Republic of Serbia (http://www.zso.gov.rs/english/medjunarodni-ugovori.htm, accessed 31 January 2011).

18. Libyan Arab Jamahiriya – Agreement on social insurance between the Socialist Federal Republic of Yugoslavia and the Socialist People's Libyan Arab Jamahiriya. Note: for pension and disability insurance only (*Official Gazette of SFRY*, 1990. International agreements No.1/90).

19. Egypt – Agreement on social insurance between the Socialist Federal Republic of Yugoslavia and the Arab Republic of Egypt (*Official Gazette of SFRY*, 1988. International agreements No.12/88).

20. Panama – Agreement in the field of social insurance between the Socialist Federal Republic of Yugoslavia and the Republic of Panama. Note: for pension

and disability insurance only (*Official Gazette of SFRY*, 1977. International agreements No.11/77).

21. Romania - Agreement between Government of the Socialist Federal Republic of Yugoslavia and Government of the Socialist Republic of Romania on cooperation in the field of health insurance. Note: for health insurance only (*Official Gazette of SFRY*, 1977. International agreements No.13/77).

22. Turkey – Agreement in the field of social insurance between Republic of Turkey and Republic of Serbia, ratified in 2006 but has not come into force (*Official Gazette of SaM*, 2006. International agreements No. 4/2006).

Agreements signed by countries of the former Yugoslavia

1. The Former Yugoslav Republic of Macedonia – Agreement between Federal Republic of Yugoslavia and The Former Yugoslav Republic of Macedonia on social insurance. Implemented 1 April 2002 (*Official Gazette of SRY*, 2001. International agreements No. 1/2001).

2. Croatia – Agreement between Federal Republic of Yugoslavia and the Republic of Croatia on social insurance. Implemented 1 May 2003 (*Official Gazette of SRY*, 2001. International agreements No. 1/2001).

3. Bosnia and Herzegovina – Agreement between Federal Republic of Yugoslavia and Bosnia and Herzegovina on social insurance. Implemented 1 January 2004 (*Official Gazette of SaM*, 2003. International agreements No. 7/2003).

4. Montenegro – Agreement between the Republic of Serbia and the Republic of Montenegro on social insurance. Signed 17 December 2006 (*Official Gazette of RS*, 102/07).

5. Slovenia – Social insurance agreement between the Republic of Slovenia and Republic of Serbia, November 2010. Institute for Social Insurance, Republic of Serbia (http://www.zso.gov.rs/english/medjunarodni-ugovori.htm, accessed 31 January 2011).

Chapter 17

International mobility of health professionals in the context of Turkey: a one way street

Hasan Hüseyin Yıldırım, Sıdıka Kaya

1. Introduction

With a population of nearly 71.5 million, Turkey is strategically located between Europe and Asia and has a dynamic and developing market economy. The current health system is a mix of public and private sectors; the General Health Insurance Scheme is the predominant provider of social security coverage to the population (Resmi Gazete 2006a). Turkey obtained candidate status within the European Union (EU) at the Helsinki Summit of 1999 and started accession negotiations in December 2005. This requires preparations for the mobility of health professionals and therefore an investigation of the dimension, profile and impact of their cross-border mobility should provide useful inputs for medium- and long-term policies in both Turkey and the EU (Yıldırım 2009).

Currently, restrictive domestic labour laws ensure that health professional mobility in Turkey is all one way. Health professionals may leave the country to seek employment elsewhere but foreigners face serious difficulties establishing themselves and working in Turkey. There are no robust data on the foreign-born, foreign-trained and foreign-national health professionals in Turkey but it is assumed that health professional mobility adds to the human resource issues facing the Turkish health system, including insufficient planning, problematic skill mix, unbalanced specializations, underproduction and maldistribution of professionals etc. The current government sees health professional mobility as a remedy to some of these issues. With a view to potential EU accession, the government has tried to ease the labour laws in order to allow foreign doctors to establish themselves. However, this policy option is very controversial in Turkey.

The purpose of this chapter is to determine the patterns of international mobility of health professionals; the pull and push factors of such mobility; its favourable and detrimental effects on the Turkish health-care system; and initiatives to better manage mobility. Three complementary methods have been used: (i) a literature review, including grey literature; (ii) collection of data from relevant national and international sources, using data collection forms developed specifically for the purpose; and (iii) contact with relevant people/institutions by e-mail, telephone or in person.

Limitations of the study

The study entails substantial limitations. Turkey has no regular recording system for the compilation of international migration data although related organizations and institutions collect certain data in line with their administrative work. However, these data do not fit international definitions and classifications of comparability and measurability (TUİK 2009). Generally, data are crude, do not include classification by occupation and are not stored electronically. Those data that do exist are in piecemeal form at various institutions and were not made available to the authors in a complete format. Certain individuals and institutions did not respond to requests for data and administrative restrictions meant that the authors were not allowed to process the existing data manually. There are neither representative data nor any research on the mobility of international health professionals to or from Turkey.

The international mobility profile of health professionals in Turkey is presented in the following sections. This is followed by an estimate of the probable effect on mobility caused by the dynamics of EU accession and the subsequent impact on the Turkish health-care system. The chapter concludes with a discussion of the policies, regulation and interventions concerning the mobility of health professionals.

2. Mobility profile of Turkey

Analysis of the emigration and immigration mobility patterns of health professionals in Turkey shows that most emigration results from three main types of personal initiative: (i) going abroad for education; (ii) staying and/or working abroad after completion of education; and (iii) going abroad for work. It is frequently stated that considerable numbers of health professionals emigrate, in parallel to emigration of the general population, but there are not sufficient reliable data with which to assess the magnitude of flows.

Very little inflow is expected, given the restrictive Turkish laws on immigration. Theoretically, there are seven main mechanisms/ways by which foreign health professionals can establish themselves in Turkey: (i) bilateral agreements; (ii) marriage; (iii) dual citizenship; (iv) EU legislation on free movement; (v) being of Turkish descent; (vi) education; and (vii) illegal work. In practice, the existing legislation makes immigration for foreign health professionals possible only if they are of Turkish descent, have dual citizenship or choose to work illegally. Consequently, the inflow figures cover people of Turkish origin and/ or dual citizenship.

It has not been possible to carry out qualitative and quantitative analysis of the stock of international health professionals in Turkey with the data available. This study analyses the limited national and international data and relevant literature due to the lack of complete, accurate data on the international and (especially) EU-related emigration and immigration of health professionals from and to Turkey.

2.1 *Outflows*

There is a long history of emigration from Turkey to Europe but it was particularly important (especially for unqualified emigrants) in the 1960s, largely to Germany and the Netherlands. Since the mid 1970s, most emigrants have been those with qualifications (Yıldırım 2009), including health professionals. There are no data to show the numbers of Turkish health professionals currently working abroad but some limited, piecemeal and isolated studies and data may give an indication. The first research on the emigration of highly qualified health professionals from Turkey was conducted in 1962–1963 with the cooperation of Ankara Hıfzıssıhha School and Johns Hopkins University. Of the 1257 medical doctors selected by sampling, 230 (18.3%) were abroad during the time of the study. It was estimated that 2248 Turkish medical doctors were resident abroad in 1964 (Taylor et al. 1968), many in the Federal Republic of Germany.

The three most prominent destination countries for emigrating Turkish-trained medical doctors and nurses were the United States of America (63%), Germany (28%) and the United Kingdom (6%) (Table 17.1).

The Organisation for Economic Co-operation and Development (OECD) countries to which most Turkish-born health professionals migrate are the United States, Switzerland, the United Kingdom, Austria, Greece and France. These are popular destinations for general migration too as they offer

Table 17.1 *OECD destination countries of Turkish-educated health professionals, 2004–2007*

Destination country	Medical doctors	Nurses	Total
Canada (2005)	5	-	5
Denmark (2005)	13	1	14
Finland (2005)	14	-	14
France (2004)	32	-	32
Germany (2005)	884	-	884
Netherlands (2007)	8	5	13
United Kingdom (2007)	187	-	187
United States (2006)	1 974	-	1 974
Total	**3 117**	**6**	**3 123**

Source: OECD 2007.

the possibility of better education, higher incomes and improved working conditions in countries with high numbers of settled Turkish citizens (Table 17.2).

2.2 Inflows

Migration to Turkey is primarily guided by descent. OECD data show a total of 21 foreign-trained medical doctors and 51 foreign-trained nurses working in Turkey in 2005 (Table 17.3), constituting 0.02% of all medical doctors (107 347) and 0.1% of nurses (83 926) (Dumont & Zurn 2007). Almost all nurses and nearly half of the medical doctors who migrated to Turkey were trained in Bulgaria, a country with historical ties. Other OECD data show that foreign-born medical doctors residing in Turkey are generally from Germany, Greece, the United States, the Netherlands and the United Kingdom[1] (Table 17.4). In addition to general features which may make destination countries attractive, Turkish descent is the main factor that causes foreign health professionals to migrate to Turkey.

The restrictive labour laws make it difficult for foreign health professionals to be employed officially and may explain why 2158 foreign-born medical doctors were *residing* in Turkey around 2000 (Table 17.4) but just 141 were permitted to *work* over 2004–2008 (Table 17.5). Work permits are issued by the Ministry of Labour and Social Security (ÇSGB). Official data from this ministry show that 309 work permits were issued to foreign health professionals between 2004 and 2008, nearly half of which (45.6%) were given to medical doctors (ÇSGB

---

1 No data available for nurses.

Table 17.2 *Turkish-born doctors and nurses by country of residence (selected OECD countries), circa 2000*

Country of residence	Medical doctors	Nurses	Total
Australia	55	51	106
Austria	106	53	159
Canada	35	15	50
Denmark	16	16	32
Finland	10	-	10
France	102	9	111
Greece	98	38	136
Hungary	1	-	1
Luxembourg	1	2	3
Mexico	2	-	2
Portugal	2	-	2
Spain	6	1	7
Sweden	51	55	106
Switzerland	62	164	226
United Kingdom	103	70	173
United States	1 080	400	1 480
Total	**1 730**	**874**	**2 604**

Source: OECD 2007.

2009). It is noteworthy that the majority of those authorized to work in Turkey do not practise their profession (Table 17.5).

Foreign students arrive to study health-related degrees in Turkey. Between 2003 and 2008, newly enrolled foreign students represented around 4% of total enrolments in faculties of medicine, of dentistry and of pharmacy (reaching 6% in medicine in 2008). Foreign enrolments in nursing studies remained below 1% in 2003–2006 (ÖSYM 2004–2009, Sağlık Bakanlığı ve Yükseköğretim Kurulu 2008).

Table 17.3 *Foreign-trained medical doctors and nurses in Turkey, by country of training, 2005*

Country of training	Medical doctors	Nurses	Total
Azerbaijan	2	1	3
Bulgaria	9	48	57
China	-	1	1
Georgia	1	-	1
Germany	1	1	2
Iran	3	-	3
Russian Federation	1	-	1
Tajikistan	1	-	1
Uzbekistan	2	-	2
Former Yugoslavia	1	-	1
Total	**21**	**51**	**72**

Source: OECD 2007.

3. Vignettes on health professional mobility[2]

Immigrant to permanent resident

Nurse X is 46 years old, of Turkish origin but was born in Bulgaria. Having completed her nursing education she worked as a nurse in Bulgaria for four years, specializing in paediatrics. In 1989, her husband was expelled for political opposition and sent to Turkey; X emigrated in 1991 when her husband was issued with an immigration visa. She applied to the Council of Higher Education and passed their examination to confirm parity. She works as a nurse in a hospital in Turkey. Despite being of Turkish origin and learning Turkish prior to migration, X experienced language difficulties at first. She has now been living in Turkey with her family for almost twenty years, her husband works there and her last child was born in Turkey. X has both Bulgarian and Turkish citizenship but is not considering going back to Bulgaria.

Immigrant to permanent resident

Dr Y is of Turkish origin but was born in Azerbaijan. She graduated from medical school in Azerbaijan and is now an internal medicine specialist. At the beginning of the 1990s, poor working conditions and inadequate pay led her husband to submit migration applications to Turkey, the United States and Canada. Turkey was the first to accept

2 From interviews with authors in May and June 2009.

Table 17.4 *Foreign-born (selected OECD countries) doctors residing in Turkey, circa 2000*

Country of birth	Medical doctors
Australia	9
Austria	65
Belgium	52
Canada	13
Czech Republic	9
Denmark	22
Finland	8
France	67
Germany	1 130
Greece	217
Hungary	5
Ireland	4
Italy	67
Japan	8
Korean peninsula[a]	3
Netherlands	109
Norway	22
Poland	39
Spain	33
Sweden	38
Switzerland	28
United Kingdom	98
United States	112
Total	**2 158**

Source: OECD 2007. *Note*: [a] Democratic People's Republic of Korea and Republic of Korea.

his application and he found employment with the help of the Azerbaijani Association. Three years later Y gained Turkish citizenship and moved with her children to join her husband. Y worked as a doctor in Azerbaijan for 10 years and has now worked in Turkey for 15 years. She is not considering going back.

Table 17.5 *Foreign[a] health professionals with Turkish work permits, by employment status, 2004–2008*

	Employment status		Total
	Practising profession	Practising as manager, trading partner, etc.	
Medical doctors	50	91	141
Dentists	11	12	23
Midwives/nurses	5	84	89
Pharmacists	20	36	56
Total	**86**	**223**	**309**

Source: ÇSGB 2009. *Note*: [a] foreign-born, foreign-trained and foreign-national.

Permanent immigrant maintains links with birth country

Nurse Z is 51 years old and was born in Bulgaria of Turkish descent. She trained as a nurse and then worked in Bulgaria for 10 years. When the family were obliged to change their names they decided to emigrate. In 1990, they emigrated to Turkey (considering it their motherland) and had no difficulty obtaining Turkish citizenship. Z applied to the Council of Higher Education for parity and was granted a health worker diploma. Having successfully completed a Ministry of Health oral exam that examined her level of knowledge and proficiency in Turkish, she was given a document stating that she could work in Turkey. She worked as a contract (not on the main staff) nurse for two years at a hospital affiliated to the Ministry of Health and then moved to a university hospital. Having worked at the university hospital for twenty years, Z earned the right to retire. Z and her family have retained their property in Bulgaria and visit every year.

Temporary migrant

Dr T is 28 years old and unmarried. He was born and graduated from the faculty of medicine in Kazakhstan but moved in 2005 for specialist training under the scope of an agreement between Kazakhstan and Turkey. He was attracted by the reputation of certain hospitals in Turkey and by the climate. After a year of Turkish language courses he passed the exam of a general surgery department in a university hospital and started his specialist training. His greatest problem is that he does not receive a salary because he does not have a work permit. He finds that his scholarship is not sufficient to make ends meet and when he finishes his specialist training will return to his home country.

4. Dynamics of enlargement

A complete lack of data makes it impossible to assess whether the EU accessions in 2004 and 2007 had positive or negative impacts on health professional mobility or produced any change in emigration patterns to the new Member States. However, as in many other spheres, it may be stated that the dynamics of accession have triggered Europeanization of the health professions since Turkey became a candidate country in 1999.

Firstly, Turkey has started to align its legislation with that of the EU – for example, revising and updating the legislation for health professionals (originally introduced over 70 years ago) in approximation to EU standards and starting to revise the legislation restricting/prohibiting immigration. Secondly, in 2003 the Health Transformation Programme (HTP), a framework of ongoing Turkish health-care reforms, noted that there was evidence to indicate that Turkey had started to take account of EU dynamics in health reforms, including health workforce planning (Sağlık Bakanlığı 2003).

EU accession would increase the migration potential of health professionals in parallel with free movement in general. In Turkey, disputes about opening up the health-care system to foreign medical doctors began in 2006. These have been exacerbated by concerns about the size of the Turkish population, the youth ratio[3] and the high unemployment rate. This is supported in the few studies on this issue – Yıldırım and Yıldırım (2005) found that 53% of their 93 key informants[4] anticipated that EU accession might prompt health professionals to emigrate. Also, it is suggested that brain drain would be a major problem following accession (Yıldırım 2004).

Health professionals (medical doctors and nurses) participating in recent research were asked "whether they would consider emigrating to an EU country if Turkey were to become an EU member under the present circumstances". Among 1054 participants, 65% responded that they might emigrate (Yıldırım 2009). These findings agree with the results of studies from past accession countries. Before the 2004 accession, there was concern that health professional outflows would increase markedly once movement became easier (Borzeda et al. 2002). However, the initial records show that the outflow of medical doctors and nurses from Estonia, Poland and Lithuania in the first 12 to 18 months

---

3 Turkey has a large population with a high proportion of young people. Concern that EU membership will enable far too much emigration to the EU has led the EU Commission to consider certain transition regulations (such as periods, derogations and specific regulation) to prevent or manage massive immigration. The EU may even suspend the free movement of persons from Turkey in order to protect the EU labour market (Commission of the European Communities 2004, Yıldırım 2009). Such measures were put in place for the 2004 and 2007 accession countries but some Member States allowed derogations for certain highly qualified groups, including health professionals.

4 Managers, experts, bureaucrats of relevant institutions, politicians and academics. The questionnaire was issued between January and July 2003.

of EU accession were not as high as the authorities in these countries had anticipated (Buchan & Perfilieva 2006).

5. Impact of health professional mobility

Data on the mobility of health professionals on the international scale is very limited and almost non-existent in Turkey. Hence it is very difficult to provide an accurate analysis of its effect on the functions and aims of the health-care system. However, despite the absence of any sound research evidence, it may be stated that health professional outflows (see section 2) from Turkey outweigh immigration. This implies the loss of domestic human capital produced through national resources but no evidence is available to identify the geographical regions or specialties in which these outflows have occurred.

6. Relevance of cross-border health professional mobility

6.1 *Distributional issues influencing composition of the health workforce*

As in many other countries, the Turkish health-care system is experiencing two main problems: (i) a lack of human resources for health; and (ii) an imbalanced distribution of health-care workers (both geographically and by profession). There are two basic opposing views on whether there are deficiencies or surpluses in the health workforce in Turkey. A group headed by the Ministry of Health holds that there is an important deficit, specifically regarding medical doctors. A group led by the Turkish Medical Association (TMA) asserts that the main problem is not a shortage but rather unbalanced distribution of health professionals (Yıldırım 2009).

Turkey is separated into seven regions and, despite considerable improvements in recent years, there are still geographical imbalances in health workforce distribution (Sağlık Bakanlığı 2007a). A large majority of health professionals work in urban areas and medical doctors are distributed unevenly between the west and east of the country, with significantly higher proportions in the former. For example, in 2003 the number of specialist medical doctors per 100 000 population was calculated at 95.0 in the Marmara region but at 23.5 in South Eastern Anatolia (Table 17.6).

Fig. 17.1 shows the distribution of medical doctors in the selected three richest and three poorest provinces of Turkey in 2006. The three poor and undeveloped provinces (Van, Muş, Ağrı) have much lower numbers of medical doctors per 100 000 population than the three rich and developed provinces (İstanbul,

Table 17.6 *Health professionals per 100 000 population in Turkey, by geographical region, 2003*

Region	Specialist doctors	Practitioner doctors[a]	Dentists	Pharmacists	Health officers	Nurses	Midwives
Marmara	95.0	69.0	37.3	40.4	48.9	105.4	48.8
Aegean	80.0	88.6	31.7	44.2	75.1	147.2	81.7
Mediterranean	48.3	64.6	20.1	32.0	67.5	107.6	75.0
Central Anatolia	85.1	105.4	35.4	45.3	127.0	168.2	65.5
Black Sea	50.4	77.6	17.2	26.9	90.5	144.1	69.5
Eastern Anatolia	38.0	61.9	10.7	13.2	70.9	86.6	47.3
South Eastern Anatolia	23.5	40.7	7.7	18.4	39.6	59.9	32.0

Sources: Sağlık Bakanlığı 2005, TÜİK 2005, Yıldırım 2009. *Note*: [a] In Turkey, physicians who complete the basic six-year medical education but do not specialize further are called practitioners. Specialists in family medicine complete a three-year residency programme in family medicine after graduating from medical school (Güneş & Yaman 2008).

Fig. 17.1 *Medical doctors per 100 000 population in selected three richest and three poorest provinces of Turkey, 2006*

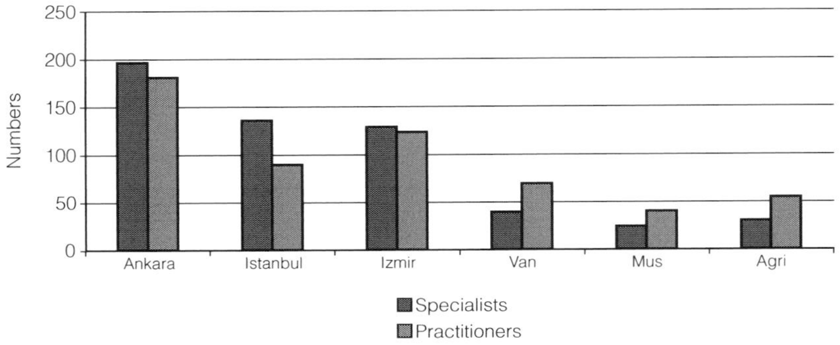

Sources: Sağlık Bakanlığı2007a, Yıldırım 2009. *Note*: Practitioners are physicians who complete the basic six-year medical education but do not specialize further.

Ankara, İzmir). There is no evidence to indicate whether or to what extent the movement of health professionals has influenced this geographical imbalance. However, the government considers the employment of foreign health professionals (particularly medical doctors) to be a solution to this imbalance. No particular country has been identified but it is implicitly understood that Turkic republics are seen as potential source countries (İstanbul Dişhekimleri Odası 2007). However, it can be argued that the recruitment of foreign health professionals is unlikely to remedy uneven geographical internal distribution as foreigners are likely to prefer work in richer areas and provinces.

In addition to geographical imbalances, there are also shortages in certain specialties. There are very low (0.02) ratios of active specialists per 100 000 population in paediatric infectious diseases, paediatric immunology and oncological surgery (Sağlık Bakanlığı ve Yükseköğretim Kurulu 2008). Foreign specialists may be recruited to fill these vacancies.

There are also imbalances within and between the different professions – for example, Ministry of Health statistics show that there are more medical doctors than nurses (see also Table 17.6). Fig. 17.2 shows the changing numbers of health professionals in Turkey between 1995 and 2006. There are very few nurses and midwives in comparison to medical doctors (Savaş et al. 2002, Thomson & Saka 2003) and similar imbalances between specialists and practitioners (Thomson & Saka 2003). Despite increases over the years, imbalances in the distribution of health professionals are still observed. The authorities acknowledge the existence of this problem but so far it has not been solved (Yıldırım 2009).

Fig. 17.2 *Health professional in Turkey, 1995–2006*

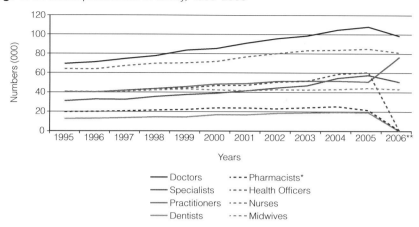

Sources: Sağlık Bakanlığı 2007a, Yıldırım 2009.
Note: * including residents; ** does not include permanent staff serving in the central organization of the health and other ministries, Turkish armed forces, Red Crescent and the Hygiene Center Presidency.

Fig. 17.3 shows that there were almost twice as many specialist doctors as practitioner doctors before 1985 but numbers of the latter have increased rapidly in recent years. In addition to the increases in the number of students and schools, the policy change towards primary care services provision (based on the model of family medicine) in the scope of the HTP has been a strong factor in the rise of practitioner numbers in recent years.

Fig. 17.3 *Specialists and practitioners in Turkey, 1950–2006*

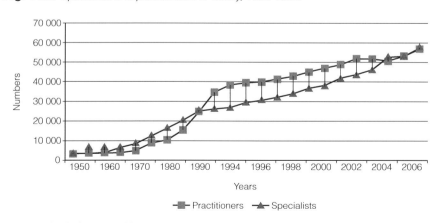

Sources: Sağlık Bakanlığı 2007a, Yıldırım 2009.

Dentists and pharmacists are employed mostly in the private sector; specialist and practitioner doctors, nurses and midwives are employed mostly in the public sector. Specialists usually have dual employment – some work in public hospitals and run their own private practices; others may work at public hospitals and be employed by private organizations or institutions (such as hospitals, polyclinics or laboratories). Furthermore, university lecturers may carry out private practice within their hospitals.

The liberal policies implemented since the 1990s and pursued particularly within the framework of the HTP (such as the possibility for everyone to be treated in private hospitals) initiated in 2003 have gradually increased the private health sector's contribution and role in service delivery. Increasing demand for private health services has caused the private sector to recruit health manpower, particularly medical doctors, from the public sector by offering higher salaries and better working conditions. As in most other countries, this has accelerated outflows from the public sector (WHO 2006).

The state has used the Ministry of Health's regulatory role and power to instigate some measures to reduce brain drain from the public sector. Firstly, private health sector capital investments were restricted. Published early in 2008, new planning regulations were set out to rationalize the joint public and private sector capacity standards for new private hospitals and outpatient diagnosis and treatment centres (OECD & World Bank 2008). Secondly, user charges were limited in the private sector. Finally, the Performance Based Supplementary Payment System was introduced as an addition to salaries in the public sector. It is reported that there has been a decline in the number of medical doctors with dual practice (working in both public and private sectors). In 2004, 2300 (15%) of 15 000 specialist doctors working for the Ministry of Health closed their private medical offices (Sağlık Bakanlığı 2008). These measures led to a substantial increase in the rate of full-time specialist doctors in Ministry of Health organizations (Sağlık Bakanlığı 2007b).

6.2 *Factors within the system influencing size and composition of the health workforce*

Educational system

The education system is one of the fundamental elements in determining the size and composition of the health workforce. In Turkey, students seeking admission to university must take the national university entrance exam; the number of university places is specified by the Council of Higher Education in cooperation with the health and education ministries. Practitioners applying for medical specialization training are required to pass the medical specialization exam that is held twice per year. However, the shortage of medical doctors is illustrated by the fact that there have been unfilled specialization places since 2001. Vacancies reached a peak in 2005–2006 but showed a decline in 2006–2007 (Table 17.7).

Table 17.7 *Specialist training places and medical faculty graduates in Turkey, 2001–2007*

Years	Medical faculty graduates in previous year	Specialist training places		
		Total	Filled	Vacant
2001–2002	4 755	4 438	3 689	749
2002–2003	4 380	4 949	4 035	914
2003–2004	4 487	4 453	4 117	336
2004–2005	4 494	6 077	4 810	1 267
2005–2006	4 532	6 513	4 376	2 137
2006–2007	4 899	6 386	5 262	1 124

Source: Sağlık Bakanlığı ve Yükseköğretim Kurulu 2008.

The number of medical, dentistry and pharmacy faculties and vocational schools of nursing and the numbers of students and faculty members have increased continuously (Table 17.8). This is a product of a deliberate policy. In fact, there has been a recent increase in medical graduates' uptake of assistant positions that enable them to train as specialists. This may well be a response to the relatively high remuneration for specialists in Turkey (OECD & World Bank 2008).

The increased demand from enhanced coverage and a flourishing private health-care sector in some parts of Turkey have exacerbated the growing workforce shortages among medical doctors and nurses. The government has responded by announcing a plan to increase annual medical school intakes from about 4500 students to about 6000. This will increase medical school intake by 30% but will have no impact on the services delivered within the next five years as it takes at least six years to train new medical doctors in Turkey (OECD & World Bank 2008).

Retirement

It was not possible to obtain any data on health professional retirement in Turkey and therefore there could be no assessment of its scale. However, it should be noted that currently there are no plans for an early or partial retirement policy. On the contrary, the retirement age is being raised and therefore it appears likely that forthcoming retirements will not drain the health professional workforce.

Health professionals retire under one of three schemes: (i) the Government Employees Retirement Fund for public sector employees; (ii) the Social Insurance Institution for private sector employees; and (iii) the Social Security Institution for the self-employed (Bağ-Kur). Until 9 September 1999, retirement age was based on the number of premium payment days. This offered some

Table 17.8 *Health education faculties, students and staff in Turkey, 1988–2007*

	Academic years	Faculties/schools	Students			Faculty members	Student/faculty member ratio
			New enrolment	Total	Graduate		
Medicine	1988–1989	24	5 148	33 686	4 138	2 560	13.2
	2002–2003	44	4 945	31 719	4 380	7 172	4.4
	2004–2005	46	5 090	32 552	4 494	7 881	4.1
	2006–2007	47	5 117	33 537	4 899	8 512	3.9
Dentistry	1988–1989	9	886	4 725	690	534	8.7
	2002–2003	14	975	5 256	813	1 410	3.7
	2004–2005	14	994	5 422	849	1 397	3.9
	2006–2007	18	1 078	5 873	763	1 480	4.0
Pharmacy	1988–1989	7	915	4 243	741	376	11.3
	2002–2003	9	855	4 149	695	803	5.2
	2004–2005	11	967	4 266	792	804	5.3
	2006–2007	12	995	4 572	785	826	5.5
Nursing	1988–1989	5	886	2 662	479	139	20.6
	2002–2003	11	3 940	16 423	2 586	427	38.5
	2004–2005	10	4 091	17 887	3 285	409	43.7
	2006–2007	12	4 361	18 630	3 782	709	26.3

Source: Sağlık Bakanlığı ve Yükseköğretim Kurulu 2008.

health professionals and other workers the possibility to retire while still in their forties (TUSİAD 2004). However, the retirement age has been raised to 58 (female) and 60 (male) for those who began work after 9 September 1999. The retirement ages will be increased gradually to 65 by 2048 (ÇSGB 2008a & 2008b). This may seem low in comparison to other European countries but is considered reasonable given that Turkish life expectancy at birth is 70.

Health professionals leaving or returning to the profession

No data could be obtained on those leaving and/or returning to the health professions yet it is possible to draw inferences by comparing the numbers of specialists who work actively and those whose diplomas have been registered. In March 2008, there were 50 828 actively working specialists; diplomas were registered for 67 312 specialists between 1 January 1966 and 14 December 2007 (Sağlık Bakanlığı ve Yükseköğretim Kurulu 2008). This indicates that 16 484 medical doctors with specialization diplomas were not working as specialists. They may have been waiting to be appointed; practising illegally in the private sector; working in another sector; or have retired, resigned, emigrated or even died.

6.3 *What does cross-border mobility mean for Turkey?*

The unavailability of healthy data makes it impossible to make a sound judgement on whether or not there is extensive cross-border health professional mobility in Turkey. However, having evaluated the data available and taken account of the legal restrictions on internal migration, it may be concluded that Turkey is a source country. The loss of educated human capital to other countries is detrimental as Turkey already has low proportions of health professionals per capita. Given that most medical education is state funded, the emigration of medical doctors has been a costly phenomenon for Turkey with effects that are felt in the long term (Gökbayrak 2006).

It is important to note that, for the time being, health professional mobility in Turkey is not as important as other human resource issues such as maldistribution and a lack of human resources for health.

7. Factors influencing health professional mobility

Only a few studies consider the factors influencing health professionals' decisions on internal or external migration. The first was conducted in 1962–1963 (Hıfzıssıhha Mektebi & Johns Hopkins University 1966). This indicated that the reasons for emigration included low income (68%); the desire to increase knowledge and experience and difficulties with specialization (12.3%); and unethical competition and bad relations among colleagues (6.2%). The data show that the level of professional income and difficulties with specialization were the primary factors in determining emigration at the time.

A recent study by Yıldırım (2009) provides certain data on potential emigration to EU countries and the reasons for it. The study population comprised medical doctors and nurses working in Ministry of Health hospitals in Ankara (one of the most developed provinces) and Muş (one of the most underdeveloped provinces). In Ankara, the hospitals were selected by a stratified cluster sampling method; the medical doctors and nurses were selected by a stratified random sampling method. Samples were not taken in Muş as there were only two hospitals.

A total of 1054 doctors (485) and nurses (569) took part in the study. Asked whether they would settle in an EU country temporarily or permanently, assuming that "Turkey became a member of the EU today under present conditions and that there is no obstacle to the free movement of persons", 65.7% of participants answered positively. Table 17.9 summarizes the most important factors influencing potential emigration of these participants. It is noteworthy that income was the most important reason for medical doctors wishing to leave Turkey in 1963. Almost 50 years later, this was not among the most important activating factors for health professionals but was reported to be the least satisfying aspect of their work. The most important factor inducing emigration was the desire for better working conditions, indicating that it may not be sufficient if policies to manage emigration include only improved wages. Better working conditions are also important considerations.

Table 17.9 *Factors influencing potential emigration of medical doctors and nurses, Ankara and Muş provinces, 2008*

Instigating factors	Dissatisfaction with current salary, working conditions, promotion opportunities
Activating factors	Desire for better working conditions; access to enhanced technology, equipment and health facilities for medical practice; better education and specialization facilities
Facilitating factors	na
Mitigating factors	Leaving family and friends, inadequate language skills, complicated and/or inconvenient paperwork/administration

Source: Yıldırım 2009. *Note*: na – not available.

8. Policy, regulation and interventions

To date, Turkey has implemented some policies to address the problems of inadequate numbers of health professionals, internal brain drain and the imbalanced distribution of human resources for health. These have included: (i) opening new faculties and increasing student intakes in order to increase the number of medical doctors; (ii) reintroducing compulsory service for practitioners in 2003 in order to address shortages in less developed areas; (iii) employing human resources for health on a contractual basis; and (iv) introducing strategies to balance the public-private sector (Yıldırım 2009). Active recruitment of foreign medical doctors is also being discussed.

8.1 *Policies and policy development on health professional mobility*

There are two ways by which a country may procure the health workforce it needs. The first uses internal resources – the country's own production. Yet changes to internal dynamics produced by the four main measures mentioned above have not yet remedied the lack of personnel or the imbalanced geographical distribution and skills composition in Turkey. The second method is to import health professionals. International recruitment of health-care workers usually results from an inability to attain the desired result through the first approach or because the first approach is not preferred (Bach 2003, WHO 2006).

The Turkish government has started work on the necessary legal regulation for international recruitment but the legislation process is proving rather problematic. In 2006, during the first term of the Erdoğan government (2002–2007), the import of medical doctors was the subject of lengthy and heated debates. In February 2007 the Turkish Grand National Assembly passed Law 5581 (TBMM 2007) that included an article to remove obstructions preventing foreign medical doctors from practising in Turkey. The stated justification for the law was to: (i) contribute to increasing the number of medical doctors in Turkey; (ii) remove obstacles preventing foreign medical doctors from working in Turkey; and (iii) remove obstacles to the free movement of persons and services from the perspective of full membership of the EU. The EU membership process and the membership requirements (mutual recognition) require the free movement of health professionals under the scope of the four freedoms (Yıldırım 2009). The law deleted "and being Turkish" from Article 1 of the law on the practice of medicine (Resmi Gazete 1928). The President vetoed the law on the grounds that the amendments in Articles 6 and 8 were inappropriate for public health requirements and it was announced that the law would be suspended for a while. However, the second Erdoğan government (2007–ongoing) frequently states that the issue of imported medical doctors is on their agenda. It is interesting to note that this does not extend to the nursing workforce.

8.2 *Workforce planning and development*

The planning and development of human resources for health does not occur within a systematic, homogenous and independent structure. Despite various official attempts, it is generally the result of knee-jerk reactions rather than strategic and systematic planning (Özcan et al. 1995). To date, no planning has taken account of international mobility (Yıldırım 2009). However, in recent years and particularly within the HTP, it has been stated that Turkey will prepare and implement policy strategies to plan and develop the health workforce in a way that is compatible with the EU integration process. Accordingly, a Draft Strategic Plan for 2023 was initiated in 2009 in order to determine a new strategy for human resources for health.

Currently, there is divided responsibility for the education and management of the human resources for health in Turkey. The State Planning Organization, The Council of Higher Education and the Ministry of Health are the three main institutions that formulate and implement health workforce policies. The Ministry of Finance and the State Personnel Department are also stakeholders (Sağlık Bakanlığı 2007a). There is a lack of effective coordination between these institutions and organizations (Sağlık Bakanlığı 2003).

8.3 *Regulatory frameworks and interventions*

The ÇSGB has been responsible for issuing work permits to foreigners since 2003. Procedures and principles are set out in the law on work permits which stipulates that "provisions which are included in other laws concerning the jobs and professions in which the foreigners will not be entitled to work are reserved" (Resmi Gazete 2003). Thus, it upholds Law 1219 that requires "doctors, dentists, midwives and medical attendants to be Turkish nationals and to have a diploma from a relevant education institution in Turkey" (Resmi Gazete 1928) and Law 6283 in which the exercise of the profession of nursing is restricted to Turkish citizens (Resmi Gazete 1954).

Some clauses in existing laws permit the employment of foreign health professionals although it is not known how many foreigners, if any, are employed on these legal bases. Law 1219 (Resmi Gazete 1928) stipulates that "those foreign medical doctors, dentists and midwives whose vested rights based on laws have been recognized are allowed to practise their professions within the provisions of this law". In addition, Law 3359 stipulates that "Turkish nationals or foreigners who have a needed special professional knowledge and speciality may be employed on contract" (Resmi Gazete 1987).

Law 2527 (amended by Law 4817) concerning foreigners of Turkish descent includes the clause: "For foreigners of Turkish origin to work and be employed in professions, arts and trades which Turkish citizens can be employed or work in, they should have the qualifications and complete the obligations specified in specific laws" (Resmi Gazete 1981). The ÇSGB is responsible for granting permission following consultation with the Ministry of Internal Affairs, the Ministry of Foreign Affairs and other relevant ministries. Yet, officials working in these organizations have reported that very few people, mostly Turkish descendents of Greek origin, are issued with work permits within this context.[5]

People married to Turkish citizens and residing in Turkey are permitted to work there under an exceptional work permission. This does not extend to foreign health professionals because of the restrictions in Law 1219 (Resmi Gazete 1928). Foreign citizens have the right to apply for naturalization when they have been married to a Turkish citizen for three years (İçduygu 2009). This confers the right to work since holders of dual citizenship can work in Turkey. People with dual citizenship or Turkish citizens who obtain diplomas in a foreign country must request recognition of their diplomas from the Council of Higher Education.

Mutual recognition of diplomas in the European Community

Since gaining candidacy status in 1999 and, more importantly, since starting accession talks in 2005, Turkey has made progress in aligning its health legislation with that of the EU. Preparatory work has been started within the context of EU accession[6] (free movement of workers, mutual recognition of professional qualifications and diplomas). Within the scope of the ongoing alignment process, the Vocational Qualifications Authority was established in 2006 (Resmi Gazete 2006b).

The Turkish government has prepared draft legislation to transpose EU Directive 2005/36/EC (European Parliament and Council of the European Union 2005) on the free movement of health professionals into Turkish law. There is continuing work and internal discussion on the Draft Law on the Regulation and Recognition of Professional Qualifications but it is expected that it will enter into force by the end of 2013. The Council of Higher Education has the authority to render compatible the minimum educational requirements for regulated professions. In this context, a regulation on the harmonization of the minimum training requirements for regulated professions (medicine, nursery, midwifery, dentistry, veterinary medicine, pharmacy and architecture) has been adopted and published in the *Official Gazette* (Commission of the European Communities 2008, Resmi Gazete 2008).

---

5 Personal interview with employee of General Directorate of Security, Ankara, 13 May 2009.

6 The EU Council Summit in December 2006 suspended accession negotiations with Turkey on eight chapters (free movement of goods, right of establishment and freedom to provide service, financial services, agriculture and rural development, fisheries, transport policy, customs union and external relations) due to lack of progress and closed those that were opened on the grounds that Turkey had failed to fulfil its obligations arising from the Additional Protocol to the Ankara Agreement.

Notwithstanding these advances, the EU Commission reported:

no progress can be reported on mutual recognition of professional qualifications and its differentiation from the recognition of academic qualifications. The current administrative structures allow the recognition of academic qualifications only. Reciprocal recognition still applies to a number of regulated professions. Nationality and language requirements persist. A contact point for implementation of Directive 2005/36/EC on the recognition of professional qualifications has yet to be designated (Commission of the European Communities 2009).

Bilateral agreements

Turkish law prohibits the employment of foreign health professionals and therefore there are no bilateral agreements on health professional mobility between Turkey and other countries. However, Turkey started the Great Student Project (GSP) in 1992–1993 with the aims of: (i) helping Turkic republics, Turks and relative communities (TR&TRC)[7] to meet their educated workforce needs; (ii) training a generation of young people with a good relationship to Turkey and building a permanent/sustainable bridge of brotherhood and friendship with the Turkic world; (iii) teaching the Turkish language and promoting Turkish culture; and (iv) enhancing the relationships between these countries within one large-scale project. The GSP is carried out within the framework of cooperation agreements, protocols and relevant legislation. Turkey provides scholarships to students according to these agreements and, as of 9 September 2009, the GSP had enabled a total of 5347 students to study there (Milli Eğitim Bakanlığı 2009). However, it was not possible to access detailed Ministry of National Education statistics on the numbers of student health professionals by years and home countries.

8.4 Political force field of regulating and managing health professional mobility

As noted before, the international migration of health professionals is highly controversial in Turkey and the policy strategies are heavily influenced by conflicts among stakeholders. The Minister of Health has stated that the greatest obstacle to health-care reform in Turkey is the lack of medical doctors, asserting that at least 100 000 more medical doctors are required in order to match EU average levels. The Ministry of Health holds that some of this gap can be filled by actively recruiting foreign health professionals but there is great public debate about this. For instance, the TMA heads a group that opposes the Ministry of Health's position and contends that human resources for health do

---

7 TR&TRC includes: *Turkic republics:* Azerbaijan, Kazakhstan, Kyrgyzstan, Turkmenistan, Uzbekistan. *Balkan and Asian countries*: Afghanistan, Bosnia and Herzegovina, Bulgaria, Iran, Iraq, Lebanon, Romania, Syria, The Former Yugoslav Republic of Macedonia *Russian Federation:* over 60 communities (Kavak & Baskan 2001).

not have a significant deficiency. The TMA estimated that Turkey should have had 109 446 medical doctors in 2008 and compared this figure with the number of actively working medical doctors (103 177) given in a report published jointly by the Ministry of Health and the Council of Higher Education (Sağlık Bakanlığı ve Yükseköğretim Kurulu 2008). The TMA noted that the difference was just 6269 doctors and concluded that this was not a major deficit. The TMA objects to opening up the Turkish health-care system to immigration, claiming that there are already sufficient numbers of medical doctors and that the main problem is their unbalanced distribution (TTB 2008).

9. Conclusion

As can be seen, there have been significant constraints on this research – Turkey's special circumstances in relation to the EU and a lack of data. Despite unavailable and/or incomplete data, this case study is a first in its field. By presenting a systematic (but limited) picture of the present situation it is hoped that it will lead the way for other studies.

While not representative of the entire Turkish health workforce, a few studies have revealed that EU accession would lead a considerable number of health professionals to consider working in other EU Member States. This indicates the need for government policies to manage outmigration in order to avoid further and serious losses from the health workforce. Inflows of foreign health professionals are currently expected to be very limited due to legal restrictions but work is under way to remove these obstacles within the context of alignment with EU legislation. Furthermore, the present government considers foreign medical doctors to be a remedy for the problem of insufficient health professionals although there is heated public debate about this.

Finally, the analysis carried out in this case study has revealed that Turkey is in need of policy and research related not only to the international mobility of health professionals but also to all policy dimensions related to health professionals. These include planning, designing planning scenarios, policy implementation, building databases and studying health professional students' professional expectations and emigration intentions in terms of the health workforce. Moreover, domestic issues such as geographical distribution across the vast territory and underproduction of some health professionals are as important as international mobility. As stated by the Ministry of Health and the Council of Higher Education, these issues can be overcome through the effective use of technology and information as well as political will and support (Sağlık Bakanlığı ve Yükseköğretim Kurulu 2008).

References

Bach S (2006). *International migration of health workers: labour and social issues*. Geneva, International Labour Office (ILO Working Paper 209) (www.ilo.org/public/ english/dialogue/sector/papers/health/wp209.pdf, accessed 3 December 2009).

Borzeda A et al. (2002). *European enlargement: do health professionals from candidate countries plan to migrate? The case of Hungary, Poland and the Czech Republic*. Paris, Ministry of Social Affairs, Labour and Solidarity.

Buchan J, Perfilieva G (2006). *Health worker migration in the European Region: country case studies and policy implications*. Copenhagen, WHO Regional Office for Europe (http:/www.euro.who.int/document/e883666.pdf, accessed 2 October 2008).

Commission of the European Communities (2004). *Communication from the Commission to the Council and the European Parliament. Recommendation of the European Commission on Turkey's progress towards accession*. Brussels (http:// eur-lex.europa.eu/LexUriServ/LexUriServ.do?uri=COM:2004:0656:FIN:EN: PDF, accessed 6 December 2009).

Commission of the European Communities (2008). *Turkey 2008 progress report*. SEC (2008) 2699, Brussels, 5/11/2008 (http://ec.europa.eu/enlargement/ pdf/press_corner/key-documents/reports_nov_2008/turkey_progress_report_ en.pdf, accessed 6 December 2009).

Commission of the European Communities (2009). *Turkey 2009 progress report*. SEC (2009) 1334, Brussels, 14/10/2009 (http://ec.europa.eu/enlargement/ pdf/key _documents/2009/tr_rapport_2009_en.pdf, accessed 6 December 2009).

ÇSGB (2008a). *Sosyal Güvenlik Reformu* [*Social security reform*]. Ankara, Çalışma ve Sosyal Güvenlik Bakanlığı [Ministry of Labour and Social Security].

ÇSGB (2008b). *Sosyal Güvenlik Reformu'nda Merak Edilen 50 Soru 50 Cevap* [*50 questions and 50 answers about social security reform*]. Ankara, Çalışma ve Sosyal Güvenlik Bakanlığı [Ministry of Labour and Social Security].

ÇSGB (2009). *Yönetsel Kayıtlar* [Administrative records]. Ankara, Çalışma ve Sosyal Güvenlik Bakanlığı [Ministry of Labour and Social Security].

Dumont J-C, Zurn P (2007). Migrant health workers in OECD countries in the broader context of highly skilled migration. In: *International migration outlook, SOPEMI*. Paris, Organisation for Economic Co-operation and Development (http://www.oecd.org/dataoecd/43/43/41522822.xls, accessed 24 February 2011). European Parliament and Council of the European Union

(2005). Directive 2005/36/EC of the European Parliament and of the Council of 7 September 2005 on the recognition of professional qualifications. *Official Journal of the European Union*, 255(48):22–142 (http://eur-lex.europa.eu/LexUriServ/LexUriServ.do?uri=OJ:L:2005:255:0022:0142:en: PDF, accessed 6 December 2009).

Gökbayrak Ş (2006). *Gelişmekte Olan Ülkelerden Gelişmiş Ülkelere Nitelikli İşgücü Göçü ve Politikalar – Türk Mühendislerinin "Beyin Göçü" Üzerine Bir İnceleme* [*Skilled labour migration from developing to developed countries and policies: a study on "brain drain"*] [PhD thesis]. Ankara, Ankara Üniversitesi Sosyal Bilimler Enstitüsü Çalışma Ekonomisi ve Endüstri İlişkileri Anabilim Dalı [Ankara University Institute of Social Sciences Discipline of Labour Economics and Industrial Relations].

Güneş ED, Yaman H (2008). Transition to family practice in Turkey. *Journal of Continuing Education in the Health Professions*, 28(2):106–112.

Hıfzıssıhha Okulu and Johns Hopkins University (1966). *Türkiye'de Sağlık Alanında İnsangücü Araştırması, Bulgular-Ön Rapor* [*Health manpower survey in Turkey: results – preliminary report*]. Ankara, Hıfzıssıhha Okulu [School of Public Health].

İçduygu A (2009). *International migration and human development in Turkey.* United Nations Development Programme (Human Development Research Paper 2009/52) (http://hdr.undp.org/en/reports/global/hdr2009/papers/HDRP_2009_52.pdf, accessed 6 December 2009).

İstanbul Dişhekimleri Odası (2007). *İthal Ucuz Hekim* [*Imported cheap physicians*] (http://www.ido.org.tr/dergiarsiv096.asp?ID=1048, accessed 23 August 2010).

Kavak Y, Baskan GA (2001). Türkiye'nin Türk Cumhuriyetleri, Türk ve Akraba Topluluklarına Yönelik Eğitim Politika ve Uygulamaları [Educational policies and applications of Turkey towards Turkic republics and communities]. *Hacettepe Üniversitesi Eğitim Fakültesi Dergisi* [*Journal of Hacettepe University Faculty of Education*], 20:92–103.

Milli Eğitim Bakanlığı (2009). *Büyük Öğrenci Projesi* [*Great student project*] (http://yeogm.meb.gov.tr/projeler/uygulanmaktaolanprj/bop.html, accessed 4 December 2009).

OECD (2007). *International migration outlook 2007.* Paris, Organisation for Economic Co-operation and Development.

OECD and World Bank (2008). *OECD reviews of health systems: Turkey.* Paris, Organisation for Economic Co-operation and Development.

ÖSYM (2004). *2003–2004 Öğretim Yılı Yükseköğretim İstatistikleri Kitabı* [*2003–2004 academic year higher education statistics book*]. Ankara, Öğrenci Seçme ve Yerleştirme Merkezi [Student Selection and Placement Centre for Turkey].

ÖSYM (2005). *2004–2005 Öğretim Yılı Yükseköğretim İstatistikleri Kitabı* [*2004–2005 academic year higher education statistics book*]. Ankara, Öğrenci Seçme ve Yerleştirme Merkezi [Student Selection and Placement Centre for Turkey].

ÖSYM (2006). *2005–2006 Öğretim Yılı Yükseköğretim İstatistikleri Kitabı* [*2005–2006 academic year higher education statistics book*]. Ankara, Öğrenci Seçme ve Yerleştirme Merkezi [Student Selection and Placement Centre for Turkey].

ÖSYM (2007). *2006–2007 Öğretim Yılı Yükseköğretim İstatistikleri Kitabı* [*2006–2007 academic year higher education statistics book*]. Ankara, Öğrenci Seçme ve Yerleştirme Merkezi [Student Selection and Placement Centre for Turkey].

ÖSYM (2008). *2007–2008 Öğretim Yılı Yükseköğretim İstatistikleri Kitabı* [*2007–2008 academic year higher education statistics book*]. Ankara, Öğrenci Seçme ve Yerleştirme Merkezi [Student Selection and Placement Centre for Turkey].

ÖSYM (2009). *2008–2009 Öğretim Yılı Yükseköğretim İstatistikleri Kitabı* [*2008–2009 academic year higher education statistics book*]. Ankara, Öğrenci Seçme ve Yerleştirme Merkezi [Student Selection and Placement Centre for Turkey]

Özcan S et al. (1995). Shaping the health future in Turkey: a new role for human resource planning. *International Journal of Health Planning and Management*, 10:305–319.

Resmi Gazete (1928). Tababet ve Şuabatı San'atlarının Tarzı İcrasına Dair Kanun. Kanun No: 1219 [Law on Practice of Arts of Medicine. Law number: 1219]. Ankara, *Resmi Gazete* [*Official Gazette*], Issue 863, 14 April 1928.

Resmi Gazete (1954). Hemşirelik Kanunu Kanun No: 6283 [Nursing Law. Law number: 6283]. Ankara, *Resmi Gazete* [*Official Gazette*], Issue 8647, 25 February 1954.

Resmi Gazete (1981). Türk Soylu Yabancıların Türkiye'de Meslek ve Sanatlarını Serbestçe Yapabilmelerine, Kamu, Özel Kuruluş veya İşyerlerinde Çalıştırılabilmelerine İlişkin Kanun. Kanun No: 2527, Sayı: 17473 [Law Enabling Foreigners of Turkish Descent to Exercise their Professions in the

Workplace in Public and Private Institutions and Enterprises in Turkey. Law number: 2527]. Ankara, *Resmi Gazete* [*Official Gazette*], Issue 17473, 29 September 1981.

Resmi Gazete (1987). Sağlık Hizmetleri Temel Kanunu Kanun No: 3359 [Basic Law on Health Care Services. Law number: 3359]. Ankara, *Resmi Gazete* [*Official Gazette*], Issue 19461, 15 May 1987.

Resmi Gazete (2003). Yabancıların Çalışma İzinleri Hakkında Kanunun Uygulama Yönetmeliği [Regulation on the Application of the Law on Work Permits for Foreigners]. Ankara, *Resmi Gazete* [*Official Gazette*], Issue 25214, 29 August 2003.

Resmi Gazete (2006a). Sosyal Sigortalar ve Genel Sağlık Sigortası Kanunu. Kanun No: 5510 [Law on Social Insurances and General Health Insurance. Law number: 5510]. Ankara, *Resmi Gazete* [*Official Gazette*], Issue 26200, 16 June 2006.

Resmi Gazete (2006b). Mesleki Yeterlilik Kurumu Kanunu. Kanun No: 5544 [Law on Professional Qualifications Institution. Law number: 5544]. Ankara, *Resmi Gazete* [*Official Gazette*], Issue 26312, 7 October 2006.

Resmi Gazete (2008). Doktorluk, Hemşirelik, Ebelik, Diş Hekimliği, Veterinerlik, Eczacılık ve Mimarlık Eğitim Programlarının Asgari Eğitim Koşullarının Belirlenmesine Dair Yönetmelik [Regulation on the Determination of the Minimum Education Requirements for the Education Programmes of Medicine, Nursing, Midwifery, Dentistry, Veterinary Medicine, Pharmacy and Architecture]. Ankara, *Resmi Gazete [Official Gazette]*, Issue 26775, 2 February 2008.

Sağlık Bakanlığı (2003). *Sağlıkta Dönüşüm Porgamı* [*Health transformation programme*]. Ankara, Sağlık Bakanlığı [Ministry of Health].

Sağlık Bakanlığı (2005). *Sağlık İstatistikleri 2005* [*Health statistics 2005*]. Ankara, Sağlık Bakanlığı [Ministry of Health].

Sağlık Bakanlığı (2007a). *Türkiye'de Sağlığa Bakış 2007 [Health at a glance in Turkey 2007]*. Ankara, Sağlık Bakanlığı [Ministry of Health].

Sağlık Bakanlığı (2007b). *Nereden Nereye. Türkiye Sağlıkta Dönüşüm Programı* [*From where to where? Health transformation programme in Turkey*]. Ankara, Sağlık Bakanlığı [Ministry of Health].

Sağlık Bakanlığı (2008). *Türkiye Sağlıkta Dönüşüm Programı İlerleme Raporu* [*Progress report: health transformation programme in Turkey*]. Ankara, Sağlık Bakanlığı [Ministry of Health] (Publication number 749).

Sağlık Bakanlığı ve Yükseköğretim Kurulu (2008). *Türkiye Sağlık İnsangücü Durum Raporu.* [*Turkey health manpower status report*]. Ankara, Sağlık Bakanlığı ve Yükseköğretim Kurulu [Ministry of Health and the Council of Higher Education] (Publication number: 739).

Savaş BS et al. (2002). *Health care systems in transition: Turkey.* Copenhagen, WHO Regional Office for Europe on behalf of the European Observatory on Health Systems and Policies.

Taylor CE et al. (1968). *Health manpower planning in Turkey. An international research case study.* Baltimore, The Johns Hopkins Press.

TBMM (2007). Bazı *Kanun ve Kanun Hükmünde Kararnamelerde Değişiklik Yapılmasına Dair Kanun.* Kanun No: 5581, Kabul Tarihi: 15/12/2007, [*Law on the Amendment of Certain Laws and Decrees.* Law number: 5581, accepted 15 December 2007], Ankara, Türkiye Büyük Millet Meclisi [Grand National Assembly of Turkey] (http://www.tbmm.gov.tr/kanunlar/k5581.html, accessed 10 December 2008).

Thomson S, Saka O (2003). Health and health care in Turkey. *Euro Observer*, 5(1):5–6.

TTB (2008). *Sağlık Emek-Gücü: Sayılar ve Gerçekler* [*Health labour force: facts and figures*]. Ankara, Türk Tabipleri Birliği [Turkish Medical Association].

TÜİK (2005). *Sağlık İstatistikleri 2005* [Health statistics 2005]. Ankara, Türkiye İstatistik Kurumu [Turkish Statistical Institute].

TUİK (2009). *Resmi İstatistik Programı Bilgi Sistemi [Information system for the official statistics programme].* Ankara, Türkiye İstatistik Kurumu [Turkish Statistical Institute] (http://www.tuik.gov.tr/rip/temalar/2_13.html, accessed 2 June 2009).

TÜSİAD (2004). *Türk Emeklilik Sisteminde Reform. Mevcut Durum ve Alternatif Stratejiler* [*Reform in the Turkish pension system: current situation and alternative strategies*]. İstanbul, Türk Sanayici ve İş Adamları Derneği [Turkish Industry and Business Association] (Publication number: TÜSİAD-T/2004-11/382)

WHO (2006). *Migration of health workers.* Geneva, World Health Organization (Fact Sheet No. 301) (http://who.int/mediacentre/factsheets/fs301/en/print.html, accessed 30 November 2009).

Yıldırım HH, Yıldırım T (2005). *Avrupa Birliği'ne Uyum ve Katılım Sürecinde Türk Sağlık Sektörü Açısından Değerlendirmeler [Evaluations about the Turkish health sector in the process of conformity and accession to the European Union].* Birinci Baskı and Ankara, Ankara Ticaret Odası [Ankara Chamber of Commerce].

Yıldırım T (2004). *Avrupa Birliği Genişlemesi ve Sağlık: Türkiye'nin Avrupa Birliği'ne Uyum Sürecinde Sağlık Sisteminin Karşılaşabileceği Sorunlar Hakkında Değerlendirmeler* [*The European Union enlargement and health: evaluations of problems likely to be faced by the Turkish health system during the process of harmonization with the European Union*] [MSc thesis]. Ankara, Hacettepe Üniversitesi Sağlık Bilimleri Enstitüsü [Hacettepe University Institute of Health Sciences].

Yıldırım T (2009). *Avrupa Birliği'nde Serbest Dolaşım ve Sağlık Hizmetleri: Ankara ve Muş İllerinde Sağlık Bakanlığı'na Bağlı Hastanelerde Çalışan Hekim ve Hemşirelerin Serbest Dolaşıma İlişkin Görüşleri ve Potansiyel Göç* [*Free movement in the European Union and health services: opinions of physicians and nurses working in the hospitals belonging to the Ministry of Health on free movement and potential migration*] [PhD thesis]. Ankara, Hacettepe Üniversitesi Sağlık Bilimleri Enstitüsü (Yayınlanmamış Doktora Tezi) [Hacettepe University Institute of Health Sciences].